CHARACTERISTICS AND POTENTIALS OF BLOOD STEM CELLS

ISBN 1-880854-21-X (Hardbound)
ISBN 1-880854-25-2 (Softbound)
ISSN 1066-5099
Library of Congress Catalog Card Number 97-73746

STEM CELLS® is published bimonthly by AlphaMed Press, One Prestige Place, Suite 290, Miamisburg, Ohio 45342-3758 USA.

The STEM CELLS Journal is regularly indexed by Current Contents/Life Sciences, Science Citation Index, BIOSIS, Index Medicus and MEDLINE on the MEDLARS system, Excerpta Medica/EMBASE, Chemical Abstracts, CABS (Current Awareness in Biological Sciences).

The STEM CELLS Journal is printed in the United States of America on paper that adheres to the requirements for library/archival stability.

While every effort is made by the Publisher and Editorial Office to see that no inaccurate or misleading data, opinion or statement appear in this publication, the data and opinions appearing in the chapters and advertisements herein are the responsibility of the contributor or advertiser concerned. Accordingly, the Publisher, the Editor and respective employees, officers and agents accept no liability whatsoever for the consequences of any such inaccurate or misleading data, opinion or statement. While every effort is made to ensure that drug doses and other quantities are presented accurately, readers are advised that new methods and techniques involving drug usage, and described within this publication, should only be followed in conjunction with the drug manufacturer's own published literature.

Cover photograph: Schloss Reisensburg castle*. First mentioned by the geographer of Ravenna in the 7th century, Schloss Reisensburg is one of the oldest castles in southern Germany, located on a hill which shows signs of human settlements dating back 5,000 years. The present building was restored after partial destruction in the 17th century, and the castle served as a country home of nobility until the end of World War II. Its guesthouse was donated in 1968-70 by the Volkswagen Foundation to the newly founded University of Ulm for use as a faculty retreat and conference center.*

CHARACTERISTICS AND POTENTIALS OF BLOOD STEM CELLS

EDITED BY

THEODOR M. FLIEDNER
DIETER HOELZER

Published as a supplement to STEM CELLS

AlphaMed Press

ACKNOWLEDGMENTS

This volume reports the proceedings of the International Stem Cell Workshop on "Pathophysiology, Diagnostic and Therapeutic Implications of Blood Stem Cells," which was held at the International Institute for Scientific Cooperation Schloss Reisensburg of the University of Ulm from July 9-12, 1997. This Workshop was carried out under aegis of the Searle-Foundation for Medical Prevention and Epidemiology and was made possible with generous support by AMGEN, which also helped sponsor the publication of this volume.

The Editors would like to express their appreciation for AMGEN's generosity, especially to *Dr. Hellein,* and for the cooperation of the authors who contributed their data, experience and enthusiasm. Furthermore, they acknowledge gratefully the expert and dedicated editorial assistance of *Dr. Ann Murphy*, *Edie McBride*, and *Christina Martin*, without whom this volume would not have been published so quickly. Special thanks are due *Dr. Martin J. Murphy, Jr.,* our Editor-in-Chief, for his continuous friendship, encouragement and support.

THEODOR M. FLIEDNER
DIETER HOELZER
CHAIRMEN
INTERNATIONAL STEM CELL WORKSHOP

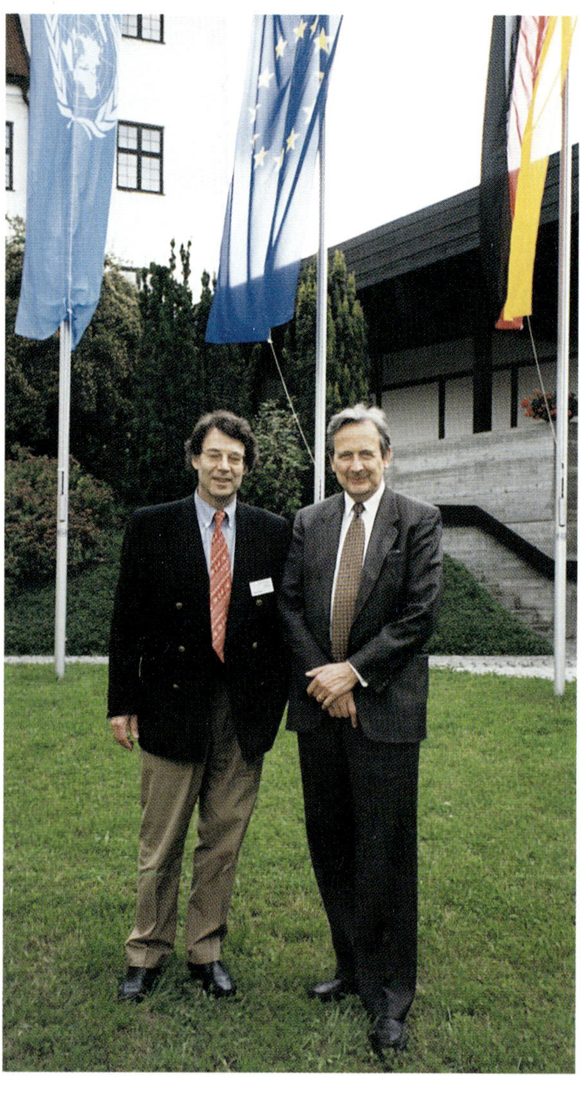

Dieter Hoelzer   *Theodor M. Fliedner*

CHARACTERISTICS AND POTENTIALS OF BLOOD STEM CELLS

VOLUME 16, SUPPLEMENT 1, 1998

CHAPTER I
KEYNOTE ADDRESSES

CHAPTER II
CHARACTERIZATION AND PROPERTIES OF BLOOD STEM CELLS

CHAPTER III
BLOOD STEM CELLS IN NORMAL AND LEUKEMIC STATES

CHAPTER VII

BLOOD STEM CELLS: TARGETS FOR GENE TRANSFER

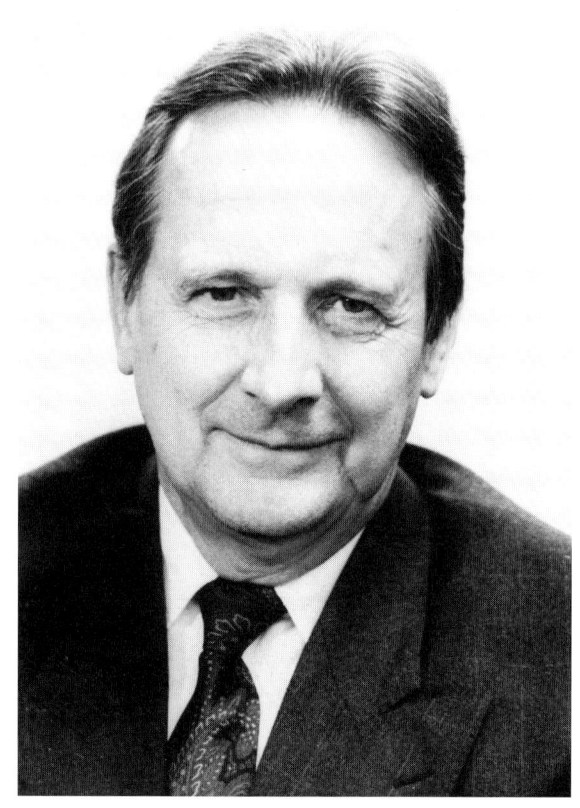

Professor Theodor M. Fliedner

A Tribute to Theodor M. Fliedner

DIETER HOELZER

Klinikum der Johann Wolfgang Goethe-Universität Frankfurt am Main,
Zentrum der Inneren Medizin, Medizinische Klinik III, Frankfurt, Germany

This issue of STEM CELLS is dedicated to *Theodor M. Fliedner,* who in 1997 retired from his active scientific work at the University of Ulm. The topic of the symposium, "Characteristics and Potentials of Blood Stem Cells," covers the breadth of his outstanding research and highlights the many contributions which he and his colleagues have made to experimental hematology during the past 45 years.

Theodor M. Fliedner was born in 1929 in Hamburg to a well-known family of distinguished Protestant missionaries. This proud heritage imbued him with a sense of mission in his own life and became a great force which propelled his scientific life's work. He began his scientific career as a student when he worked in the Radiation Department of the Cancer Therapy Hospital in Heidelberg. There he studied structural alterations and blood cell regeneration in the bone marrow of rats following single-dose irradiation with fast electrons. After he graduated as a licensed physician in 1955, he performed postdoctoral research from 1957 to 1963 at the Medical Research Center of the Brookhaven National Laboratory, New York, USA. Working under his great and always admired teachers *Dr. E.P. Cronkite* and *Dr. V.P. Bond,* he explored the sequence of radiation injury and regeneration of bone marrow in dogs and man after single radiation exposure, including studies of radiation accident victims. The understanding of bone marrow injury, the re-establishment of the integrity of the vascular architecture, as well as the seeding of circulating hemopoietic stem cells, led to his lifelong interest in the blood stem cell.

The innovative early scientific pursuits of *T.M. Fliedner* were recognized and appreciated by *Prof. Ludwig Heilmeyer,* the famous hematologist in Freiburg, and, soon thereafter, *Ted* was appointed Director of the Institute of Hematology of the Society of Radiation Research in association with EURATOM in Freiburg. Here with his research group he established animal models using ^{3}H-thymidine continuous labeling methods which helped to characterize pluripotent and committed stem cells. By labeling all cells with ^{3}H-TdR before and early after birth he demonstrated that the few remaining labeled marrow lymphocytes were associated with or identical to pluripotent stem cells—actually the first time a stem cell was recognized.

A recurrent theme he has long considered is the inquiry of what experimental research could reveal to the clinician, using the ^{3}H-TdR labeling model, for example. How are resting stem cells affected by a transplantable leukemia, or how do the kinetics of leukemic blast cells differ from their normal counterparts? He also found, using ^{3}H-cytidine labeling, that extended proliferation of leukemic cells prolongs the life of malignant cells, yielding even more tumor cells which further contribute to the leukemic cell load.

Ted Fliedner was not only an enthusiastic and leading research hematologist, but also he had visions of how to improve and create new medical education. He was one of the eight founding professors of the new University of Ulm and soon became the founding Dean of the Faculty of Theoretical Medicine. It was in Ulm that he developed the concept of blood stem cell banks with which to treat bone marrow failure. Since the blood of all species so far tested is known to contain pluripotent hemopoietic stem cells, he established a preclinical canine model suitable for autologous blood stem cell transplantation. This work, in collaboration with his co-worker *Martin Körbling,* led to one of the first clinical autologous blood stem cell transplantations in human beings.

Ted Fliedner's enthusiasm, power of conviction, and honesty were soon recognized by his peers and for eight years he was *Rector Magnificus* and President of the University of Ulm, with his crowning achievement the creation in 1987 of the first "Science City" in Germany comprised of the University (with its Biomedical and Natural Sciences as well as Engineering and Computer Sciences) and a number of high-tech industrial research institutes plus "joint venture" research establishments in a "Science Park." International recognition of his prominence is evidenced by his election as President of the International Society of Experimental Hematology (1988) and his three doctoral degrees *Honoris Causa* in Science and Medicine. But his most profound—and fulfilling—achievements are to be appreciated by his countless friends all over the world, and especially by his long-standing dedication to his sponsorship and patronage of young German research scientists. It can rightfully be claimed that "all of *Ted's* young men did well." In short, he fostered the growth of many of Germany's finest experimental hematology laboratories.

Last, but not least, his enthusiasm was not confined to the realm of science. When he came to Ulm, he and his Founding Rector *Heilmeyer* discovered the ruins of the 14th century Castle Reisensburg. It was in a disastrous state. By his persistent and prodigious efforts with politicians, private sponsors, and the University, he lovingly restored this unique place which is now the site of outstanding international symposia, such as the one published in this volume. From the parapets of its lofty towers it proclaims to the horizon that nothing in the world can take the place of vision and determination—two of *Ted's* greatest virtues.

Now, after retiring from his active professorial life at the University of Ulm, he remains the patron of Castle Reisensburg and embarks on his next new career with the World Health Organization. For his many, many contributions we send him our thanks, and for his new challenges and future achievements we send him our heartiest "good luck!"

Profile of Theodor M. Fliedner

Department of Clinical Physiology, Occupational and Social Medicine,
University of Ulm, Ulm, Germany

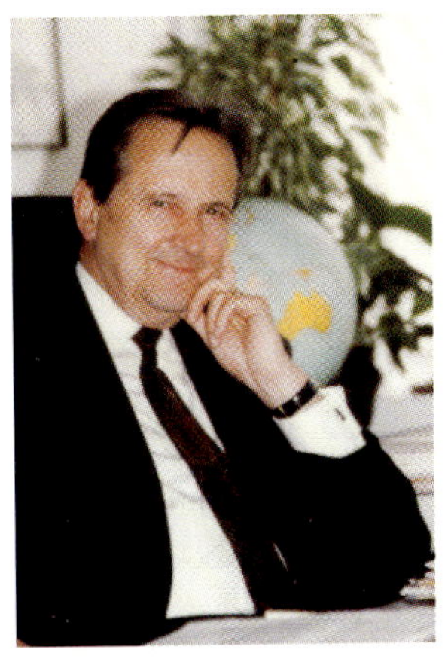

Dr. Theodor M. Fliedner is Professor of Clinical Physiology and Occupational Medicine at the University of Ulm, Germany. He earned his doctoral degree in medical sciences at the University of Heidelberg (*summa cum laude*) in 1957. Between 1957 and 1963 he worked as associate scientist at the Brookhaven National Laboratory in the group of *Dr. E. P. Cronkite* and as a fellow in hematology under the late *Dr. C. V. Moore* at Washington University, School of Medicine, in St. Louis, Missouri. During these years, he contributed extensively to experimental hematology by elucidating the cellular kinetics of normal and leukemic hemopoietic cell renewal using tritiated thymidine and single cell autoradiography. He also contributed extensively to the analysis of the pathophysiology of the acute and chronic radiation syndromes. After returning to Germany in 1963, he became the director of a EURATOM-Institute for Radiation Hematology. In 1967 he was one of the eight founding professors of the University of Ulm, characterizing a new approach to an integrated teaching and research in medicine, science and engineering. From 1983 to 1991 he served as president of Ulm University and initiated its key role as the core in the first "Science City" of Germany. During these years (1969-1985) *Dr. Fliedner* and his group (consisting of associates from Europe and from many parts of the world) paved the way for the characterization, physiology and pathophysiology of hemopoietic stem cells in the peripheral blood and to their mobilization, collection, cryopreservation and utilization for hemopoietic reconstitution after total body irradiation both in the canine model and, in the early 1980s, in human beings (in collaboration with the University of Heidelberg). In recent years, he and his group established a database for the clinical signs and symptoms as well as course and follow-up for radiation accident victims (containing now over 500 individual case histories) as a basis for the pathophysiological characterization and analysis of radiation, especially of the responses of the hemopoietic system. His group is in the process of establishing a telecommunications linkage between the University of Ulm and the Ural Research Center for Radiation Medicine in Chelyabinsk, Russia, to support the clinical and hematological management of chronically radiation exposed inhabitants as a consequence of mismanagement of radioactive waste in the Techa River region.

Dr. Fliedner received several honors: Member of the Academies of Sciences in Heidelberg as well as in Milano; Foreign Member (Academician) of the Academy of Medical Sciences of the Ukraine; Honorary Member of the American, Italian and Hungarian Society of Hematology, Honorary Doctor of Medical Sciences of the Mahidol University, Bangkok (Thailand), the Medical University of Debrecen (Hungary) and LB-University of Uppsala (Sweden). At the present time, he serves as the Chairman of the Global Advisory Committee for Health Research of the World Health Organization (WHO), Geneva, a body entrusted with the challenge to develop, by 1998, a Research Agenda for Science and Technology to support the renewed strategy of the WHO for health development.

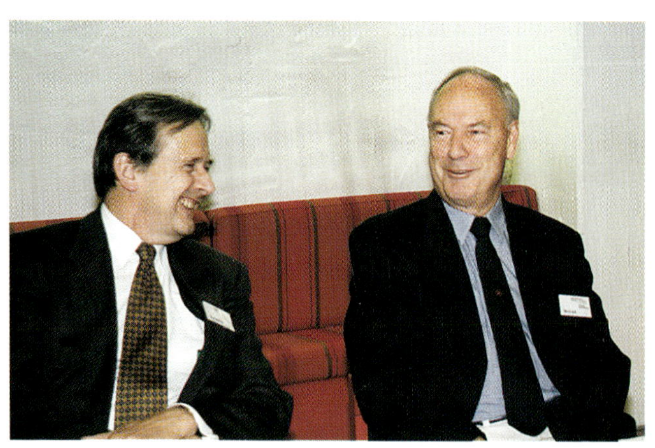

Theodor M. Fliedner, Donald Metcalf

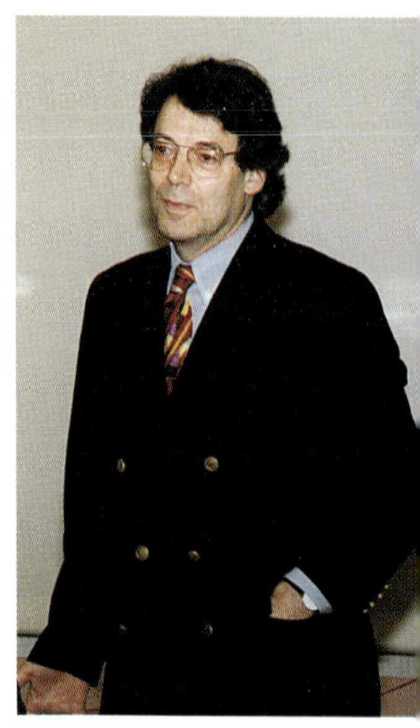

Dieter Hoelzer

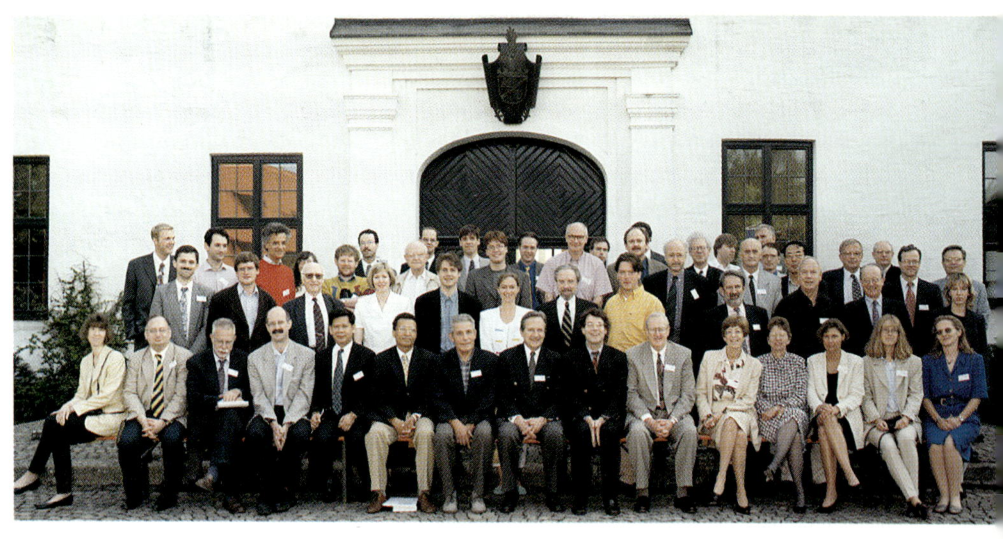

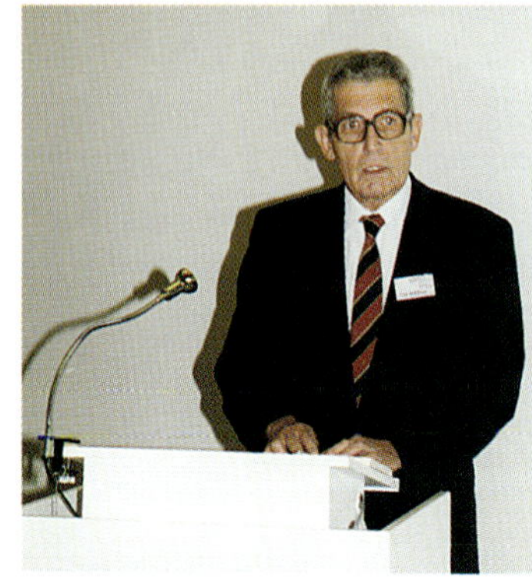

Dirk W. van Bekkum

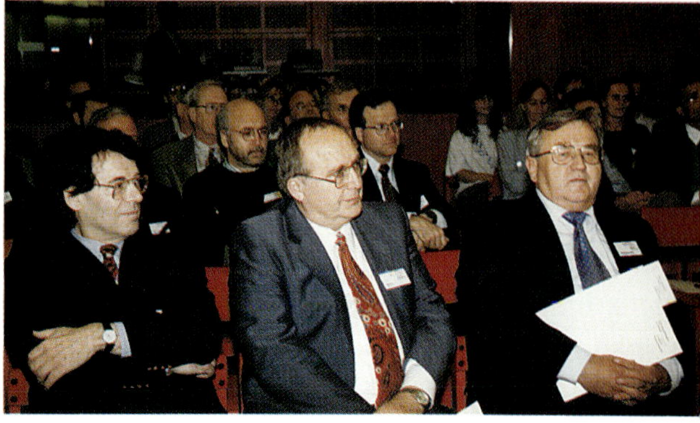

Opening ceremony

Prologue

THEODOR M. FLIEDNER

Department of Clinical Physiology, Occupational and Social Medicine,
University of Ulm, Ulm, Germany

The center of this monograph—based on the International Stem Cell Workshop on Pathophysiology, Diagnostic and Therapeutic Implications of Blood Stem Cells held at the International Institute for Scientific Cooperation, Schloss Reisensburg, Germany—is the

Blood Stem Cell.

This term was used in the scientific literature as a "key word" only in the 1960s. It appeared intermittently between 1970 and 1985, but gained the attention of a large number of physicians and scientists when the first publications came out in the middle of the 1980s on the clinical use of blood stem cells to restore hematopoiesis in patients rendered aplastic as a consequence of extensive radiation and/or chemotherapy [1-4].

However, the discussion about the physiological as well as pathophysiological significance of circulating pluripotent stem cells is lagging behind. Therefore, it has been the purpose of the International Workshop to assemble a group of leading international scientists and physicians to exchange views on the "Characteristics and Potentials of Blood Stem Cells."

It appears of interest in these introductory remarks to trace the scientific steps that eventually led to the recognition of the blood stem cell as an important entity of its own.

For decades, the notions of *Alexander Maximow* remained "dormant." It is fascinating to recognize that this investigator, working in St. Petersburg, presented conclusions of his studies at an extraordinary session of the Hematological Society of Berlin on June 1, 1909, which turned out to be pioneering work in the best sense of the word. The title of his lecture was "The Lymphocyte as Common Stem Cell of the Different Blood Elements during Embryonic Development and in the Post-Fetal Life of Mammals" (Fig. 1) [5]. His paper comprised almost 15 pages in which he described the studies he had performed using stained histological preparations. And he concluded:

> "In the mammalian organism exists one cell type, the lymphocyte in the widest sense of the word, which may look different according to the site of residence as well as to the local conditions and which can produce different products of cellular differentiation. The lymphocytes are "ubiquitär," of equal value everywhere. Histogenic and hematogenic cannot be distinguished. In the adenoidal tissue they produce by homoplastic proliferation again and again lymphocytes. The easily transportable form, the small lymphocyte, circulates with the blood- and lymph stream throughout the organism and is able to regain after a sufficient timelag of inactivity its full developmental potential."

Characteristics and Potentials of Blood Stem Cells
STEM CELLS **1998;16(suppl 1):xiii-xvii** ©AlphaMed Press. All rights reserved.

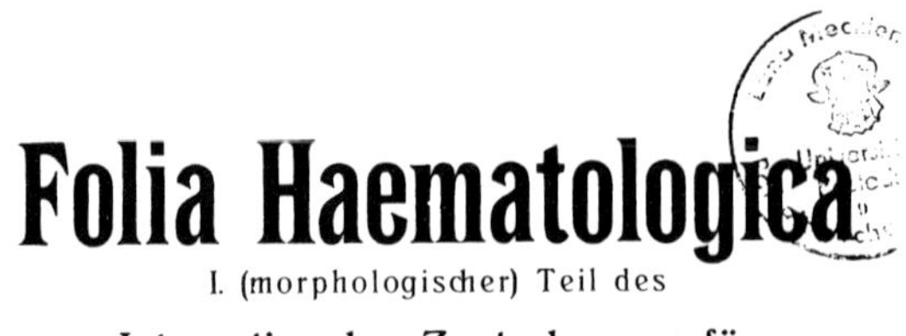

Folia Haematologica

I. (morphologischer) Teil des

Internationalen Zentralorgans für
Blut- und Serumforschung

**Der Lymphozyt als gemeinsame Stammzelle
der verschiedenen Blutelemente in der embryonalen
Entwicklung und im postfetalen Leben der Säugetiere.**[1])

Von

Prof. Dr. **A. Maximow.**

Die ersten Blutelemente entstehen bekanntlich aus den sog. Blutinseln, aus unregelmässig begrenzten, miteinander netzartig verbundenen Zellansammlungen des peripheren mesenchymatösen Mesoblasts, im Bereiche der Area opaca. Die peripherischen Zellen der Blutinseln platten sich ab, werden zu Endothelzellen, die inneren runden sich ab und schwimmen als die ersten Blutzellen frei in einer Flüssigkeit, die man Blutplasma nennen kann. Ich habe nun gefunden, dass diese primitiven Blutzellen, wie ich sie nenne, keineswegs Erythroblasten vorstellen, wie es nach der geläufigen Vorstellung sein sollte, sondern vollkommen indifferente Elemente, mit rundem hellem Kern und schmalem basophilem Protoplasma; es sind weder rote, noch weisse Blutkörperchen; eher dürften sie noch weisse Blutkörperchen genannt werden, da sie manchmal, besonders z. B. beim Hühnchen, sofort amöboid und den grossen Lymphozyten sehr ähnlich sind. Sie wuchern weiter, in der ersten Zeit vergrössert sich ihre Zahl auch noch durch

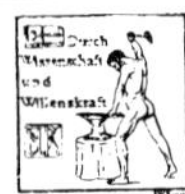

Leipzig 1909
Verlag von Dr. Werner Klinkhardt
Paris, 2, rue Bonaparte, Frédéric Gittler   New York. G. E. Stechert & Co.
Librairie   129—133 West 20 the Street

Figure 1. Announcement of Professor Maximow's lecture, June 1, 1909.

Thus, it was *Alexander Maximow* who had the vision of a "blood stem cell," the potential of which would be to replicate, proliferate and differentiate into different cell lineages depending on local tissue conditions.

This early notion of a "monophyletic" theory of blood cell formation and the role of circulating stem cells remained in the texts of hematology as an option next to other theories, called "dualistic" (*Ehrlich, Schridde, Naegeli*), "trialistic" (*Schilling*) or "polyphyletic" (*Sabin*) (fully discussed [6]).

In the classical hematological textbooks of the 1950s (such as in *Karl Rohr* [7] and *Maxwell M. Wintrobe* [8]), it was assumed that in the circulating blood of hematological healthy individuals, no immature cells are present in the blood stream. Extramedullary hematopoiesis was considered at that time to be a return of certain tissues (spleen, liver, lymph nodes) to an embryonic state and, hence, pathological. *Karl Rohr* [7] writes:

> "As far as the myeloid metaplasia is concerned, it has to be seen as an expression of potential of blood cell formation at an abnormal site..... The colonization by cells that emigrated from the blood is possible only under extraordinary circumstances such as identical twins or after roentgen-irradiation of the bone marrow. The immature cell forms that appear in the blood in cases of myeloid metaplasia are a natural consequence of abnormal foci of blood formation and not their cause. If the myeloid metaplasia regresses simultaneously with the normalization of the bone marrow activity, then the immature cells disappear from the blood."

But this phase of a rather "static" hematology resting on cellular morphology only was replaced by a "dynamic phase" of experimental hematology which was greatly influenced by experimental radiobiology research. *Swift, Taketa* and *Bond* (at the Naval Radiological Defense Laboratory, San Francisco, CA) performed in the early 1950s an experimental study of exposing mice by whole-body irradiation, but given in a sequential way [9]. Considerably lower mortality resulted from 875 rad X-irradiation of the entire body in mice if the abdomen was exposed 90 min prior to, or following, exposure of the remainder of the body. Results were similar regardless of the order in which the exposures were carried out, and the degree of protection so obtained was similar to that afforded by shielding the exteriorized spleen during total-body irradiation. It is by now of science-history interest to note the care that the authors used to evaluate and discuss their findings. It also showed clearly that at that time the idea of a functioning blood stem cell system was by no means established:

> "The finding that whole-body irradiation mortality can be substantially reduced by the exposure method employed in these studies furnishes presumptive evidence in support of the theory that the factor responsible is humoral in nature. However, it appears theoretically possible that whole-body irradiation by means of regionally fractionated exposures could result in a certain proportion of circulating blood, reticuloendothelial, or other, cells receiving a roentgen dose greater or lesser, by varying amounts, than that received by the fixed cells of the body. It is conceivable that a few such cells might receive very little radiation at all by virtue of being fortuitously retained within shielded body regions during most of the two exposures. One cannot entirely exclude the possibility, therefore, that the decreased radiation effect obtained in the present study by regionally fractionated exposure is associated with the activity of such spared cells, and hence might conceivably be the result of "seeding" rather than of the activity of a humoral agent. This factor cannot be assessed on the basis of the data available at the present time."

These studies were followed just a few years later by the discovery that DNA synthesizing cells are normal constituents of the peripheral blood (*V.P. Bond, E.P. Cronkite, T.M. Fliedner* and *P. Schork* at the Brookhaven National Laboratory in New York, NY [10]). The authors summarized their discoveries by the following remarks:

> "The findings that histiocytes, or specific cells of the reticuloendothelial system, may be multipotential in character, and may be transported to needed sites normally via the blood stream, are pertinent in connection with protection against X-radiation by parabiosis and by regionally fractionated exposures. In the later experiments, exposure of one-half of the body only was followed in a few minutes by exposure of only the other half of the body. Mortality was less than it was in animals that received equivalent single-dose total-body irradiation. Normally circulating multipotential cells would explain these findings. The hypothesis is supported by estimates that only a very few intact cells are required to repopulate a radiation-depleted marrow population."

In the early 1960s it was *Joan Goodman* and *George Hodgson* who published their pacemaking paper "Evidence for Stem Cells in the Peripheral Blood of Mice" [11]. This paper in conjunction with the earlier papers of the Brookhaven group and with the methodological development of the "spleen colony assay method" as developed by the Toronto group around *Till* and *McCulloch* [12], as well as of the in vitro colony-forming unit assay as initiated by *Bradley* and *Metcalf* (Melbourne) [13], and by *Pluznik* and *Sachs* (Jerusalem) [14], paved the way for the development of the studies on the physiology and pathophysiology of "blood stem cells" as an integral system of the homeostasis of blood cell formation. It must be mentioned at this point that it was the group around *Yoffey* in Bristol (United Kingdom) who maintained the importance of considering the multipotentiality of lymphocytes (see his classical paper "The Fourth Circulation" in [15]).

Thus, in their book on "Hemopoietic Cells," *Metcalf* and *Moore* [16] in 1970 were able to review the "state of the arts" of that time. They recognized fully the fact that circulating stem cells are of primary importance for the embryonic development of hematopoiesis in the bone marrow and of lymphopoiesis in the appropriate organs and suspected that they do play a role in the maintenance of hemopoiesis in the adult in which hematopoiesis is distributed throughout the skeletal bones. These authors expressed their conclusions in the following way:

> "The existence of stem cell migration in adult life is presumably the price to be paid for homeostasis and flexibility of haemopoietic response in the face of fluctuating demands. Excessive differentiation pressure may produce local exhaustion of the stem cell populations which can only be circumvented by migration of additional stem cells into the region. Furthermore, adaptation to situations of chronic demand for haemopoiesis involves the colonization by circulating stem cells of potential haemopoietic microenvironments existing in the fatty marrow spaces, the spleen, and, to a lesser extent, the liver. One may also speculate that, as haemopoiesis places a continuous proliferative demand on the stem cell population, safeguards are required to avoid excessive proliferation of stem cell clones since their reproductive integrity may be impaired by known limitations on the division capacity of somatic cells. Stem cell circulation and equilibration may therefore ensure equalization of proliferative pressure throughout the entire stem cell population."

With their monograph, *Metcalf* and *Moore* opened the door for extensive further experimental and clinical research on the physiological role of blood stem cells and their pathophysiology in diseased states. This area still offers unlimited opportunities for research especially to utilize the determination of quantity and quality of circulating stem cells as an aid in the diagnosis of hematological perturbations in a way similar to the use of numbers and qualities of red cells, granulocytes and platelets in hematological practice.

This brief survey on the scientific steps that had to be taken to recognize the circulating stem cell as an essential cellular element for the homeostatic mechanisms of an inexhaustible blood cell formation indicates that it is not enough to have an "evidence-based vision" (*Maximow*), but that the time has to be appropriate to test visions and hypotheses by experimental studies.

It was *Lord Kelvin* who expressed this notion in a masterly fashion:

> "I often say that when you can measure what you are speaking about, and express it in numbers, you know something about it, but when you cannot express it in numbers your knowledge is of a meagre and unsatisfactory kind: it may be the beginning of knowledge, but you have scarcely, in your thoughts, advanced to the stage of science, whatever the matter may be."

REFERENCES

1 Körbling M, Dörken B, Ho AD et al. Autologous transplantation of blood derived hemopoietic stem cells after myeloablative therapy in a patient with Burkitt's lymphoma. Blood 1986;67:529-532.

2 Juttner CA, To LB, Haylock DN et al. Circulating autologous stem cells collected in very early remission from acute non-lymphoblastic leukemia produce prompt but incomplete haemopoietic reconstitution after high dose melphalan or supralethal chemoradiotherapy. Br J Haematol 1985;61:739-745.

3 Reiffers J, Bernard PH, David B et al. Successful autologous transplantation with peripheral blood hemopoietic cells in a patient with acute leukemia. Exp Hematol 1986;14:312-315.

4 Kessinger A, Armitage JO, Landmark JD et al. Reconstitution of human hematopoietic function with autologous cryopreserved circulating stem cells. Exp Hematol 1986;14:192-196.

5 Maximow A. Der Lymphozyt als gemeinsame Stammzelle der verschiedenen Blutelemente in der

embryonalen Entwicklung und im postfetalen Leben der Säugetiere. Folia Haematol (Leipz) 1909;8:125-141.

6 Downey H, ed. Handbook of Hematology. New York: Harper and Row Publishers, 1938.

7 Rohr K. Das menschliche Knochenmark. Stuttgart: Georg Thieme Verlag, 1960:126-130.

8 Wintrobe M, ed. Clinical Hematology. Philadelphia: Lea and Febinger, Fifth Edition, 1961.

9 Swift MN, Taketa ST, Bond VP. Regionally fractionated x-irradiation equivalent in close to total body exposure. Radiat Res 1954;1:241-252.

10 Bond VP, Cronkite EP, Fliedner TM et al. Deoxyribonucleic acid synthesizing cells in peripheral blood of normal human beings. Science 1958;128:202-203.

11 Goodman JW, Hodgson GS. Evidence for stem cells in the peripheral blood of mice. Blood 1962;19:702-714.

12 Till JE, McCulloch EA. A direct measurement of the radiation sensitivity of normal mouse bone marrow cells. Radiat Res 1961;14:213-222.

13 Bradley TR, Metcalf D. The growth of mouse bone marrow cells in vitro. Austr J Exp Biol Med Sci 1966;44:287-300.

14 Pluznik DH, Sachs L. The cloning of normal mast cells in tissue culture. J Cell Comp Physiol 1965;66:319-324.

15 Yoffey JM. The fourth circulation. In: Yoffey JM, ed. The Lymphocyte in Immunology and Haemopoiesis. London: Edward Arnold Ltd., 1967.

16 Metcalf D, Moore MAS. Haemopoietic Cells. Frontiers of Biology. Amsterdam-London: North Holland Publishing Co., 1971.

CHAPTER I

KEYNOTE ADDRESSES

REGULATORY MECHANISMS CONTROLLING HEMATOPOIESIS: PRINCIPLES AND PROBLEMS

Donald Metcalf

THE ROLE OF BLOOD STEM CELLS IN HEMATOPOIETIC CELL RENEWAL

Theodor M. Fliedner

Regulatory Mechanisms Controlling Hematopoiesis: Principles and Problems

DONALD METCALF

The Walter and Eliza Hall Institute of Medical Research, Royal Melbourne Hospital, Victoria, Australia

Key Words. *Hematopoiesis · Hematopoietic regulators · Proliferation · Differentiation commitment*

ABSTRACT

Hematopoiesis is regulated by the combined action of specialized stromal cells and a consortium of hematopoietic regulatory factors. The multiplicity of these regulatory controls does result in overlapping regulator action, but multiple regulators are required to stimulate stem cell proliferation and are more efficient than single regulators when stimulation of progenitor cells is required. Gene inactivation studies have indicated that despite overlapping actions each hematopoietic regulator does have unique functions. Delayed elevations of stem and progenitor cells in the blood are a feature of enhanced hematopoiesis induced by the injection of regulators. These cells are not a random sample of marrow cells in such situations and may well be selected to rapidly amplify hematopoiesis by seeding previously inactive hematopoietic regions. *Stem Cells 1998;16(suppl 1):3-11*

INTRODUCTION

Ted Fliedner and I are close contemporaries who as young medical graduates entered experimental hematology but by somewhat different routes. In *Ted's* case it was via studies on the consequences of irradiation on hematopoiesis and the associated biology of marrow transplantation. My entry was via studies on leukemogenesis and the evident necessity to understand the nature of normal hematopoiesis. Both of us were to make extensive use of tritiated thymidine as the most elegant tool available in the late 1950s and early 1960s for analyzing cell kinetics and the overall nature of the stepwise production of blood cells. That this tedious autoradiography is no longer used in such studies no doubt is a cause of regret for us both. It is also a source of not a little wry amusement as one sees fluorescence-activated cell sorter analysis misused to produce some very silly misinformation on cell kinetics in the multiplicity of wonderful transgenic and gene inactivation models now available to experimental hematologists.

No doubt we made equally silly mistakes when young but in this period of youthful energy and self-confidence we also both tried hard in our different ways to promote the development of experimental hematology in Germany. Our efforts were to come together firmly in 1973 with a training course for experimental hematologists held for the World Health Organization in Schloss Reisensberg. It is therefore a particular pleasure for me to participate in this celebratory symposium for *Ted Fliedner* in the same location in which we introduced modern hematopoietic research methods to our students about a quarter of a century ago.

In retrospect, the mid-1960s saw the birth of the modern hematology, the 1970s its flowering, the 1980s its transfer via molecular biology from the bench to the clinic and the 1990s its mature status as the most advanced area of cell biology with exciting possibilities for exploitation but still many problems for resolution.

Characteristics and Potentials of Blood Stem Cells
STEM CELLS 1998;16(suppl 1):3-11

Hematopoiesis

Hematopoiesis is the continuous process by which the production of the eight major lineages of mature blood cells is achieved from a small population of multipotential hematopoietic stem cells. The regulatory systems controlling this process normally operate with high precision and have the ability in situations of stress to greatly amplify cell production within days. The cellular events are complex with the stepwise generation by stem cells of committed progenitor cells, then the formation by these cells of immature dividing cells in the various lineages with concurrent maturation of the cells and their eventual release from the major producing organ—the bone marrow. A number of qualitatively different cellular processes are involved (cell division, differentiation commitment, maturation induction, cellular trafficking and mature cell activation) often with more than one of the first three occurring simultaneously in individual cells.

Three decades of investigation have identified two types of regulatory system operating on hematopoietic populations: A) local control by microenvironmental stromal cells in the marrow and spleen, often appearing to involve or require close cell proximity or contact, and B) molecular regulators, most often secreted but sometimes membrane-displayed, that may be produced locally in hematopoietic tissues or distant tissues, in which case they operate in a humoral manner.

Local Stromal Control

From a combination of studies on spleen colony formation in irradiated recipients [1], long-term culture of cells with stromal underlayers [2, 3] and short-term clonal cultures, it has become conventional to regard stromal control as playing a dominant role in regulating stem cell behavior and progenitor cell formation while molecular regulators are viewed as primarily controlling the generation of maturing cells from progenitor cells. There is little experimental basis for this appealing model with its neat division of labor. Molecular regulators are now known with undoubted actions on stem cells. Conversely, there is no real evidence that excludes stromal cells from having a regulatory role in the more mature stages of hematopoiesis. Indeed, stromal cells are a known, but not exclusive, source of many molecular regulators acting on more mature hematopoietic precursor cells [4]. The two control systems are better regarded as probably operating simultaneously at most stages of hematopoiesis.

While stromal cells undoubtedly play a key role in determining the restricted location of hematopoiesis to the bone marrow, spleen, thymus and lymph nodes, why this role is special is becoming increasingly less clear. More and more molecular regulators are being identified, many as products of stromal cells. The difficulty however is that none have been identified as exclusive products of stromal cells, and the answer may be merely that local membrane display of regulatory factors can sometimes be more efficient, as is the case for stem cell factor (SCF) [5], or that local production of secreted regulators achieves higher concentrations than achievable by circulating regulators.

The availability of a network of active stromal cells does appear to set physical limits to the number of hematopoietic cells able to be supported in a particular region, but adjacent dormant regions in an organ like the human marrow can readily be reactivated when additional hematopoiesis is required. The notion that individual stromal cells may be specialized to promote hematopoiesis of a particular type arose from early studies on colony-forming units, spleen-derived colony formation in irradiated mice where erythroid colony formation was prominent in the spleen, while granulocyte colony formation was the dominant pattern in the bone marrow [6]. This may still be a correct view but is in need of more substantiation. Cloned stromal cell lines have a fairly unselective and variable capacity to support various types of hematopoiesis in culture [7] while nonhematopoietic fibroblast cell lines can often function equally well. If there is specificity in the function of various stromal cells, this appears to be readily able to be overridden. For example, administration of G-CSF can entirely suppress erythropoiesis in the marrow with displacement of these populations to the spleen [8, 9]. Is this simply the consequence of overcrowding by one hematopoietic population physically displacing another or are the putative "erythroid" stromal niches able to be functionally suppressed by regulator action? The original striking differences between spleen erythroid colonies and marrow granulocytic colonies were in fact deceptive because analysis showed that erythroid colonies contained progenitor cells of other lineages [10]. At best, what was being observed was selective amplification of more mature cell elements to produce the appearance of a pure erythroid colony. These are a more mature series of cellular events than are normally assigned to stromal control in the above-mentioned conventional model.

Hematopoietic Regulators

Work in the past 20 years has led to the characterization of more than 20 molecular regulators of hemopoiesis and this has led to considerable progress in understanding the control of hematopoiesis, at least in terms of identifying key processes susceptible to regulation and in characterizing unresolved problems requiring further study.

Figure 1 shows the molecular regulators identified as likely to play a role in controlling the formation of granulocytes and macrophages. The pattern revealed can be reproduced for cells of other lineages and so the granulocyte-macrophage regulators can be considered as a useful model for discussing some of the questions at issue.

What is evident from Figure 1 is that multiple regulators are available to achieve either progenitor cell production by stem cells or mature cell production from progenitor cells. The cellular basis permitting this situation is the simultaneous display on various cells of receptors for more than one regulator. The resulting arrangement is more complex than would appear necessary and has been regarded by some as exhibiting redundancy. Certainly there is obvious potential overlap in the actions of various regulators but gene inactivation studies (with the arguable exception of interleukin 3 [IL-3]) have indicated unique roles for each regulator that are not able to be taken over by other regulators with partially overlapping actions [11, 12]. The multiplicity of available regulators therefore needs to be regarded as having a valid design purpose [13], either by achieving a more efficient, flexible, or subtle control system, and some of these features have already been verified.

One characteristic of hematopoietic regulators, now well-recognized, is that none exhibit absolute lineage specificity [4]. Regulators such as G-CSF, erythropoietin (EPO) or thrombopoietin (TPO) may exhibit lineage-dominant actions respectively on granulocytic, erythroid or megakaryocytic cells, but all have actions on cells of at least some other lineages and many have actions on cells in the heterogeneous stem cell compartment. There is also increasing evidence for actions of many on non-hematopoietic cells, but the physiological relevance of many of these actions has not yet been firmly established.

In terms of proliferative stimulation, there is now a repeatedly documented major apparent difference between stem cells and progenitor cells. Stem cells require simultaneous signaling by multiple regulators before proliferating [14-16] while, in sharp contrast, progenitor cells can respond well to proliferative signaling by a single regulator. It may be that this peculiar responsiveness pattern of stem cells is designed to protect them from wasteful expenditure of their possibly finite proliferative potential by stress situations requiring merely the increased production of one particular type of blood cell, such as erythroid cells or granulocytes.

However, what is this revealing about the intracellular mitotic signaling pathways in stem cells that differ from those in progenitor cells? In various experiments in this laboratory in recent years, we have inserted cDNA encoding a variety of receptors into the continuous murine cell lines FDC-P1 or Ba/F3 [17-19] (Fig. 2). FDC-P1 cells normally express receptors

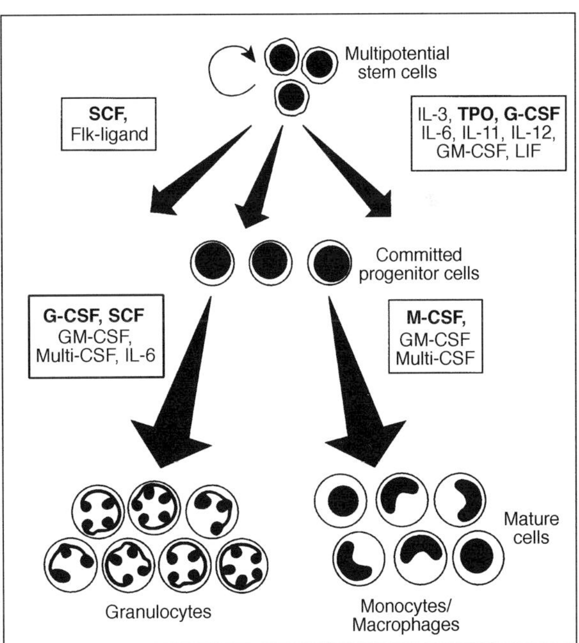

Figure 1. Multiple hematopoietic regulators have been identified as being able to stimulate progenitor cell formation by stem cells or the formation of maturing progeny by progenitor cells. For stem cell proliferation, stem cell factor and Flk ligand are of special importance when acting in collaboration with one or more of the regulators listed on the right of the diagram. From gene inactivation studies, the regulators in bolded type are of special importance in controlling the numbers of cells produced.

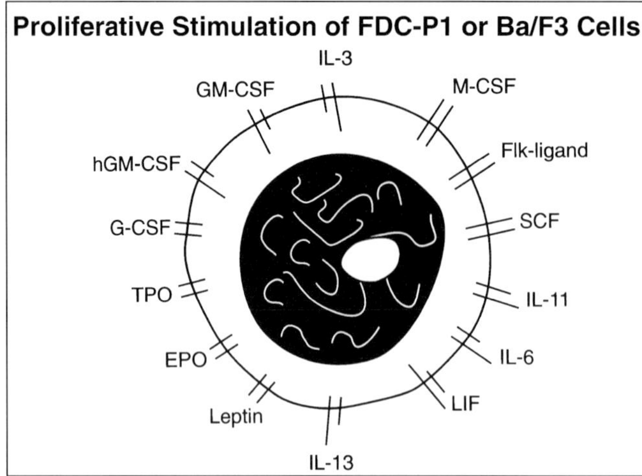

Figure 2. A composite diagram of experiments inserting individual receptors of many types into FDC-P1 or Ba/F3 cells. Expression of the receptor allows these cells to respond to proliferative stimulation by the relevant growth factor, strongly indicating that there is likely to be a final common mitotic signaling pathway.

for GM-CSF and IL-3 and depend on mitotic signaling by either of these two regulators, while Ba/F3 cells express receptors only for IL-3. When these cells are modified to express receptors for M-CSF, SCF or Flk-ligand (homodimeric tyrosine kinase receptors), G-CSF or TPO (homodimeric nontyrosine kinase receptors of the cytokine family) or IL-6, IL-11, leukemia inhibitory factor or oncostatin M (heterodimeric nontyrosine kinase, gp130-containing receptors of the cytokine receptor family) they can then be stimulated to exhibit comparable proliferation with usually unremarkable concentrations (10 to 100 pg/ml) of the appropriate regulator. The initial signaling events clearly differ between these receptor groups yet the cells exhibit apparently complete promiscuity in their ability to exhibit a proliferative response to inappropriate types of receptor signaling, even that from inserted human GM-CSF receptors [20].

These observations argue strongly for a final common pathway for proliferative signaling, there presumably only being a single set of genes to be activated to achieve passage of a cell through the cell cycle.

It is in this context that the requirement of stem cells for multiple regulator signaling becomes puzzling unless restricted numbers of any one type of receptor make it impossible to achieve the necessary concentrations of required transcription factors, regardless of the concentration of the single regulator used. The alternative, that in certain cells there are multiple possible terminal signaling cascades which must act in concert to achieve activation of the complex of mitotic genes, seems inherently improbable but cannot be dismissed.

What at first seemed to be a unique problem posed by stem cells is now not likely to be so. There are many examples now recognized of superadditive synergy between regulators acting on individual progenitor cells. These raise the same question. Why do two regulators achieve greater proliferation than twice the concentration of either regulator [21]? For some progenitors, combined stimulation appears mandatory to achieve colony formation. The clearest example encountered by us in which this problem is raised was seen when using a combination of GM-CSF with M-CSF to stimulate mouse bone marrow cells. Although the combination was inhibitory for many macrophage progenitors, it is necessary to induce the formation by special progenitor cells of certain very large macrophage or granulocyte-macrophage colonies [21], a situation comparable to that existing for stem cells.

Hematopoietic regulators, as typified by the colony stimulating factors, are now known to be polyfunctional and control not only mitotic activity but differentiation commitment, maturation initiation, cell viability and functional activity in various responding cells [4]. This initially raised the question of how these multiple cellular processes could be regulated by a single type of activated receptor. Resolution of this question has come from the identification of distinct functional regions in the receptor chains initiating signals for cell division, differentiation commitment and maturation [22-25]. While the distinctness of the subsequent signaling pathways from these separate regions has yet to be fully documented, there are good grounds for presuming these are indeed distinct. The separateness of these response pathways has been verified in normal cells, where induced expression of anomalous receptors allows inappropriate regulator stimulation of proliferation but without altering the differentiation program of the responding cells. For example, macrophage progenitors engineered to express EPO receptors can then be stimulated to colony formation by EPO but the colonies are macrophage in composition, not erythroid [26]. Similarly, the pattern of maturation of leukemic cells expressing aberrant receptors is dictated by the cell, not the actual receptor used to activate the program. The nature of these host cell-determined mechanisms remains unknown, as does the nature of the program differences allowing a myeloblast to respond to GM-CSF stimulation by cell division while a neutrophil with similar receptor numbers responds merely by functional activation.

The general pattern of promiscuity of hematopoietic cells to initially differing signaling cascades has been reinforced by studies using receptor insertion into leukemic cell lines. As shown in Figure 3, a wide variety of receptors has been expressed in this laboratory in two murine leukemic cell lines, permitting the relevant regulators to initiate differentiation commitment or maturation [25, 27]. This indicates the permissiveness of cells, in this case for maturation induction, with again the likelihood of a common final signaling pathway. Nevertheless, the type of maturation exhibited by the cell is again unrelated to the ligand/receptor system used to activate the program.

What is missing in our present knowledge is any clue to what allows a particular differentiation program to be activatable in the cell. The newly recognized SOCS gene family [28] encodes molecules that seem able to modulate cell signaling and might be of

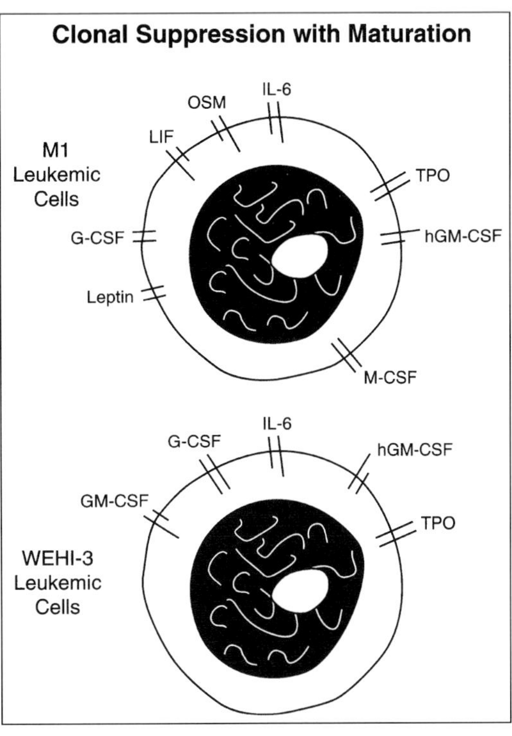

Figure 3. Composite diagrams summarizing various experiments in which receptors of different types have been inserted into WEHI-3B or M1 leukemic cell lines. In each case, after receptor expression, the cells can be induced by the relevant growth factor to suppress their self-renewing proliferative activity and/or exhibit maturation to macrophages.

relevance to this question. The SOCS proteins were identified as being able to block cytokine-induced maturation in leukemic cell lines. Those members so far studied only inhibit cell proliferation in a minor manner and therefore have a certain selectivity of action. They also do not block the capacity of the cells to mature in response to other agents such as dexamethasone. While they appear to act early in signaling to block phosphorylation and activation of certain JAKS and STATS [28, 29], some selectivity of action seems likely and potentially they might be relevant modulators of actual gene programs able to be activated. In this context, the SOCS genes are induced by cytokine signaling [28, 30] but the pattern of induction varies with time, cell type and the cytokine used, which raises the possibility of some subtlety in modulating action.

The maturation programs, once activated, almost certainly need to be autocatalytic to ensure the fidelity of maturation normally observed and the orderly sequence in which the necessary events occur. It would be a seemingly impossible control system if each separate event needed to be independently regulated in such a tightly coordinated manner.

Action of Regulators In Vivo

Daily injection of regulators such as G-CSF, GM-CSF, TPO or EPO to mice or man results in stimulation of the proliferation of the expected hematopoietic populations, resulting in elevated levels of the relevant mature cells [31-34]. These responses have indicated that the prior in vitro characterization of these regulators had given valid information on their likely action in vivo. Pessimistic predictions had been that: A) a single injected agent would not elicit measurable responses because of the potentially complex nature of the regulatory network controlling hematopoiesis and B) responses would not be sustained because all progenitor cells would expend themselves in generating maturing progeny.

The concerns raised in A) have some validity if only that an injected regulator is not likely to be operating independently of other regulators already present in vivo. Indeed, the larger than expected responses to G-CSF are likely to be the consequence of a synergistic action of resident SCF with the injected G-CSF, since responses to G-CSF in W^v or Sl^d mice (lacking in SCF receptors or the ability to produce SCF) are considerably lower than in other mice [35]. This is supported by the strong synergy demonstrable in vitro when combinations of SCF and G-CSF are used [36]. What remains puzzling is why other agents such as IL-6 or IL-3, which have equally strong synergistic interactions with SCF in vitro, should be relatively inactive in stimulating granulopoiesis in vivo. The concerns raised in B) proved to be unfounded for the simple reason that replacement of expended progenitor cells was able to be achieved rapidly by stem cells in the responding animal.

Regulator-Induced Rises in Purified Blood Stem and Progenitor Cells

The earliest in vivo experiments involving the injection of crude CSF-containing preparations into mice noted a major rise in blood progenitor cells in the animals [37]. It was not particularly surprising therefore when major rises in progenitor and stem cells were observed in the blood in man and mice following the injection of CSFs, particularly G-CSF [38, 39]. In view of the facts that synergy with SCF is probably occurring in vivo and that, in vitro, this synergy leads to increased progenitor cell formation in all myeloid lineages [40], it was also not surprising that G-CSF should elevate levels of a broad range of progenitor and stem cells. These cells have proved highly effective in transplantation [31] and seem likely to replace marrow cells as the transplanted population of choice in the future.

What remains unclear are the mechanisms responsible for this rise in so-called "peripheral blood stem cells." It is widely assumed that these cells are released from the bone marrow although this has never been formally proved. Spleen progenitor and stem cell levels rise equally spectacularly during these cytokine-induced responses [9] and again it is assumed without proof that these cells also are mainly of marrow origin rather than being locally generated.

What is clear however in both mouse and man is that when G-CSF induces such rises in precursor cells in the peripheral blood, the process cannot be due to random release of cells from the marrow. Progenitor cell rises in the blood in man are characteristically delayed to six or eight days following commencement of injections [41, 42] in comparison to the earlier rises in mature cells, a curious inverse of what might have been expected. Furthermore, the cells are noncycling, unlike progenitor cells in the marrow [43], and the relative frequency of different subsets of progenitor cells not only changes with time but at no stage matches those present in the marrow [9]. It is also characteristic that the most mature precursors, day 7 GM-CFC and CFU-E, are underrepresented or not present in the blood. There are also unexplained 10-fold interindividual variations in progenitor cell responses, a feature in mice that has been shown to be genetically determined [44].

These features indicate that CSF-induced marrow release is likely to be a complex process involving a number of components. Alterations in the expression by various hematopoietic cells of adherence molecules is likely to be an important determinant [45] but CSF-induced changes in sinus vascular endothelial channels may also occur. One component receiving little consideration so far is the intrinsic motility of progenitor and stem cells. It seems to be assumed by many that primitive cells such as stem or progenitor cells are likely to be nonmotile. This could be a mistaken view and it is relevant to consider the implications of some familiar patterns of clonal proliferation in vitro.

In semisolid agar cultures, some progenitor cells form highly compact colonies such as immature granulocytic colonies where cell migration only occurs following maturation to more mature forms. This implies that the progenitor cell concerned and its initial progeny are nonmotile. This contrasts sharply with the behavior of BFU-E and stem cells, both of which characteristically form multicentric (burst) colonies. As shown in Figure 4, the basis for a multicentric colony is the rapid motility of the initial progeny, for example of a BFU-E, followed then by the immobility of subsequent progeny. From this it can be deduced that BFU-E and their initial progeny are in fact highly motile cells in contrast to CFU-E and their progeny which are nonmotile. Similar conclusions can be drawn about the stem cell-generated blast colonies composed of progenitor cells. Again these are multicentric in nature and again, the conclusion is that at least this stem cell and its initial progeny are in fact highly motile cells. These conclusions introduce another variable into the process of cytokine-induced release of cells to the blood. Some of the cells appearing in the blood are in fact highly motile cells and this might well be enhanced by the injected cytokine. Certainly it provides an

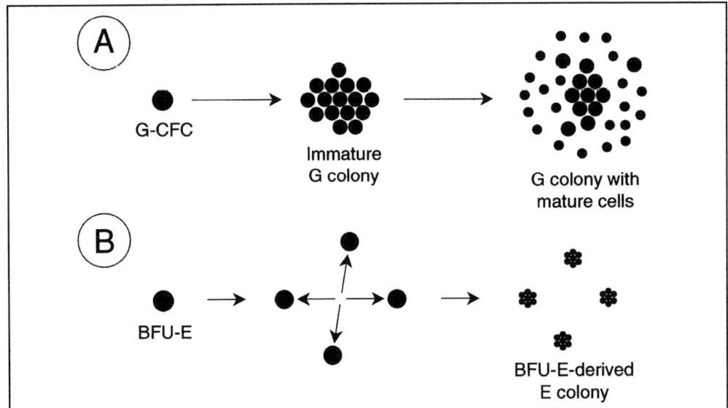

Figure 4. In (A) colonies composed of immature granulocytes exhibit no motility of colony cells until some of the cells mature to neutrophils. In contrast in (B), in developing burst-erythroid colonies derived from BFU-E, the initial progeny move widely apart, demonstrating their active motility. When they have matured to CFU-E, these cells and their progeny exhibit no further motility.

intriguing possible explanation of why BFU-E but not CFU-E appear in the peripheral blood in these responses.

The appearance of large numbers of stem and progenitor cells in situations involving increased hematopoiesis could be regarded as a trivial accompaniment of increased hematopoietic population size and proliferative activity. It is more likely, however, that this event has a design purpose and the most likely is that it serves as a rapid method for extending regions of active hematopoietic tissue in the spleen and marrow. In humans, it may well be more efficient to seed distant, dormant regions of the marrow, by blood-borne seeding than to rely on simple expansion into adjacent dormant regions. Whether the cells involved are in any way selected for exceptional homing efficiency could be checked experimentally in mice by determining seeding factor efficiencies compared to unselected marrow cells.

ACKNOWLEDGMENT

The work from the author's laboratory was supported by the Carden Fellowship Fund of the Anti-Cancer Council of Victoria, the National Health and Medical Research Council, Canberra, the AMRAD Corporation, Melbourne and the National Institutes of Health, Bethesda, Grant No. CA22556.

REFERENCES

1 Trentin JJ. Hemopoietic microenvironments. In: Tavassoli M, ed. Handbook of the Hemopoietic Microenvironment. Clifton: Humana Press, 1989:1-86.

2 Dexter TM, Spooncer E, Simons P et al. Long-term marrow culture: an overview of techniques and experience. In: Wright DG, Greenberger JS, eds. Long-Term Bone Marrow Culture. New York: Alan R Liss, 1984:57-96.

3 Coulombel L, Eaves AC, Eaves CJ. Enzymatic treatment of long-term human marrow cultures reveals preferential location of primitive progenitors in the adherent layer. Blood 1983;62:291-297.

4 Metcalf D, Nicola NA. The Hemopoietic Colony Stimulating Factors. Oxford: Cambridge University Press, 1995.

5 Toksoz D, Zsebo KM, Smith KA et al. Support of human hematopoiesis in long-term bone marrow cultures by murine stromal cells selectively expressing the membrane-bound and secreted forms of the human homolog of the Steel gene product, stem cell factor. Proc Natl Acad Sci USA 1992;89:7350-7354.

6 Wolf NS, Trentin JJ. Hemopoietic colony studies. V. Effect of hemopoietic organ stroma on differentiation of pluripotent stem cells. J Exp Med 1968;127:205-214.

7 Cicuttini FM, Martin M, Salvaris E et al. Support of early human cord blood progenitor cells on human stromal cell lines transformed by SV40 large T antigen under the influence of an inducible metallothionein promoter. Blood 1992;80:102-112.

8 de Haan G, Loeffler M, Nijhof W. Long-term recombinant human granulocyte colony-stimulating factor (rhG-CSF) treatment severely depresses murine marrow erythropoiesis without causing an anemia. Exp Hematol 1992;20:600-604.

9 Roberts AW, Metcalf D. Granulocyte colony-stimulating factor induces selective elevations of progenitor cells in the peripheral blood of mice. Exp Hematol 1994;22:1156-1163.

10 Johnson GR, Metcalf D. The commitment of multipotential hemopoietic stem cells: studies in vivo and in vitro. In: Le Douarin N, ed. Cell Lineage, Stem Cells and Cell Determination. INSERM Symposium No. 10. Amsterdam: Elsevier/North-Holland, 1979:199-213.

11 Metcalf D. The granulocyte-macrophage regulators: reappraisal by gene inactivation. Exp Hematol 1995;23:569-572.

12 Metcalf D. Suppression or overexpression of genes encoding myeloid growth factors or their receptors. Hematol Cell Ther 1997;39:98-101.

13 Metcalf D. Hemopoietic regulators: redundancy or subtlety? Blood 1993;82:3515-3523.

14 Li CL, Johnson GR. Rhodamine 123 reveals heterogeneity within murine Lin⁻, Sca-1⁺ hemopoietic stem cells. J Exp Med 1992;175:1443-1447.

15 Galli SJ, Zsebo KM, Geissler EN. The kit ligand, stem cell factor. Adv Immunol 1994;55:1-96.

16 Jacobsen SE, Okkenhaug C, Myklebust J et al. The FLT3 ligand potently and directly stimulates the growth and expansion of primitive murine bone marrow progenitor cells in vitro: synergistic interactions with interleukin (IL) 11, IL-12, and other hematopoietic growth factors. J Exp Med 1995;181:1357-1363.

17 Metcalf D, Willson T, Rossner M et al. Receptor insertion into factor-dependent murine cell lines to develop specific bioassays for murine G-CSF and M-CSF and human GM-CSF. Growth Factors 1994;11:145-152.

18 Hilton DJ, Hilton AA, Raicevic A et al. Cloning of a murine IL-11 receptor α-chain; requirement for gp130 for high affinity binding and signal transduction. EMBO J 1994;13:4765-4775.

19 Hilton DJ, Zhang J-G, Metcalf D et al. Cloning and characterization of a binding subunit of the interleukin 13 receptor that is also a component of the interleukin 4 receptor. Proc Natl Acad Sci USA 1996;93:497-501.

20 Metcalf D, Nicola NA, Gearing DP et al. Low-affinity placenta-derived receptors for human granulocyte-macrophage colony-stimulating factor can deliver a proliferative signal to murine hemopoietic cells. Proc Natl Acad Sci USA 1990;87:4670-4674.

21 Metcalf D, Nicola NA. The clonal proliferation of normal mouse hemopoietic cells: enhancement and suppression by CSF combinations. Blood 1992;79:2861-2866.

22 Sato N, Sakamaki K, Terada N et al. Signal transduction by the high-affinity GM-CSF receptor: two distinct cytoplasmic regions of the common beta subunit responsible for different signalling. EMBO J 1993;12:4181-4189.

23 Dong F, Van Buitenen C, Pouwels K et al. Distinct cytoplasmic regions of the human granulocyte colony-stimulating factor receptor involved in induction of proliferation and maturation. Mol Cell Biol 1993;13:7774-7778.

24 Fukunaga R, Ishizaka-Ikeda E, Nagata S. Growth and differentiation signals mediated by different regions in the cytoplasmic domain of granulocyte-stimulating factor receptor. Cell 1993;74:1079-1087.

25 Smith A, Metcalf D, Nicola NA. Cytoplasmic domains of the common β-chain of the GM-CSF/IL-3/IL-5 receptors that are required for inducing differentiation or clonal suppression in myeloid leukaemic cell lines. EMBO J 1997;16:451-464.

26 McArthur GA, Longmore GL, Klingler K et al. Lineage restricted recruitment of immature hemopoietic cells in response to erythropoietin after transfection of normal hemopoietic cells with the erythropoietin receptor. Exp Hematol 1995;23:645-654.

27 Gainsford T, Willson TA, Metcalf D et al. Leptin can induce proliferation, differentiation, and functional activation of hemopoietic cells. Proc Natl Acad Sci USA 1996;93:14564-14568.

28 Starr R, Willson TA, Viney EM et al. A family of cytokine-inducible inhibitors of signalling. Nature 1997;387:917-921.

29 Endo TA, Masuhara M, Yokouhi M et al. A new protein containing an SH2 domain that inhibits JAK kinases. Nature 1997;387:921-924.

30 Yoshimura A, Ohkubo T, Kiguchi T et al. A novel cytokine-inducible gene CIS encodes an SH2-containing protein that binds to tyrosine-phosphorylated interleukin 3 and erythropoietin receptors. EMBO J 1995;14:2816-2826.

31 Welte K, Gabrilove J, Bronchud MH et al. Filgrastim (r-metHuG-CSF): the first 10 years. Blood 1996;88:1907-1929.

32 Lieschke GJ, Maher D, Cebon J et al. Effects of bacterially-synthesized recombinant human granulocyte-macrophage colony-stimulating factor in patients with advanced malignancy. Ann Int Med 1989;110:357-364.

33 O'Malley CJ, Rasko JEJ, Basser RL et al. Administration of pegylated recombinant human megakaryocyte growth and development factor to humans stimulates the production of functional platelets that show no evidence of in vivo activation. Blood 1996;88:3288-3298.

34 Adamson JW, Eschbach JW. The use of recombinant human erythropoietin in humans. In: Bock G, Marsh G, eds. Molecular Control of Haemopoiesis. Chichester: John Wiley and Sons, 1990:186-200.

35 Cynshi O, Satoh K, Shimonaka Y et al. Reduced response to granulocyte colony-stimulating factor in W/Wᵛ and Sl/Slᵈ mice. Leukemia 1991;5:75-77.

36 Metcalf D, Nicola NA. Direct proliferative actions of stem cell factor on murine bone marrow cells in vitro. Effects of combination with colony-stimulating factors. Proc Natl Acad Sci USA 1991;88:6239-6243.

37 Bradley TR, Metcalf D, Sumner M et al. Characteristics of in vitro colony formation by

cells from haemopoietic tissues. In: Farnes P, ed. Hemic Cells In Vitro. In Vitro 1969;4:22-35.

38 Dührsen U, Villeval J-L, Boyd J et al. Effects of recombinant human granulocyte-colony stimulating factor on hemopoietic progenitor cells in cancer patients. Blood 1998;72:2074-2081.

39 Villeval J-L, Dührsen U, Morstyn G et al. Effect of recombinant human granulocyte-macrophage colony-stimulating factor on progenitor cells in patients with advanced malignancies. Brit J Haematol 1990;74:36-44.

40 Metcalf D. The cellular basis for enhancement interactions between stem cell factor and the colony stimulating factors. STEM CELLS 1993;11(suppl 2):1-11.

41 DeLuca E, Sheridan WP, Watson D et al. Prior chemotherapy does not prevent effective mobilisation by G-CSF of peripheral blood progenitor cells. Br J Cancer 1992;66:893-899.

42 Grigg AP, Roberts AW, Raunow H et al. Optimising dose and scheduling of filgrastim (granulocyte colony-stimulating factor) for mobilization and collection of peripheral blood progenitor cells in normal volunteers. Blood 1995;86:4437-4445.

43 Roberts AW, Metcalf D. Noncycling state of peripheral blood progenitor cells mobilized by granulocyte colony-stimulating factor and other cytokines. Blood 1995;86:1600-1605.

44 Roberts AW, Foote S, Alexander WS et al. Genetic influences determining progenitor cell mobilization and leukocytosis induced by granulocyte colony-stimulating factor. Blood 1997;89:2736-2744.

45 Simmons PJ, Leavesley DI, Levesque J-P et al. The mobilization of primitive hemopoietic progenitors into the peripheral blood. In: Murphy MJ, ed. Polyfunctionality of Hemopoietic Regulators: The Metcalf Forum. Stem Cells 1994;12(suppl 1):187-202.

The Role of Blood Stem Cells in Hematopoietic Cell Renewal

THEODOR M. FLIEDNER

Department of Clinical Physiology, Occupational and Social Medicine,
University of Ulm, Ulm, Germany

Key Words. *Blood stem cells · Hematopoiesis · Cell renewal · Stem cell migration streams · Hematopoietic recovery · Progenitor cells*

ABSTRACT

It has been the purpose of this keynote address to review available evidence for the notion that the stem and progenitor cells circulating in the peripheral blood play a decisive role in the homeostasis of blood cell formation distributed throughout dozens of bone marrow units in the skeleton. Furthermore, if this notion is correct, one could speculate that the quantity and quality of stem and progenitor cells in the blood should reflect the functional state of the hematopoietic stem cell system throughout the skeletal bone marrow and provide a new tool for the evaluation of alteration in blood cell production. On this basis, the following questions are considered: A) What do we know about the quality and quantity of blood stem cells in steady state conditions? B) In what way do blood stem cells respond to perturbations of the "steady state" of blood cell formation? C) Which role do blood stem cells play during hemopoietic development

assuming that the establishment of bone marrow hemopoiesis requires the "seeding" of blood stem cells into an appropriate cellular environment? D) What is the role of blood stem cells in hemopoietic regeneration after partial body irradiation with a small volume of marrow (and hence stem cells) protected? and E) What are the mechanisms and/or kinetics of hemopoietic recovery if stem cells introduced into the circulation were collected from exogenous (autologous or allogeneic) sources? In this review presentation, experimental work of our group and of other members of the scientific community is summarized. It becomes obvious that blood stem and progenitor cells play a key role in hematopoietic homeostasis. Furthermore, their physiology and pathophysiology deserve rigorous experimental studies in order to develop a novel tool in the diagnosis and prognosis of neoplastic and non-neoplastic disorders of blood cell formation. *Stem Cells 1998;16(suppl 1):13-29*

INTRODUCTION: SCOPE AND PURPOSE

It is the purpose of this presentation to examine and discuss two statements with respect to their experimental evidence and to suggest that the assessment of the quantity and quality of blood stem cells may well be useful as indicators of health and health impairments in the mammalian organism and, in particular, its blood-cell-forming tissues.

- The hematopoietic stem cell pool is distributed through the sites of hematopoietic cell renewal in a large number of bone marrow units distributed throughout the skeleton. That the hematopoietically active bone marrow sites act and respond as one organ system is due to the stem cell migration

Characteristics and Potentials of Blood Stem Cells
STEM CELLS 1998;16(suppl 1):13-29

streams which connect via the blood stream all sites and assure a local stem cell concentration sufficient to maintain a balance between cell production and cell removal.

- The quality and quantity of stem cells in the peripheral blood should reflect the quality and quantity of the extravascular stem cell pools and the balance between the sites of hematopoietic cell renewal. Hence, a systematic investigation of blood stem cell changes in health and disease may well contribute to the arsenal of methods guiding the work of clinical hematology.

Alexander Maximow, while working in St. Petersburg as a military doctor in 1909, was the first to suggest that there was a hematopoietic stem cell with the morphological appearance of a "lymphocyte" capable of migrating through the blood to microecological niches that would allow them to proliferate and differentiate along lineage specific pathways [1]. Since then, many hematologists have contributed to the debate about the origin and mechanisms of homeostasis in hematopoietic cell renewal, and many decades have passed during which the "monophyletic" versus the "polyphyletic" origin of blood cell formation was discussed [2]. Today, we have to acknowledge the fact that *Maximow*, in principle, was right to suggest the origin of hematopoiesis in one stem cell capable of migrating from one site of hematopoiesis to the other via the blood stream and settling in tissue sites in which the microenvironment is conducive to differentiation and proliferation of blood progenitor and precursor cells.

The experimental evidence for the significance of blood stem cells in research and clinical practice can be derived from the developmental dynamics of scientific publications that are devoted in one way or the other to "blood stem cells." The International Database DIMDI for 1996 lists 314 references under the key word "blood stem cells." A search for the use of this term for 1970 showed only one reference (Fig. 1). The first scientists to use or imply this term in experimental hematology were *Goodman* and *Hodgson* in 1962 [3].

Thus, it may be useful to review the experimental evidence of the physiology and pathophysiology of blood stem cells and to ask—even without being able to give final answers—what role they might play in the study and evaluation of hemopoietic cell renewal in health and disease.

In this presentation, stem cell migration streams will be examined using five key examples:

A) steady-state situation in the adult;

B) "physiological" perturbations of the steady state;

C) hemopoietic development during embryogenesis;

D) hematopoietic reconstitution after partial-body irradiation or chemotherapy, and

E) hematopoietic recovery introducing stem cells into blood from exogenous sources.

It will become apparent that the stem and progenitor cells migrating in the blood stream may have a much higher significance for hematopoietic cell renewal than was assumed until recently. They do not appear to be "waste products" of bone marrow cell production [4] and require extensive research to further elucidate their physiological role in hematopoietic cell renewal and their diagnostic and therapeutic potentials.

STEM CELL MIGRATION STREAMS IN THE ADULT

The bone marrow in the adult organism is distributed throughout the skeleton which contains, according to the textbooks of anatomy, up to 206 bones, many of which house active blood-cell-forming tissue, and most of them can be activated to blood cell production under pathophysiological situations (leukemia, myelofibrosis,

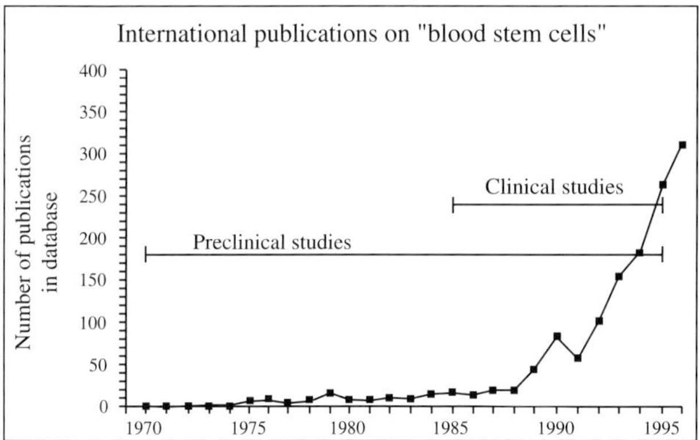

Figure 1. Numbers of scientific publications with the key word "blood stem cells" in the International DIMDI Database.

etc.). The amount of active bone marrow is known to amount to about 2,600 g, with about 126×10^{10} marrow cells and a turnover of 18.8×10^7/kg/h [5].

The question that comes up repeatedly is, "How is it possible that such a hematopoietic tissue which is 'disseminated' throughout so many skeletal bone cavities can act as one organ system?" If the clinician examines bone marrow aspirates taken from sternum, iliac crests, or other sites actively engaged in blood cell production, he can be certain to find a more or less identical cellular composition. It is the message of this presentation to suggest

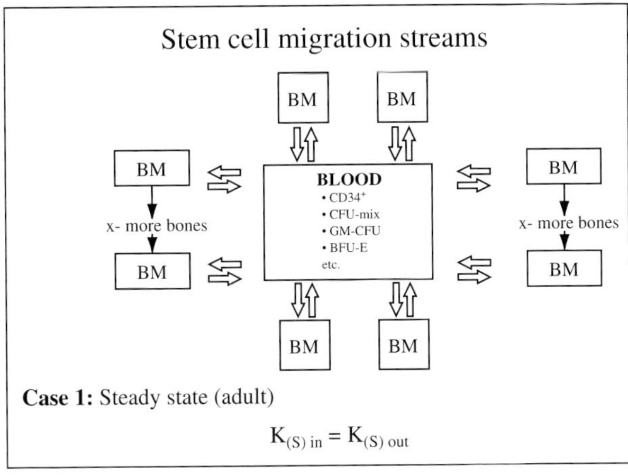

Figure 2. Case 1 for stem cell migration streams: steady state (adult).

that it is due to stem cell migration via the peripheral blood that all bone marrow sites actively participating in blood cell production have and maintain a sufficient local concentration of hematopoietic stem cells as a prerequisite for humeral and nerval regulatory actions.

Let us review briefly what we know about stem and progenitor cells in the blood under steady-state conditions. The peripheral blood contains hematopoietic stem and progenitor cells that have been and are measurable as CD34+ cells, as colony-forming units (based on the pioneering work of *Metcalf* and his group [6]) or, as in the mouse, as CFU-S (colony-forming units in the mouse spleen) [7]. In the steady-state situation, it can now be assumed that they are in an equilibrium with the stem and progenitor pools in the bone marrow. As will be shown later, the stem and progenitor cells in the blood are not just random samples of the bone marrow stem and progenitor cells but subsets with surface properties that enable them to circulate and to seed in environments suitable for their replication and/or differentiation.

In the steady state, we can assume that the relationship is correctly described as

$$K_{(S)\ in} = K_{(S)\ out}$$

meaning that the rate of stem and progenitor cells entering the blood stream from the bone marrow sites is equal to the rate of their leaving the blood stream (Fig. 2).

What is the concentration of stem and progenitor cells in the circulating blood? Table 1 summarizes current knowledge. It is obvious from this table that several mammalian species, including man, show a definite presence of stem and progenitor cells in the peripheral blood, the concentration depending on the method of assessment that was used. However, the concentrations reported are in the range of several hundred to a few thousand/ml blood.

Table 1. Stem and progenitor cells in peripheral blood (steady-state conditions of hemopoiesis)					
Test Systems/Adult	**CD34+**	**CFU-Mix**	**GM-CFU**	**BFU-E**	**DNA Synth.C.**
Mouse		(as CFU-S) 20-50/ml			
Dog			27-325/ml (x = ±18%)		
Monkey	19×10^3 (1-62)/ml				
Man	9.7×10^3 (1.9-34.7)/ml	32 ± 18/ml	92.5 ± 44/ml	591 ± 228/ml	3.6×10^3/ml

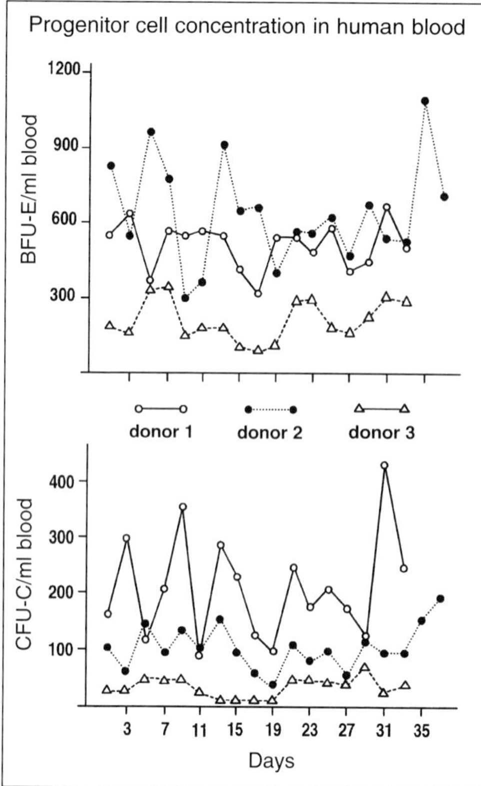

Figure 3. Day-to-day concentration of BFU-E and CFU-C/ml blood in three volunteer donors: ○ = *donor 1;* ● = *donor 2;* ▲ = *donor 3. For donor 1: the mean values ± standard deviation were for BFU-E 501 ± 98, for CFU-C/ml blood 209 ± 95 (n=17). For donor 2: BFU-E/ml blood 200 ± 81, CFU-C/ml blood 29 ± 12 (n=17). For donor 3: BFU-E/ml blood 624 ± 202 and CFU-C/ml blood 102 ± 40 (n=19).*

Studies have been performed to measure the concentration of stem and progenitor cells during several days and weeks in order to examine variations and oscillations. *Micklem* [8] noted in mice a twofold diurnal variation in circulating numbers of CFU-S in mice. In the five dogs examined during more than 11 weeks, *Nothdurft et al.* [9] could show that the concentration of colony-forming unit-culture (CFU-C) fluctuated around 181-341 CFU-C/ml. It was of interest to note that each dog appeared to have its personal CFU-C concentration similar to the common clinical knowledge that the "normal" level of blood cells can well be an "individual" characteristic. In human beings, *Kreutzmann* and *Fliedner* [10] could show in three normal volunteers, studied three times a week for 70 days, that the numbers of CFU-C were 255 ± 108, 125 ± 82, and 222 ± 87/ml, respectively, and that there was evidence for significant oscillation with periods of 23, 19, and 25 days (which is about twice the transit time from the granulocytic progenitor level to granulocyte release into the peripheral blood). Another 35-day study of our group revealed a mean concentration of CFU-C and of BFU-E of between 29 and 209/ml and 200 and 624/ml respectively [11] (Fig. 3).

The residence time of stem and progenitor cells in the blood stream is not very well known. However, some information is available for the mouse, using the CFU-S assay. Half-times between six min and 6-10 h were calculated [12, 13]. In the dog, *Raghavachar et al.* studied the disappearance rate of granulocytic progenitor cells (CFU-C) of normal recipient dogs and found a blood transit time of 11.8 to 13.0 min [14]. *Nothdurft et al.* used the CFU-C decline after dextran sulfate mobilization to calculate the blood transit time to be 1.4 ± 0.5 h and the T 1/2 to be 1.0 ± 0.4 h [15].

Thus, being well aware of all inherent methodological limitations, we conclude that the blood transit time of circulating progenitor cells is about one to two h, which is short in comparison to other "leukocytes."

The data obtained so far are not in contradiction to the following notions:

- Stem and progenitor cells are normal constituents of the "leukocyte population" in the peripheral blood of man as well as experimental animals studied.
- Their concentration, as measured by a considerable spectrum of methods, is characteristic of the method used but also of the individual organism.
- The tentative evidence of regular oscillations found for specific subpopulations is suggestive for a feedback regulation of their concentration.
- Their residence time in blood appears to be short, even shorter than that of granulocytes. Their fate after leaving the blood remains to be determined in detail; possibilities are intravascular apoptosis, seeding to appropriate environments (medullary and extramedullary), and changing "recognition" criteria.

STEM CELL MIGRATION STREAMS AFTER PERTURBATIONS

Let us now examine in what way the blood stem cell pool reacts to specific perturbations. In the next scheme (Case 2) (Fig. 4), a continuous-flow centrifugation (CFC) is depicted as it was performed in dogs [16] and in man [17]. From these experiments, two examples appear to be of characteristic importance for the topic of our presentation. A CFC was performed in a dog for 12.5 h

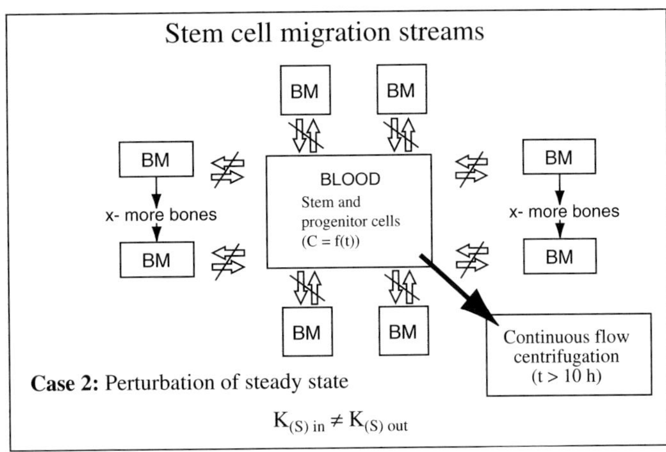

$$K_{(S)\,in} \neq K_{(S)\,out}$$

Figure 4. Case 2: Perturbation of steady state in stem cell migration streams by measures such as continuous-flow centrifugation.

(Fig. 5). During this time, the CFU-C concentration in the blood decreased to 30% of normal. At the same time, it was evident that 60 times the number of CFU-C normally present in the blood stream could be collected from the blood. This was explained by the assumption that these cells were drained from extravascular sites. It can also be seen that after the end of CFC, the blood concentration of CFU-C rose above normal levels by day 5 and returned to normal levels only after more than 20 days. This type of experiment was repeated three times with, in essence, the same results. These results suggested to us that the concentration of blood stem and progenitor cells is a feedback-controlled number and that there is in extravascular sites a "reserve pool" of progenitor cells prepared to be released into the circulation. This notion was further substantiated by studying the physical properties of the progenitor cells released into the blood after dextran sulfate mobilization and/or after CFC mobilization.

In our group, relevant canine studies were performed by *Gerhartz et al.* [18]. In these studies, the physical characteristics of circulating CFU-C were compared to those in the bone marrow. It was found that a four-to-eight-h CFC after dextran sulfate mobilization resulted in a selective release of CFU-C from the marrow into the blood with a velocity sedimentation profile of 4.65 ± 0.64 mm/h (range 3.6-5.5 mm/h), which is the same as that of unperturbed CFU-C blood population. However, when the CFC was prolonged to eight h or more, there were already more than eight h of evidence for a release of CFU-C with a sedimentation profile resembling more closely that of bone marrow CFU-C. This is

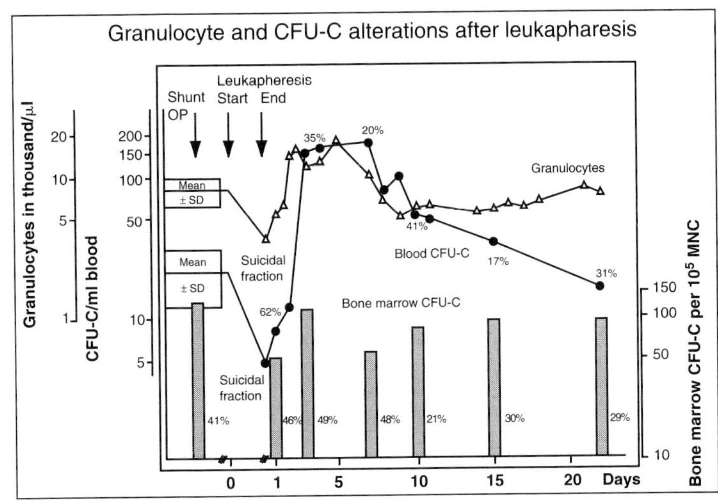

Figure 5. 12.5 hours of leukocytapheresis in a dog. The CFU-C show a decrease toward the end of leukapheresis, an overshoot between day 1 and day 10, and a return to normal levels by day 23.

similar to the sedimentation profile of CFU-C in the bone marrow of the same dogs, which was 5.54 ± 54 mm/h (range 3.8-6.2 mm/h). These studies were taken to indicate that the bone marrow releases a specific subpopulation of progenitor cells which is considerably smaller than the average of bone marrow progenitor cells. It was shown by *Raghavachar* [19] in our group that the bone marrow progenitor cells characterized by the slow sedimentation rate of < 5.1 mm/h result in a more pronounced hematopoietic regeneration than equal numbers of bone marrow progenitor cells characterized by a faster sedimentation rate (> 7.1 mm/h).

In human beings, it was shown by our group in initial studies in 1980 that one CFC results (without mobilization) in the collection of some $8.7 \pm 4.3 \times 10^5$ CFU-C (mean of 35 leukaphereses), which is 20 times the number of CFU-C in the circulation. Repeated CFC resulted in a collection of 1.5 times the number of CFU-C in the circulation [17, 20]. More recent studies using CD34$^+$ cells as an indicator for stem and progenitor cell properties indicated that the administration of recombinant colony stimulating factors (CSF) increases the concentration of CD34$^+$ cells from $3.8 \pm 0.8 \times 10^3$ to $61.9 \pm 11.3 \times 10^3$/ml blood [21]. A subsequent leukocytapheresis is then capable of collecting about 5×10^8 CD34$^+$ cells, which is about 26 times the number of CD34$^+$ cells normally in the blood stream. There is also evidence that such "perturbations" of the pool of circulating stem and progenitor cells can only be explained by a selective release of such cells from the bone marrow into the blood. It is evident that the perturbance is temporary and that after several days the system returns to its steady-state situation [22].

STEM CELL MIGRATION STREAMS DURING BONE MARROW DEVELOPMENT

Evidence for the important role of stem and progenitor cells in the peripheral blood for hematopoietic cell renewal comes from the studies on embryonic and fetal development of hematopoiesis. It is now accepted, in contrast with the classical views of hematopoietic development [23], that hematopoiesis in the bone marrow cavity is the result of the seeding of hematopoietic stem cells onto a matrix characterized by a very specific innervated vascular and cellular structure within a firm bony capsule [24]. This process has been studied in detail in rats [25, 26], in dogs [27], and in man [28]. In these mammalian organisms, there is a characteristic development of hematopoiesis in each bone cavity. The cartilage in the skeletal part becomes necrobiotic, leaving a cavity in which the mesenchymal elements of the perichondrium penetrate followed by blood vessels and nerves. All these elements form the stroma or matrix of the marrow in which blood-borne stem cells find the adequate microenvironment to divide, replicate, and/or differentiate [29, 30].

In dogs, it can be shown that there is in each skeletal bone an identical sequence: from cartilage (C) to a prehemopoietic stroma (S) to hemopoiesis (H) (Table 2). The time for the first bones in the dog to develop a prehematopoietic stroma is day 37 to 38 of gestation, and it takes the entire fetal development to colonize all bone cavities. In man, the stromal matrix becomes established in the clavicle as early as six to eight weeks of gestation. Fifteen out of 38 weeks of human development are needed to establish "the" bone marrow distributed throughout the entire skeleton [24, 28].

It is now of interest to examine the hematopoietic development in the bone marrow from the viewpoint of blood stem cell physiology. The concept can be described as follows (Fig. 6): it is possible to conceive the establishment of hematopoiesis in the marrow as a consequence of the introduction of hemopoietic stem and progenitor cells into the blood entering and leaving the vascular system of the marrow matrix. These embryonic stem and progenitor cells in the blood can be measured. *Nothdurft et al.* [27] were able to show that the blood of a dog on its 35th day of gestation, when the liver contains already some 50×10^5 GM-CFC, shows a concentration of some 31×10^3 GM-CFC per ml (Fig. 7). Thereafter, the numbers decline to reach about 4×10^3 pre-partum (adult dog about 200-300/ml). In other words, the blood stem and progenitor cell concentration during hemopoietic development is at a factor of 30 or more higher than in the adult steady-state situation. Hence it is likely that the stem cell egress from the blood into the marrow matrix exceeds by far the egress of stem cells from the marrow into the blood until the marrow sites have established a suitable stem cell concentration.

Table 2. Development of bone marrow in dogs and in human fetuses

| | Development of bone marrow in dogs (beagle) | | | | | | |
| | Days of gestation[*] | | | | | | |
Bones	34 - 35	37 - 38	41 - 42	43 - 44	46 - 48	50	56
Humerus	C	S	H	H	H	H	H
Femur	C	S	H	H	H	H	H
Radius	C	S	H	H	H	H	H
Tibia	C	S	H	H	H	H	H
Metacarpal bone	C	C	S	H	H	H	H
Metatarsal bone	C	C	S	H	H	H	H
Vertebrae (Th.)	C	C	S	S	S	H	H
Ribs	C	C	S	S	S	H	H
Sternum	C	C	C	S	S	H	H
Phalanx (3rd)	C	C	C	C	C	S	H
Carpal bones	C	C	C	C	C	C	C
Tarsal bones	C	C	C	C	C	C	C

| | Development of bone marrow in the human fetus | | | | | | |
| | Weeks | | | | | | |
Bones	6 - 8	9 - 10	11 - 12	13 - 14	15 - 16	17 - 18	19 - 20	21 - 22
Clavicle	S	H	H	H	H	H	H	H
Humerus	C	S	H	H	H	H	H	H
Tibia	C	S	H	H	H	H	H	H
Rib	C	S	S	H	H	H	H	H
Vertebra	C	C	S	S	II	H	H	H
Sternum	C	C	C	C	C	C	S	H

[*] Time of gestation = 63 days.
Abbreviations: C: cartilage; H: hemopoiesis; S: prehemopoietic stroma.

In the human being, the pattern of hemopoietic development in relation to blood stem cell migration is identical in principle. During weeks 10 and 11 of gestation, the blood contains about 134 CFU-C/ml. At this time, only a few bones are ready to accept immigrating stem cells. During weeks 16 to 18 of gestation, when bones in all parts of the skeleton are ready to allow seeding of stem cells, the concentration of stem and progenitor cells reaches a peak value of as many as 65,000 CFU-C/ml. At the time of birth when it can be assumed that all suitable bone marrow sites have been seeded with stem and progenitor cells, their concentration is down to about 10,000 CFU-GM/ml [24].

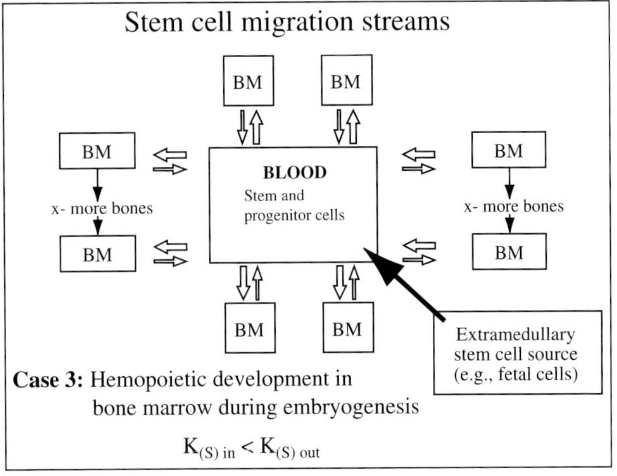

Figure 6. Case 3: Hemopoietic development of stem cell migration during embryogenesis. There is evidence for the migration of stem and progenitor cells through the blood stream into the bone marrow.

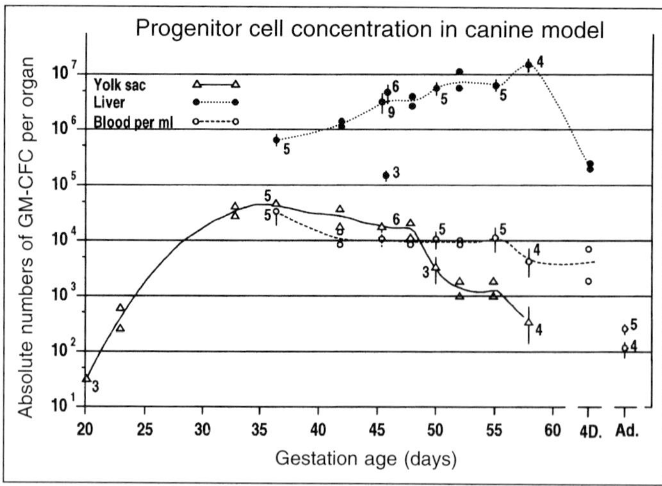

Figure 7. Absolute numbers of GM-CFC in the yolk sac and liver and their concentration per ml blood in canine fetuses between days 20 and 57 to 59 of gestation. Values are also shown for two pups on day 4 post partum and two collectives of adult dogs [27].

It is, therefore, concluded that the embryonic and fetal development of hematopoiesis in the bone marrow can be compared to the seeding of stem cells to a suitable, well-prepared, and biochemically characterized bone matrix environment showing at the time of the colonization the microscopic picture of an "aplastic" marrow. In this morphological and functional sense, it may be speculated that a blood stem cell transfusion results in essentially the same pattern of hemopoietic development as seen during embryogenesis.

STEM CELL MIGRATION STREAMS AFTER PARTIAL-BODY IRRADIATION

A classical example of stem cell migration streams comes from radiobiological research. Evidence for the fact that intact stem cells can migrate from one part of the bone marrow to the other was derived from studies in mice in which radiation was given in the lethal range but in a way that one part of the body was shielded during irradiation. This resulted in a significant decrease of the (LD) 50/30 days. *Hartweg* [31], as early as 1954, showed the protective effect of shielding a femur in an otherwise lethally irradiated rat. In shielding experiments, several authors have demonstrated that a lethally irradiated organism could be saved if the cell migration streams would be established from the nonirradiated to the irradiated part of the body [32-34]. In human beings, it is well known that bone marrow sites receiving therapeutic exposure doses up to several 1,000 cGy can recover by endogenous stem cell migration [35].

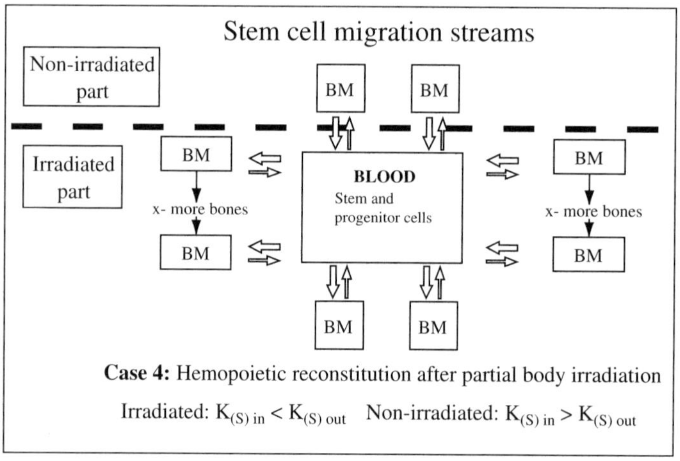

Thus we can, in principle, depict the following scheme (Case 4, Fig. 8). If a fraction of bone marrow is shielded (upper part), then one would postulate that a migration of stem cells would commence from this part of the bone marrow to bone marrow parts irradiated highly enough [36, 37]. One would then expect an emigration from stem and progenitor cells from blood into irradiated bone marrow sites until a new steady state occurs.

Figure 8. Case 4: Hemopoietic reconstitution after partial-body irradiation. It is assumed that in the nonirradiated part of the body, there is an influx of stem and progenitor cells from the blood derived from nonirradiated parts of the bone marrow.

In our own group, we have studied associated problems both in rats [38] and in dogs [39, 40]. In the rat, we were interested in finding out whether "resting bone marrow mononuclear cells" that had been shown in transfusion experiments to be associated with hemopoietic restoration potential and that were labeled by tritiated thymidine using the "complete thymidine labeling method" [41] would start to proliferate when distant bone marrow parts were irradiated. This indeed was the case; the resting mononuclear cells of the protected bone marrow sites were recruited to proliferate and differentiate at the time when stem and progenitor cells were needed to repopulate the irradiated bone marrow sites. In a smilar way, *Micklem* and *Ford* were able to demonstrate in mice, using chromosomal markers, under what circumstances stem and progenitor cells can be recruited to migrate from a protected marrow site into an irradiated marrow area [42].

These problems of stem cell migration were studied most extensively by *Nothdurft et al.* [39, 40]. It is sufficient here to point out that a myeloablative dose to 70% of the bone marrow while 30% was shielded results in a perturbation of the GM-CFU fraction of the shielded marrow. In the irradiated parts, obviously, virtually all GM-CFU were destroyed within one day after irradiation (Fig. 9A). The blood

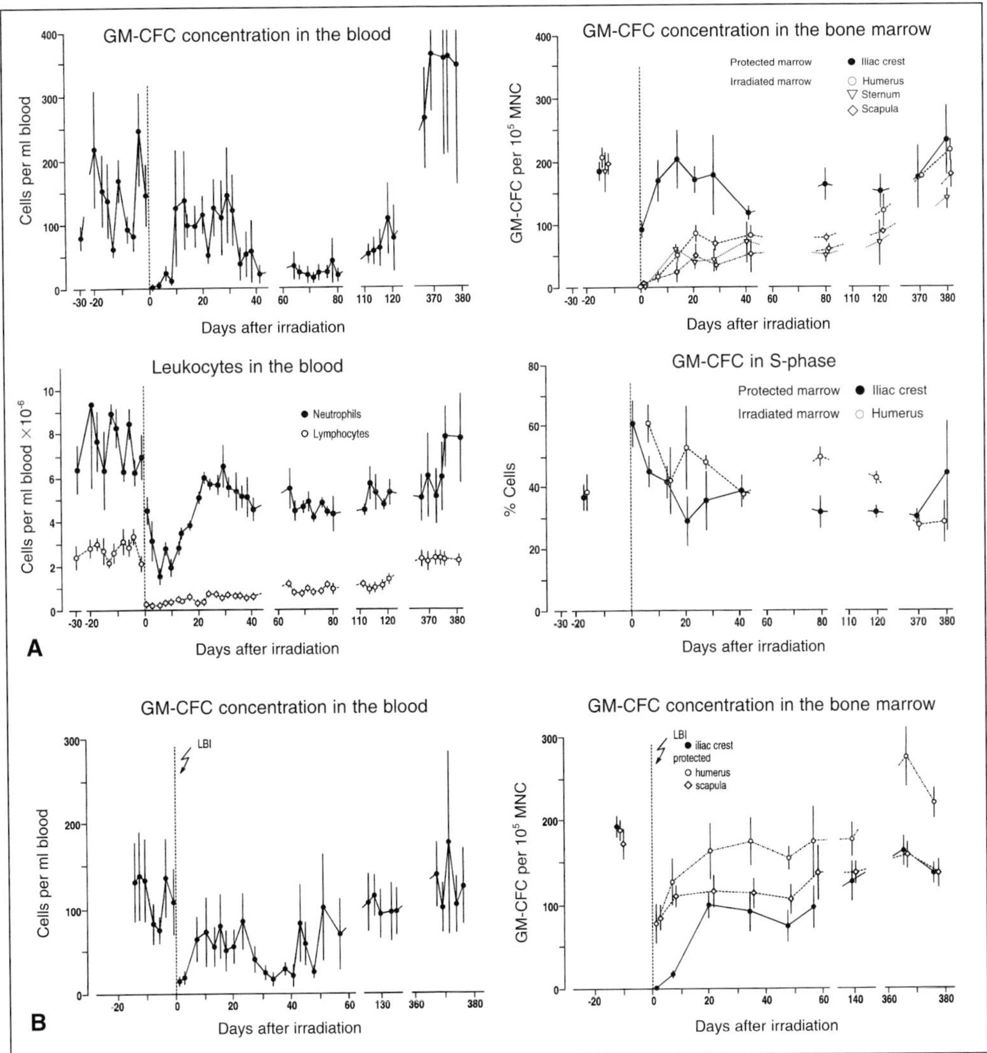

Figure 9. Blood cell changes after partial-body irradiation. *(A) 70% irradiation of the bone marrow and 30% shielded. (B) 30% irradiation of the bone marrow and 70% shielded. Used with permission from [39, 40].*

pool of GM-CFU showed a decrease after partial-body irradiation and "overshoot values" between days 10 and 35 after irradiation—which means during the time of hemopoietic reconstitution in the irradiated marrow parts.

If 30% of the total marrow mass were irradiated and 70% protected [40], one could again observe an initial decrease of circulating GM-CFC immediately after partial-body exposure, but then during the re-establishment of hemopoiesis in the irradiated bone marrow sites an overshooting reappearance of circulating GM-CFC associated with a gradual return of hematopoiesis in the irradiated sites (Fig. 9B).

In summary, the observations are in agreement with the assumption that blood stem cell migration plays a crucial role in re-establishing a sufficient level of stem cells in bone marrow units that were rendered aplastic by irradiation or other means, for instance, mechanical depletion as shown by *Meyer-Hamme et al.* [43].

STEM CELL MIGRATION TO RECONSTITUTE HEMATOPOIESIS

The role of blood stem and progenitor cells can also be considered and appreciated in all those cases in which bone marrow hematopoiesis is damaged or eradicated by total body radiation exposure or after myeloablative chemotherapy. In all these cases, the following scheme might help to elucidate the problems on hand.

In a situation schematically depicted in Figure 10 (Case 5), hematopoietic stem and progenitor cells are introduced into the blood pool derived from exogenous stem cell sources.

In our group, back in the days of collaboration between the Brookhaven Laboratory and the Mary Imogene Basset Hospital in Cooperstown, we studied the disappearance rate of transfused bone marrow precursor cells in dogs labeled in vitro in their DNA with tritiated thymidine [44]. The bulk of labeled cells disappeared from the circulating blood within two to three h but could not be traced to bone marrow sites. Today we know that the bulk of pluripotent stem cells is not in DNA synthesis but at rest [45], and it was only in studies using the reverse approach—activation of thymidine-labeled resting mononuclear cells by partial-body irradiation and/or by their transfusion into lethally irradiated recipient animals—that we came to the appropriate assumption that the pluripotent stem cell is a resting cell capable of migration through the blood [46], but not recircling through the lymph [47], that can home in hematopoietic stroma prepared to accept this seeding process in medullary but also in appropriate extramedullary sites [48].

This notion is in accordance with studies of other groups in mice [49], dogs [50], and monkeys [51], supporting the concept that it is the role of blood stem cells to replenish the stem cell pool of hematopoietic tissue in case of a stem cell concentration deficit.

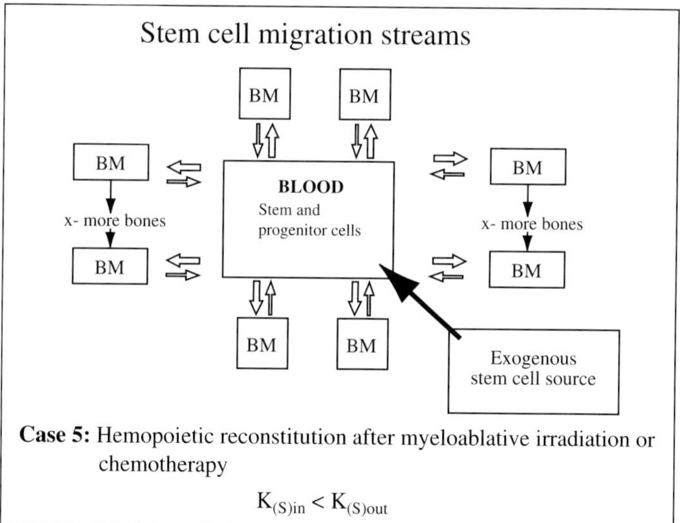

Figure 10. Case 5: Hemopoietic reconstitution after myeloablative irradiation or chemotherapy. The objective of blood stem cell transplantation is the hemopoietic reconstitution which can only occur by stem cell migration.

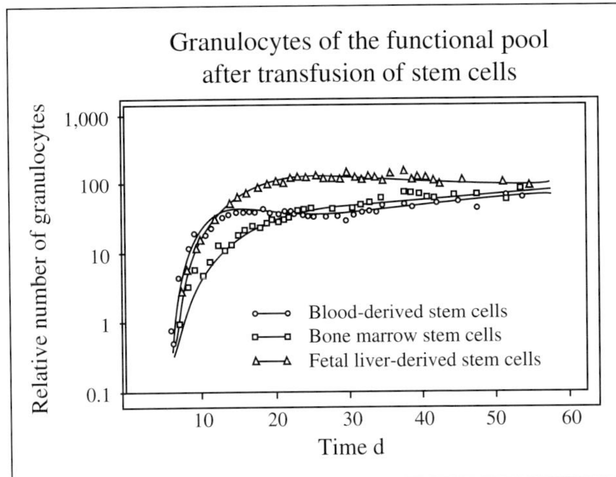

Figure 11. The immigration of stem cells from blood, from bone marrow, and from fetal liver in dogs was analyzed on the basis of the recovery of blood granulocytes after total-body irradiation and stem cell transfusion. Blood-derived stem cells have a similar initial course of granulocyte recovery in comparison to fetal liver cells. However, fetal liver cell transfusion allows the granulocyte concentration to return to normal and even to overshoot within 20 days.

This was substantiated by our previous studies in dogs. In the first experiments studying blood stem cell transplantation using CFU-C as an indicator for the presence of progenitor cells in the transfusate, it was quite evident that the number of CFU-C in the transfusate determined the quality and quantity of bone marrow restoration. The histology of dog bone marrow 10 days after a lethal whole-body exposure and transfusion of blood mononuclear cells containing 7.5×10^5 CFU-C showed only a few spongiosa niches with full hemopoietic recovery while adjacent spongiosa niches were completely aplastic. If 15×10^5 CFU-C were in the transfusate, more niches were filled but others were still completely empty. It was only after administration of some 30×10^5 CFU-C that all niches were completely recovered within 10 days [52-54].

This prompted us to examine the quality and quantity of stem cells collected from different sources, including blood, in terms of their regenerative potential. Comparing transfusates of mononuclear cells from fetal liver, bone marrow, and peripheral blood containing equal numbers of CFU-C, it was found that the recovery of blood granulocytes was very quick when fetal liver cells and blood mononuclear cells were used in comparison to bone-marrow-derived cells. However, the complete recovery of blood granulocytes after blood stem cell transplantation was delayed in comparison to fetal liver transplantation [55, 56] (Fig. 11).

We developed and used a biomathematical model [57] to try to understand these differences and found that the fetal cells must have a replicative power that exceeds that of bone-marrow- and blood-derived stem cells. While the computer model could fit the recovery data of bone-marrow- and blood-derived stem cells utilizing a replication probability value of 0.63 [58], it was necessary to assume a replication probability of 0.95 for fetal stem cells [57].

The same biomathematical model was used to study the relationship between the number of blood stem cells in a transfusate measured as CD34$^+$ cells and hematopoietic recovery in patients with multiple myeloma treated with cyclophosphamide, busulfan, and thiotepa at the M.D. Anderson Hospital under the leadership of *Dr. M. Körbling* and his colleagues [59-61]. The simulation model developed first by *Steinbach* [62] and extended by *Hofer* and *Tibken* [63] consists of eight cellular and two regulatory compartments [64] (Figs. 12A, 12B). It assumes a homeostatic equilibrium which has to guarantee that for each granulocyte leaving the circulation by senescence or emigration one granulocyte enters the circulation from the bone marrow (compartment F). For each cell leaving the extravascular bone marrow sites there has to be a net gain of one granulocyte through cell division (compartments S, CBM, and P). The life spans of the cells involved and their proliferation rates as well as cell cycle characteristics are largely known [65]. It can also be assumed that there are feedback regulatory mechanisms

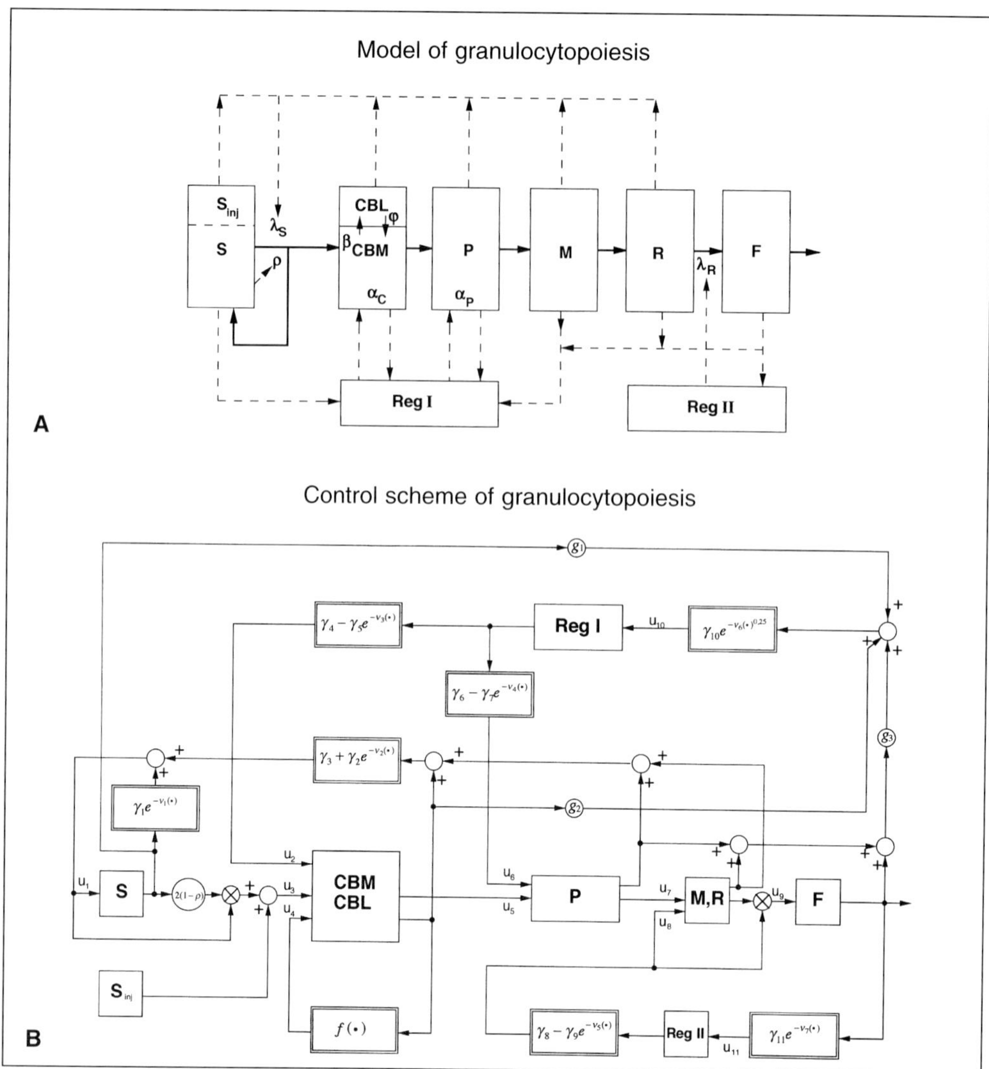

Figure 12. (A) Model of granulocytopoiesis used as the basis for a biomathematical model to assess radiation effects. (B) Control scheme of granulocytopoiesis (the details of the differential equations used are given in [63, 64, 68, 69]).

mediated through regulatory molecules such as cytokines [66, 67]. For this model, two regulatory compartments are assumed, and each of them would contain a balance of stimulatory and inhibitory effects (Reg. I and II). The control scheme of granulocytopoiesis is given in Fig. 12B (and the essential differential equations are described in mathematical detail elsewhere) [68, 69]. It is sufficient here to indicate that the model consists, in terms of regulation technology, of bilinear subsystems which are connected with each other by nonlinear static transfer linkages. This type of bilinear system is very useful in order to describe the cell proliferation and fluxes in the different cell compartments. Changes in the input values of a bilinear system are able to describe increases as well as decreases of cell numbers. The modeling of cell regulatory processes becomes a very natural way of using bilinear systems but requires no fewer than 37 differential equations.

This model was used to simulate the blood granulocyte recovery in five multiple myeloma patients given autologous blood stem cell transfusates containing between 0.24 and 17.54×10^6 CD 34$^+$ cells per kg body weight [61]. It was possible to simulate the recovery pattern and calculate the number of "biomathematical stem cell units" that must have been in the transfusate to achieve this type of recovery (Patients No. 20 and No. 11) (Figs. 13A, 13B). It was gratifying to see that there was a linear relationship between the number of CD 34[+] blood cells in the transfusate and the number of calculated (mathematical) stem cells. This indicated a new approach to relate the quality as well as the quantity of blood stem cell suspensions to the pattern of hemopoietic recovery and hence also to its quality and quantity (Fig. 14).

From such concepts and experimental studies, it appears justified to conclude that blood-derived stem cells must have qualitative properties that enable them to circulate in the peripheral blood without necessarily being "trapped" but capable of migrating to sites of tissue within which they can "home." Apparently, this property of entering and remaining in the blood stream has to do with adhesion receptors, especially of the integrin family [70-72]. Their homing within tissues (medullary and extramedullary matrix such as in liver and/or spleen) is likely to depend on "local tissue" conditions (as described by a number of authors [69]) and also from stem cell surface properties as described by others [73-75]. Thus, it will be of great importance to study in detail the physiological and pathophysiological properties of blood stem cells that were introduced into the circulation and to follow their fate and function and their transforming potentials.

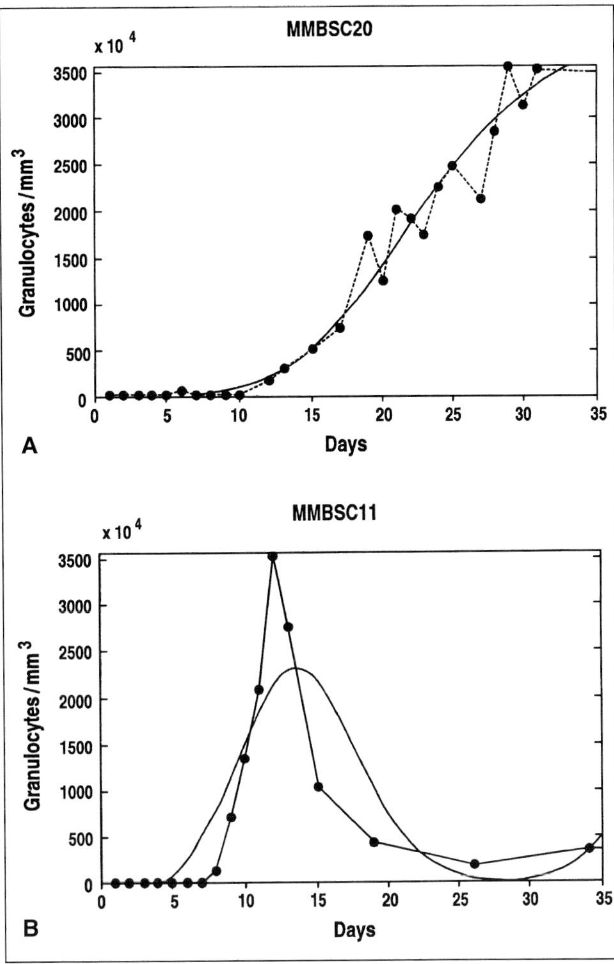

Figures 13A, 13B. Computer simulation curves of the granulocyte recovery in two patients (No. 20 and No. 11) with multiple myeloma treated with high-dose chemotherapy and showing rapid granulocyte recovery.

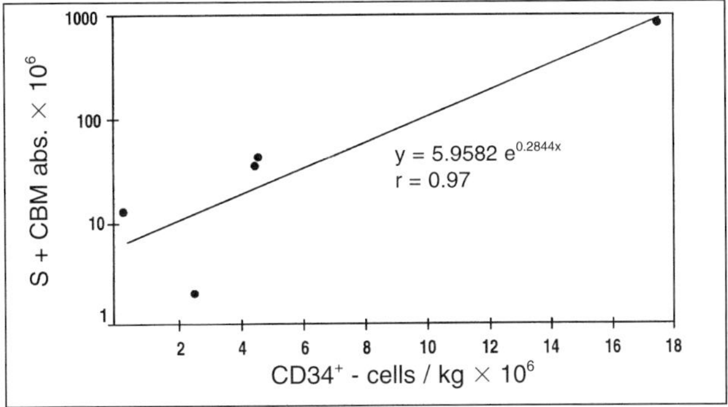

Figure 14. The correlation is shown between the number of CD positive cells/kg body weight $\times 10^6$ as used in the multiple myeloma treatment scheme [6] in relation to the number of stem and progenitor cells calculated from the biomathematical model [59] by means of simulating the granulocyte recovery curve.

THE ROLE OF BLOOD STEM CELLS IN HEMATOPOIETIC CELL RENEWAL

This keynote presentation for the International Workshop on "Pathophysiology, Diagnostic and Therapeutic Implications of Blood Stem Cells" served the purpose of reviewing the present concepts regarding the role of blood stem cells in hematopoietic cell renewal.

A number of conclusions might be appropriate:

A) In the steady-state situation of blood cell production and removal, there are stem and progenitor cells present in the circulation. They can be identified by their surface properties, clonogenic potentials, and biophysical properties, while their morphology is indistinguishable from the bulk of cells called "lymphocytes." Additional work is necessary before one begins to understand their life cycle, their migratory properties, and their fate after immigrating into the circulation.

B) Blood stem cells are apparently in an equilibrium with extravascular sites; leukocytapheretic procedures indicate that there is an extravascular reserve of an easily mobilizable pool of stem and progenitor cells which can even be further expanded by the administration of specific stimulatory molecules. Under steady-state and conditions "early" after apheresis, the physical properties of blood stem cells are similar to those of the easily mobilizable cells. It remains to be determined in what way the quality of blood stem cells changes as a function of time after recombinant cytokine stimulation. The type of perturbations after CFC indicates that blood stem cells are in a feedback regulated equilibrium with bone marrow stem cells.

C) Blood stem cells are of decisive importance for the establishment of hematopoiesis in all skeletal bones. Apparently, the hematogenous seeding of fetal stem cells results in a "filling-up" of the local (semiautonomous) hematopoietic sites in the bone marrow. If there is additional need for hematopoiesis, such as in certain disease states (polycythemia, thalassemia, etc.) then "fatty marrow" can become hematopoietic, most likely as a result of stem cell seeding.

D) The blood stem cell migration streams become most obvious in "enforced" migration, as observed in partial body irradiation, but also in the process of establishing extramedullary hematopoiesis.

E) If hematopoietic stem cells are introduced into the circulating blood, it is obvious that "blood-derived" stem cells have migratory potentials most suitable for "homing" in appropriate hematopoietic microenvironments. More work is needed to characterize the migration properties and streams in the steady-state situation of hematopoiesis and in diseased conditions, especially "stem cell disorders."

ACKNOWLEDGMENTS

Throughout the years, the following scientists (among others) have contributed in particular to the experimental work of our group: *W. Calvo, F. Carbonell, H.D. Flad, H.H. Gerhartz, G. Grilli, R.J. Haas, E.B. Harriss, E. Herbst, D. Hoelzer, S. Issaragrisil, M. Körbling, P. Kovacs, H. Kreutzmann, W. Nothdurft, H. Pflieger, O. Prümmer, A. Raghavachar, W.M. Ross, H.J. Seidel, K.H. Steinbach,* and *B.L. Ziegler.*

The research work was supported by the European Commission, Brussels, the Ministries of the Federal Government of Germany, and the State of Baden-Wuerttemberg.

REFERENCES

1 Maximow A. Der Lymphozyt als gemeinsame Stammzelle der verschiedenen Blutelemente in der embryonalen Entwicklung und im postfetalen Leben der Säugetiere. Folia Haematologica VIII 1909;8:125-134.

2 Lee GR et al. Wintrobe's Clinical Hematology. Philadelphia, London: Lea and Febiger, 1993.

3 Goodman JW, Hodgson G. Evidence for stem cells in the peripheral blood of mice. Blood 1962;19:702-714.

4 Micklem HS, Anderson N, Ross E. Limited potential of circulating haemopoietic stem cells. Nature 1975;256:41-43.

5 Fliedner TM, Steinbach KH, Hoelzer D. Adaptation to environmental changes: the role of cell-renewal systems. In: Finckh, ed. The Effects of Environment

on Cells and Tissue. Amsterdam/Oxford: Excerpta Medica, 1976:20-38.

6 Metcalf D, Moore MAS. Haemopoietic Cells. Amsterdam: North-Holland Publishing Co, 1971.

7 Till JE, McCulloch EA. A direct measurement of the radiation sensitivity of normal mouse bone marrow cells. Radiat Res 1961;14:213-222.

8 Micklem HS. Effect of phytohemagglutinin-M (PHA) on the spleen-colony-forming capacity of mouse lymph node and blood cells. Transplantation 1966;4:732-741.

9 Nothdurft W, Fliedner TM. The response of the granulocytic progenitor cells (CFU-C) of blood and bone marrow in dogs exposed to low doses of x-irradiation. Radiat Res 1992;89:38-52.

10 Kreutzmann H, Fliedner TM. Studies on the presence and possible oscillation of granulocytic progenitor cells (CFU-C) in human blood. Scand J Haematol 1979;23:360-366.

11 Grilli G, Carbonell F, Fliedner TM. Variations in erythroid and myeloid progenitor cell numbers in normal human peripheral blood. Br J Haematol 1980;44:679-681.

12 Hodgson G, Guzman E, Herrera C. Characterization of the stem cell population of phenyl hydrazine treated rodents. In: Doyle E, ed. Effects of Radiation on Cellular Proliferation and Differentiation. Vienna: IAEA, 1968:163-170.

13 Moloney MA, Patt HM. Marrow stem cell release in the autorepopulation assay. Exp Hematol 1978;6:227-232.

14 Raghavachar A, Steinbach KH, Prümmer O et al. Survival of transfused cryopreserved granulocytic progenitor cells (CFU-C) in recipient circulation. Cell Tissue Kinet 1983;16:303-311.

15 Nothdurft W, Steinbach KH, Ross WM et al. Quantitative aspects of granulocytic progenitor cell (CFUc) mobilization from extravascular sites in dogs using dextran sulfate. Cell Tissue Kinet 1982;15:331-340.

16 Fliedner TM, Calvo W, Körbling M et al. Hematopoietic stem cells in blood: characteristics and Potentials. In: Golde DW, Cline MJ, Metcalf D et al., eds. Hematopoietic Cell Differentiation. ICN-UCLA Symposia on Molecular Biology. New York: Academic Press 1978:193-212.

17 Körbling M, Fliedner TM, Pflieger H. Collection of large quantities of granulocyte/macrophage progenitor cells (CFUS) in man by continuous flow leukapheresis. Scand J Haematol 1980;24:22-28.

18 Gerhartz HH, Fliedner TM. Velocity sedimentation and cell cycle characteristics of granulopoietic progenitor cells (CFU-C) in canine blood and bone marrow: influence of mobilization and CFU-C depletion. Exp Hematol 1980;8(suppl 2):209-218.

19 Raghavachar A, Prümmer O, Calvo W et al. Repopulating potential of canine bone marrow cells: differences between large and small cells separated by velocity sedimentation. Br J Haematol 1985;60:33-40.

20 Fliedner TM, Körbling M, Arnold R et al. Collection and cryopreservation of mononuclear blood leukocytes and of CFU-C in man. Exp Hematol 1979;7(suppl 5):398-408.

21 Körbling M, Anderlini P, Durett A et al. Delayed effects of rhG-CSF mobilization treatment and apheresis on circulating $CD34^+$ and $CH34^+Thy-1^{dim}$ $CD38^+$ progenitor cells, and lymphoid subsets in normal stem cell donors for allogeneic transplantation. Bone Marrow Transplant 1996;18:1073-1079.

22 Nothdurft W, Fliedner TM. Stem cell migration after irradiation. In: Okada S et al., eds. Radiation Research. Tokyo: Toppan, 1979:657-663.

23 Doan CA. On the origin and developmental potentialities of blood cells. Acad Med 1939;15:668-697.

24 Fliedner TM, Calvo W. Hematopoietic stem cell seeding of a cellular matrix: a principle of initiation and regeneration of hematopoiesis. In: Clarkson B. et al., eds. Cold Spring Harbor Conferences on Cell Proliferation. Cold Spring Harbor Laboratory 1978;5:757-773.

25 Calvo W, Haas RJ. Die Histogenese des Knochenmarkes der Ratte. Z Zellforsch 1969;95:377-395.

26 Haas RJ, Hoelzer D, Kurrle E et al. Experimental analysis of developing haematopoiesis in fetal bone marrow. Pediat Res 1976;10:164-168.

27 Nothdurft W, Braasch E, Calvo W et al. Ontogeny of the granulocyte/macrophage progenitor cell (GM-CFV) pools in the beagle. J Embryol Exp Morph 1984;80:87-103.

28 Keleman E, Calvo W, Fliedner TM. Atlas of Human Hemopoietic Development. Berlin: Springer-Verlag 1979:

29 Tavassoli M. Embryonic and fetal hemopoiesis: an overview. Blood Cells 1991;1:269-281.

30 Zon LI. Developmental biology of hematopoiesis. Blood 1995;86:2876-2891.

31 Hartweg H. Die Wirkung geschützten homologen Knochenmarks auf die Regeneration des haemopoetischen Systems nach dem Strahleninsalt. Strahlentherapie 1954;95:594-604.

32 Swift MN, Takta ST, Bond VP. Regionally fractionated x-irradiation equivalent in dose to total body exposure. Radiat Res 1954;1:241-252.

33 Hanks GE. In vivo migration of colony forming units from shielded bone marrow in the irradiated mouse. Nature 1964;203:1393-1395.

34 Croizat H, Frissdal E, Tubiana M. The effects of partial body irradiation on haemopoietic stem cell migration. Cell Tissue Kinet 1980;13:319-325.

35 Chone B. Knochenmarkveränderungen im Rahmen der Strahlentherapie in morphologischer und elektronenoptischer Sicht. Nucl Med 1963;2:425-433.

36 Micklem HS, Ford CE, Evans EP et al. Compartments and cell flows within the mouse haemopoietic system. I. Restricted interchange between haemopoietic sites. Cell Tissue Kinet 1975;8:219-232.

37 Micklem HS, Ogden DA, Evans EP et al. Compartments and cell flows within the mouse haemopoietic system. II. Estimated rates of interchange. Cell Tissue Kinet 1975;8:233-248.

38 Haas R, Bone F, Fliedner TM. Cytokinetic analysis of slowly proliferating bone marrow cells during recovery from radiation injury. Cell Tissue Kinet 1971;4:31-45.

39 Nothdurft W, Calvo W, Klinnert V et al. Acute and long-term alterations in the granulocyte/macrophage progenitor cell (GM-CFC) compartment of dogs after partial body irradiation. Irradiation of the upper body with a single myeloablative dose. Int J Radiat Oncol 1986;12:949-957.

40 Baltschukat K, Fliedner TM, Nothdurft W. Hematological effects in dogs of the lower part of the body with a single myeloablative dose. Radiother Oncol 1989;14:239-246.

41 Fliedner TM, Haas RJ, Stehle H et al. Complete labeling of all cell nuclei in new-born rats. A tool for the evaluation of rapidly and slowly proliferating cell systems. Lab Invest 1968;18:249.

42 Micklem HS, Ford CD, Evans EP et al. Interrelationships of myeloid and lymphoid cells: studies with chromosome-marked cells transfused into lethally irradiated mice. Proc Roy Soc 1966;165:78-102.

43 Meyer-Hamme K, Haas RJ, Fliedner TM. Cytokinetics of bone marrow stroma cells after stimulation by partial depletion of the medullary cavity. Acta Haematol 1971;46:349-361.

44 Fliedner TM, Thomas ED, Meyer LM et al. The fate of transfused H3-thymidine labeled bone marrow cells in irradiated recipients. Ann NY Acad Sci 1964;114:510-526.

45 To LB, Haylock DN, Döwse T et al. A comparative study of the phenotype and proliferative capacity of peripheral blood CD34+ cells mobilized by four different protocols and those of steady-phase PB and bone marrow CD34+ cells. Blood 1994;84:2930.

46 Haas RJ, Flad HD, Fliedner TM et al. Correlation between cytokinetically resting lymphocytes and bone marrow restoration: experiments using a discontinuous albumin gradient. Blood 1973;42:209-218.

47 Storb R, Epstein RB, Thomas ED. Marrow repopulating ability of peripheral blood cells compared to thoracic duct cells. Blood 1968;32:662-667.

48 Fliedner TM, Wandl UB, Calvo W. Medulläre und extramedulläre Haemopoese im Hund nach Ganzkörperbestrahlung und Transfusion von aus dem Blut gewonnenen Stammzellen. Schweizer Medizinische Wochenschrift 1982;112:1423-1429.

49 Barnes DW, Loutit JF. Effects of irradiation and antigenic stimulation on circulating haemopoietic stem cells of the mouse. Nature 1967;213:1142-1143.

50 Abrams RA, McCormack K, Bowles C et al. Cyclophosphamide treatment expands the circulating hematopoietic stem cell pool in dogs. J Clin Invest 1981:67:1392-1399.

51 Storb R, Graham TC, Epstein RB et al. Demonstration of hemopoietic stem cells in the peripheral blood of baboons by cross circulation. Blood 1977;5:537-542.

52 Calvo W, Fliedner TM, Herbst E et al. Regeneration of blood-forming organs after autologous leukocyte transfusion in lethally irradiated dogs. II. Distribution and cellularity of the marrow in irradiated and transfused animals. Blood 1967;47(suppl 4):593-601.

53 Fliedner TM, Flad HD, Bruch CH et al. Treatment of aplastic anemia by blood stem cell transfusion: a canine model. Haematologica 1976;61:141-156.

54 Nothdurft W, Bruch CH, Fliedner TM et al. Studies on the regeneration of the CFUc-population in blood and bone marrow of lethally irradiated dogs after autologous transfusion of cryopreserved mononuclear blood cells. Scand J Haematol 1977;19:470-481.

55 Prümmer O, Raghavachar A, Werner C et al. Fetal liver transplantation in the dog. I. Restoration of haemopoiesis with cryopreserved fetal liver cells from DLA-identical siblings. Transplantation 1985;39;349-355.

56 Prümmer O, Werner C, Raghavachar A et al. Fetal liver transplantation in the dog. II. Repopulation of the granulocyte-macrophage progenitor cell compartment by fetal liver cells from DLA-identical siblings. Transplantation 1985;40:498-503.

57 Fliedner TM, Steinbach KH. Simulationsmodelle von Perturbationen des Granulozytären Zellerneuerungssystems. In: Doerr W, Schipperges H, eds. Modelle der Pathologischen Physiologie. Berlin, Heidelberg, New York: Springer-Verlag, 1987:89-106.

58 Vogel H, Niewisch H, Matioli G. The self renewal probability of hemopoietic stem cells. J Cell Physiol 1968;72:221-228.

59 Paul W. Die Analyse der Regeneration der Granulopoese nach Stammzelltransplantationen mit Hilfe einer Regelungstechnischen Implementation eines Biomathematischen Modells. Inaugural-Dissertation Universität Ulm, 1997.

60 Körbling M, Huh YO, Durrett A et al. Allogeneic blood stem cell transplantation: peripheralization and yield of donor-derived primitive hematopoietic progenitor cells (CD34$^+$Thy-1^{dim}) and lymphoid subsets, and possible predictors of engraftment and GVHD. Blood 1995;86:2842-2848.

61 Alexanian R, Dimopoulos MA, Hester J et al. Early myeloablative therapy for multiple myeloma. Blood 1994;84:4278-4282.

62 Steinbach KH, Raffler H, Pabst G. A mathematical model of canine granulocytopoiesis. J Math Biol 1980:10:1-12.

63 Hofer EP, Tibken B, Fliedner TM. Modern control theory as a tool to describe the biomathematical model of granulopoiesis. In: Möller DPF, Richter O, eds. Analyse Dynamischer Systeme in Medizin, Biologie und Ökologie. Informatik-Fachberichte. Berlin: Springer Verlag, 1991;275:33-39.

64 Fliedner TM, Tibken B, Hofer EP et al. Stem cell responses after radiation exposure: a key to the evaluation and prediction of its effects. Health Physics 1996:70;787-797.

65 Cronkite EP, Fliedner TM. Granulopoiesis. New Engl J Med 1964;270:1347, 1403.

66 Golde DW. Hematopoietic growth factors - An Overview. In: Murphy MJ, Rizzoli V, eds. Blood Cell Growth Factors: Their Biology and Clinical Application. Int J Cell Cloning 1990;8:4-10.

67 Broxmeyer HE. Biomolecule-cell interaction and the regulation of myelopoiesis: an update. In: Murphy MJ, ed. Concise Reviews in Clinical and Experimental Hematology. Dayton: AlphaMed Press, 1992:119-147.

68 Tibken B, Hofer EP. A biomathematical model of granulocytopoiesis for estimation of stem cell numbers. STEM CELLS 1995;13(suppl 1):282-289.

69 Tibken B, Hofer P. Constrained optimization algorithms and automatic differentiation for parameter estimation with applications to granulocytic models. In: Dolezal J, Fidler J, eds. System Modelling and Optimization. Proc 17th IFIP TC7 Conf on System Modelling and Optimization. Prag. London: Chapman and Hall, 1996:115-119.

70 To LB, Haylock DN, Simmons PJ et al. The biology and clinical uses of blood stem cells. Blood 1997;89:2223-2258.

71 Papayannopoulou T, Nakamoto B. Peripheralization of hemopoietic progenitors in primates treated with anti-VLA4 integrin. Proc Natl Acad Sci USA 1993;90:9374-9378.

72 Tavassoli M, Hardy CL. Molecular basis of homing of intravenously transplanted stem cells. Blood 1990;76:1059-1070.

73 Turner ML. Regulation of hematopoietic progenitor cell migration, mobilization and homing. STEM CELLS 1994:12:227-229.

74 Levesque JP, Haylock DN, Simmons PJ. Cytokine regulation of proliferation and cell adhesion are correlated events in human CD34+ hemopoietic progenitors. Blood 1996;88:1168-1176.

75 Long MW. Blood cell cytoadhesion molecules. Exp Hematol 1992;20:288-301.

Chapter II

Characterization and Properties of Blood Stem Cells

Phenotype of the Engrafting Stem Cell in Mice

P.J. Quesenberry, P. Becker, F.M. Stewart

Comparative Effects of Retroviral-Mediated Gene Transfer into Primary Human Stromal Cells of Flt3-Ligand, Interleukin 3 and GM-CSF on Production of Cord Blood Progenitor Cells in Long-Term Culture

Alessandra Balduini, Stephen E. Braun, Kenneth Cornetta, Stewart Lyman, Hal E. Broxmeyer

Unilineage Hematopoietic Differentiation in Bulk and Single Cell Culture

Benedikt Ziegler, Ugo Testa, Gianluigi Condorelli, Luigi Vitelli, Mauro Valtieri, Cesare Peschle

Phenotype of the Engrafting Stem Cell in Mice

P.J. QUESENBERRY, P. BECKER, F.M. STEWART

Cancer Center, University of Massachusetts Medical Center, Worcester, Massachusetts, USA

Key Words. *Phenotype · Engraftment · Host-donor ratios · BALB/c mice*

ABSTRACT

The present data on engraftment into non-myeloablated mice strongly suggest that engraftment is determined by host-donor ratios as opposed to opening space. Theoretically, if the ratios of donor to host stem cells could be altered, especially without causing toxicity to the host animal, then the phenotypic readout could be increased in a clinically applicable manner.

To research this further, we investigated low-dose irradiation (100 cGy) for its effects on marrow, spleen and peripheral blood counts, as well as engrafting stem cell levels. We found a transient but significant depression in the white blood cell and platelet counts in the peripheral blood which returned to normal by two weeks, with no apparent deleterious effect on the animals. However, the same irradiation dose after two months impaired marrow repopulation and reduced engraftment potential to less than 20% capacity. These results suggested that we could obtain much higher phenotypic readouts after engraftment with this model; thus, we assessed the engraftment of 40 million male BALB/c marrow cells into female hosts exposed to 100 cGy at two, five and eight months after cell infusion. The resultant high levels of chimerism, reaching 100% in many cases, strongly suggest that the key to engraftment in these models is host-donor stem cell ratios.

One important issue relative to the above finding is whether cytokine-stimulated proliferating stem cells have irreversibly lost engraftment capacity or whether changes in the engraftment capacity are of a plastic nature, possibly related to cell cycle transit. A number of experiments following engraftment have shown that the engraftment defect is reversible and can be repeatedly lost and regained during the initial portions of a cytokine-stimulated culture.

The above results suggest that, at least at the more primitive stem cell level, hematopoietic stem cell regulation may in part be based on a cell cycle model rather than a hierarchical system. *Stem Cells 1998;16 (suppl 1):33-35*

We have assessed engraftment of male marrow into normal nonmyeloablated BALB/c female mice and found very high levels of engraftment at the stem cell level with the final differentiated phenotype appearing to be dependent upon competition between hosts and donor stem cells [1-5]. Characteristics of engraftment into normal murine marrow are presented in Table 1.

Cells engrafting into this model are quiescent as determined by hydroxyurea suicide techniques, and induction into active cell cycle by in vivo treatment with 5-fluorouracil (5-FU) results in a marrow defective in long-term engraftment; this defect reverses over time. The cells, which engraft rapidly, migrate to the endosteal surface (six weeks) as determined by fluorescence in situ hybridization on marrow section

Characteristics and Potentials of Blood Stem Cells
STEM CELLS 1998;16(suppl 1):33-35

Table 1. Engraftment into normal hosts

▲ High levels of chimerism — appears quantitative

▲ Engraftment is multilineage

▲ Engraftment is persistent

▲ Engraftment occurs in marrow, spleen and thymus

mapping [6]. In addition, we have now demonstrated engraftment into normal mice of highly purified lineage-negative Rho^{lo} Ho^{lo} cells, albeit at a much lower level than would be anticipated by the number of starting marrow cells.

When murine BALB/c marrow cells are induced to proliferate in vitro by exposure to interleukin 3 (IL-3), IL-6, IL-11 and steel factor for 48 h, there is an expansion of high proliferative potential and total colony-forming cells by 48 h, but at this time point in culture there is a marked diminishment in engraftment potential and thus a discordance between the in vitro progenitor results and the in vivo engraftment results [7-8]. Studies of murine lineage-negative Rho^{lo} Ho^{lo} stem cells purified from whole male BALB/c marrow cells and cultured in the same cytokine cocktail indicate that the cells, in a relatively synchronized fashion, enter cell cycle, progress to S phase within 16 to 20 h and to mitosis by approximately 40 h [9]. Subsequent doublings of this population occur every 12 h, thus indicating an extraordinarily short G$_1$ after the first cell cycle transit. During the first cell cycle, the cells are highly synchronized with at least partial synchrony being maintained thereafter. The data on in vivo 5-FU effect and in vitro cytokine effect suggest that induction of proliferation by murine hematopoietic stem cells is associated with the acquisition of an engraftment defect discordant with the continued expansion of in vitro progenitor cells. This defect with in vivo 5-FU or in vitro cytokines has also been seen in irradiated hosts. The phenotype of stem cells engrafting into nonmyeloablated mice is presented in Table 2.

The present data on engraftment into nonmyeloablated mice strongly suggested that engraftment was determined not by opening space but by host-donor ratios. The potential application of these studies to clinical therapies in transplantation or gene therapy is limited in part by the relatively large number of cells needed for high level of expression of differentiated cells from the transplanted cell. Theoretically, if the ratios of donor to host stem cells could be altered, especially without toxicity to the host animal, then the phenotypic readout could be increased in a clinically applicable manner. Accordingly, we investigated low-dose irradiation for its effects both on marrow, spleen and peripheral blood cell counts, as well as engrafting stem cell levels [10]. After exposure to 100 cGy whole body irradiation from a gamma cesiom source, we found a transient, albeit significant, depression in the white blood cell count and platelet count in the peripheral blood which returned to normal by two weeks; there is no apparent deleterious effect on the animals. Marrow cellularity was only marginally and variably affected. However, the ability of murine male BALB/c marrow to repopulate and engraft at two months after marrow infusion was markedly impaired by exposure to 100 cGy either in vitro or in vivo; less than 20% of the engrafting capacity remained after this low level of radiation. These data suggested that 100 cGy could provide an approach with nontoxic and minimal myeloablation, but with significant stem cell ablation, and that, if our hypothesis was correct, we should be able to obtain much higher phenotypic readouts after engraftment in this model. Accordingly, we assessed the engraftment of 40 million male BALB/c marrow cells into 100 cGy exposed female hosts at two, five and eight months after cell infusion. We found extraordinarily high levels of chimerism approaching 100% in many instances and suggesting, again, that the key to engraftment in these models is simply host-donor stem cell ratios.

An important issue relates to whether the cytokine-stimulated proliferating stem cells have irreversibly lost engraftment capacity or whether changes in engraftment capacity might be of a plastic nature, possibly related to cell cycle transit. A number of experimens following engraftment at two to four-h time intervals from 24 to 48 h of IL-3, IL-6, IL-11 and steel factor-stimulated in vitro liquid culture have shown that the engraftment defect is in fact reversible and that engraftment may be lost, regained, lost and regained again during the initial portions of a cytokine-stimulated culture [11].

The above results have important implications for our basic understanding of hematopoietic stem cell regulation. They suggest that, at least at the more primitive stem cell level, regulation may in part be based on a cell cycle model rather than a hierarchical system. In addition, these data suggest strategies for stem cell transplantation and gene therapy approaches. One area of investigation will be the use of minimal therapy to create allochimeric states in nonmalignant diseases such as sickle cell anemia and thalassemia. It is clear that high rates of engraftment can be obtained, and the major challenges in this area will be approaches to tolerize the animal and prevent graft-versus-host-disease. In addition, stem cell expansion approaches and the potential to use different populations for engraftment need to be carried out with a full understanding of the engraftment potential of cells at different points in cell cycle and in cytokine-stimulated culture. Lastly, many of the failures of gene therapy approaches which have been assumed to be due to the nature of the vectors, or promoter shut-off of the vectors, may in fact be due to failures of engraftment of transduced marrow stem cells. Strategies to maximally transduce stem cells in vitro and then infuse them in an engraftable state may well improve our approaches to gene therapy.

Table 2. Phenotype of stem cells engrafting in nonmyeloablated mice

▲ Quiescent

▲ Easily induced into cell cycle by cytokines

▲ Induced into cell cycle within 24 h of engraftment

▲ Six weeks after engraftment has moved to bone surface

▲ May need the interactions of a facilitator cell for full engraftment

▲ Acquires an engraftment defect when transiting cell cycle after either in vitro cytokine exposure or in vivo 5-FU exposure

REFERENCES

1 Stewart FM, Crittenden R, Lowry PA et al. Long-term engraftment of normal and post-5-fluorouracil murine marrow into normal nonmyeloablated mice. Blood 1993;81:2566-2571.

2 Ramshaw HS, Rao SS, Crittenden RB et al. Engraftment of bone marrow cells into normal unprepared hosts: effects of 5-fluorouracil and cell cycle status. Blood 1995;86:924-929.

3 Ramshaw H, Crittenden RB, Dooner M et al. High levels of engraftment with a single infusion of bone marrow cells into normal unprepared mice. Biol Blood Marrow Trans 1995;1:74-80.

4 Rao SS, Peters SO, Crittenden RB et al. Stem cell transplantation in the normal nonmyeloablated host: relationship between cell dose, schedule and engraftment. Exp Hematol 1997;25:114-121.

5 Blomberg ME, Rao S, Reilly JL et al. Repetitive bone marrow transplantation in nonmyeloablated recipients. Exp Hematol 1997 (in press).

6 Nilsson S, Dooner M, Tiarks C et al. Potential and distribution of transplanted hematopoietic stem cells in a nonablated mouse model. Blood 1997;89:4013-4020.

7 Peters SO, Kittler EL, Ramshaw HS et al. Murine marrow cells expanded in culture with IL-3, IL-6, IL-11, and SCF acquire an engraftment defect in normal hosts. Exp Hematol 1995;23:461-469.

8 Peters SO, Kittler ELW, Ramshaw HS et al. Ex vivo expansion of murine marrow cells with interleukin-3, interleukin-6, interleukin-11, and stem cell factor leads to impaired engraftment in irradiated hosts. Blood 1996;87:30-37.

9 Reddy GPV, Tiarks CY, Pang L et al. Synchronization and cell cycle analysis of pluripotent hematopoietic progenitor stem cells. Blood 1997;90:2293-2299.

10 Stewart FM, Zhong S, Quesenberry PJ. Minimal myeloablation of the host increases the competitive dominance of donor stem cells: implications for human gene therapy. Exp Hematol 1997;25:872a.

11 Habibian HK, Peters SO, Quesenberry PJ. Fluctuating engraftment potential of cytokine stimulated murine marrow stem cells in liquid culture. Blood 1997;90:3365a.

Comparative Effects of Retroviral-Mediated Gene Transfer into Primary Human Stromal Cells of Flt3-Ligand, Interleukin 3 and GM-CSF on Production of Cord Blood Progenitor Cells in Long-Term Culture

ALESSANDRA BALDUINI,[a] STEPHEN E. BRAUN,[a,b] KENNETH CORNETTA,[b,c] STEWART LYMAN,[d] HAL E. BROXMEYER[a-c]

[a]Walther Oncology Center, [b]Departments of Microbiology/Immunology, and [c]Medicine (Hematology/Oncology), Indiana University School of Medicine and the Walther Cancer Institute, Indianapolis, Indiana, USA; [d]Immunex Corporation, Seattle, Washington, USA

Key Words. *Gene transfer · Stromal cells · Long-term culture · Flt3-ligand · Progenitor cells*

ABSTRACT

The effects of different cytokines on growth of human cord blood CD34^{+++} cells was studied by performing long-term culture (LTC) with primary human stromal cells transduced with genes for either Flt3-ligand (L) (human transmembrane, murine soluble or murine membrane-bound forms), human interleukin 3 (IL-3) or human GM-CSF. Molecular analysis of genomic DNA from transduced stromal cells using neo-specific polymerase chain reaction demonstrated gene transfer of G418-selected stromal cell populations. Enzyme-linked immunosorbent assay and biological assays of conditioned media from transduced stromal cells indicated expression and release of soluble cytokines. Numbers of both immature and more mature progenitors (colony-forming unit-granulocyte, erythroid, macrophage, megakaryocyte; CFU-GEMM, BFU-E, CFU-GM) were increased threefold compared to control in the Flt3-L (transmembrane) LTC throughout five weeks of culture. IL-3 and GM-CSF feeders increased progenitor cell output also, but these effects were significantly lower than Flt3-L feeders. The two Flt3-L isoform engineered feeders, Ex6 (soluble isoform) and 5H (membrane-bound isoform), showed a decreased effect compared to the transmembrane Flt3-L feeders and, in particular, Ex6 feeders were similar to control feeders and 5H feeders were comparable to Flt3-L feeders only in the first two weeks of LTC. These results were apparent also by limiting dilution assays that showed a higher frequency of pre-CFU in the transmembrane Flt3-L feeders compared to control and the other cytokine feeders. Exogenous addition of soluble growth factors to suspension cultures without feeder layers, while superior to stromal feeders for short-term expansion of early progenitors, were inferior to the long-term maintenance/output on stromal feeders. Pre-CFU analysis supported these data. These results may be of some significance to understanding the actions of Flt3-L on blood cell production. *Stem Cells 1998;16(suppl 1):37-49*

Characteristics and Potential of Blood Stem Cells.
STEM CELLS 1998;16(suppl 1):37-49

INTRODUCTION

The defining characteristic of a stem cell is its capacity for extensive self-renewal and retention of multilineage differentiation potential. Hematopoietic stem and progenitor cell proliferation and differentiation are regulated in vivo by cellular interactions in the bone marrow microenvironment and by a number of different cytokines that can stimulate, costimulate/augment or suppress growth [1]. The in vitro long-term culture (LTC) system reproduces many features of the bone marrow microenvironment [2]. A fundamental role of stromal cells in LTC is to provide a combination of cellular interactions and growth factors that promote the proliferation and differentiation of stem and progenitor cells [1-6]. Accessory cells are known to produce cytokines such as GM-CSF and G-CSF that seem to act preferentially on later hematopoietic progenitors, while steel factor (SLF) and Flt3 ligand (Flt3-L) have effects preferentially on early, more immature subsets of stem and progenitor cells [7-9]. It has been shown that G-CSF, GM-CSF and interleukin 3 (IL-3) produced by engineered stromal layers in LTC are able to modulate hematopoietic stem and progenitor cell growth and differentiation [10-12].

Flt3-L binding to the Flt3 tyrosine kinase receptor leads to activation of intracellular signaling [13], including MAP kinase activation and proliferative signals [14]. Both murine (mu) and human (hu) Flt3-L stimulate the proliferation of hu bone marrow and cord blood stem and progenitor cells and synergize with hu cytokines such as GM-CSF, G-CSF and IL-3 [15-17]. Murine (mu) Flt3-L is expressed in transmembrane (muFlt3-L), soluble (muEx6) and membrane-bound (mu5H) isoforms by alternative splicing [18, 19]. However, the hu form is found only as transmembrane (huFlt3-L) and soluble (huEx6) forms [18]. Inclusion of exon 6 in the Flt3-L mRNA leads to translational termination before the hydrophobic transmembrane domain of Flt3-L protein and production of the soluble isoform [19]. Inclusion of intron 5 in the mRNA leads to translation of a hydrophobic domain which anchors the Flt3-L protein to the cell surface [19]. The muFlt3-L is known to be biologically active in both soluble and membrane-bound forms [15-19].

In the current study, we investigated the effects of different cytokines on the growth activity of CD34^{+++} cells from umbilical cord blood [20-22] in LTC with stromal cells from normal human LTC adherent layers transduced with genes by retroviral vectors to produce IL-3, GM-CSF, Flt3-L and the alternatively spliced isoforms of Flt3-L.

MATERIALS AND METHODS

Cell Culture

Stromal Cell Layers.

Low density cells (< 1,077 g/ml), obtained from hu bone marrow of healthy donors, were cultured in Myelocult medium (Terry Fox Laboratory; Vancouver, Canada) with hydrocortisone sodium succinate (10^{-6}M) at 37°C in 5% CO_2. The cultures were supplied with weekly half medium changes until the adherent layer had reached confluence [2].

Retroviral Vectors and Gene Transfer

The amphotropic packaging cell PA317, the ecotropic packaging cell line GP+E86, and the murine fibroblast cell line NIH 3T3 were grown in Dulbecco's modified Eagle's medium (BioWhittaker; Walkersville, MD), 10% fetal bovine serum (FBS) (Hyclone; Logan, UT), 100 U/ml penicillin and 100 µg/ml streptomycin.

Construction of the retroviral vector L (Flt3-L) SN containing the huFlt3-L coding sequence transcriptionally regulated by the LTR was described previously [14]. This gene codes for the transmembrane form of huFlt3-L which includes both the soluble and membrane forms of Flt3-L. The coding region for the 5H (membrane-bound) and Ex6 (soluble) isoforms (Immunex Corp.; Seattle, WA) of the muFlt3-L were ligated into the retroviral vector pLXSN [23]. The coding regions of the huIL-3 (Genetics Institute; Cambridge, MA) and huGM-CSF (Genetics Institute) genes were cloned into pLXSN. After $CaPO_4$ coprecipitation and transient expression of the recombinant vectors in the ecotropic packaging cell line GP+E86 [24], PA317 cells [25] were transduced with supernatant and selected in medium containing 0.4 mg/ml G418 [14]. To obtain high-titer amphotropic producer cells, clones were isolated and the virus titer determined using NIH 3T3 cells as a target population [14].

After two to three weeks culture, primary bone marrow stromal cells were trypsinized (0.25% Trypsin-EDTA, Sigma; St. Louis, MO) and replated at 2×10^6 cells/T75 flask in Myelocult medium with hydrocortisone sodium succinate (10^{-6} M) overnight at 37°C with 10 ml of supernatant from amphotropic packaging cell lines containing 8 µg/ml polybrene. Cells were cultured for two days with Myelocult medium with hydrocortisone before the addition of 0.4 mg/ml of G418 to the medium cultures for five to nine days to select for the transduced cells [10].

Analysis for Gene Transfer and Expression

The stromal cells and supernatants were used to detect proviral integration and measure the secretion and the expression of the growth factor. To demonstrate retroviral gene transfer and integration, genomic DNA from the stromal cells was isolated using the Purgene DNA Isolation Kit (Gentra Systems; Triangle Park, NC). Polymerase chain reaction (PCR) was performed using the 25 pmoles of the neo-specific primers Neo1 (5′— CAA GAT GGA TTG CAC GCA GG¬3′) and the Neo 5 (5′—CCC GCT CAG AAG AAC TCG TC—3′) with 1×PCR buffer (Promega; Madison, WI), 1.5x $MgCl_2$, 200µM dNTPs, and 1.25 U Taq in 25 µL.

Enzyme-linked immunosorbent assay (ELISA) for huIL-3 (R&D Systems; Minneapolis, MN), huGM-CSF (R&D) and huFlt3-L [26] was used to measure production of cytokines. Conditioned media from the stromal cells and the appropriate controls were collected after three days. ELISA was performed as described by the manufacture or as described previously [26]. Since an ELISA for muFlt3-L is not available, a bioassay using huAML-5 cells as a readout [14] was also done. This line responds to Flt3-L and GM-CSF. AML-5 cells (1,000/ml) were plated with 10% FBS in 0.4% agarose culture medium and colonies scored after 10 days of incubation [14].

Cells and Separation

Cells were obtained from normal cord blood scheduled for discard after delivery of the infant and after prior need of samples for clinical study had been satisfied. CD34^{+++} cells obtained from a nonadherent, low-density T lymphocyte-depleted (NALT-) cell fraction were separated using a Coulter Epics 753 dual laser flow cytometry system (Coulter Immunology; Hialeah, FL) as previously described [21]. These cells were ≥99% CD34-positive and are highly enriched for immature progenitor cells [21].

LTC

The LTCs were performed by plating 5×10^5 cells ml/well using nontransduced (NT) cells or G418-selected transduced cells. These stromal cells were either NT, transduced with a control vector (LXSN) or with this vector containing different cytokine genes (huIL-3, huGM-CSF, huFlt3-L, mu5H, muEx6) as described elsewhere [10]. For studies in which stromal cells containing the huFlt3-L gene were mixed with stromal cells containing either the gene for huGM-CSF or huIL-3, these stromal cells were each initiated at 2.5×10^5 cells/ml/well. LTCs were initiated by seeding 5,000 cord blood CD34^{++} cells in 1 ml of Myelocult medium containing hydrocortisone sodium succinate (10^{-6}M) onto confluent layers of irradiated (1500 rads) stromal cells. LTCs were maintained for five weeks, with half medium changes weekly, at 37°C in an humidified atmosphere of 5% CO_2 and lowered (5%) O_2.

Suspension Cultures without Stromal Feeders.

Liquid cultures were initiated by plating 5,000 cord blood CD34^{+++} cells in 1 ml Iscove's modified Dulbecco's medium (IMDM) containing 10% FBS, 1% Penicillin-Streptomycin (GIBCO BRL; Gaithersburg, MD) and 100 ng/ml recombinant (r) huFlt3-L, 100 U/ml rhuIL-3 and 50 ng/ml rhuSLF singularly or in combination. The cultures were maintained for up to three to five weeks, with half medium changes weekly (including the above concentrations of cytokines), at 37°C in a humidified atmosphere of 5% CO_2 and 5% O_2.

Colony Assays

After 10 days, 2, 3 and 5 weeks, LTCs were sacrificed, nonadherent cells were counted and adherent cells were harvested using trypsin (Trypsin 1x, Sigma) and these were plated in semisolid methylcellulose culture medium assays. Semisolid cultures were incubated for two weeks at 37°C in a humidified atmosphere of 5% CO_2 and lowered (5%) O_2 in the presence of recombinant human erythropoietin (rhuEpo) (2 U/ml), rhuGM-CSF (100 U/ml), rhuIL-3 (100 U/ml) and rhuSLF (50 ng/ml). Epo was purchased from Amgen (Thousand Oaks, CA) and GM-CSF, IL-3 and SLF were kind gifts of Immunex Corp. After 14 days, colony-forming unit-granulocyte-macrophage (CFU-GM), erythroid (BFU-E) and multipotential (CFU-granulocyte, erythroid, macrophage, megakaryocyte; GEMM) progenitor cell-derived colonies were scored by microscopy [17, 20].

Limiting Dilution Assays (LDA) for Pre-CFU

After five weeks of LTC, nonadherent and adherent cells from LTC initiated on stromal cell layers and cells from liquid cultures initiated without stromal cells were seeded at 600, 300, 150 and 75 cells/well in 100 µl IMDM medium containing 10% FBS, 200 ng/ml rhuSLF, 100 U/ml rhuIL-3, 100 U/ml rhuIL-6, 100 U/ml rhuGM-CSF and 2 U/ml rhuEpo into the wells of flat-bottomed 96-well plates. For every cell dilution a total of 12 replicates were prepared. Cells were cultured in a humidified atmosphere of 5% CO_2 and 5% O_2 with the addition of complete medium supplemented with cytokines on day 7. After 14 days, 120 µl of methylcellulose supplemented with growth factors as described for colony assays were added to each well. After 14 days, CFU-GM, BFU-E and CFU-GEMM colonies were scored by microscopy. Wells were considered positive, indicating the presence of at least one pre-CFU in the original cell inoculum deposited into the well, if one or more colonies were detected [27].

Statistics

Results are expressed as mean ± 1 standard deviation (SD), and the significant differences were evaluated by Student's *t* test. A *p* value of < 0.05 was considered a significant difference.

RESULTS

Generation of huCSF-Producing Layers

To study the effects of expression of various cytokines in stromal cells on the production and expansion of hematopoietic progenitor cells in LTC, retroviral vectors L(IL-3)SN, L(GM-CSF)SN, L(muEx6)SN, L(mu5H)SN and L(huFlt3-L)SN [14] were constructed based on the vector LXSN [23] containing respectively cDNA for huIL-3, huGM-CSF, the soluble (muEx6) and membrane-bound (mu5H) isoforms of huFlt3-L and the transmembrane-bound form of huFlt3-L transcriptionally regulated by the Moloney murine leukemia virus (Mo-MLV) long terminal repeat (LTR) and the neomycin phosphotransferase gene (Neo) transcriptionally regulated by the SV40 early promoter (Fig. 1). High-titer

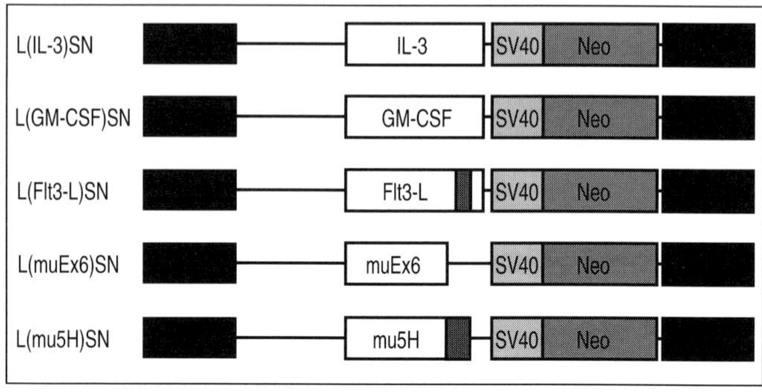

Figure 1. Retroviral vectors containing cytokine cDNAs. The SV40 early promoter transcriptionally regulates neomycin phosphotransferase gene (neo). The LTR from Moloney MLV (black box) regulates the IL-3, GM-CSF, Flt3-L, Ex6 and 5H genes (white box) with the hydrophobic membrane domain (cross-hatched box).

amphotropic packaging cells were generated by shuttle packaging through ecotopic packaging cell line GP+E86 into the amphotropic packaging cell line PA317.

To demonstrate gene transfer and integration of the provirus, PCR was performed to amplify the Neo gene from genomic DNA of the stromal cells. As shown in Figure 2, the cytokine gene-transduced stromal cells generated the 793 bp product, while the NT and negative control samples did not. The plasmid pLXSN was used as a positive control. These results demonstrate integration of the provirus in the stromal cells. To demonstrate expression of the cytokine in the stromal cells, conditioned media were collected after three days and studied for production and release of soluble cytokine. As shown in Table 1, soluble Flt3-L was detected in the conditioned media from the Flt3-L and Flt3-L + IL-3-transduced stromal layers, whereas soluble Flt3-L was undetectable (<100 pg/ml) in conditioned media from NT cells. Also, conditioned media from IL-3 and GM-CSF-transduced stroma were studied for release of soluble cytokines (Table 1). IL-3 and GM-CSF were detected in the conditioned media from the transduced stromal cells while production from the NT cells was undetectable (< 31.2 pg/ml for IL-3 and < 7.8 pg/ml for GM-CSF). These results indicate gene transfer and expression of the transduced cytokine with production of ng/ml concentrations of these cytokines in the media. It is seen that the amount of Flt3-L released was similar whether only stromal cells transduced with the Flt3-L were evaluated or these cultures had these stromal cells mixed with stromal cells containing the genes for either IL-3 or GM-CSF. Also,

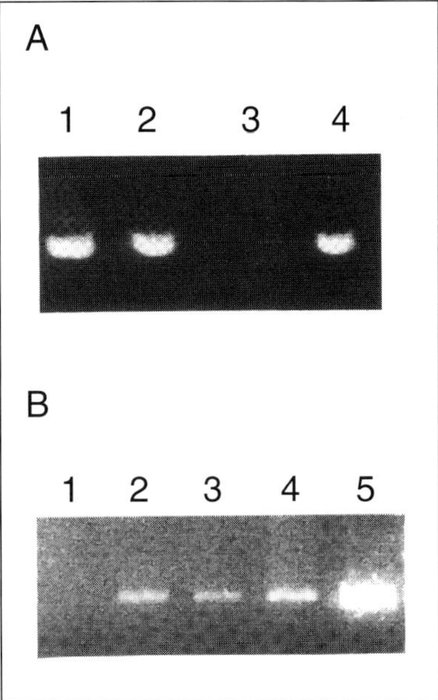

Figure 2. Molecular analysis of proviral integration in transduced stroma cells. *The 793 bp neo-specific PCR amplification from genomic DNA of stroma cells as shown by ethidium bromide straining of agarose gels. Part A: Lane 1, IL-3-transduced; Lane 2, GM-CSF-transduced; Lane 3, negative control; Lane 4, pLXSN positive control. Part B: Lane 1, NT; Lane 2, Flt3-L-transduced; Lane 3, Ex6-transduced; Lane 4, 5H-transduced; Lane 5, pLXSN positive control.*

the amount of GM-CSF or IL-3 released was not changed when stromal cells containing these cells were mixed with stromal cells containing the Flt3-L gene, suggesting that a plateau amount of cytokine release had been reached that did not increase further with increasing stromal cell numbers.

Table 1. ELISA analysis of human cytokine gene expression[a]

Feeders[b]	Flt3-L (pg/ml)	IL-3 (pg/ml)	GM-CSF (pg/ml)
NT	ND	ND	ND
Flt3-L	1,263 ± 703	–	–
IL-3	–	1,434 ± 837	–
Flt3-L + IL-3	1,310 ± 820	1,878 ± 288	–
GM-CSF	–	–	1,000 ± 752
Flt3-L + GM-CSF	–	–	970 ± 600

[a]The results are expressed as the mean ± 1 SD of four separate experiments in which different sets of cytokine gene-transduced stromal cells were evaluated for cytokine release. Medium assessed for cytokine release was conditioned for three days by confluent stromal cell layers that were at the stage in which they could be seeded by CD34[+++] cells. No CD34[+++] cells were part of the cells conditioning the culture medium. Abbreviations: NT = nontransduced; ND = not detected.
[b]Feeders refer to NT cells, those containing only cells transduced with huFlt3-L (transmembrane), huIL-3 or huGM-CSF gene, or a combination in which stromal cells transduced with huFlt3-L gene were added with stromal cells transduced with either the IL-3 or GM-CSF genes.

LTC with Engineered Stromal Cells

LTCs were performed with NT and transduced stromal cells singularly or in combination, and initiated by seeding cord blood CD34^{+++} cells. Cultures with NT stromal cells were used as controls. Results with NT stromal cells were equal to that with LXSN-transduced stromal cells (Table 2). Figure 3 shows the growth activity of cord blood CD34^{+++} cells after 10 days, 2, 3 and 5 weeks of LTC onto engineered stromal cells compared to the controls. The huFlt3-L producing feeders were able to maintain, during five weeks of LTC, a higher number of progenitor cells than the controls (Fig. 3A). huIL-3-producing feeders were also more effective than the controls in maintaining a population of progenitors (Fig. 3B), but the progenitor content was significantly less than that with the huFlt3-L-producing feeders. The combination of huFlt3-L and huIL-3-producing layers did not enhance the effect of the feeder cells containing only the huFlt3-L gene (Fig. 3C). With the huGM-CSF-producing feeders we observed a small, but significant increase of the progenitor content compared to the controls except at week 3 when the results could be compared to the controls (Fig. 3D). With respect to huFlt3-L-producing layers, the effect of huGM-CSF-producing feeders was significantly lower (Fig. 3D). The combination of huFlt3-L and huGM-CSF-transduced stromal cells did not enhance the effect of the singular huFlt3-L feeders (Fig. 3E). In some cases, when the huFlt3-L-transduced stromal cell layers were mixed with the huGM-CSF- or huIL-3-transduced stromal cell layers, the enhancement noted by the huFlt3-L stroma itself was reduced. This does not seem to reflect amounts of soluble huFlt3-L released (Table 1).

Engineered stromal cells containing the transmembrane form of the huFlt3-L gene, which expresses soluble and membrane-bound Flt3-L, were compared for activity to stromal cells containing the mu genes for the soluble isoform (Ex6) and membrane-bound isoform (5H). Flt3-L is not species-specific in action with huFlt3-L or muFlt3-L-stimulating/costimulating hu and mu

Table 2. Comparative output of progenitor cells in LTC supported by stromal cells NT versus stromal cells transducedwith control LXSN vector

Progenitor	Progenitors/well	
	NT	**LXSN-Transduced**
10 days		
CFU-GM	120 ± 26	125 ± 35
BFU-E	123 ± 50	130 ± 45
CFU-GEMM	123 ± 35	135 ± 30
2 weeks		
CFU-GM	280 ± 28	260 ± 40
BFU-E	143 ± 92	140 ± 83
CFU-GEMM	126 ± 65	130 ± 60
3 weeks		
CFU-GM	355 ± 100	360 ± 180
BFU-E	150 ± 68	160 ± 52
CFU-GEMM	310 ± 52	280 ± 70
5 weeks		
CFU-GM	180 ± 100	185 ± 100
BFU-E	123 ± 40	135 ± 70
CFU-GEMM	176 ± 75	180 ± 60

Results shown are the mean ± 1 SD of two experiments in which CD34^{+++} cord blood cells were initiated into culture at time zero as described in **Materials and Methods**. There is no statistical difference between progenitors produced from NT stromal cells and LXSN-transduced at any time point ($p > 0.05$).

progenitors, with no apparent different dose-response effects based on Flt3-L or progenitor cell species [8, 9, 15-17].

The LTCs with feeders expressing huFlt3-L were more effective than the feeders transduced with either of its two isoforms (Fig. 4). The stromal cells engineered with Flt3-L gene were able to maintain progenitor cells at a higher level with respect to each of the two isoforms. The effects of the soluble form (muEx6)-producing feeders were similar to controls during the entire five weeks of culture (Fig. 4B). The stromal cells containing the gene that produces only soluble Flt3-L did not sustain progenitor cell production any better than the NT feeders (Fig. 4B). That soluble Flt3-L was being produced by these stromal cells was determined by assessing conditioned medium from these cells on colony formation by AML-5 cells, a human cell line that grows somewhat without added growth factors, but whose growth is significantly enhanced by Flt3-L [14]. Colony formation by 100

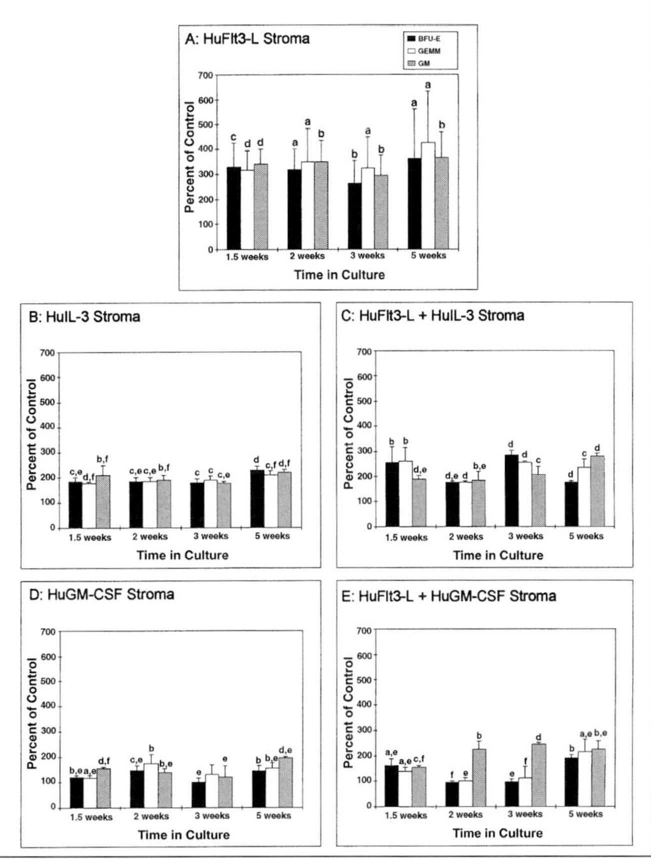

Figure 3. Total progenitor cell content (both adherent and nonadherent layer cell populations) of LTCs with feeders transduced with genes producing growth factors compared to normal LTCs with NT feeders. Each bar represents the mean ± 1 SD of three to four experiments. The absolute numbers for control NT layer LTC represented as 100% on the figure were: BFU-E = 123 ± 50, CFU-GEMM = 123 ± 35, CFU-GM = 120 ± 26 at week 1.5; BFU-E = 143 ± 92, CFU-GEMM = 126 ± 65, CFU-GM = 280 ± 28 at week 2; BFU-E = 150 ± 68, CFU-GEMM = 310 ± 52, CFU-GM = 355 ± 200 at week 3; BFU-E = 123 ± 40, CFU-GEMM = 176 ± 75, CFU-GM = 180 ± 100 at week 5 for 5,000 cord blood $CD34^{+++}$ cells initially seeded. Significant differences are designated as follows:
versus NT feeders: [a]p<0.05; [b]p<0.01; [c]p<0.005; [d]p<0.001;
versus Flt3-L feeders: [e]p<0.05; [f]p<0.01; [g]p<0.005

AML-5 cells/ml in the absence of conditioned medium was 58 ± 3 (mean ± 1 SD). This growth was not significantly altered by 40% conditioned medium from NT stromal cells (62 ± 3), but was significantly enhanced by 40% conditioned medium from Ex6-transduced stromal cells (105 ± 21, $p < 0.05$), an effect equivalent to that of 100 U/ml rhuFlt3-L (90 ± 11, $p < 0.05$). The membrane-bound form (mu5H) engineered stromal cells maintained a higher number of progenitor cells compared to the controls, but their effect decreased during the five weeks of LTC (Fig. 4C); by the third week, we observed a significant difference between 5H and Flt3-L stromal cells.

All the LTC conditions were able to maintain all types of progenitor cells (CFU-GM, BFU-E, CFU-GEMM).

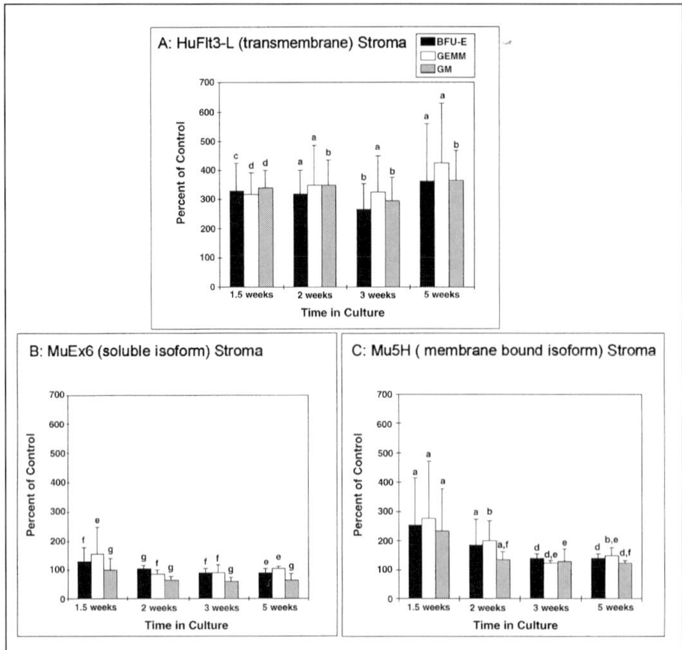

Figure 4. Total progenitor content (both adherent and nonadherent layer cell populations) of LTCs with feeders producing growth factors compared to normal LTCs with NT feeders. Each bar represents the mean ± 1 SD of three of four experiments. The absolute numbers for control NT layer LTC are represented as 100% on the figure and the significant difference designation are reported in the legend of Figure 3.

Suspension Culture

The effects of engineered and nonengineered stromal cells were then compared to that of soluble recombinant human cytokines for growth activity. Liquid cultures were initiated by seeding cord blood CD34^{+++} cells, at the same concentrations used for LTC (5,000 cells/ml), in complete medium supplemented with cytokines singularly or in combinations. No preformed stromal cell layers were used in these experiments. The cultures were maintained for three to five weeks under the same conditions of LTC as for the stroma-initiated cultures.

Figure 5 shows the progenitor cell contents of the different cytokine-initiated nonstromal suspension cultures after 10 days, 2, 3 and 5 weeks as a percent of control of NT stromal cell cultures. An increase of the progenitor cell output after 10 days of culture is noted for all the added cytokine culture conditions and especially when Flt3-L, SLF and IL-3 were used in combination (Fig. 5F). However, by the second week of culture we noticed a significant decrease of the progenitor cell content, in particular for BFU-E and CFU-GEMM. At week 3 only CFU-GM-derived colonies were present in most of the cultures. In all cases, by the third week of culture, the numbers of BFU-E and CFU-GEMM were less than in the stroma cell controls. With the combination of Flt3-L, SLF and IL-3, the number of progenitor cells was higher than in the other culture conditions, but we observed the same significant decrease of the colony output after the second week of culture, and in the third and fifth week we observed only the presence of CFU-GM. CFU-GM output at five weeks in the culture with added IL-3 + SLF + Flt3-L was greater than that of mock-transduced stroma.

LDA

To determine effects of engineered stroma compared to that of NT stroma or to addition of recombinant cytokines on progenitors more immature than CFU-GM, BFU-E and CFU-GEMM, we studied the frequency of the pre-CFU by harvesting cells after five weeks at different LTC and suspension culture conditions and assaying them by LDA. As seen in Table 3, the results confirmed those obtained with the colony assays after five weeks of culture. The frequency of pre-CFU was higher in the LTC with the transmembrane huFlt3-L-producing stromal layers compared to the control stromal layers. With the IL-3-producing stromal cells we did not observe a significant difference with respect to controls. Moreover we noticed a difference between the two muFlt3-L isoforms. The soluble isoform (muEx6)-producing feeders were similar to the controls, while the membrane-bound isoform (mu5H)-producing feeders were significantly more active than

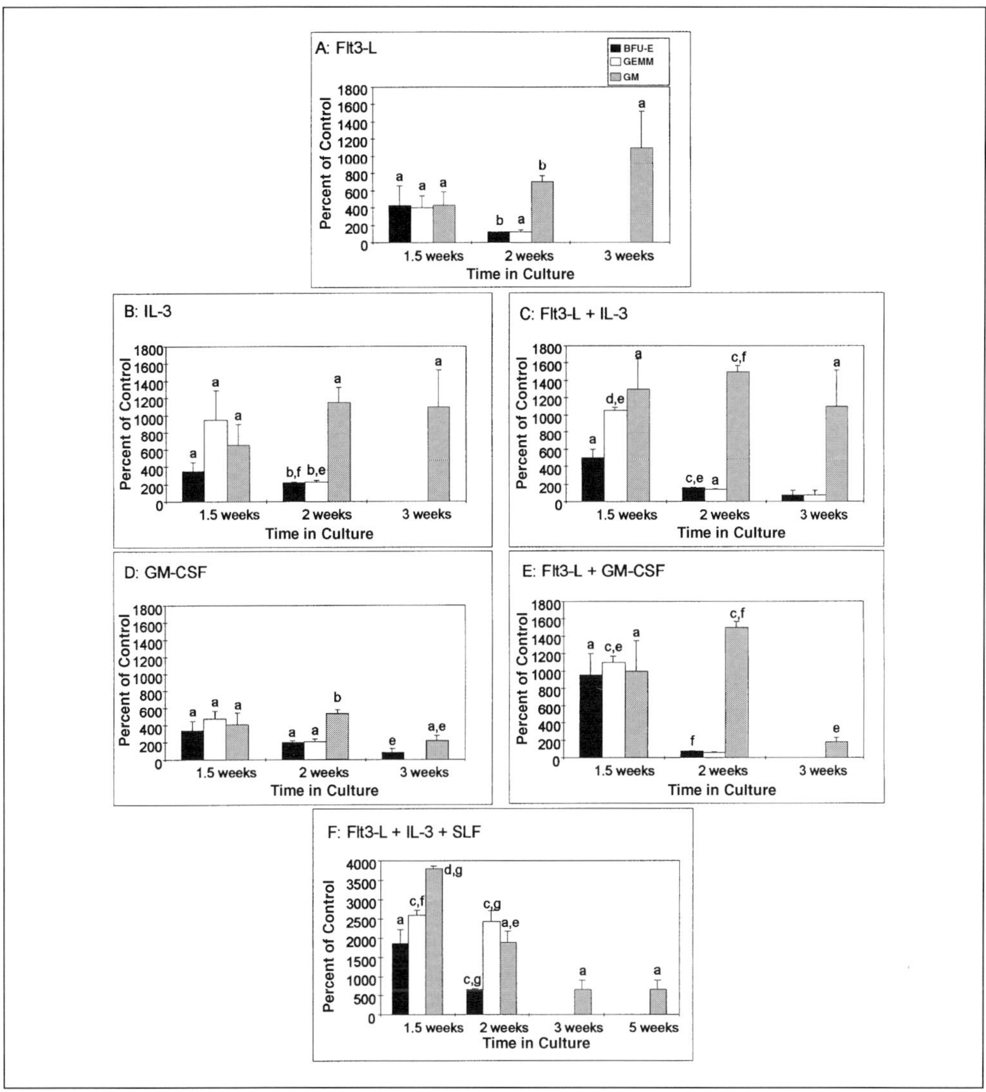

Figure 5. Total progenitor content of suspension cultures performed with different added soluble growth factors compared to normal LTC with NT feeders. Each bar represents the mean ± 1 SD of three experiments. The absolute numbers for control NT layer LTC is represented as 100% on the figure, and the significant difference designations are the same as those reported in the legend of Figure 3.

the controls. Finally, the pre-CFU frequency after five weeks of suspension culture in the presence of Flt3-L, SLF and IL-3 was significantly lower than with the control stromal layers.

DISCUSSION

The most primitive cells in the hematopoietic system represent a quiescent reserve population with the capability, when activated, of self-renewal and differentiation into lineage-committed progenitor cells. In vivo, this process is sustained by the bone marrow microenvironment, while in vitro the LTC system represents many features of the bone marrow microenvironment. In the LTC system the fundamental role of the stromal cells is to regulate the activity of stem and progenitor cells by providing a combination of proteins in soluble- or membrane-bound form that can stimulate or suppress the growth activity of the cells. The protein interactions represent an important key in the regulation of the stem/progenitor cell growth

Table 3. Frequency of pre-CFU after five weeks of LTC

	NT feeders	IL-3 feeders	Flt3-L feeders	Ex6 feeders	5H feeders	Suspension culture (IL-3 + Flt3-L + SLF)
	3.5 ± 1.2	5.1 ± 1.5	9.4 ± 4.2a	3.9 ± 1.0	5.8 ± 1.6[a]	0.6 ± 0.08[b]
Fold Change Compared to NT	1.0	1.4 ± 0.06	2.6 ± 0.3	1.0 ± 0.06	$1.7 \pm 0.60.$	2 ± 0

Frequency of pre-CFU (mean $\pm$ 1 SD) per 1,000 cells after five weeks of LTC with different gene-transduced stromal layers. The results are represented as the mean $\pm$ 1 SD for four experiments for feeders and two experiments for suspension cultures and the fold change with respect to LTC with NT feeders is shown. [a]Significant differences compared to NT feeders. [a]$p < 0.01$; [b]$p < 0.001$.

activity. It has been shown that GM-CSF-engineered feeders are able to modulate the hematopoietic activity in LTC system, in particular of more differentiated progenitor cells [10]. IL-3 increases production of both early erythroid and granulopoietic progenitors and the more mature granulocyte and macrophage output whether IL-3 is secreted by engineered stromal cells or added as soluble factor [11]. Moreover, the cotransplantation of hu bone marrow stromal cells engineered with the IL-3 gene and huCD34$^+$ cells in immunodeficient mice [28] or transplantation of hu cord blood or bone marrow into transgenic severe combined immunodeficiency (SCID) mice engineered to express human forms of certain cytokines (GM-CSF, IL-3 and SLF)[29] results in enhanced growth of human cells.

Among the many cytokines now known to be involved in blood cell production, Flt3-L is considered to be especially involved early in hematopoiesis of the myeloid and lymphoid lineages [30]. It acts as a growth factor, a survival factor and as a potent costimulating cytokine [8, 9, 15-17, 31-45]. However, little is known regarding the activity of Flt3-L in the microenvironment, and it is in the context of cells of the microenvironment that Flt3-L may be most efficient and relevant for long-term hematopoiesis. This possibility is evident in the present studies, where it is clear that under the conditions of the engineered stroma layers, Flt3-L production was more effective than either GM-CSF or IL-3 production in the long-term proliferation of early progenitors, including pre-CFU, CFU-GEMM and BFU-E. This activity was greater than that of NT stromal cells or stromal cells transduced with an empty LXSN control vector, and was not enhanced by combinations of cytokine-engineered feeders, including those producing Flt3-L plus either GM-CSF or IL-3. Combinations of soluble recombinant factors such as Flt3-L, SLF and IL-3 work in additive to greater-than-additive fashion with each other [8, 9, 15-17, 31-45] and when added to nonstroma cell-initiated cultures, had potent progenitor cell expansion effects short-term in comparison to control stromal cell feeders. However, long-term support of continuously produced early cells such as pre-CFU, BFU-E and CFU-GEMM was best accomplished by a pre-established stromal cell layer, and this production was most enhanced with stromal cells engineered to express the transmembrane Flt3-L gene.

While some information is known regarding intracellular signaling events of Flt3-L for established factor-dependent cell lines [13, 14], little is known regarding the mechanisms of action of Flt3-L for long-term maintenance of primary blood cell production. The use of stromal cells expressing Flt3-L may be useful in this context when compared to the effects of a soluble recombinant Flt3-L molecule. How the membrane and soluble forms of Flt3-L may interact to regulate long-term hematopoiesis of early cells is also an area of much interest, especially in light of the physiological relevance of the membrane-bound form of SLF [7]. Soluble, but not membrane-bound, SLF is produced by the Steel Dickie mouse (Sl/Sl^d) which manifests abnormalities in blood cell production. Our studies in LTC suggest that maximal long-term production of early progenitors required stromal cell production of both the membrane-bound and soluble Flt3-L. The expression of transmembrane Flt3-L was more potent than that of the membrane-bound (5H) Flt3-L, especially at week 2 (for CFU-GEMM), week 3 (for BFU-E and CFU-GEMM) and week 5 (for BFU-E and CFU-GEMM, and with a trend for LTC-initiating cell [LTC-IC]). Interestingly, stromal cells engineered to express only the soluble form of Flt3-L (Ex6) had no significant activity above that of control stromal cells. In these experiments, the transmembrane form of Flt3-L was of hu origin, while that for Ex6 and 5H were of mu origin. Since Ex6 is a mu gene, and there is no ELISA for muFlt3-L, we could not quantitate the exact amount of Flt3-L released by the muEx6-transduced stromal cells. However, lack of activity of Ex6-transduced stromal cells on LTCs did not appear to be due to the lack of production of a bioactive form of soluble Flt3-L. Medium conditioned by muEx6-transduced stroma was biologically active on AML-5 cells in an amount equivalent in activity to that of 100 ng/ml rFlt3-L, a plateau amount of material for stimulation/costimulation of progenitor cell proliferation. Studies with muFlt3-L on human progenitor cell proliferation, in which no differences between mu and huFlt3-L were seen, [8, 9, 15-17] and the studies herein, in which the mu membrane-bound form (5H) of Flt3-L was active in LTC do not seem to point to species differences in Flt3-L as a reason for the activities of stromal cells that had been engineered to express different isoforms of Flt3-L. However, until the mu Flt3-L transmembrane form is compared to the mu soluble and mu membrane-bound forms, it cannot be definitively ruled out that the differences observed are at least in part due to species differences. As noted, the hu form of Flt3-L is only found in transmembrane and soluble (hu Ex6) forms [18]. While it is clear that more studies are needed to define the roles of membrane and soluble Flt3-L in production of blood cells long-term in vivo and in LTC in vitro, the studies reported here are suggestive that both forms may be necessary for optimal effects.

In order to more precisely and definitively define the comparative short versus long-term growth effects in LTC due to stromal components or soluble cytokines, it will be necessary to assess the combined effects of human soluble, exogenously added Flt3-L to stromal cells transduced with mock-virus, or the Flt3-L, Ex6, or 5H gene. It will also be important to analyze the stability of Flt3-L, GM-CSF and IL-3 production over time in cultures from the cytokine gene-transduced and selected stromal cell population. While it is likely that these cytokines were continuously produced over time in culture, the present studies only assessed cytokine production at the time of initial seeding of CD34^{+++} cells on to the LTC stromal feeders, and the amount of cytokine produced at different times is not known. Moreover, we used a modified LTC-IC assay in which cells were seeded for two weeks, in comparison to the more standard LTC-IC assays of five weeks or longer, prior to plating in semisolid medium assays for a cell more immature than a progenitor (pre-CFU) but perhaps not as immature as an LTC-IC. Assessment of effects of LTC on LTC-IC or even more primitive cells as detected in a hu SCID mouse model is warranted.

ACKNOWLEDGMENTS

We thank *Nancy Hague* and *Scott Cooper* for technical assistance, *Susan Grisby* and *Jon McMahel* for assistance in operating the FACS; and *Becki Miller* for typing the manuscript.

These studies were supported by U.S. Public Health Service Grants R01 HL54037, R01 HL46416, a project in P01 HL53586, and training program T32 DK07519 from the NIH to *H.E.B. S.E. Braun* is a Fellow of the Leukemia Society of America.

REFERENCES

1 Broxmeyer HE, Williams DE. The production of myeloid blood cells and their regulation during health and disease. CRC Crit Rev Oncol/Hematol 1988;8:173-226.

2 Eaves CJ, Cashman JD, Eaves A. Methodology of long term culture of human hemopoietic cells. J Tiss Cult Meth 1991;13:55-62.

3 Migliaccio AR, Migliaccio G, Johnson G et al. Comparative analysis of hematopoietic growth factors released by stromal cells from normal donors or transplanted patients. Blood 1990;75:305-312.

4 Kittler ELW, Megrath H, Temeles D et al. Biological significance of constitutive and subliminal growth factor production by bone marrow stroma. Blood 1992;79:3168-3178.

5 Eaves CJ, Cashman JD, Kay RJ et al. Mechanisms that regulate the cell cycle status of very primitive hematopoietic cells in long-term human marrow cultures. Analysis of positive and negative regulators produced by stromal cells within the adherent layer. Blood 1991;78:110-117.

6 Verfaille CM. Soluble factor(s) produced by human bone marrow stroma increase cytokine-induced proliferation and maturation of primitive hematopoietic progenitors while preventing their terminal differentiation. Blood 1993;82:2045-2051.

7 Broxmeyer HE, Maze R, Miyazawa K et al. The Kit receptor and its ligand, steel factor, as regulators of hemopoiesis. Cancer Cells 1991;3:480-487.

8 Lyman SD, Williams DE. Biology and potential clinical applications of flt3 Ligand. Current Opin Hematol 1995;2:177-180.

9 Lyman SD. Biology of flt3 ligand and receptor. Int J Hematol 1995;62:63-73.

10 Hogge DE, Cashman JD, Humphries RK et al. Differential and synergistic effects of human granulocyte-macrophage colony stimulating factor and human granulocyte-colony stimulating factor on hematopoiesis in human long-term marrow cultures. Blood 1991;77:493-497.

11 Otsuka T, Thacker JD, Eaves CJ et al. Differential effects of microenvironmentally presented interleukin 3 versus soluble growth factor on primitive human hematopoietic cells. J Clin Invest 1991;88:417-421.

12 Sutherland HJ, Eaves CJ, Lansdorp PM et al. Differential regulation of primitive human hematopoietic cells in long-term cultures maintained on genetically engineered murine stromal cells. Blood 1991;78:666-672.

13 Dosil M, Wang S, Lemischka IR. Mitogenic signalling and substrate specificity of the Flk2/Flt3 receptor tyrosine kinase in fibroblasts and interleukin 3-dependent hematopoietic cells. Mol Cell Biol 1993;13:6572-6585.

14 Braun SE, Aronica SM, Ge Y et al. Retroviral-mediated gene transfer of Flt3 ligand enhances proliferation and MAP kinase activity of AML5 cells. Exp Hematol 1997;25:51-56.

15 Lyman SD, James L, Vanden Bos T et al. Molecular cloning of a ligand for the flt3/flk-2 tyrosine kinase receptor: a proliferative factor for primitive hematopoietic cells. Cell 1993;75:1157-1167.

16 Lyman SD, James L, Johnson L et al. Cloning of human homologue of murine flt3 Ligand: a growth factor for early hematopoietic progenitor cells. Blood 1994;83:2795-2801.

17 Broxmeyer HE, Lu L, Cooper S et al. Flt-3-ligand stimulates/co-stimulates the growth of myeloid stem/progenitor cells. Exp Hematol 1995;23:1121-1129.

18 Lyman SD, Stocking K, Davison B et al. Structural analysis of human and murine flt3 ligand genomic loci. Oncogene 1995;11:1165-1172.

19 Lyman SD, James L, Escobar S et al. Identification of soluble and membrane bound isoforms of the murine flt3 ligand generated by alternative splicing of mRNAs. Oncogene 1995;10:149-157.

20 Broxmeyer HE, Hangoc G, Cooper S et al. Growth characteristics and expansion of human umbilical cord blood and estimation of its potential for transplantation of adults. Proc Natl Acad Sci USA 1992;89:4109-4113.

21 Lu L, Xiao M, Shen RN et al. Enrichment, characterization and responsiveness of single primitive $CD34^{+++}$ human umbilical cord blood hematopoietic progenitor with high proliferative and replating potential. Blood 1993;81:41-48.

22 Carow CE, Hangoc G, Broxmeyer HE. Human multipotential progenitor cells (CFU-GEMM) have extensive replating capacity for secondary CFU-GEMM: an effect enhanced by cord blood plasma. Blood 1993;81:942-949.

23 Miller AD, Rosman GJ. Improved retroviral vectors for gene transfer and expression. BioTechniques 1989;7:980-982.

24 Markowitz DG, Goff SP, Bank A. Safe and efficient ecotropic and amphotropic packaging lines for use in gene transfer experiments. Trans Assoc Am Physicians 1988;101:212-218.

25 Miller A, Buttimore C. Redesign of retrovirus packaging cell lines to avoid recombinant leading to helper virus production. Mol Cell Biol 1986;6:2895-2899.

26 Lyman SD, Seaberg M, Hanna R et al. Plasma/serum levels of flt3 ligand are low in normal individuals and highly elevated in patients with Fanconi anemia and acquired aplastic anemia. Blood 1995;86:4091-4096.

27 Traycoff CM, Kosak ST, Grigsby S et al. Evaluation of ex vivo expansion potential of cord blood and bone marrow hematopoietic progenitor cells using cell tracking and limiting dilution analysis. Blood 1995;85:2059-2068.

28 Nolta JA, Hanley MB, Kohn DB. Sustained human hematopoiesis in immunodeficient mice by cotransplantation of marrow stroma expressing human interleukin-3: analysis of gene transduction of long-lived progenitors. Blood 1994;83:3041-3051.

29 Bock TA, Orlic D, Dunbar CE et al. Improved engraftment of human hematopoietic cells in severe combined immunodeficient (SCID) mice carrying human cytokine transgenes. J Exp Med 1995;182:2037-2043.

30 Mackarehtschian K, Hardin JD, Moore KA et al. Targeted disruption of the flk2/flt3 gene leads to deficiencies in primitive hematopoietic progenitors. Immunity 1995;3:147-161.

31 Hannum C, Culpepper J, Campbell D et al. Ligand for flt3/flk2 receptor tyrosine kinase regulates growth of haematopoietic stem cells and is encoded by variant RNAs. Nature 1994;368:643-648.

32 Muench MO, Roncarolo MG, Menon S et al. Flk-2/flt-3 ligand regulates the growth of early myeloid progenitors isolated from human fetal liver. Blood 1995;85:963-972.

33 Jacobsen SEW, Okkenhaug C, Myklebust J et al. The flt3 ligand potentially and directly stimulates the growth and expansion of primitive murine bone marrow progenitor cells in vitro: synergistic interactions with interleukin (IL) 11, IL-12, and other hematopoietic growth factors. J Exp Med 1995;181:1357-1363.

34 Hirayama F, Lyman SD, Clark SC et al. The flt3 ligand supports proliferation of lymphohematopoietic progenitors and early B-lymphoid progenitors. Blood 1995;85:1762-1768.

35 Hudak S, Hunte B, Culpepper J et al. Flt3/Flk2 ligand promotes the growth of murine stem cells and the expansion of colony-forming cells and spleen colony-forming units. Blood 1995;85:2747-2755.

36 Hunte BE, Hudak S, Campbell D et al. flk2/flt3 ligand is a potent cofactor for the growth of primitive B cell progenitors. J Immunol 1995;156:489-496.

37 McKenna HJ, de Vries P, Brasel K et al. Effect of flt3 ligand on the ex vivo expansion of human CD34$^+$ hematopoietic progenitor cells. Blood 1995;86:3413-3420.

38 Takahira H, Lyman SD, Broxmeyer HE. Flt3-ligand prolongs survival of CD34^{+++} human umbilical cord blood myeloid progenitors in serum-free culture medium. Ann Hematol 1996;72:131-135.

39 Rusten LS, Lyman SD, Veiby OP et al. The flt3 ligand is a direct and potent stimulator of the growth of primitive and committed human CD34$^+$ bone marrow progenitor cells in vitro. Blood 1996;87:1317-1325.

40 Namikawa R, Muench MO, de Vries JE et al. The flk2/flt3 ligand synergizes with interleukin-7 in promoting stromal-cell-independent expansion and differentiation of human fetal Pro-B cells in vitro. Blood 1996;87:1881-1890.

41 Shah AJ, Smogorzewska EM, Hannum C et al. Flt3 ligand induces proliferation of quiescent human bone marrow CD34$^+$CD38$^-$ cells and maintains progenitor cells in vitro. Blood 1996;87:3563-3570.

42 Jacobsen SEW, Veiby OP, Myklebust J et al. Ability of flt3 ligand to stimulate the in vitro growth of primitive murine hematopoietic progenitors is potently and directly inhibited by transforming growth factor-β and tumor necrosis factor-α. Blood 1996;87:5016-5026.

43 Veiby OP, Jacobsen FW, Cui L et al. The flt3 ligand promotes the survival of primitive hemopoietic progenitor cells with myeloid as well as B lymphoid potential. J Immunol 1996;157:2953-2960.

44 Brasel K, McKenna HJ, Morrissey PJ et al. Hematologic effects of flt3 ligand in vivo in mice. Blood 1996;88:2004-2012.

45 Petzer AL, Zandstra PW, Piret JM et al. Differential cytokine effects on primitive (CD34$^+$CD38$^-$) human hematopoietic cells: novel responses to flt3-ligand and thrombopoietin. J Exp Med 1996;183:2551-2558.

Unilineage Hematopoietic Differentiation in Bulk and Single Cell Culture

BENEDIKT ZIEGLER,[a] UGO TESTA,[b] GIANLUIGI CONDORELLI,[c]
LUIGI VITELLI,[b] MAURO VALTIERI,[b] CESARE PESCHLE[b,c]

[a]Department of Medicine, Division of Hematology and Oncology, Eberhard-Karls
University Tübingen, Tübingen, Germany; [b]Department of Hematology-Oncology, Istituto
Superiore di Sanità, Rome, Italy; [c]T. Jefferson University, Kimmel Cancer Center,
Philadelphia, Pennsylvania, USA

Key Words. *Hematopoietic progenitors · Unilineage hematopoietic differentiation culture*

ABSTRACT

The rarity of hematopoietic stem and progenitor cells (HSCs, HPCs) has hampered the analysis of cellular and molecular mechanisms underlying early hematopoiesis. Methodology for HPC purification has partially offset this limitation. A further hurdle has been represented by the heterogeneity of the analyzed HPC/precursor populations: recently, development of unilineage HPC differentiation cultures has provided homogeneous populations of hematopoietic cells, particularly in the early differentiation state, i.e., populations pertaining to a single lineage and a restricted stage of differentiation/maturation, but sufficiently large for cellular/molecular analysis.

This report focuses on the development and characterization of the unilineage HPC differentiation culture systems. A section is devoted to selected cellular and molecular mechanisms underlying hematopoiesis, which have been investigated by the HPC unilineage culture approach. Finally, recent advances in the development of HPC unilineage cultures at single cell level are discussed. *Stem Cells 1998;16(suppl 1):51-73*

INTRODUCTION

The rarity of hematopoietic stem and progenitor cells (HSCs, HPCs) has hampered the analysis of cellular and molecular mechanisms underlying early hematopoiesis. Methodology for HPC purification has partially offset this limitation. A further hurdle has been represented by the heterogeneity of the analyzed HPC/precursor populations: recently, development of unilineage HPC differentiation cultures has provided homogeneous populations of hematopoietic cells, particularly in the early differentiation stage, i.e., populations pertaining to a single lineage and a restricted stage of differentiation/maturation, but sufficiently large for cellular/molecular analysis.

This report focuses on the development and characterization of the unilineage HPC differentiation culture systems. A section is devoted to selected cellular and molecular mechanisms underlying hematopoiesis which have been investigated by the HPC unilineage culture approach. Finally, recent advances in the development of HPC unilineage cultures at the single cell level are discussed.

Characteristics and Potentials of Blood Stem Cells
STEM CELLS 1998;16(suppl 1):51-73 ©AlphaMed Press. All rights reserved.

THE MODEL OF EARLY HEMATOPOIESIS

Hematopoietic proliferation and differentiation is sustained by a pool of HSCs which feed into HPCs differentiated precursors and terminal cells circulating in peripheral blood (PB) [1, 2].

HSCs feature three important properties: A) extensive self-renewal capacity, B) broad differentiation potential and C) prolonged maintenance in a noncycling state in adult life [1, 2].

The HSC self-renewal potential is apparently limited and heterogeneous. Thus, serial transplantation of murine bone marrow (BM) cells leads to a decreasing long-term reconstitution ability (LTRA) [3].

The HSC differentiation potential may also be heterogeneous. Studies with murine HSCs marked by unique radiation-induced chromosomal aberrations showed that pluripotent HSCs repopulate the entire hematopoietic system, while other putative HSCs feed either the myeloid or the T lymphoid system, i.e., they are functionally restricted to repopulate selected hematopoietic compartments [4].

Due to their prolonged noncycling state, adult HSCs are resistant to cycle-specific cytotoxic agents; this provided the basis for purification of murine HSCs [5] and putative human HSCs [6] by treatment with 5-fluorouracil. In spite of these advances, purification of human HSCs with LTRA still represents a crucial unresolved issue.

HSCs/primitive HPCs give rise to a hierarchy of committed HPCs, functionally defined as BFUs or colony-forming units (CFUs). The earliest HPCs are multipotent and generate mixed colonies (CFU-GEMM; CFU-granulocytic, erythroid, macrophage, megakaryocyte). Multipotent HPCs differentiate and become gradually committed to specific lineages, i.e., HPCs of the erythroid series (early and late, BFU-E and CFU-E), the megakaryocytic lineage (BFU-MK, CFU-MK) and the granulomonocytic lineage (CFU-GM, CFU-G, CFU-M).

BM hematopoiesis is at least in part regulated by a network of hematopoietic growth factors (HGFs) and related cytokines. The HGFs may be classified according to the spectrum of their biological activity on HSCs/HPCs in three different categories:

A) Early-acting HGFs include KL (c-kit receptor ligand or stem cell factor) [7, 8], the FLT3 receptor ligand (FL) [9, 10], basic fibroblast GF (bFGF) [11, 12], interleukin 6 (IL-6) [13], leukemia inhibitory factor (LIF) [14] and IL-11 [15]. These HGFs are characterized by a stimulatory action largely restricted to the early stages of hematopoiesis (as a notable exception, IL-6 also exerts pleiotropic effects on a variety of mature hematopoietic cells [16]).

B) A second category is represented by multilineage HGFs, whose prototypes are IL-3 and GM-CSF [17]. Both stimulate early HPCs (CFU-GEMM, BFU-E, BFU-MK and CFU-GM) to proliferate and differentiate. Furthermore, these cytokines stimulate the proliferation and survival of late CFU-GM, CFU-G/CFU-M and their progeny through terminal maturation [17].

C) A third category is represented by unilineage HGFs, which mainly induce the proliferation and differentiation of unilineage committed HPCs. Thus, erythropoietin (Epo) [18], G-CSF [19], IL-5 [20], M-CSF [21] and thrombopoietin (Tpo) [22] promote the production of differentiated and terminal precursors of the erythroid, neutrophilic, eosinophilic, monocytic and megakaryocytic lineages, respectively (in addition, TPO directly stimulates multilineage HPCs and potentiates the KL and FL effects on early hematopoiesis [23]).

UNILINEAGE HPC DIFFERENTIATION CULTURES

Limitations of Current Experimental Tools

As previously mentioned, the rarity of HSCs and early HPCs (which together represent <0.1% and <0.01% of human BM [1] and PB [11, 24-26] mononuclear cells, respectively) has hindered analysis of the cellular/molecular mechanisms underlying early hematopoiesis.

Studies on unpurified HSC/HPC in semisolid culture led to the identification of the main HPC categories. However, this approach bears intrinsic limitations: A) the culture contains a large majority of accessory cells, which release biologically significant and variable amounts of endogenous HGFs, thus obscuring the effects of exogenous cytokines, and B) the recovery and analysis of early hematopoietic cells is hardly possible.

Leukemia cell lines and immortalized murine HPC lines (32D, FCDP-Mix [27, 28]) provide important, extensively utilized tools: however, these cell models reflect, in part, selected stages and lineages of normal hematopoiesis, which have become partially or totally independent of HGF(s) and other physiological control mechanisms.

Introduction of the genetically engineered murine models, i.e., transgenic and knock-out mice, has represented a fundamental innovation to investigate the molecular basis of blood cell development. The latter approach has provided crucial insight into mechanisms underlying hematopoiesis [29]; however, it bears significant limitations [29-31], particularly with respect to A) lack of a phenotype due to generation of gene redundancy; B) multiple phenotypes, due to positional effects of the disrupted gene on adjacent genes [30]; C) lethal effects in early ontogenesis; D) lack of tissue specificity, and E) murine versus human species differences [31]. These limitations are partially offset by (a) generation of chimeric knock-out mice via introduction of mutant embryonic stem (ES) cells into the normal murine blastocyst [32], (b) in vitro analysis of primitive/definitive (but not adult) hematopoiesis generated by the knock-out ES cells [32, 33] and (c) development of tissue-specific and time-restricted [34] knock-out techniques.

New experimental tools, which complement the currently available methodology, are needed to investigate cellular/molecular mechanisms underlying human adult hematopoiesis. Recently, analysis of these aspects has been facilitated by development of unilineage HPC differentiation in liquid suspension culture [10, 35-41]. In the bulk systems a sufficiently large population of purified early HPCs/HSCs are induced into a wave of gradual differentiation/maturation along a specific lineage(s). A further approach is based on HPC unicellular culture followed by daughter cell analysis at cellular and/or molecular level.

HPC Purification

The intensive efforts devoted to development of purification methods for human early HPCs/HSCs have provided a high level of HPC enrichment, usually coupled with relatively low recovery (5%-20%) [11, 42-44].

The methodology developed by our group [11], recently potentiated [10, 35-41], provides stringent purification and abundant recovery of early HPCs (CFU-GEMM, BFU-E, BFU-MK, CFU-GM) together with a minority of primitive HPCs/putative HSCs (see below) from normal adult PB. The Step IIIP cells obtained by the modified purification procedure are characterized by 90%-95% HPC frequency and 70% HPC recovery (mean values) [45 and unpublished results]. With respect to membrane antigen phenotype, Step IIIP cells are 90% CD34$^+$/HLA-DR$^+$/CD38$^+$ (only 5%-10% of CD34$^+$ cells are lin$^+$, e.g., CD4$^+$): 5%-10% are CD34$^+$/CD38^{low} and CD34$^+$/HLA-DR-/^{low} cells, while 5%-15% are Thy-1$^+$ and gp170$^+$ (MDR1) [45]. In line with this phenotype, Step IIIP cells comprise primitive HPCs, i.e., 3-6% CFU-B, (blast colony-forming unit [46]), 10%-15% HPP-CFCs (high proliferative potential colony-forming cells, 47]), and putative HSCs, i.e., 0.3%-1.5% LTC-ICs (long-term culture initiating cell [48]) [10 and unpublished results].

Unilineage HPC Differentiation/Maturation in Liquid Suspension Culture

We have developed a strategy to induce purified HPCs into unilineage erythroid (E) (Fig. 1A, B), granulopoietic-neutrophilic (G) (Fig. 2A, B) or -eosinophilic (Eo) (not shown), megakaryopoietic

(MK) (Fig. 3A, B) and monopoietic (M) (Fig. 4A, B) differentiation/maturation in liquid suspension culture [10, 35-41, 45]. In these culture systems, HPCs are stimulated by a unilineage HGF (Epo, G-CSF, IL-5, Tpo or M-CSF, respectively) at a saturating level combined with appropriate dosages of multilineage or early-acting HGF(s). The unilineage dendritic (Den) cell culture system is currently under development. Finally, HPC cultures generating 80%-90% basophilic cells have been established.

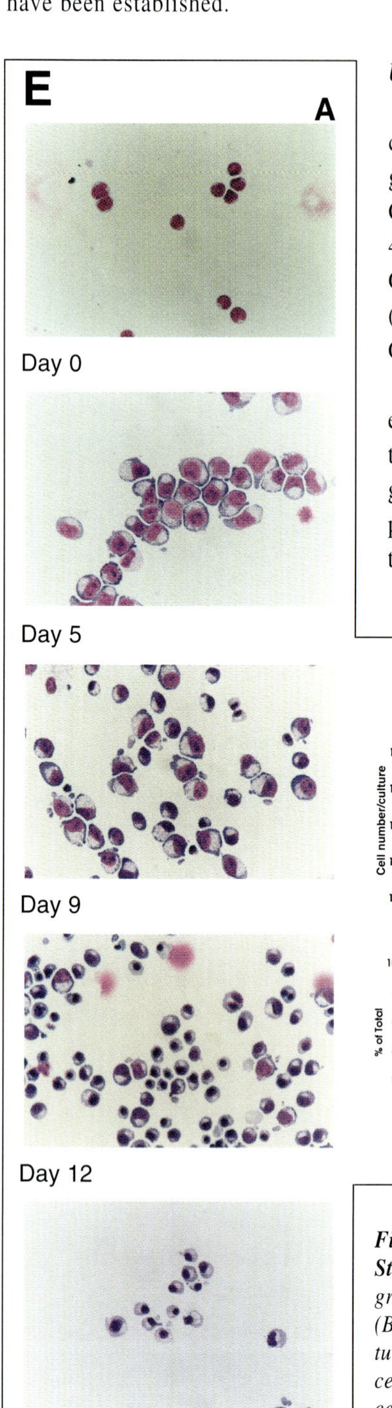

Unilineage E, G or Eo Growth (Figs. 1A, B, 2A, B and results not shown)

In these fetal calf serum-free (FCS⁻) liquid suspension cultures, purified HPCs are induced to A) selective E growth by very low dosages of IL-3 (0.01 U/ml) and GM-CSF (0.001 ng) and a saturating Epo level (3 U) [35-41, 45], B) unilineage G growth by low-dose IL-3 (1 U) and GM-CSF (0.1 ng) combined with plateau level of G-CSF (500 U) [37, 38] or C) unilineage Eo growth by replacing G-CSF with IL-5 (10 ng) (unpublished results).

In the first week of culture, HPCs show a high proliferative activity (Fig. 1B and 2B) which is associated with their progressive differentiation; this is shown by the gradual decrease of CD34⁺ and blast cell frequency, coupled with a decline of the size of colonies generated by the HPCs replated in secondary semisolid culture.

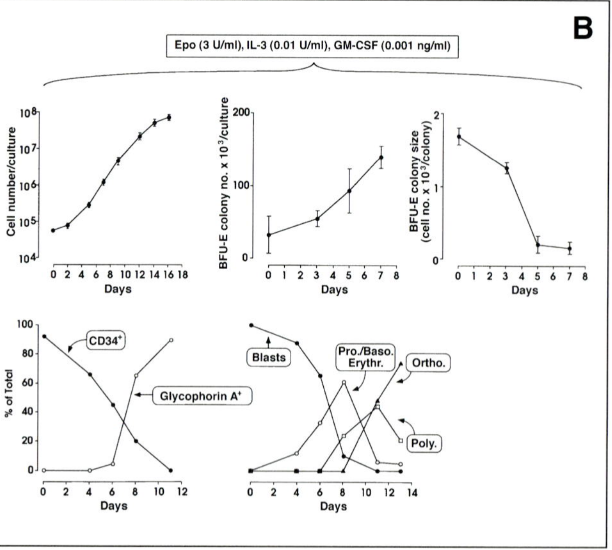

Figure 1. (A) Cell morphology in E unilineage cultures of purified Step IIIP HPCs, as evaluated at sequential days. A color photograph for each culture day (original magnification × 630) is shown. (B) Cell growth curve (top panel, left), BFU-E colony number/culture (top panel, middle), BFU-E colony size (top panel, right), percentage of CD34⁺ and glycophorin A⁺ cells (bottom panel, left) and cell type composition classified according to the differentiation/maturation stage (bottom panel, right). Mean ± SE values (top) or representative results (bottom) are presented.

In the second week we observed the disappearance of CD34$^+$ cells and blasts and the progressively increasing expression of specific membrane markers for E and G precursors (e.g., glycophorin A and CD11b, respectively); cell morphology analysis showed a gradual wave of maturation along the E or G pathway to terminal cells, i.e., at day 14-16 ≥ 97% erythroid cells (largely orthochromatic normoblasts) in E culture, and ≥ 98% granulopoietic cells in G or Eo culture (largely neutrophils or eosinophils, respectively) (Figs. 1, 2 and results not shown).

Altogether, these findings suggest that highly purified HPCs grown in FCS⁻ liquid suspension cultures undergo a gradual and homogeneous wave of differentiation specifically along the E lineage or G, Eo pathway.

Basophilic Culture System

In addition to its potentiating effect on early-acting HGFs, KL stimulates in vitro fetal HPCs to generate basophils/mast cells, while favoring mast cell survival [49]. In line with these studies, purified Step IIIP HPCs grown in FCS⁻ liquid suspension culture supplemented with KL alone (10 or 100 ng/ml) develop a progeny comprising a majority (80%-90%) of basophils and a minority of neutrophils [10 and unpublished data]. This culture system allows only an ~10-fold expansion of total cell number after 14 days of culture, seemingly due to the low frequency of basophilic HPCs. Furthermore, addition of the HGFs stimulating granulopoiesis (e.g., IL-3 and/or GM-CSF) reduces the frequency of basophils and increases that of neutrophils and/or eosinophils.

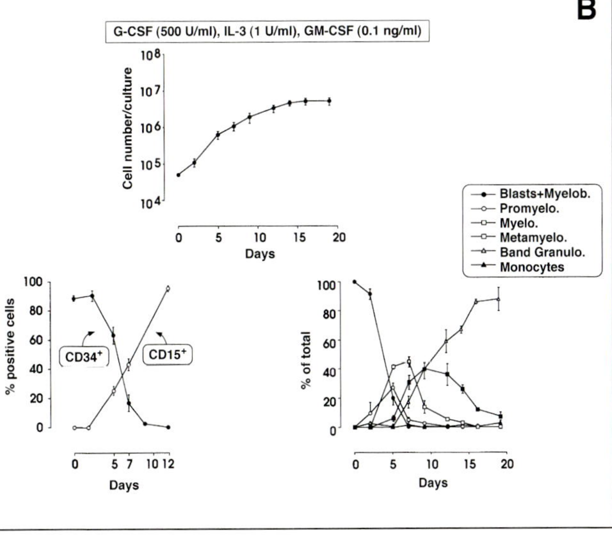

Figure 2. (A) Cell morphology in G unilineage cultures of purified Step IIIP HPCs, as evaluated at sequential days. A color photograph for each culture (original magnification × 630) is shown. (B) Cell growth curve (top panel), percentage of CD34$^+$ and CD15$^+$ cells (bottom panel, left) and cell type composition classified according to the differentiation/maturation stage (bottom panel, right). Mean + SE values are presented.

Unilineage MK Growth (Fig. 3A, B)

Early studies suggested that megakaryocytopoiesis is regulated at two different levels [50]: early-acting GFs (IL-3, KL and GM-CSF) may stimulate the proliferation of BFU-MK/CFU-MK; late "thrombopoietin-like" factors (IL-6, LIF or Epo) may stimulate later stages of thrombopoiesis.

The c-*mpl* proto-oncogene plays a key role in megakaryocytopoiesis, as indicated by antisense oligonucleotide [51] and knock-out [52] reports. The murine and human mpl ligand (Tpo), recently cloned [53-55], exerts in vivo and in vitro a stimulatory activity restricted to the MK lineage [22, 53-56] at both early [56] and late [22] differentiation stages.

Liquid suspension cultures of partially purified PB HPCs grown in the presence of recombinant Tpo generated a cell progeny enriched in MKs (37%-41%), but still contaminated by a majority of G cells [55].

To bypass these limitations we have developed culture systems for HPC unilineage MK differentiation. Thus, Step IIIP HPCs were grown in FCS⁻ liquid suspension cultures in the presence of either an HGF cocktail (IL-3, KL and IL-6) and/or recombinant Tpo [41]: A) the HGF cocktail induced the growth of a 40% purified MK population; B) further addition of Tpo increased the MK purity level to 80% with a final yield of 4×10^5 MKs starting from 4×10^4 purified HPCs at day 0 of culture, and C) treatment with Tpo alone resulted in a 97%-99% MK population with a slight increase of cell number (to 6×10^5 cells).

In Tpo-supplemented culture, morphological evaluation indicated the presence of putative mononuclear MK precursors and then mature polynucleated platelet-forming MKs peaking at days 5 and 12, respectively (Fig. 3B). In the first week of culture,

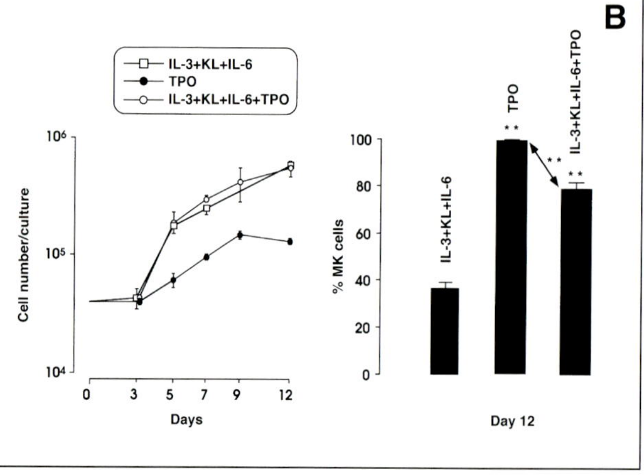

*Figure 3. (A) Cell morphology in MK unilineage cultures of purified Step IIIP HPCs, as evaluated at sequential days. A color photograph for each culture day (original magnification ✕ 630) is shown. (B) Cell growth curve (left) and % MK cells (right) using different HGF combinations. Mean ± SE values are presented. **p < 0.01 when compared to control values, as well as when comparing second and third bars. Reprinted, with modifications, with permission from [41].*

HPCs show a moderate proliferative activity, as indicated by the cell growth curve, which is associated with their progressive differentiation (i.e., here again, gradual decrease of CD34$^+$ and blast cell frequency were coupled with a decline of the size of colonies generated by the HPCs replated in secondary semisolid culture). In the second week the disappearance of CD34$^+$ cells was associated with the progressively increasing expression of MK-specific antigens (e.g., CD61/CD62/CD42b), which precedes the appearance of mature MKs, as evaluated by morphology analysis (Fig. 3A).

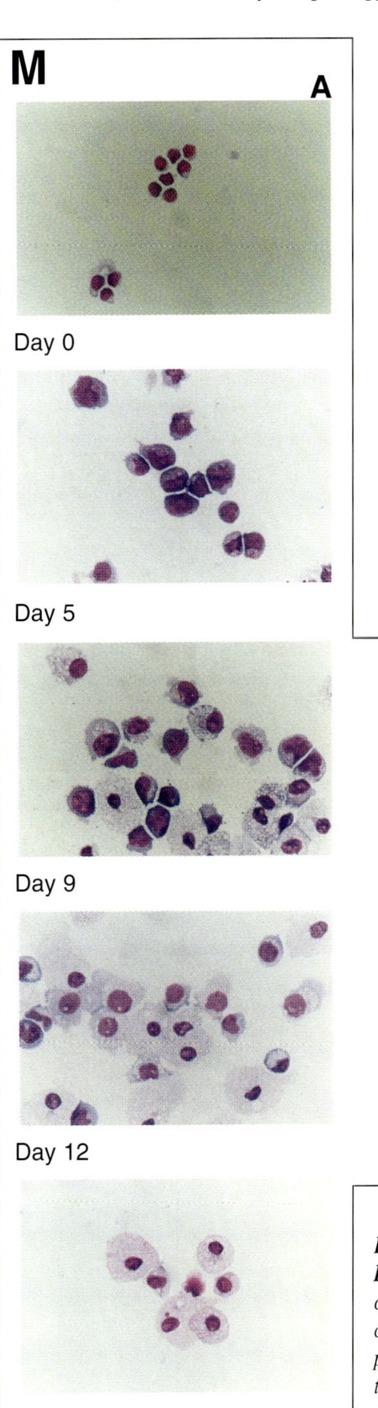

Unilineage M Growth (Fig. 4A, B)

Despite extensive studies on monocytopoiesis [57], methodology for selective proliferation/differentiation of HPCs along the M lineage has not been available. In clonogenic and liquid suspension culture, M-CSF, IL-3 and GM-CSF induce BM/PB HPCs to M colony formation [58] and differentiation [59]; in both cases, however, a large number of contaminant G colonies or cells was observed.

We have recently developed a culture system for unilineage M growth of Step IIIP HPCs stimulated by saturating M-CSF and FL dosages [10] (M-CSF alone causes predominant, 90%, M differentiation associated with limited growth; FL alone generates a cell progeny composed of a majority of monocytes/macrophages, 78%, and a minority of basophilic granulocytes). This combined cytokine treatment causes both HPC proliferation (i.e., 15-20-fold amplification

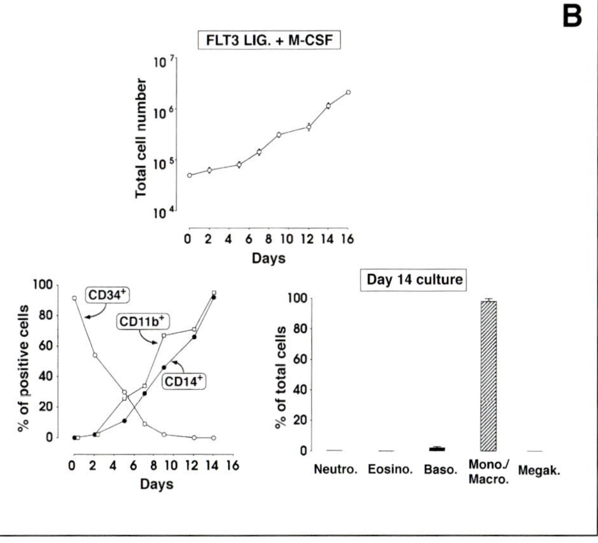

Figure 4. (A) Cell morphology in M unilineage cultures of purified Step IIIP HPCs, as evaluated at sequential days. A color photograph for each culture day (original magnification × 630) is shown. (B) Cell growth curve (top), percentage of CD34$^+$, CD11b$^+$ and CD14$^+$ cells (bottom panel, left) and cell type composition classified according to the differentiation/maturation stage (bottom panel, right). Mean ± SE values are presented; a representative experiment is shown for membrane antigen markers.

of cell number) and selective M differentiation/maturation (i.e., in 14-16 day culture 95%-100% monocytes/macrophages). The positive interaction of FL and M-CSF to induce M differentiation is seemingly related to the structural homologies between FL and M-CSF as well as FL and M-CSF receptors [9].

In the first week of culture, HPCs proliferate and progressively differentiate, as shown by the progressive decline of both CD34$^+$ cell frequency and the size of the M colonies generated in secondary semisolid culture (in the M lineage the decline of colony size was less rapid than for other lineages; in the second culture week the survival of a minuscule CFU-M population, e.g., ~3% of total cells on day 12, is seemingly related to the capacity of FL to stimulate the proliferation of primitive HPCs and CFU-GM [8]) (Fig. 4A and results not shown).

In the second week of culture, disappearance of CD34$^+$ cells is coupled with the gradual acquisition of monocytic-specific membrane antigen (i.e., CD14), properties (i.e., the capacity to bind bacterial lipopolysaccharide) and functions (i.e., phagocytosis) typically expressed in mature phagocytes (Fig. 4B).

Unilineage Den Cell Growth (results not shown here)

Unilineage M cultures comprise < 2% Den cells, which are morphologically similar to macrophages, but partially differ for membrane phenotype, i.e., loss of CD14 and expression of CD1a and CD80 [60]. The differentiation of Den cells from either BM or PB CD34$^+$ cells requires the presence of GM-CSF and one of the cytokines which exerts a suppressive effect on monocytopoiesis, i.e., tumor necrosis factor-α (TNF-α) [60], IL-4 [61] or IL-13 [62]. Using an optimized combination of cytokines (low-dose GM-CSF, 0.001 ng/ml; intermediate FL, KL dosage, 1 ng/ml; high-dose IL-4, IL-6, IL-7, 10 ng/ml) we induced Step IIIP HPCs to generate a progeny composed by ≥ 90% Den cells, as determined by morphologic and immunologic criteria (see below), with an ~50-fold amplification of the initial cell number [63 and unpublished observations].

HPCs induced to Den cell differentiation undergo early and intermediate stages of Den cell maturation, characterized by the progressive acquisition of immunophenotypical (notably, CD1a, CD80, CD86 and HLA-DR antigen expression) and functional properties (high capacity of macropinocytosis and receptor-mediated endocytosis). Upon TNF-α addition the cells undergo terminal maturation associated with downmodulation of both macropinocytosis and receptor-mediated endocytosis, upmodulation of HLA-class II and high capacity of inducing lymphocyte alloreactivity

Development of Alternative HPC Unilineage Differentiation Culture

An alternative strategy to the development of HPC unilineage differentiation cultures may be provided by HPC fractionation studies. In this context: A) CD34$^+$/CD45RA^{++} and CD34$^+$/CD45RA$^-$ cells are enriched (95% and 80%) in CFU-GM and BFU-E, respectively [64]; B) CD34$^+$/CD13$^+$ cells preferentially generate CFU-GM colonies [65]; C) CD34$^+$/CD38$^+$/CD64$^+$ cells are greatly enriched in CFU-GM (98%), while CD34$^+$/CD38$^+$/CD64$^-$/CD71^{++} cells comprise almost exclusively BFU-E [66]. In liquid suspension cultures supplemented with saturating doses of HGFs (i.e., IL-6, bFGF, KL, GM-CSF, IL-3, Epo), CD34$^+$/CD38$^+$/CD64$^+$ or CD64$^-$ cells generate a progeny composed of 83% GM cells or 81% E cells, respectively, while CD34$^+$/CD38$^+$/CD64$^+$/CD71^{++} cells generate 95% erythroblasts [66]; D) CD34$^+$/c-kit^{hi} simian [67] and human [68] cells are highly enriched (~90%) in BFU-E, while CD34$^+$/c-kit^{low} cells were enriched in CFU-GM (~75%), and E) finally, CD34^{lo}/CD71^{++}, but not CD34^{hi}/CD71^{++} cells generate a large majority of BFU-E, while both CD34^{hi}/CD64$^+$ cells generate almost exclusively CFU-GM [69].

These fractionation studies, while providing novel insight into HPC subsets, do not yet provide a basis for development of HPC unilineage differentiation systems. Thus, A) the E cultures comprise 5%-20% contaminating cells [67], while the studies mentioned above do not report unilineage G, MK and M cultures; B) the differentiation capacities of the HPC subsets have not been evaluated using E-, MK-, G- or M-specific HGF combinations; it is hence unclear whether the fractionated HPCs have strictly unilineage differentiation potential, and C) the yield for the HPC subsets is low, particularly for multisort experiments, thus hampering their utilization for studies on the cellular/molecular basis of early hematopoiesis.

CELLULAR/MOLECULAR MECHANISMS UNDERLYING HEMATOPOIESIS: STUDIES IN HPC UNILINEAGE DIFFERENTIATION CULTURE

Expression and Modulation of HGF Receptors (HGFRs)

Elucidation of HGFR expression and control mechanisms is obviously crucial in unveiling the cellular/molecular basis of hematopoiesis, particularly at the level of HPCs.

We initially showed that purified PB HPCs express diverse high-affinity HGFRs, mainly IL-3R, IL-6R and GM-CSFR and barely detectable levels of EpoR [70]. These observations were confirmed by subsequent studies. Thus, double-labeling of total human [71] or simian BM cells [72, 73] with anti-CD34 and either anti-IL-3R or anti-GM-CSFR monoclonal antibodies (mAbs) showed that a subset of CD34$^+$ HPCs express on their membrane IL-3R and/or GM-CSFR. Furthermore, small-sized CD34$^+$ cells possess a higher IL-6R, IL-3R, GM-CSFR and c-kit density than large ones [74]. In this regard, the c-kit$^+$ fraction of BM CD34$^+$/HLA-DR$^-$ cells generates HPCs after 10 weeks in culture [75]; however, the majority of BM LTC-ICs is c-kit^{low}, while more distal HPCs are c-kit^{high} [76 and our unpublished observations]. Furthermore, CD34$^+$ human BM c-kit^{low} cells are enriched for long-term repopulating cells in fetal sheep [77]. Finally, flow cytometric studies have shown that: A) TpoR is expressed on ~0.5% BM CD34$^+$ cell subset which contains CFU-MK, but not primitive HPCs [78], and B) EpoR is expressed on erythroid HPCs (CD34$^+$/CD38$^+$/CD71^{++} cells) but not CFU-GM (CD34$^+$/CD38$^+$/CD64$^+$) purified from fetal BM [69].

Recently, we have investigated the expression of diverse HGFRs on purified Step IIIP HPCs. Receptors for both early-acting HGFs (FL, KL, IL-6 and bFGF) and multilineage HGFs (IL-3 and GM-CSF) are expressed, whereas HGFRs for late-acting unilineage HGFs (Epo, G-CSF, M-CSF and TPO) are not or only barely expressed [45]. These studies were carried out by both reverse transcriptase-polymerase chain reaction (RT-PCR) assay for HGFR mRNAs and flow cytometry analysis using anti-HGFR mAbs.

A second set of studies was aimed at evaluating the modulation of HGFR expression on purified HPCs induced to proliferation/differentiation.

Initially [70], we incubated HPCs with HGF(s) for 24-48 h and then analyzed heterologous HGFR expression: IL-6, IL-3 and GM-CSF induce the receptor(s) for distal GF(s), i.e., IL-6 enhances the expression of IL-3R, but not of GM-CSFR or EpoR; IL-3 causes rapid upmodulation of GM-CSFR and EpoR; finally, GM-CSF induces EpoR expression. Based on these data, we proposed a model of cascade transactivation of HGFRs in the initial steps of hematopoiesis, whereby the action of the early-acting HGFs enhances the effect of the distal-acting HGFs by a multistep chain-potentiation mechanism.

Taking advantage of unilineage differentiation systems, we have investigated the expression of HGFRs during HPC differentiation/maturation along the E, G, M and MK lineages [45]. In all differentiation pathways, expression of early-acting cytokine receptors shows a progressive decline, more rapidly for bFGFR-1 and FLT3 than for c-kit and IL-6R (as a partial exception, IL-6Rs are still detected through the early and late stages of maturation in the MK and M lineage, respectively, while FLT3 is still expressed in mature CD14$^+$ monocytes but not in granulocytes [10, 79]). IL-3Rs are progressively downmodulated during differentiation along all four lineages; the decline is rapid in the E and MK series, whereas it is slower in the G and M lineages. The expression pattern of GM-CSFRs is similar to that of IL-3Rs, in that it is maintained through the G and M lineages, while it significantly decreases at late stages of E and MK differentiation. As expected, the expression of receptors for late-acting unilineage cytokines (Epo, G-CSF, Tpo and M-CSF) is specific for the corresponding series: all these receptors are: A) barely detected in quiescent HPCs; B) initially slightly induced in specific and nonspecific lineages, but C) sustainably expressed according to a unilineage-restricted pattern. Thus, EpoR mRNA expression is maintained in the E series, while suppressed in the other lineages; G-CSFR, TpoR and M-CSFR show a sustained expression in the G, MK and M series, respectively, but are suppressed in all the other lineages.

These observations suggest a two-step model for HGFR regulation (Fig. 5), which involves first the activation of multilineage HGFRs and then the sustained expression of the receptors for unilineage HGFs, via molecular mechanism(s) triggered by interaction of each receptor with its specific ligand.

Altogether, these results are compatible with a hybrid model of hematopoietic differentiation including both stochastic and inductive events (Fig. 5). Following this model: A) the differential expression of receptors for early-acting HGFs on quiescent HPCs may reflect a stochastic process in early commitment; B) the quiescent HPCs consistently express multilineage HGFRs and are induced into cycling by IL-3/GM-CSF; C) the cycling HPCs may express unilineage HGFRs according to a stochastic process, and D) the sustained expression of each unilineage HGFR through the corresponding differentiation/maturation pathway represents an inductive process, mediated by the pertinent unilineage HGF. The unilineage HGF prevailing in each microenvironmental niche may channel HPCs expressing its receptor into the corresponding lineage; unipotent HPCs growing in the absence of a sufficient level of the pertinent unilineage HGF seemingly undergo apoptosis.

Expression and Function of Erythroid TFs

It is generally conceded that HSC/HPC differentiation is mediated by a complex network of transcription factors (TFs), which orchestrate specific differentiative gene programs at the transcriptional level [29]. The TFs may be subdivided in two groups, which are related to either the E/MK or the G/M lineages; this subdivision is in line with observations indicating that E and MK lineages derive from a common precursor [80], while both G and M-specific HPCs derive from CFU-GM [81]. This section is mainly focused on erythroid/megakaryocytic TFs in HPC unilineage culture systems.

Knock-out studies have provided evidence that in murine development, E/MK TFs orchestrate E/MK differentiation according to a hierarchical model [29]; thus, GATA-2 and tal-1 act at early stages of HSC/HPC differentiation, while GATA-1 and NF-E2 exert their action at later developmental stages. With respect to human adult hematopoiesis, a similar model is suggested by studies on TF expression and function in HPC unilineage differentiation cultures. This section comparatively discusses results from knock-out mice, in vitro ES cell studies and adult HPC unilineage cultures.

GATA TFs

The GATA motif, present in *cis*-regulatory elements of erythroid-expressed and other genes, is recognized by the GATA TFs (comprising six members, GATA-1 to GATA-6); GATA-1 and -2 play key functional roles in hematopoiesis [29].

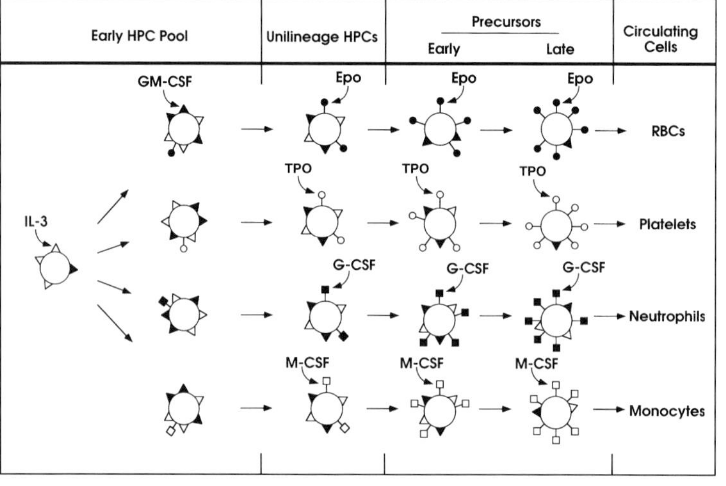

Figure 5. Multistep expression of multilineage (IL-3R and GM-CSFR) and unilineage (EpoR, TpoR, G-CSFR and M-CSFR) growth factor receptors in unilineage differentiation culture of purified Step IIIP HPCs. In this model, A) early HPCs express the receptors for multilineage HGFs, but barely or not those for unilineage HGFs [108], B) IL-3 triggers HPCs to proliferate and upmodulates GM-CSFRs [70], C) IL-3/GM-CSF induce early HPCs to express a low number of receptors for unilineage HGF(s) [70], and D) stimulation of a lineage-committed HPC by the pertinent unilineage HGF induces further upmodulation of the homologous HGFR [108], thus channeling the HPCs into the corresponding unilineage differentiation pathway. (Early-acting growth factor receptors are not included in the model).

GATA-2

Mice rendered GATA-2⁻ die in embryonic life with widespread defects in yolk sac (YS) hematopoiesis: A) 50-fold depletion of primitive erythroblasts, and B) deficit in lymphopoiesis (GATA-2$^{-/-}$ ES cells fail to reconstitute T and B lymphocyte populations in recombinant activating gene-2 [RAG-2]-deficient mice) [82]. In vitro differentiation of GATA-2⁻ ES cells shows reduced formation of primitive E and M colonies and a drastic reduction of KL-dependent definitive E, mast cell and M colonies [82]. More recently, this issue was investigated using a two-step assay; it was apparent that GATA-2 is strictly required for proliferation and/or survival of multipotent HPCs and generation of mast cells, while it is dispensable for maturation of erythroid cells and macrophages [83]. In line with these observations, GATA-2 is rapidly phosphorylated in HPCs triggered by HGFs via the mitogen-activated protein kinase pathway [84].

In HPC unilineage cultures GATA-2 mRNA and protein, already expressed in ~30% quiescent progenitors, are rapidly induced as early as three h after HGF stimulus, but then decline in advanced E, G, M and MK differentiation and maturation ([41] and Fig. 6A). Treatment of purified HPCs with antisense oligomer targeting GATA-2 mRNA causes a decrease of both BFU-E and CFU-GM colony number [41]. This pattern is consistent with the hypothesis that in human adult hematopoiesis, GATA-2 plays a key role in the early HPC proliferation/differentiation mechanisms.

GATA-1

Initial knock-out studies have shown that mice rendered GATA-1⁻ fail to generate mature definitive E cells in fetal liver [85]. In vitro, GATA-1⁻ ES cells give rise to abortive E colonies which deteriorate due to differentiation block and apoptosis of resident proerythroblasts [86]. Subsequent knock-out studies carried out with a strategy allowing the generation of mice with selective loss of MK GATA-1 expression allowed to define a functional role for GATA-1 in MK differentiation/maturation [87]; in fact GATA-1$^{-/-}$ mice generated a markedly reduced number of platelets and produced MK exhibiting severely impaired cytoplasmic maturation [87].

Expression in HPC unilineage E, G, M and MK cultures [35, 36, 38] showed that GATA-1 mRNA and protein, while barely or not detected in quiescent HPCs, are gradually induced at 24-48 h in E, G, MK and M cultures; starting at late differentiation/early maturation stage, GATA-1 is accumulated in E and MK pathways, whereas it is suppressed in G and M series (Fig. 6B). The transient induction of GATA-1 in G and M cultures may be related to the expression in multipotent E/GM HPCs whose proliferation and survival is initially stimulated by HGFs contained in G and M cultures, respectively. Antisense oligomer treatment targeting GATA-1 mRNA showed selective impairment of BFU-E colony formation [38].

NF-E2

The NF-E2 heterodimer comprises the hematopoietic-restricted p45, a basic region-leucine zipper, and the ubiquitous p18, constituted by one of the small Maf family proteins (MafF, MafG or MafK) [88]. Mice rendered NF-E2 p45⁻ fail to produce platelets, secondary to a maturational arrest in the MK lineage, and die of hemorrhage [89]; in contrast, the effect on the erythroid lineage is surprisingly mild in that the surviving adult animals exhibit only a mild decrease in the Hb content per cell [90].

In all HPC unilineage culture systems, NF-E2 mRNA and protein, barely or not detected in quiescent HPCs, are gradually induced at 24-48 h; starting from day 5-7, i.e., at late differentiation/early maturation stages, NF-E2 is accumulated in the E and MK pathways, whereas it is suppressed in the G and M series ([38] and Fig. 6B). Treatment of purified HPCs with antisense oligomers suppressing NF-E2 mRNA causes a dose-related inhibitory effect on BFU-E but not CFU-GM colony formation [38], thus indicating that NF-E2 is selectively required for human adult erythropoiesis. Accordingly, expression of both p18/p45 subunits is required for optimal hemoglobinization and erythroid maturation of MEL cells [91, 92].

In conclusion, these studies consensually indicate that NF-E2 is required for MK differentiation and plays an important role in erythropoiesis; in the E series of NF-E2⁻ mice, other erythroid TF(s) may partially replace NF-E2 function.

TAL-1

TAL-1 encodes a bHLH protein which interacts with class A bHLH proteins (E12 and E47, encoded by the E2A locus) to form heterodimeric complexes (tal-1/E12 and tal-1/E47) binding E-box promoter sequences [93]. Initial knock-out studies have demonstrated that TAL-1 gene expression is essential for primitive erythropoiesis in YS blood islands [94, 95]; subsequent observations have shown that tal-1 is also required for HSC development into all hematopoietic lineages [96, 97]. In tal-1⁻ YS, normal levels of GATA-2 mRNA are associated with lack of GATA-1 mRNA [94, 95]; in vitro, tal-1⁻ ES cells express GATA-2, CD34 and c-kit, but not GATA-1, EKLF and PU.1 [98]. It is hence apparent that tal-1 acts at an intermediate developmental stage between that of GATA-2 and GATA-1.

Studies in HPC unilineage cultures focused on the expression and functional role of tal-1/E2A heterodimer in adult hematopoiesis.

In unilineage E, G, MK and M differentiation/maturation ([40] and unpublished results): A) RT-PCR analysis showed that TAL-1 and E2A mRNAs, barely or not expressed in quiescent HPCs, are induced and sustainedly expressed in E differentiation/maturation, while they are transiently induced in the first week of G differentiation [40]; B) this expression pattern is consistent with that of the tal-1/E2A heterodimer, evaluated by mobility shift assay [40], and tal-1 protein,

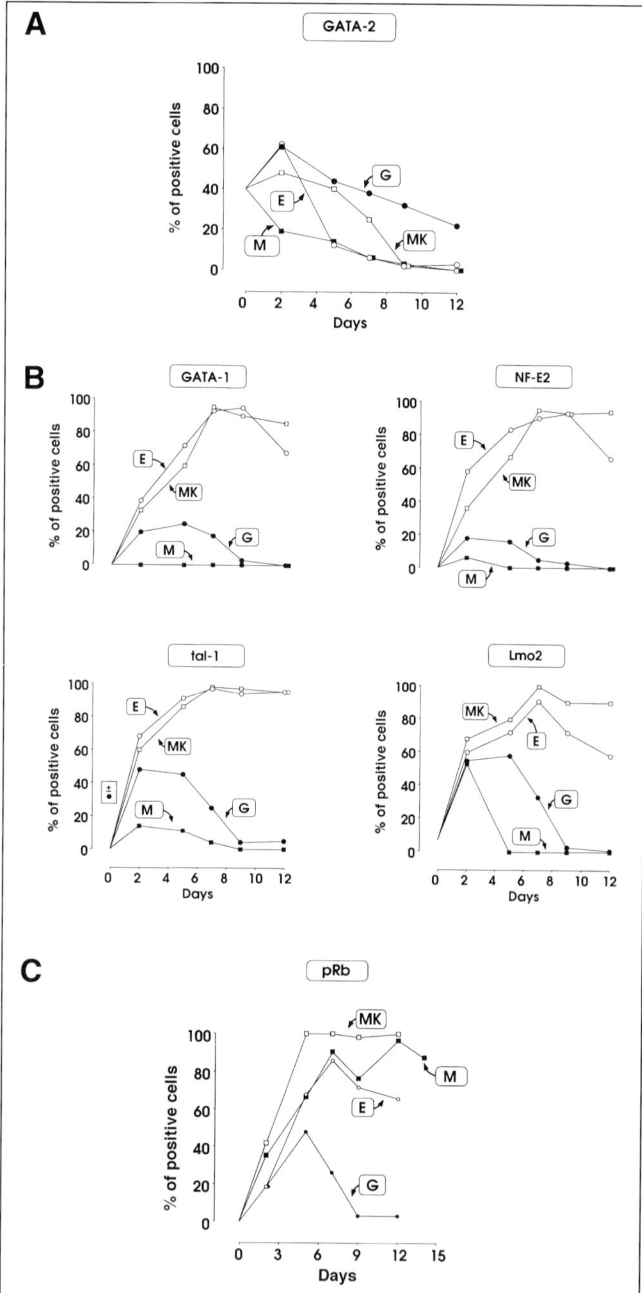

Figure 6. Kinetics of expression of GATA-2. (A) GATA-1, NF-E2, tal-1 and Lmo2 (B) and pRb (C) in unilineage E, G, M and MK cultures. The expression of these TFs was assessed by indirect immunofluorescence using specific mAbs. The percentage of tal-1± "dim" cells on day 0 is also indicated. Representative experiments are presented.

monitored by Western blot [40] and immunofluorescence (Fig. 6B). Particularly, the latter analysis showed a discrete population of tal-1^{dim} quiescent HPCs (Fig. 6B, see ± group), and C) Recent immunofluorescent studies have shown that the tal-1 expression pattern in unilineage MK and M differentiation culture is similar to that reported in the E and G series, respectively (Fig. 6B).

Functional experiments were carried out on purified HPCs treated with antisense oligomer targeting TAL-1 mRNA [40]; consistent with the expression studies, anti-TAL-1 oligomer induces a dose-related inhibitory effect on erythroid but not GM colonies. Furthermore, TAL-1 retroviral transfer in HPCs resulted in: A) an increase of BFU-E colony number and size and CFU-MK colony number; B) an inhibition of CFU-GM and CFU-G, but not CFU-M colony number, and C) a proliferative stimulus on primary and secondary HPP-CFC colonies [99].

Altogether, these findings indicate that tal-1 plays an important role in both early (HSCs and primitive HPCs) and late (erythropoiesis and possibly megakaryocytopoiesis) stages of hematopoiesis. Interestingly, recent studies indicate that different mechanisms regulate the TAL-1 promoter region in CD34$^+$ primitive myeloid cells and differentiating erythroid cells [100].

Id Proteins

Id HLH proteins lack the basic domain necessary for DNA binding: they sequester the ubiquitous E proteins, thus preventing the formation of an active transcriptional complex between E and tissue-specific bHLH proteins [101]. In HPC unilineage differentiation [40] Id2 mRNA, expressed in quiescent HPCs, is downmodulated in E culture from the onset of HPC differentiation through late precursor maturation, whereas its expression is maintained in G culture. Functional experiments carried out with antisense oligomer to Id2 mRNA showed a moderate dose-dependent increase of BFU-E colony formation. Finally, murine and human GST-Id2 polypeptides complete the tal-1/E2A-specific DNA binding when added to the nuclear extracts derived from erythroid culture cells, thus indicating biochemical and suggesting functional interaction of Id2 with the tal-1/E2A complex [40]. Altogether, these observations indicate a coordinate expression and function of the inhibitory Id2 protein and the stimulatory tal-1/E2A heterodimer in normal E and possibly MK differentiation.

Tal-1/E2A Multi-Component Transcriptional Complex

Growing evidence suggests that the tal-1/E2A heterodimer is part of a multicomponent transcriptional complex, which may comprise diverse proteins including Lmo2 and pRb. These aspects are briefly outlined here.

LMO2

The LMO2/RBTN2 gene is essential for erythroid differentiation: mice rendered Lmo2$^-$ show blockage of primitive YS erythropoiesis, associated with a marked decline of E, but not GM HPCs [102] (further studies, however, suggest that myelopoiesis is also affected [29]). Immunofluorescence analysis indicates that Lmo2 expression in HPC unilineage cultures (Fig. 6B) is similar to that of tal-1 and GATA-1. The phenotypes of the Lmo2, tal-1 and GATA-1 null mutations, as well as the pattern of expression of these TFs during adult hematopoietic differentiation, suggest that they are closely related in erythroid differentiation. Indeed, recent observations in erythroid cell lines indicate that: A) Lmo2 binds to both tal-1 and GATA-1 in erythroid cell lines (these two interactions may occur simultaneously with Lmo2 bridging between tal-1 and GATA-1) [103]; B) Lmo2 is part of a DNA binding complex involving tal-1, E47, GATA-1 and LIM domain-binding factor-1 (Ldb1) proteins [104], and C) our studies in HPC-generated erythroblasts indicate that Lmo2 is bound in complex with both tal-1 and E2A (see below).

RB

Gene knock-out studies have indicated a role for pRb in ontogenetic development of the hematopoietic system. pRb⁻ mice die in early gestation due to gross defects of both the central nervous and hematopoietic systems [105-107]. The latter abnormalities involve reduced embryonic liver erythropoiesis due to hampered CFU-E differentiation [100-102]. pRb may also play a role in MK differentiation: in transgenic mice, a functional blockade of pRb in the MK lineage by overexpression of E2F-1 blocks terminal differentiation and causes proliferation of MKs [108].

The expression/function of pRb in normal adult hematopoiesis was investigated in HPC unilineage E, G, M and MK cultures ([39] and Fig. 6C). During the initial HPC differentiation stages, the pRb gene is gradually induced at mRNA and protein levels in both E and G cultures. During late HPC differentiation and precursor maturation, pRb expression is sustained in the E lineage, whereas it is sharply downmodulated in the G series. In MK and M lineages, the pRb expression pattern is similar to that observed in the E series (Fig. 6C). In agreement with the expression pattern, treatment with antisense oligomer targeting Rb mRNA selectively causes a dose-dependent inhibition of late erythroid colony formation.

It is conceivable that pRb controls erythroid differentiation via interaction with lineage-specific TFs. A similar model has been established in myogenic cell lines, where pRb interacts with the protein-binding domain of the bHLH MyoD TF, thereby potentiating transcription of muscle-specific genes by MyoD-E2A heterodimers [109]. Our studies on HPC unilineage cultures (*L. Vitelli et al.*, submitted) have shown by immunological and biochemical assays that early erythroblasts contain a protein complex comprising tal-1/E2A linked to both Lmo2 and pRb. Furthermore, pRb potentiates the E-box binding activity of the tal-1/E2A/Lmo2 protein complex, i.e., addition of synthetic full-length pRb induces a dose-dependent increase up to 10-fold of the tal-1/E2A/Lmo2 trimer binding to its recognition sequence. Finally, we have explored the functional significance of the interaction between pRb and the tal-1/E2A/Lmo2 complex by evaluating the effect of pRb on an artificial reporter plasmid (E1bLuc-E6) containing six binding sites for tal-1/E2A heterodimers in the transiently transfected pRb⁻ SAOS-2 cell line: results showed that pRb enhances up to eightfold the transcriptional activity of the tal-1/E2A/Lmo2 trimer, but not of the tal-1/E2A. Altogether, these findings suggest a positive role of pRb in erythroid differentiation via modulation of the activity of the erythroid-specific tal-1/E2A/Lmo2 complex.

THE SINGLE HPC ANALYSIS APPROACH

Although HPC unilineage differentiation in bulk cultures allows investigation of the hematopoietic control mechanisms, the HPC population is heterogeneous, i.e., as mentioned above it initially comprises a minority of putative HSCs (LTC-ICs) and primitive HPCs (CFU-B, HPP-CFC) and a majority of early HPCs (CFU-GEMM, BFU-E, CFU-GM, CFU-MK). To offset this heterogeneity, we have developed a novel approach based on a single HPC unilineage culture followed by daughter cell analysis (Fig. 7A). The single HPC culture approach has been successfully applied to demonstrate that all-*trans* retinoic acid (RA) induces FL HPCs to shift from the erythroid/monocytic/ multipotent to the granulocytic differentiation program (Fig. 7B) [110].

The following section briefly describes recent studies carried out at cellular and molecular level based on this novel strategy.

Molecular Studies: RT-PCR Analysis of Sibling Cells in Unilineage Culture

We have developed RT-PCR analysis of sibling cells generated in single HPC unilineage culture. In the standard protocol, A) a single HPC generates four sibling cells in unilineage culture; B) two siblings are analyzed by RT-PCR, while another sibling is grown in liquid or semisolid medium to verify its capacity to generate a control unilineage colony, and C) the last sibling generates a second round of four daughter cells and so forth (Fig. 7A). This approach may be successfully applied if four experimental conditions are met: (1) asymmetric mitoses, (2) asynchronous cell divisions and (3) apoptotic cell death are largely absent, and (4) the single cell RT-PCR methodology is well-controlled. Also, (5) quantitative competitive RT-PCR analysis may add to this approach.

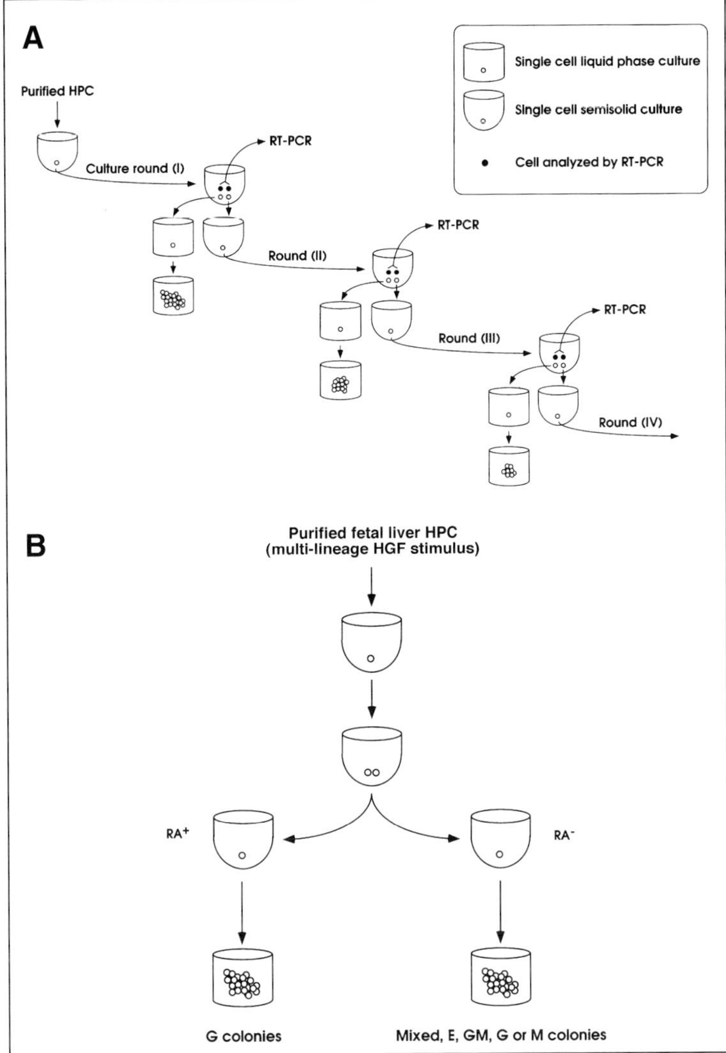

Figure 7. Single cell culture for purified HPCs. (A) Single HPC unilineage differentiation culture: sibling cell analysis (clonogenic capacity and gene expression, as evaluated by single cell RT-PCR) after sequential rounds of cell division. Modified from [Ziegler et al., manuscript in preparation]. (B) Schematic representation of paired daughter cell analysis in RA+ versus RA- fetal liver HPC culture (see results in [110]): addition of RA reprograms CFU-GEMM, BFU-E, CFU-GM and CFU-M to shift to the granulopoietic differentiation program.

(1) In single HPC unilineage culture, analysis of colonies generated by sibling cells did not reveal asymmetric divisions (unpublished results). However, when the HPCs are grown in cultures supplemented with saturating levels of early-acting, multilineage and unilineage HGFs, asymmetric divisions are observed in a minority of cases (unpublished data), as originally reported in [111].

(2) Although HPCs have different cycling times, the unicellular-unilineage culture system provides daughter cells that have emerged after an identical number of cell divisions, i.e., at each culture round four cells have been generated by two mitoses from the initiating cell. Thus, the number of cell divisions performed is known for each analyzed cell. Since proliferation is linked to differentiation, individual cells at each culture round are expected to express the same differentiation-specific mRNAs. Indeed, analysis of E differentiation culture showed that single cells from the same culture round were characterized by the same mRNA phenotype, as evaluated by RT-PCR for stage-specific expressed genes, i.e., CD34, CD36, GPA, EpoR or β-globin [Ziegler et al., manuscript in preparation]. These data strongly suggest that each culture round comprises four daughter cells that represent an identical stage of E development.

Conversely, cells within colonies in semisolid culture are heterogeneous at the mRNA level even when grown under unilineage HGF stimulus (unpublished observations). This phenomenon is likely due to the difference in cycling times of the generated cells, which is not controlled as in the unicellular unilineage culture system described here; therefore, colonies comprise a heterogeneous cellular population in which individual cells have emerged after different numbers of cell divisions.

(3) Under the described unilineage E culture conditions, HPCs may undergo apoptosis (programmed cell death; [PCD]) due to HGF starvation. This aspect is particularly relevant in that genes involved in the apoptotic program may interact with developmentally regulated genes. Although freshly seeded CD34$^+$/Lin$^-$ and CD34$^+$/CD38$^-$ cells displayed a high frequency of PCD (55% and 97.5%, respectively) in unicellular-unilineage E cultures, the frequency of apoptotic cells was low (0-7-3.5%) among cycling cells from both populations. It follows that interaction of PCD genes with developmentally regulated genes in this culture system is negligible.

(4) Single-cell RT-PCR [112] has been successfully applied to analyze different genes in single cells, e.g., macrophages [112, 113], HSCs/HPCs [6] and hematopoietic cell lines [114]. However, this approach is still under development and diverse aspects deserve discussion.

A) Since RT-PCR analysis of RNA is often obscured by copurified genomic DNA, we have applied single-cell RT-PCR methodology that allows detection of mRNA transcripts in the absence of genomic sequences [113, 115, 116]. This was achieved first by DNase digestion [113, 115] and more recently by mRNA purification via utilization of biotinylated oligo(dT) and streptavidin-conjugated paramagnetic particles [116]. To verify the validity of these methodologies, we comparatively evaluated expression of membrane antigens at mRNA and protein level in sorted cord blood (CB) CD34$^+$ HPCs [117]. Thus, RT-PCR of single sorted CD34$^+$/CD18$^-$, CD34$^+$/CD33$^-$, CD34$^+$/CD36$^-$, CD34$^+$/CD38$^-$, CD34$^+$/Thy-1$^-$ and CD34$^+$/c-kit$^-$, as well as corresponding double-positive cells, demonstrated that their antigenic phenotype corresponded to their mRNA profile [*Ziegler et al.*, manuscript in preparation]. This correlation was confirmed by a limiting dilution RT-PCR approach aimed to determine the frequency of lineage marker-positive cells in negative sort fractions [118]. Therefore, it is possible to link expression of lineage-specific markers with that of other genes in single sibling cells at specific stages of differentiation.

B) The limited amount of RNA in individual or small numbers of cells has led to the development of strategies for the sequence-independent (SIP) amplification of RNA by RT-PCR to enable analysis of multiple mRNA species [6, 114, 119]. Thus, the cDNA has been A-tailed or G-tailed at its 3′ end and then amplified by oligo(dT) alone or oligo(dT) and oligo(dC), respectively. Using SIP-RT-PCR, detection of gene expression in single hematopoietic cells has been achieved by Southern blot hybridization using specifically labeled target gene probes [6, 114] or by sequence-specific PCR of SIP-RT-PCR product using primers recognizing the gene of interest [*Ziegler et al.*, manuscript in preparation].

Three limitations, however, hamper the SIP-RT-PCR approach. A) In our experience, genomic DNA is not removed in one-tube reactions [6, 114], thus obscuring SIP-RT-PCR results [*Ziegler et al.*, manuscript in preparation]. To avoid this bias, it would be necessary to eliminate genomic DNA prior to processing of RNA for RT-PCR, to isolate pure, i.e., DNA-free, mRNA [113, 115, 116] and/or to reamplify SIP-RT-PCR products using target gene-specific primers or even primers recognizing different exons of the target gene to distinguish between cDNA and genomic DNA; B) Furthermore, SIP-RT-PCR analysis may be hampered by underrepresentation of long sequences; these are competed out by short ones, which are amplified more efficiently [120], thus rendering difficult detection of long mRNAs. This problem was tentatively addressed by differential amplification, i.e., reamplification of size-separated SIP-RT-PCR products [120], or cDNA synthesis conditions designed to limit the length of first strand cDNA [6, 114], and C) In addition, hybridization of SIP-RT-PCR products using target gene-specific probes may result in unspecific detection of related genes.

To overcome the technical limitations inherent to SIP-RT-PCR, we developed an alternative methodology based on mRNA purification by biotinylated oligo(dT) (as indicated above) followed by sequence-specific RT-PCR; this approach allowed analysis of the mRNA expression of two to four genes in a single cell (alternatively, we performed single-cell SIP-RT-PCR on mRNA followed by sequence-specific RT-PCR of SIP-RT-PCR products). Thereby, we evaluated multiple gene expression in single CB CD34$^+$/lin$^-$ (purity, >99% for CD34, lin$^-$ markers not detectable) or CD34$^+$/CD38$^-$ HPCs induced to unilineage E differentiation ([*Ziegler et al.*, manuscript in preparation], Fig. 8).

Figure 8. Single-cell RT-PCR analysis in unilineage E culture generated by individual CD34+/CD38- HPCs. Single CD34+/CD38- cells were induced to unilineage E differentiation (Fig. 7A). When the four-cell stage was reached (at round I, II, III and IV) two individual daughter cells were removed from culture and processed separately for RT-PCR (Fig. 7A). mRNA was isolated from each cell and reverse transcribed into cDNA. The cDNA was divided into two to four aliquots that were processed in separate PCR reactions using primers that recognize GATA-

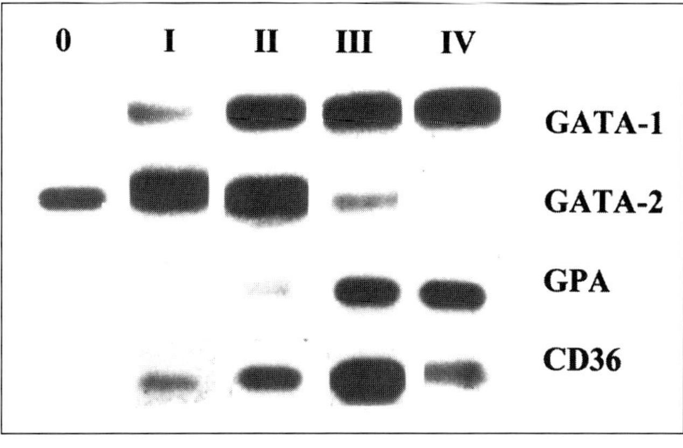

1, GATA-2, glycophorin A (GPA) or CD36. Lane 0: Gene expression pattern of freshly isolated single CD34+ CD38- cells. Lane I: Single daughter cell (first round). Lane II: Single daughter cell (second round). Lane III: Single daughter cell (third round). Lane IV: Single daughter cell (fourth round). Note that only GATA-2 is expressed in freshly sorted CD34+/CD38- cells. At round I, GATA-1, GATA-2 and CD36 are expressed. Round II cells are characterized by additional expression of GPA. In separate experiments copurification of genomic DNA with mRNA from single cells was not detected by RT-PCR using intron-spanning primers for β2-microglobulin (not shown). Modified from [Ziegler et al., manuscript in preparation].

Freshly sorted CD34+/CD38- cells or CD34+/lin- cells express CD34, c-kit and GATA-2, but not glycophorin A, CD36 or EpoR (Fig. 8 and results not shown). In the unicellular E culture (Fig. 7A), early to intermediate stages of differentiation are characterized by expression of CD34/GATA-2/c-kit mRNA accompanied by GATA-1, which precedes expression of EpoR and CD36 followed by glycophorin A upregulation (Fig. 8 and data not presented). Expression of GATA-2 was not detected at late stages of erythroid differentiation (Fig. 8). It is noteworthy that this sequence of gene expression is strictly coherent with that observed in HPC bulk cultures underlying unilineage E differentiation, as outlined above.

(5) It is noteworthy that wild-type mRNA transcripts can be quantitated at the single cell level [Ziegler et al., manuscript in preparation] by competitive RT-PCR [121] using cRNA deletion constructs in a one-tube reaction. Utilizing this methodology, we observed that the CD34 mRNA is gradually down-regulated in CB CD34+/CD38- HPCs induced to unilineage E differentiation ([*Ziegler et al.,* manuscript in preparation], Fig. 9).

Altogether, it is postulated that availability of HPC unilineage-unicellular culture systems and RT-PCR methodology for mRNA analysis/quantitation at the single cell level paves the way to future investigations aimed to elucidate mechanisms underlying hematopoiesis. Particularly, this novel approach may eliminate ambiguities derived from molecular analysis of heterogeneous populations of hematopoietic progenitors/precursors growing in culture, particularly in the initial stages of development.

CONCLUSIONS

The HPC unilineage differentiation/maturation cultures may provide an important tool to explore mechanisms underlying human hematopoiesis. These culture systems allow not only gene expression analysis [35-40], but also functional studies based on gene transfer [25 and unpublished results] or antisense oligodeoxynucleotide treatment [37-40].

It is crucial to establish whether these culture systems reflect in vivo hematopoiesis. The evidence available so far indicates that each unilineage system recapitulates the corresponding in vivo HPC differentiation/maturation events (**HPC Purification**, above). It is noteworthy that each culture system is supplemented with a saturating dosage of the appropriate unilineage HGF, which is

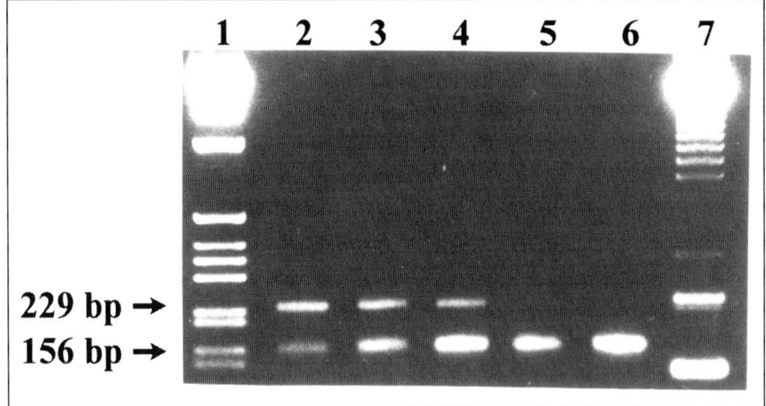

Figure 9. Competitive single-cell RT-PCR of sibling cells induced to unilineage E differentiation. Single CD34⁺/CD38⁻ cells were seeded into E differentiation culture (Fig. 7A). When the four-cell stage was reached (at round I, II, III and IV) a single daughter cell was isolated and the RNA corresponding to 0.8 cell equivalents processed for competitive RT-PCR to semiquantitate the CD34 mRNA. To each RT-PCR cRNA CD34 deletion construct corresponding to 100 transcripts (based on prior titration) was added and coprocessed with the isolated wild-type mRNA. Ethidium bromide-stained RT-PCR products were separated over a 2.5% agarose gel (MetaPhor, Biozym; The Netherlands) and photographed. Each band was excised from the gel and the radioactive counts determined. Based on Cerenkov counts of excised bands, round I, II, III and IV daughter cells contain 60%, 20%, 3% and 0.01%, respectively of the CD34⁻ mRNA transcripts present in a freshly sorted CD34⁺ CD38⁻ cell. Lane 1: size marker. Lane 2: single sorted CD34⁺CD38⁻ cell prior to culture. Lane 3: single daughter cell (first round). Lane 4: single daughter cell (second round). Lane 5: single daughter cell (third round). Lane 6: single daughter cell (fourth round). Lane 7: size marker. Note that the wild-type CD34 mRNA message is gradually downregulated from round I to IV. Products corresponding to β2-microglobulin mRNA, but not to genomic sequences, were detected when the RNA corresponding to 0.2 cell equivalent from each daughter cell was processed for RT-PCR using β2-microglobulin primers (not shown). Modified from [Ziegler et al., manuscript in preparation].

associated with low-dose IL-3/GM-CSF to optimize E, G or Eo differentiation. This dosage combination may reflect a physiologic pattern: in BM regeneration following autologous HSC transplantation, the serum cytokine levels feature an elevated concentration of unilineage HGFs (Epo, Tpo, G-CSF, IL-5, M-CSF) and a markedly lower level of multilineage HGFs (IL-3/GM-CSF) [122, 123 and our unpublished observations].

As mentioned above, both selective/apoptotic and inductive mechanisms may underlie cell differentiation/maturation in HPC unilineage cultures. However, further studies are required to elucidate the relative impact of these mechanisms in the first culture week, particularly via single HPC unilineage culture followed by RT-PCR analysis of HGFR and apoptotic gene expression in single daughter cells.

Theoretically, unilineage HPC differentiation cultures may be developed on the basis of preliminary sorting of HPC subsets with restricted commitment (see above). This approach, while feasible for unilineage-restricted HPCs, may be difficult for oligopotent or multipotent HPCs. Furthermore, the preliminary sorting does not allow full investigation of the instructive events following HGF addition on unseparated oligo-/multipotent HPCs, unless the appropriate unilineage HGF combinations are applied in culture. Finally, the sorting procedure usually results in cell loss, thus limiting analysis of cultured cells. Altogether, it is apparent that preliminary separation of unipotent or oligo-/multipotent HPC subsets, coupled with utilization of the appropriate unilineage HGF combinations, may further improve the HPC unilineage culture systems described here.

An attractive approach is represented by single HPC unilineage cultures, followed by sibling cell analysis at the cellular and molecular levels through sequential stages of HPC differentiation-maturation; this approach may be applied to preliminarily sorted HPC subsets and combined with gene transfer or antisense oligodeoxynucleotide treatment of parental or daughter cells [79].

REFERENCES

1 Harrison DE. Evaluating functional abilities of primitive hematopoietic stem cell populations. In: Müller-Sienburg C, Torok Storb B, Visser J et al., eds. Hematopoietic Stem Cells. Heidelberg: Springer Verlag, 1992:13-30.

2 Ogawa M. Differentiation and proliferation of hematopoietic stem cells. Blood 1993;81:2844-2853.

3 Harrison DE, Stone M, Astle CM. Effects of transplantation on the primitive immunohematopoietic stem cell. J Exp Med 1990;172:431-437.

4 Abramson S, Miller RG, Phillips RA. The identification in adult bone marrow of pluripotent and restricted stem cells of the myeloid and lymphoid systems. J Exp Med 1977;145:1567-1579.

5 Ogata H, Bradley WG, Inaba M et al. Long-term repopulation of hematolymphoid cells with only a few hemopoietic stem cells in mice. Proc Natl Acad Sci USA 1995;92:5945-5949.

6 Berardi AC, Wang A, Levine JD et al. Functional isolation and characterization of human hematopoietic stem cells. Science 1995;267:104-108.

7 Bernstein ID, Andrews RG, Zsebo KM. Recombinant human stem cell factor enhances the formation of colonies by CD34$^+$ and CD34$^+$ lin$^-$ cells, and the generation of colony-forming cell progeny from CD34$^+$ lin$^-$ cells cultured with interleukin-3, granulocyte colony-stimulating factor, or granulocyte-macrophage colony-stimulating factor. Blood 1991;77:2316-2321.

8 Peschle C, Gabbianelli M, Testa U et al. c-kit ligand reactivates fetal hemoglobin synthesis in serum-free cultures of stringently purified normal adult burst-forming unit-erythroid. Blood 1993;81:328-336.

9 Lyman SD, James L, Johnson L et al. Cloning of the human homologue of the murine flt3 ligand: a growth factor for early hematopoietic progenitor cells. Blood 1994;83:2795-2801.

10 Gabbianelli M, Pelosi E, Montesoro E et al. Multi-level effects of FLT3 ligand on human hematopoiesis: expansion of putative stem cells and proliferation of granulomonocytic progenitors/monocytic precursors. Blood 1995;86:1661-1670.

11 Gabbianelli M, Sargiacomo M, Pelosi E et al. "Pure" human hematopoietic progenitors: permissive action of basic fibroblast growth factor. Science 1990;249:1561-1564.

12 Berardi AC, Wang A, Abraham J et al. Basic fibroblast growth factor mediates its effects on committed myeloid progenitors by direct action and has no effect on hematopoietic stem cells. Blood 1995;86:2123-2129.

13 Leary AG, Ikebuchi K, Hirai Y et al. Synergism between interleukin-6 and interleukin-3 in supporting proliferation of human hematopoietic stem cells: comparison with interleukin-1α. Blood 1988;71:1759-1763.

14 Leary AG, Wong GG, Clark SC et al. Leukemia inhibitory factor differentiation-inhibiting activity/human interleukin for DA cells augments proliferation of human hematopoietic stem cells. Blood 1990;75:1960-1964.

15 Du XX, Scott D, Yang ZX et al. Interleukin-11 stimulates multilineage progenitors, but not stem cells, in murine and human long-term marrow cultures. Blood 1995;86:128-134.

16 Van Snick J. Interleukin-6: an overview. Annu Rev Immunol 1990;8:253-278.

17 Metcalf D. Hematopoietic regulators: redundancy or subtlety? Blood 1993;82:3515-3523.

18 Krantz SB. Erythropoietin. Blood 1991;77:419-434.

19 Demetri GD, Griffin JD. Granulocyte colony-stimulating factor and its receptor. Blood 1991;78:2791-2808.

20 Sanderson CJ. Interleukin-5, eosinophils and disease. Blood 1992;79:3101-3109.

21 Sherr CJ. Colony-stimulating factor-1 receptor. Blood 1990;75:1-12.

22 Kaushansky K, Lok S, Holly RD et al. Promotion of megakaryocyte progenitor expansion and differentiation by the c-Mpl ligand thrombopoietin. Nature 1994;369:568-571.

23 Ramsfjell V, Borge OJ, Cui L et al. Thrombopoietin directly and potently stimulates multilineage growth and progenitor cell expansion from primitive (CD34$^+$ CD38$^-$) human bone marrow progenitor cells: distinct and key interactions with the ligands for c-kit and flt3, and inhibitory effects of TGF-beta and TNF-alpha. J Immunol 1997;158:5169-5177.

24 Udomsakdi C, Lansdorp PM, Hogge DE et al. Characterization of primitive hematopoietic cells in normal human peripheral blood. Blood 1992;80:2513-2521.

25 Valtieri M, Schirò R, Chelucci C et al. Efficient transfer of selectable and membrane reporter genes in hematopoietic progenitor and stem cells purified from human peripheral blood. Cancer Res 1994;54:4398-4404.

26 Sawada K, Krantz SB, Dai CH et al. Purification of human blood burst-forming units-erythroid and demonstration of the evolution of erythropoietin receptors. J Cell Physiol 1990;142:219-230.

27 Greenberger JS, Sakakeeny MA, Humpries RK et al. Demonstration of permanent factor-dependent multipotential (erythroid/neutrophil/basophil) hematopoietic progenitor cell lines. Proc Natl Acad Sci USA 1983;80:2931-2935.

28 Spooncer E, Heyworth CM, Dunn A et al. Self-renewal and differentiation of interleukin-3-dependent multipotent stem cells are modulated by stromal cells and serum factors. Differentiation 1986;31:111-118.

29 Shivdasani RA, Orkin SH. The transcriptional control of hematopoiesis. Blood 1996;87:4025-4039.

30 Olson EN, Arnold H-H, Rigby PWJ et al. Know your neighbors: three phenotypes in null mutants of the myogenic bHLH gene *MRF4*. Cell 1996;85:1-4.

31 Hakem R, De La Pompa JL, Sirard C et al. The tumor suppressor gene Brca 1 is required for embryonic cellular proliferation in the mouse. Cell 1996;85:1009-1023.

32 Weiss MJ, Orkin SH. In vitro differentiation of murine embryonic stem cells. New approaches to old problems. J Clin Invest 1996;97:591-595.

33 Nakano T, Kodama H, Honjo T. In vitro development of primitive and definitive erythrocytes from different precursors. Science 1996;272:722-724.

34 Kühn R, Schwenk F, Aguet M et al. Inducible gene targeting in mice. Science 1995;269:1427-1429.

35 Sposi NM, Zon LI, Carè A et al. Cell cycle-dependent initiation and lineage-dependent abrogation of GATA-1 expression in pure differentiating hematopoietic progenitors. Proc Natl Acad Sci USA 1992;89:6353-6357.

36 Labbaye C, Valtieri M, Testa U et al. Retinoic acid downmodulates erythroid differentiation and GATA-1 expression in purified adult progenitor culture. Blood 1994;83:651-656.

37 Giampaolo A, Sterpetti P, Bulgarini D et al. Key functional role and lineage-specific expression of selected *HOXB* genes in purified hematopoietic progenitor differentiation. Blood 1994;84:3637-3647.

38 Labbaye C, Valtieri M, Barberi T et al. Differential expression and functional role of GATA-2, NF-E2 and GATA-1 in normal adult hematopoiesis. J Clin Invest 1995;95:2346-2358.

39 Condorelli GL, Testa U, Valtieri M et al. Modulation of retinoblastoma gene in normal adult hematopoiesis: peak expression and functional role in advanced erythroid differentiation. Proc Natl Acad Sci USA 1995;92:4808-4812.

40 Condorelli GL, Vitelli L, Valtieri M et al. Coordinate expression and developmental role of Id2 protein and TAL1/E2A heterodimer in erythroid progenitor differentiation. Blood 1995;86:164-175.

41 Guerriero R, Testa U, Gabbianelli M et al. Unilineage megakaryocytic proliferation and differentiation of purified hematopoietic progenitors in serum-free liquid culture. Blood 1995;86:3725-3736.

42 Sawada K, Krantz SB, Dai CH et al. Purification of human blood burst-forming units-erythroid and demonstration of the evolution of erythropoietin receptors. J Cell Physiol 1990;142:219-230.

43 Lu L, Xiao M, Shen RN et al. Enrichment, characterization, and responsiveness of single primitive CD34^{+++} human umbilical cord blood hematopoietic progenitors with high proliferative and replating potential. Blood 1993;81:41-48.

44 Huang S, Terstappen LWMM. Lymphoid and myeloid differentiation of single human CD34^{+}, HLA-DR^{+}, CD38^{-} hematopoietic stem cells. Blood 1994;83:1515-1526.

45 Testa U, Fossati C, Samoggia P et al. Expression of growth factor receptors in unilineage differentiation culture of purified hematopoietic progenitors. Blood 1996;88:3391-3406.

46 Leary AG, Zeng HQ, Clark SC et al. Growth factor requirements for survival in G0 and entry into the cell cycle of primitive human hemopoietic progenitors. Proc Natl Acad Sci USA 1992;89:4013-4017.

47 McNiece IK, Stewart FM, Deacon DM et al. Detection of a human CFC with a high proliferative potential. Blood 1989;74:609-612.

48 Sutherland HJ, Lansdorp PM, Henkelman DH et al. Functional characterization of individual human hematopoietic stem cells cultured at limiting dilution on supportive marrow stromal layers. Proc Natl Acad Sci USA 1990;87:3584-3588.

49 Irani AM, Nilsson G, Miettinen U et al. Recombinant human stem cell factor stimulates differentiation of mast cells from dispersed human fetal liver cells. Blood 1992;79:3009-3021.

50 Wendling F, Vainchenker W. Thrombopoietin and its receptor, the proto-oncogene c-mpl. Curr Opin Hematol 1995;2:231.

51 Methia N, Louache F, Vainchenker W et al. Oligodeoxynucleotides antisense to the proto-oncogene c-*mpl* specifically inhibit in vitro megakaryocytopoiesis. Blood 1993;82:1395-1401.

52 Gurney AL, Carver-Moore K, De Sauvage FJ et al. Thrombocytopenia in c-mpl-deficient mice. Science 1994;265:1445-1447.

53 Lok S, Kaushansky K, Holly RD et al. Cloning and expression of murine thrombopoietin cDNA and stimulation of platelet production in vivo. Nature 1994;369:565-568.

54 De Sauvage FJ, Hass PE, Spencer SD et al. Stimulation of megakaryocytopoiesis and thrombopoiesis by the c-Mpl ligand. Nature 1994;369:533-538.

55 Bartley TD, Bogenberger J, Hunt P et al. Identification and cloning of a megakaryocyte growth and development factor that is a ligand for the cytokine receptor mpl. Cell 1994;77:1117-1124.

56 Wendling F, Maraskovsky E, Debili N et al. c-Mpl ligand is a humoral regulator of megakaryocytopoiesis. Nature 1994;369:571-574.

57 Gordon S, Clarke S, Greaves D et al. Molecular immunobiology of macrophages: recent progress. Curr Opin Immunol 1995;7:24-33.

58 Caracciolo D, Shirsat N, Wong GG et al. Recombinant human M-CSF requires subliminal concentration of GM-CSF for optimal stimulation of human macrophage colony formation in vitro. J Exp Med 1987;166:1851-1860.

59 Egeland T, Steen R, Quarsten H et al. Myeloid differentiation of purified CD34$^+$ cells after stimulation with recombinant human granulocyte-monocyte colony stimulating factor (CSF), granulocyte-CSF, monocyte-CSF, and interleukin-3. Blood 1991;78:3192-3199.

60 Caux C, Dezutter-Dambuyant C, Schmitt D et al. GM-CSF and TNF-α cooperate in the generation of dendritic Langerhans cells. Nature 1992;360:258-261.

61 Jansen JH, Wientjens GJ, Fibbe WE et al. Inhibition of human macrophage colony formation by interleukin 4. J Exp Med 1989;170:577-582.

62 Sakamoto O, Hashiyama M, Minty A et al. Interleukin-13 selectively suppresses the growth of human macrophage progenitors at the late stage. Blood 1995;85:3487-3493.

63 Montesoro E, Testa U, Gabbianelli M et al, Unilineage dendritic cell cultures generated by purified human hematopoietic progenitor cells. In: Proceedings of the IV International Symposium on Dendritic Cells in Fundamental and Clinical Immunology. 1997;139-143.

64 Fritsch G, Buchinger P, Printz D et al. Rapid discrimination of early CD34$^+$ myeloid progenitors using CD45-RA analysis. Blood 1993;81:2301-2309.

65 Ema H, Suda T, Miura Y et al. Colony formation of clone-sorted human hematopoietic progenitors. Blood 1990;75:1941-1946.

66 Olweus J, Lund-Johansen F, Terstappen LW. CD64/Fc gamma RI is a granulo-monocytic lineage marker on CD34$^+$ hematopoietic progenitor cells. Blood 1995;85:2402-2413.

67 De Jong MO, Wagemaker G, Wognum AW. Separation of myeloid and erythroid progenitors based on expression of CD34 and c-kit. Blood 1995;86:4076-4085.

68 Laver JH, Abboud MR, Kawashima I et al. Characterization of c-kit expression by primitive hematopoietic progenitors in umbilical cord blood. Exp Hematol 1995;23:1515-1519.

69 Olweus J, Terstappen LW, Thompson PA et al. Expression and function of receptors for stem cell factor and erythropoietin during lineage commitment of human hematopoietic progenitor cells. Blood 1996;88:1594-1607.

70 Testa U, Pelosi E, Gabbianelli M et al. Cascade transactivation of growth factor receptors in early human hematopoiesis. Blood 1993;81:1442-1456.

71 Jubinsky PT, Laurie AS, Nathan DG et al. Expression and function of the human granulocyte-macrophage colony-stimulating factor receptor alpha subunit. Blood 1994;84:4174-4185.

72 Wognum AW, Westerman Y, Visser TP et al. Distribution of receptors for granulocyte-macrophage colony-stimulating factor on immature CD34$^+$ bone marrow cells, differentiating monomyeloid progenitors, and mature blood cell subsets. Blood 1994;84:764-774.

73 Wognum AW, Visser TP, De Jong MO et al. Differential expression of receptors for interleukin-3 on subsets of CD34-expressing hematopoietic cells of rhesus monkeys. Blood 1995;86:581-591.

74 Wagner JE, Collins D, Fuller S et al. Isolation of small, primitive human hematopoietic stem cells: distribution of cell surface cytokine receptors and growth in SCID-Hu mice. Blood 1995;86:512-523.

75 Briddell RA, Broudy VC, Bruno E et al. Further phenotypic characterization and isolation of human hematopoietic progenitor cells using a monoclonal antibody to the c-kit receptor. Blood 1992;79:3159-3167.

76 Gunji Y, Nakamura M, Osawa H et al. Human primitive hematopoietic progenitor cells are more enriched in KIT^{low} cells than in KIT^{high} cells. Blood 1993;82:3283-3289.

77 Kawashima I, Zanjani ED, Almaida-Porada G et al. CD34$^+$ human marrow cells that express low levels of kit protein are enriched for long-term marrow-engrafting cells. Blood 1996;87:4136-4142.

78 Debili N, Wendling F, Cosman D et al. The Mpl receptor is expressed in the megakaryocytic lineage from late progenitors to platelets. Blood 1995;85:391-401.

79 Rappold I, Ziegler BL, Köhler I et al. Functional and phenotypic characterization of cord blood and bone marrow subsets expressing FLT3 (CD135) receptor tyrosine kinase. Blood 1997;90:111-125.

80 Debili N, Coulombel L, Croisille L et al. Characterization of a bipotent erythro-megakaryocytic progenitor in human bone marrow. Blood 1996;88:1284-1296.

81 Metcalf D. The molecular control of cell division, differentiation, commitment and maturation in hematopoietic cells. Nature 1989;339:27-30.

82 Tsai FY, Keller G, Kuo FC et al. An early haematopoietic defect in mice lacking the transcription factor GATA-2. Nature 1994;371:221-226.

83 Tsai FY, Orkin SH. Transcription factor GATA-2 is required for proliferation/survival of early hematopoietic cells and mast cell formation, but not for erythroid and myeloid terminal differentiation. Blood 1997;89:3636-3643.

84 Towatari M, Enver T, Saito H. GATA-2 phosphorylated by mitogen-activated protein kinase in response to mitogenic cytokine. Blood 1995;86(suppl 1):1000a.

85 Pevny L, Simon MC, Robertson E et al. Erythroid differentiation in chimaeric mice blocked by a targeted mutation in the gene for transcription factor GATA-1. Nature 1991;349:257-260.

86 Weiss MJ, Keller G, Orkin SH. Novel insights into erythroid development revealed through in vitro differentiation of GATA-1⁻ embryonic stem cells. Genes Dev 1994;8:1184-1197.

87 Shivdasani RA, Fujiwara Y, McDevitt MA et al. A lineage-selective knockout establishes the critical role of transcription factor GATA-1 in megakaryocyte growth and platelet development. EMBO J 1997;16:3965-3973.

88 Andrews NC, Erdjument-Bromage H, Davidson MB et al. Erythroid transcription factor NF-E2 is a haematopoietic-specific basic-leucine zipper protein. Nature 1993;362:722-728.

89 Shivdasani RA, Rosemblatt MF, Zucker-Franklin D et al. Transcription factor NF-E2 is required for platelet formation independent of the actions of thrombopoietin/MGDF in megakaryocyte development. Cell 1995;81:695-704.

90 Shivdasani RA, Orkin SH. Erythropoiesis and globin gene expression in mice lacking the transcription factor NF-E2. Proc Natl Acad Sci USA 1995;92:8690-8694.

91 Igarashi K, Itoh K, Hayashi N et al. Conditional expression of the ubiquitous transcription factor MafK induces erythroleukemia cell differentiation. Proc Natl Acad Sci USA 1995;92:7445-7449.

92 Lu SJ, Rowan S, Bani MR et al. Retroviral integration within the Fli-2 locus results in inactivation of the erythroid transcription factor NF-E2 in Friend erythroleukemias: evidence that NF-E2 is essential for globin expression. Proc Natl Acad Sci USA 1994;91:8398-8402.

93 Hsu HL, Huang L, Tsan JT et al. Preferred sequences for DNA recognition by the TAL1 helix-loop-helix proteins. Mol Cell Biol 1994;14:1256-1265.

94 Shivdasani RA, Mayer EL, Orkin SH. Absence of blood formation in mice lacking the T-cell leukemia oncoprotein tal-1/SCL. Nature 1995;373:432-434.

95 Robb L, Lyons I, Li R et al. Absence of yolk sac hematopoiesis from mice with a targeted disruption of the scl gene. Proc Natl Acad Sci USA 1995;92:7075-7079.

96 Porcher C, Swat W, Rockwell K et al. The T cell leukemia oncoprotein SCL/tal-1 is essential for development of all hematopoietic lineages. Cell 1996;86:47-57.

97 Robb L, Elwood NJ, Elefanty AG et al. The scl gene product is required for the generation of all hematopoietic lineages in the adult mouse. EMBO J 1996;15:4123-4129.

98 Elefanty AG, Robb L, Birner R et al. Hematopoietic-specific genes are not induced during in vitro differentiation of scl-null embryonic stem cells. Blood 1997;90:1435-1447.

99 Valtieri M, Tocci A, Gabbianelli M et al. Enforced tal-1 expression stimulates primitive, erythroid and megakaryocytic progenitors but blocks the granulopoietic differentiation program. Cancer Res (in press).

100 Bockamp EO, McLaughlin F, Gottgens B et al. Distinct mechanisms direct SCL/tal-1 expression in erythroid cells and CD34 positive primitive myeloid cells. J Biol Chem 1997;272:8781-8790.

101 Voronova AF, Lee F. The E2A and tal-1 helix-loop-helix proteins associate in vivo and are modulated by Id proteins during interleukin 6-induced myeloid differentiation. Proc Natl Acad Sci USA 1994;91:5952-5956.

102 Warren AJ, Colledge WH, Carlton MB et al. The oncogenic cysteine-rich LIM domain protein rbtn2 is essential for erythroid development. Cell 1994;78:45-57.

103 Osada H, Grütz G, Axelson H et al. Association of erythroid transcription factors: complexes involving the LIM protein RBTN2 and the zinc-finger protein GATA-1. Proc Natl Acad Sci USA 1995;92:9585-9589.

104 Wadman IA, Osada H, Grütz GG et al. The LIM-only protein Lmo2 is a bridging molecule assembling an erythroid, DNA binding complex which includes the TAL1, E47, GATA-1 and Ldb1/NLI complex. EMBO J 1997;16:3145-3157.

105 Clarke AR, Maandag ER, van Roon M et al. Requirement for a functional Rb-1 gene in murine development. Nature 1992;359:328-330.

106 Jacks T, Fazeli A, Schmitt EM et al. Effects of an Rb mutation in the mouse. Nature 1992;359:295-300.

107 Lee EY-HP, Chang CY, Hu N et al. Mice deficient for Rb are nonviable and show defects in neurogenesis and haematopoiesis. Nature 1992;359:288-294.

108 Guy CT, Zhou W, Kaufman S et al. E2F-1 blocks terminal differentiation and causes proliferation in transgenic megakaryocytes. Mol Cell Biol 1996;16:685-693.

109 Gu W, Schneider JW, Condorelli G et al. Interaction of myogenic factors and the retinoblastoma protein mediates muscle cell commitment and differentiation. Cell 1993;72:309-324.

110 Tocci A, Parolini I, Gabbianelli M et al. Dual action of retinoic acid on human embryonic-fetal hematopoiesis: blockade of primitive progenitor proliferation and shift from multipotent/erythroid/monocytic to granulocytic differentiation program. Blood 1996;88:2878-2888.

111 Leary AG, Strauss LC, Civin CI et al. Disparate differentiation in hemopoietic colonies derived from human paired progenitors. Blood 1985;66:327-332.

112 Rappolee DA, Wang A, Mark D et al. Novel method for studying mRNA phenotypes in single or small number of cells. J Cell Biochem 1989;39:1-11.

113 Ziegler BL, Lamping C, Thoma S et al. Single-cell cDNA-PCR: Removal of contaminating genomic DNA from total RNA using immobilized DNase I. Biotechniques 1992;13:726-729.

114 Brady G, Barbara M, Iscove NN. Representative in vitro cDNA amplification from individual hemopoietic cells and colonies. Methods Mol Cell Biol 1990;2:17.

115 Ziegler BL, Lamping C, Thoma S et al. Single-cell cDNA-PCR. Methods Neurosciences 1995;26:62.

116 Ziegler BL, Lamping CP, Thoma SJ et al. Analysis of gene expression in small numbers of purified hemopoietic progenitor cells by RT-PCR. STEM CELLS 1995;13(suppl 1):106-116.

117 Thoma S, Lamping CP, Ziegler BL. Phenotype analysis of hematopoietic CD34$^+$ cell populations derived from human umbilical cord blood using flow cytometry and cDNA-polymerase chain reaction. Blood 1994;83:2103-2114.

118 Ziegler BL, Thoma S, Lamping C et al. Surface antigen expression on CD34$^+$ cord blood cells: comparative analysis by flow cytometry and limiting dilution (LD) RT-PCR of chymopapain-treated or untreated cells. Cytometry 1996;25:46-57.

119 Tam AW, Smith MM, Fry KE et al. Construction of cDNA libraries from small numbers of cells using sequence independent primers. Nucleic Acids Res 1989;17:1269.

120 Belyavsky A, Vinogradova T, Rajewsky K. PCR-based cDNA library construction: general cDNA libraries at the level of a few cells. Nucleic Acids Res 1989;17:2919-2932.

121 Wang AM, Doyle MV, Mark DF. Quantitation of mRNA by the polymerase chain reaction. Proc Natl Acad Sci USA 1989;86:9717-9721.

122 Testa U, Martucci R, Rutella S et al. Autologous stem cell transplantation: release of early and late acting growth factors relates with hematopoietic ablation and recovery. Blood 1994;84:3532-3539.

123 Nichol JL, Hokom MM, Hornkohl A et al. Megakaryocyte growth and development factor. J Clin Invest 1995;95:2973-2978.

CHAPTER III

BLOOD STEM CELLS IN NORMAL AND LEUKEMIC STATES

DIFFERENCES BETWEEN NORMAL AND CML STEM CELLS: POTENTIAL TARGETS FOR CLINICAL EXPLOITATION

A.C. Eaves, M.J. Barnett, L. Ponchio, J.D. Cashman, A.L. Petzer, C.J. Eaves

MATURATION HIERARCHY OF LEUKEMIC STEM CELLS

Bob Löwenberg, Wim Terpstra

PANEL DISCUSSION: DEFINITION OF THE LEUKEMIC STEM CELL: AN ACHIEVABLE GOAL

P.J. Quesenberry, Ludwika Kreja

Differences Between Normal and CML Stem Cells: Potential Targets for Clinical Exploitation

A.C. EAVES, M.J. BARNETT, L. PONCHIO, J.D. CASHMAN, A.L. PETZER, C.J. EAVES

Terry Fox Laboratory and Division of Hematology, British Columbia Cancer Agency and University of British Columbia, Vancouver, British Columbia, Canada

Key Words. *Stem cells · Chronic myeloid leukemia (CML) · Cycling control · Autografting*

ABSTRACT

Chronic myeloid leukemia (CML) is a clonal myeloproliferative disorder in which there is a deregulated amplification of CML progenitors at intermediate stages of their differentiation along the myeloid, erythroid and megakaryocyte pathways. Such cell populations are routinely quantified using standard in vitro colony-forming cell (CFC) assays. The excessive production of leukemic CFC that is seen in most CML patients at diagnosis may be explained at least in part by their increased proliferative activity. An anomalous cycling behavior in vivo has also been found to extend to more primitive CML progenitor populations detectable as long-term culture-initiating cells (LTC-IC). Although the molecular basis of these changes in CML progenitor regulation is not fully understood at the level of the primitive CFC compartment, a selective inability of CML progenitors to be inhibited by certain -C-C-type chemokines has been demonstrated. Failure of the CML stem cell compartment to expand in vivo at the same rate as later progenitor cell types may be explained by their unique additional possession of an intrinsically upregulated probability of differentiation. Such a mechanism would be consistent with the observed loss of LTC-IC activity by CML cells incubated in vitro under conditions that sustain or expand normal LTC-IC populations. Initial clinical studies undertaken at our center established the feasibility of exploiting the differential behavior of primitive normal and CML cells in vitro as a potential purging strategy for reducing the leukemic stem cell content of CML marrow autografts. The results of a larger, second trial now in progress on a group of unselected patients are encouraging. Future studies of nonobese diabetic/severe-combined immunodeficiency mice engrafted with CML cells should provide another useful preclinical model for evaluating treatments that may more effectively eradicate the neoplastic clone in vivo. *Stem Cells 1998;16(suppl 1):77-83*

INTRODUCTION

This Workshop has served as a focal point to bring together many investigators who have shared *Ted Fliedner's* fascination with hematopoietic stem cells as well as his dedication to the goal of harnessing new knowledge about the behavior of these cells for clinical applications. This update on our work on chronic myeloid leukemia (CML) reflects both of these perspectives. I am, therefore, particularly pleased to be presenting our findings for discussion in this setting and to join in the recognition of *Ted's* historic leadership in experimental hematology at the difficult and challenging interface between biology and medicine.

CML offers unique opportunities for analyzing the regulation of primitive hematopoietic cell functions for several reasons. First, the biologic alterations imposed on the leukemic stem cell compartment have a common and known genetic basis in the expression of the BCR-ABL gene [1]. Second, these alterations must be relatively subtle in order to explain the documented five to seven years of growth of the clone before it becomes symptomatic [2]. Third, because overt effects on the expression of differentiation programs are not seen, all of the known progenitor assays for quantifying cells at different stages of normal hematopoietic progenitor differentiation have been found to detect phenotypically indistinguishable populations of leukemic (Philadelphia chromosome; Ph^+/BCR-ABL$^+$) progenitors [3]. What, then, has the application of these progenitor assays revealed? In most patients assessed at a time when their disease first becomes symptomatic, there appears to be a normal reservoir of primitive normal hematopoietic cells. These cells are capable of being transplanted [4] or endogenously restoring normal blood formation for transient periods after intensive chemotherapy treatments [5]. They include cells referred to as long-term culture-initiating cells (LTC-IC) because they can generate in vitro colony-forming cell (CFC) progeny when cocultured with stromal fibroblasts for periods in excess of five or six weeks [6, 7]. Until recently the latter method was the only way that quantitative changes in the number of very early normal or CML cell populations could be assessed. These indicated that the most primitive cell types are initially predominantly normal [8]. However, transplantable Ph^+ cells have also been known to exist for a long time from early experiences with transfusions of unirradiated allogeneic blood products obtained from CML donors [9]. More recently, the presence of transplantable leukemic cells has been demonstrated by retroviral marking studies of CML autografts [4]. Both Ph^+ and Ph^- cells capable of engrafting sublethally irradiated immunocompromised severe-combined immunodeficiency (SCID) [10] and nonobese diabetic (NOD)/SCID mice [11, 12] have also confirmed the existence of transplantable leukemic stem cells in the blood and marrow of CML patients at diagnosis, with the Ph^- stem cells normally predominating.

Extensive characterization of the most primitive hematopoietic cell compartment(s) in CML patients has, however, been limited in most studies to assessments of Ph^+ and Ph^- LTC-IC. These have shown that the frequency of both genotypes of LTC-IC in the total marrow cell population is often reduced by comparison to the frequency of LTC-IC in the marrow of normal individuals. However, this apparent reduction is likely to be due primarily to the increased cellularity of the marrow in patients with CML in whom there is a selective expansion in the output of terminally differentiating Ph^+ granulocytes. Among the LTC-IC that are detected in the marrow, Ph^- LTC-IC typically outnumber the Ph^+ LTC-IC to a sufficient extent that the latter are often beyond the limit of detectability [8]. In contrast to the marrow, LTC-IC frequencies in the circulation are usually elevated, presumably because they can (or are induced to) exit from the overcrowded marrow space more readily than the bulk of the terminally differentiating cells. Regardless of what the exact underlying molecular mechanism is that causes an exodus of LTC-IC into the blood of CML patients, it is interesting to note that it affects both normal and leukemic LTC-IC genotypes alike. Thus, newly presenting CML patients with highly elevated WBC counts (primarily granulocytes) indicative of the presence of a large uncontrollably expanding Ph^+ clone may, nevertheless, be found to have a large number of almost exclusively normal LTC-IC cocirculating with their Ph^+ WBC [7].

In fact, in terms of many of their properties (expression of CD34 and Thy-1; lack of expression of lineage markers such as CD71, CD45RA, CD38; type and number of CFC produced per LTC-IC), Ph^+ and Ph^- LTC-IC appear indistinguishable [6, 7, 13, 14]. Genotyping studies on their CFC progeny are therefore required to allow them to be separately quantitated when both are present. This is best accomplished by a DNA-based strategy, e.g., by cytogenetics, interphase fluorescence in situ hybridization or polymerase chain reaction (PCR) (if the position of the breakpoints in the BCR or ABL genes is known). Reverse transcriptase (RT)-PCR is also useful for identifying cells expressing BCR-ABL transcripts but this procedure may not adequately discriminate genetically normal and BCR-ABL$^+$ cells in which BCR-ABL transcripts may not be detected [15, 16].

Ph$^+$ and Ph$^-$ LTC-IC populations do, however, appear to differ in two major ways, both of which may be important to the pathogenesis of the disease in terms of understanding the observed pattern of clonal expansion in vivo. The first of these is a difference in the cycling state of Ph$^+$ and Ph$^-$ LTC-IC which is seen both when these are examined in freshly isolated samples and when their behavior in LTC is followed [3, 17]. As has been well-documented for Ph$^+$ and Ph$^-$ CFC, all members of the Ph$^+$ LTC-IC compartment appear to be continuously proliferating and do not develop a subpopulation of G_0 cells which is typical of their normal counterparts. It is therefore not surprising that most Ph$^+$ LTC-IC also display changes typical of primitive normal cells that have been activated, e.g., increased expression of HLA-DR, retention of Rhodamine-123 and increased sensitivity to 4-hydroperoxycyclophospamide [13, 18].

If this were the only difference between Ph$^+$ and Ph$^-$ LTC-IC, then one might expect a more rapid amplification of the Ph$^+$ LTC-IC population to occur, as for example, is seen at the level of the CFC compartment. In CML patients it is well-known that the CFC population becomes grossly inflated by a deregulated expansion of Ph$^+$ progenitors (on all lineages). Moreover, this is associated with a failure of primitive Ph$^+$ CFC to respond to some (but not all) of the controls that maintain an appropriate balance between proliferating and quiescent normal CFC [19-22]. The LTC system has proven a useful model for exploring the types of factors involved and in particular for identifying those that are ineffective in regulating primitive Ph$^+$ CFC cycling. Such studies have revealed two classes of candidate inhibitors, transforming growth factor-β, which can affect Ph$^+$ and Ph$^-$ CFC alike [20], and certain members of the -C-C- family of chemokines which arrest the proliferation of primitive Ph$^-$ CFC, but not of analogous Ph$^+$ CFC. Macrophage inflammatory protein-1α (MIP-1α) was the first member of the latter family of inhibitors to be shown to be differentially active on normal and Ph$^+$ CFC [21]. More recently we have shown that monocyte chemoattractant protein-1 (MCP-1) can be added to this list and MCP-1, rather than MIP-1α, has been shown to be a participant in the mechanisms operative within the adherent layer of the LTC system (*Cashman et al.*, manuscript in preparation).

Whether the deregulated cycling activity exhibited by Ph$^+$ LTC-IC involves a failure to respond to MCP-1 (or MIP-1α) is not yet known. From detailed analyses of cytokine effects on different types of responses of early hematopoietic cells, we now know that both the types and modes of activation of different cytokine receptors can differentially stimulate LTC-IC viability, mitogenesis and amplification (self-renewal) or differentiation (generation of CFC) (see accompanying article by *C.J. Eaves et al.* in this Workshop proceedings). Therefore, it would not be surprising to learn that the initiation of signals that can antagonize any of these responses might also result from, or require, the activation of different receptors, or different modes of receptor activation, in hematopoietic progenitors that are at different stages of differentiation.

What is clear is that the biological consequences of the increased proliferative activity of Ph$^+$ LTC-IC are not the same as the increased proliferative activity of Ph$^+$ CFC, both of which, nevertheless, appear to be inherent to the disease process (i.e., both changes are common to the leukemic LTC-IC and CFC of all CML patients thus far examined and they are evident even before any treatment is applied). However, at the level of the CFC compartment, these changes are associated with a gross enlargement of the population with predominantly Ph$^+$ elements. In contrast, as discussed above, the LTC-IC compartment does not appear to expand much and in some patients at diagnosis may still be predominantly Ph$^-$. We suggest that this may be explained by a second abnormal characteristic of Ph$^+$ LTC-IC which can be seen as an intrinsically determined and reduced capacity for their executing self-renewal divisions [8]. Thus, in spite of an ability to generate an equivalent number of CFC during the first wave of progeny derived from initially stimulated LTC-IC [6], this activity of Ph$^+$ LTC-IC is poorly sustained. After more prolonged periods in LTC and upon replating, the frequency of Ph$^+$ cells retaining detectable LTC-IC activity decreases much more rapidly than the rate at which normal LTC-IC decline in vitro [6]. The fact that this occurs regardless of whether the viability of the cells is being sustained by direct contact with stromal feeders, or by defined cytokines in the absence of stroma (or serum) [23], supports the concept that this behavior of CML LTC-IC is intrinsically determined and likely to be related to some activity of the BCR-ABL gene product.

One might therefore anticipate that each Ph^+ LTC-IC division (in vitro or in vivo) would favor the production of CFC and correspondingly reduce the rate of expansion of the Ph^+ LTC-IC compartment. This prediction is in fact born out by what has been observed in unperturbed CML patients. Such a model would also explain the differential ascendancy exhibited by Ph^+ and Ph^- populations under different conditions of normal stem cell activation. For example, in the absence of any perturbation, Ph^+ stem cells would have a slow but selective growth advantage due to an inherently increased proliferative activity (relative to any residual normal stem cells). On the other hand, an opposite pattern would be expected to occur under conditions where a large proportion of the normal stem cell population would be effectively activated. Thus, both in vivo (in the patient), e.g., after intensive chemotherapy, and in vitro, e.g., following exposure of the cells to stimulating cytokines or other factors that stromal cells may produce, the growth of primitive normal cells would be anticipated to be favored and this would be seen precisely in those situations where their proliferation was most effectively stimulated.

If correct, this model has a number of important implications for therapy. First, it should be possible to exploit the proposed differences in cycling control of normal and Ph^+ stem cells to eventually eradicate Ph^+ elements using agents that kill cycling but not quiescent cells. Second, it may be possible to exploit differences in the self-renewal abilities of normal and Ph^+ stem cells to devise conditions that push the latter type of cell to extinction without compromising the functional integrity of coexisting normal stem cells. These two concepts underlie the autografting trial design that we began to explore 10 years ago and for which a brief update is given below.

Use of "Culture-Purging" as a Strategy to Reduce the Ph^+ Stem Cell Content of Autografts in the Treatment of Chronic Phase CML

In 1987 we designed a clinical trial to evaluate the feasibility of using "culture-purged" marrow autografts to enable CML patients to be given myeloablative doses of chemo-radiotherapy. At the time it was not known what the side effects of such a procedure might be; whether hematologic recovery would be adequate in recipients of cultured cells, and if so, whether the initial cells regenerated would be Ph^+ or Ph^-. The results of our first study, which involved the treatment of 26 patients, addressed all of these points. We found that the procedure itself could be easily and safely carried out by a small but well-trained team of laboratory and clinical staff. Hematologic recoveries in most patients were consistent with rates obtained using other purging strategies, and the predominant population seen during the recovery phase in most patients was Ph^- and polyclonal [24-26]. A survival curve for the 23 patients in this trial who were treated in chronic or accelerated phase is shown in Figure 1.

The main criticism of this study is that all patients entered were pre-screened and selected, not

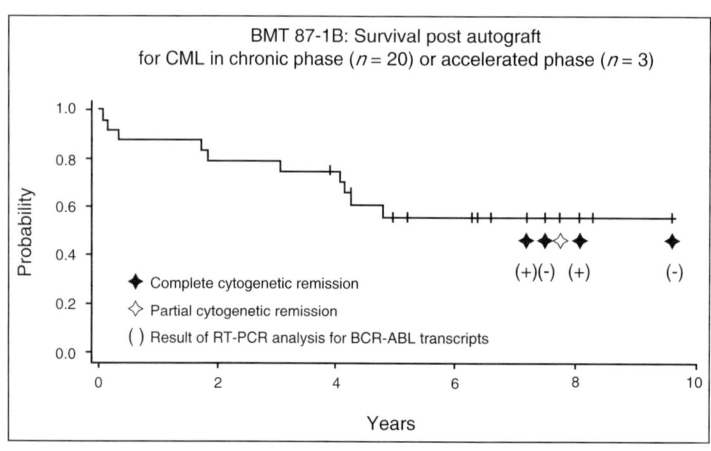

Figure 1. Survival plot of selected CML patients given myeloablative therapy and a "culture-purged" (10 days) marrow autograft. *The results shown represent an update of data published in [26].*

only for standard clinical parameters making them eligible for an autograft, but also on the basis of a preliminary laboratory study. The purpose of the latter was to try to anticipate whether the marrow autograft would contain a reasonable number of predominantly Ph^- LTC-IC after being cultured for 10 days. In retrospect this selection would likely have identified a subset of patients with relatively small Ph^+ stem cell populations and thereby have contributed a favorable bias to all outcomes considered, including survival. Therefore, when we were satisfied that the procedure would not incur significant toxicity, a second trial was started in which the prescreening selection step was eliminated in an attempt to avoid any such bias. To also overcome potential losses in vivo of the cultured cells by their nonspecific removal by the spleen, the second trial also required that all patients be splenectomized prior to being autografted. In addition, the administration of low dose α-interferon to patients as soon as their post-transplant recoveries permitted was introduced as a further modification. Accrual of patients into the second trial has been made possible by the cooperation of a number of transplant centers in Canada. All patients entered into this trial have their marrows harvested, cultured and cryopreserved in Vancouver, but the myeloablative treatment, reinfusion of the cryopreserved cells and subsequent patient follow-up is undertaken in the original referring transplant center. Table 1 shows a comparison of the results of the first trial to preliminary findings from the second trial. Although it is still too early to anticipate what long-term benefits may accrue to patients being entered into the second trial, it is already clear that the ability to obtain an initial post-transplant repopulation of the marrow and blood with Ph^- cells is not strongly dependent on the selection criteria used to select the patients entered into the first trial.

These pioneering studies with cultured CML marrow autografts have dispelled most major practical concerns about the use of such cells for clinical transplant purposes. Nevertheless, exploiting this opportunity to enhance the engrafting activity of selected normal stem cells by additional or alternative in vitro manipulations [23] remains an important future challenge. Hopefully, it will eventually also be possible to couple this kind of technology with gene transfer strategies designed to enhance the complete and permanent elimination of Ph^+ cells both in vivo and in the autograft.

Table 1. Comparison of the patient characteristics and results post-transplant for the two Vancouver CML autografting trials using "culture-purged" marrow

	Trial 1	Trial 2
Patient characteristics:		
Number of patients entered	26 (Vancouver)	21 (Vancouver 9, other 12)
Disease status at entry	20 CP-1, 6 > CP-1[*]	17 CP-1, 4 AP
Age at entry	42 (22-59) yr	49 (23-59) yr
Prior interferon	6	7
Interval from diagnosis to BMT	12 (5-64) mo	13 (6-62) mo
Post-transplant results:		
Neutrophils >0.5 $\times$ 10^9/l	26 (11-52) days	22 (12-63) days
Platelets >20 $\times$ 10^9/l	46 (16-337) days	28 (15-256) days
Ph^- BM metaphases	100% in 14,	100% in 7
	66%-99% in 5,	66%-99% in 5,
	24% in 1	19% in 1, 0% in 2, NE in 1
Graft failure	5	1
Therapy-related deaths	4	1

[*]Three in accelerated phase, one in a second chronic phase, one in a third chronic phase, one in blast crisis.

ACKNOWLEDGMENT

The authors express their gratitude to all of the staff of the Division of Hematology of the British Columbia Cancer Agency and the Vancouver Health Sciences Centre, as well as those in other centers participating in the CML clinical study described, for their assistance in making this trial possible. Appreciation is also extended to Amgen, Cangene, Immunex, Novartis, Schering-Plough and StemCell Technologies, Inc. for critical reagents. Finally, we thank *Bernadine Fox* for expert assistance in preparing the manuscript.

This work was supported by grants from the National Cancer Institute of Canada (NCIC) with funds from the Terry Fox Run and the Canadian Cancer Society, and Novartis. *L. Ponchio* was a recipient of support from the Associazione Italiana per la Ricerca sul Cancro, *A. Petzer* was funded by the E. Schrödinger Foundation and *C. Eaves* holds a Terry Fox Cancer Research Scientist Award from the NCIC.

REFERENCES

1 Maguer-Satta V, Petzer AL, Eaves AC et al. BCR-ABL expression in different subpopulations of functionally characterized Ph$^+$ CD34$^+$ cells from patients with chronic myeloid leukemia. Blood 1996;88:1796-1804.

2 Ichimaru M, Ishimaru T, Mikami M et al. Incidence of leukemia in a fixed cohort of atomic bomb survivors and controls, Hiroshima and Nagasaki October 1950–December 1978. Technical Report RERF TR 13-81. Hiroshima: Radiation Effects Research Foundation, 1981.

3 Eaves CJ, Eaves AC. Cell culture studies in CML. In: Goldman J, ed., Hinton K. Bailliere's Clinical Haematology. London: Bailliere Tindall/W.B. Saunders, 1987:931-961.

4 Deisseroth AB, Zu Z, Claxton D et al. Genetic marking shows that Ph$^+$ cells present in autologous transplants of chronic myelogenous leukemia (CML) contribute to relapse after autologous bone marrow in CML. Blood 1994;83:3068-3076.

5 Goto T, Nishikori M, Arlin Z et al. Growth characteristics of leukemic and normal hematopoietic cells in Ph1$^+$ chronic myelogenous leukemia and effects of intensive treatment. Blood 1982;59:793-808.

6 Udomsakdi C, Eaves CJ, Swolin B et al. Rapid decline of chronic myeloid leukemic cells in long-term culture due to a defect at the leukemic stem cell level. Proc Natl Acad Sci USA 1992;89:6192-6196.

7 Petzer AL, Eaves CJ, Lansdorp PM et al. Characterization of primitive subpopulations of normal and leukemic cells present in the blood of patients with newly diagnosed as well as established chronic myeloid leukemia. Blood 1996;88:2162-2171.

8 Eaves C, Udomsakdi C, Cashman J et al. The biology of normal and neoplastic stem cells in CML. Leuk Lymphoma 1993;11:245-253.

9 Levin RH, Whang J, Tjio JH et al. Persistent mitosis of transfused homologous leukocytes in children receiving antileukemic therapy. Science 1963;142:1305-1311.

10 Sirard C, Lapidot T, Vormoor J et al. Normal and leukemic SCID-repopulating cells (SRC) co-exist in the bone marrow and peripheral blood from CML patients in chronic phase while leukemic SRC are detected in blast crisis. Blood 1996;87:1539-1548.

11 Lewis ID, McDiarmid LA, Samels LM et al. Establishment of a reproducible model of chronic-phase chronic myeloid leukemia in NOD/SCID mice using blood-derived mononuclear or CD34$^+$ cells. Blood 1998;91:630-640.

12 Wang JCY, Lapidot T, Cashman JD et al. High level engraftment of NOD/SCID mice by primitive normal and leukemic hematopoietic cells from patients with chronic myeloid leukemia (CML) in chronic phase. Blood 1998 (in press).

13 Udomsakdi C, Eaves CJ, Lansdorp PM et al. Phenotypic heterogeneity of primitive leukemic hematopoietic cells in patients with chronic myeloid leukemia. Blood 1992;80:2522-2530.

14 Ghaffari S, Dougherty GJ, Lansdorp PM et al. Differentiation-associated changes in CD44 isoform expression during normal hematopoiesis and their alteration in chronic myeloid leukemia. Blood 1995;86:2976-2985.

15 Keating A, Wang X-H, Laraya P. Variable transcription of BCR-ABL by Ph$^+$ cells arising from hematopoietic progenitors in chronic myeloid leukemia. Blood 1994;83:1744-1749.

16 Bedi A, Zehnbauer BA, Collector MI et al. BCR-ABL gene rearrangement and expression of primitive hematopoietic progenitors in chronic myeloid leukemia. Blood 1993;81:2898-2902.

17 Ponchio L, Cashman J, Zoumbos N et al. Primitive CML cells show a deregulation of their cycling status both in vivo and in longterm cultures which is not normalized in the presence of interferon-α. Blood 1995;86:(suppl 1):493a.

18 Verfaillie CM, Miller WJ, Boylan K et al. Selection of benign primitive hematopoietic progenitors in chronic myelogenous leukemia on the basis of HLA-DR antigen expression. Blood 1992;79:1003-1010.

19 Eaves AC, Cashman JD, Gaboury LA et al. Unregulated proliferation of primitive chronic myeloid leukemia progenitors in the presence of normal marrow adherent cells. Proc Natl Acad Sci USA 1986;83:5306-5310.

20 Cashman JD, Eaves AC, Eaves CJ. Granulocyte-macrophage colony-stimulating factor modulation of the inhibitory effect of transforming growth factor-β on normal and leukemic human hematopoietic progenitor cells. Leukemia 1992;6:886-892.

21 Eaves CJ, Cashman JD, Wolpe SD et al. Unresponsiveness of primitive chronic myeloid leukemia cells to macrophage inflammatory protein 1α, an inhibitor of primitive normal hematopoietic cells. Proc Natl Acad Sci USA 1993;90:12015-12019.

22 Cashman JD, Eaves AC, Eaves CJ. The tetrapeptide AcSDKP specifically blocks the cycling of

primitive normal but not leukemic progenitors in long-term culture: evidence for an indirect mechanism. Blood 1994;84:1534-1542.

23 Petzer AL, Eaves CJ, Barnett MJ et al. Selective expansion of primitive normal hematopoietic cells in cytokine-supplemented cultures of purified cells from patients with chronic myeloid leukemia. Blood 1997;90:64-69.

24 Barnett MJ, Eaves CJ, Phillips GL et al. Successful autografting in chronic myeloid leukaemia after maintenance of marrow in culture. Bone Marrow Transplant 1989;4:345-351.

25 Turhan AG, Humphries RK, Eaves CJ et al. Detection of breakpoint cluster region-negative and nonclonal hematopoiesis in vitro and in vivo after transplantation of cells selected in cultures of chronic myeloid leukemia marrow. Blood 1990;76:2404-2410.

26 Barnett MJ, Eaves CJ, Phillips GL et al. Autografting with cultured marrow in chronic myeloid leukemia: results of a pilot study. Blood 1994;84:724-732.

Maturation Hierarchy of Leukemic Stem Cells

BOB LÖWENBERG, WIM TERPSTRA

University Hospital Rotterdam and Erasmus University, Rotterdam, The Netherlands

Key Words. *Acute myeloid leukemia · AML · Stem cells · Hematopoietic stem cells · Leukemia · Hematopoietic growth factors · SCID mouse*

ABSTRACT

Here we discuss the characteristics of various progenitor cell assays for human acute myeloid leukemia (AML) with emphasis on the repopulating properties of human AML progenitor cells, their potential relevance for pathophysiological studies, and treatment development in AML. *Stem Cells 1998;16(suppl 1):85-88*

Acute myeloid leukemia (AML) stem cells may be defined as the subset of leukemic cells that expresses abilities to initiate and maintain long-term growth of AML. Until recently, human AML growth has mainly been studied in culture for limited periods of time (e.g., one to two weeks). Transplantation of human AML cells in various strains of mice resulted in transient and local growth. Thus, the available in vitro and in vivo systems did not allow for study of long-term growth of AML cells. More recently, transplantation of primary human AML cells into newly developed strains of immunodeficient mice (severe combined immunodeficient [SCID] and non-obese diabetic [NOD]/SCID) has resulted in reproducible growth of AML for prolonged periods of time [1]. Furthermore, long-term bone marrow culture systems (e.g., the cobblestone area-forming cell [CAFC] assay) have become available to sustain normal and malignant hematopoiesis over periods of two to four months [2-4]. These models of growth of human leukemias have provided assays for investigating long-term growth of AML and furnished insight into the characteristics of more primitive AML stem cells.

Frequency of AML Stem Cells

The leukemic stem cell is a rare cell. Limiting dilution experiments of AML in immunodeficient mice have shown that the frequency of the cells with the ability to initiate AML in immunodeficient mice ranges between 2 and 1,000 per 10^5 AML cells [5, 6]. The frequencies of cells with the ability to produce leukemic cobblestone areas (CA) after an interval of five to eight weeks in long-term bone marrow culture vary between 4 and 2,400 per 10^5 AML cells [3, 4]. These so-called late CAFCs are assumed to represent primitive progenitors. Thus, the frequencies of cells initiating long-term growth of leukemia in vivo and cobblestone areas in culture beyond four weeks are similar. This suggests that they probably represent identical or closely related cell populations. Nevertheless, these quantitative estimations are only approximations. Due to residual graft resistance of the mouse recipients and the incomplete seeding efficiency of hematopoietic cells in culture, these values may be underestimations. The variations observed in the frequencies of the AML stem cells among individual cases are most likely exponents of the heterogeneity of clinical AML.

Are these cells capable of maintaining AML growth indefinitely? This question remains unresolved. In certain cases, leukemic growth can be maintained in SCID mice for as long as 100 days [3], and leukemia may reinitiate after transplantation of AML into secondary mouse recipients. Human AML cells recovered from the recipient bone marrow contained AML progenitor cells (colony forming unit-AML (CFU-AML)) and these progenitor cells could also be maintained in the mouse for a minimum of 100 days [3, 5-7]. Thus, the data show that human AML cells with proliferative abilities may survive without exhaustion in the murine bone marrow environment for extended periods of time. Additional experiments would be needed to define any time restriction of AML growth in these animals.

Immunophenotype of AML Stem Cells

Normal primitive hematopoietic cells may be enriched according to immunophenotype as they express CD34 brightly but do not show CD38 or lineage-associated antigens. These $CD33^{++}/CD38^-$ cells are present at a frequency of 0.01% in normal bone marrow [8]. Flow-cytometric analysis of more than 90 AML samples disclosed that $CD34^+$ cells can be identified among the leukemic cell population in 83% of cases. $CD34^{++}/CD38^-$ AML cells are demonstrable in 35% of cases. This phenotypically distinct subset of cells is present at variable frequencies [9]. These data suggest that primitive AML cells might express the normal $CD34^{++}/CD38^-$ phenotype in many instances.

The characteristics of subsets of cells can be conveniently examined following cell separation, e.g., using immunomagnetic beads or fluorescence-activated cell sorting. We have reported the detailed analysis in a case of AML that contained a significant $CD34^+/CD38^-$ subpopulation [3]. The leukemic cells were separated into $CD34^+$ and $CD34^-$ fractions. AML growth could be initiated either by the $CD34^+$ or $CD34^-$ AML cell subsets. Following transplantation into SCID mouse recipients, both cell fractions infiltrated the mouse bone marrow to a similar degree. The leukemia derived from the $CD34^-$ AML cells could be maintained for at least 100 days. Leukemic cells recovered from mice that had received $CD34^-$ grafts contained AML progenitor cells (CFU-AML). Further, leukemic cells recovered from these primary mouse recipients initiated leukemia in secondary recipients. Finally, in vitro investigations showed that the $CD34^-$ fraction contained considerable numbers of cells with the ability to produce cobblestone areas after eight weeks of culture. Taken together, the data indicate that the $CD34^-$ fraction of the leukemia expressed the abilities to initiate and maintain AML growth in vivo (>100 days) and in leukemia-initiating abilities. Thus, in this case, the primitive AML progenitors were heterogeneous and expressed a diverse $CD34^+$ or a $CD34^-$ immunophenotype which is in contrast to normal hematopoiesis. How do these data compare to the results previously reported by other investigators? The phenotype of AML cells with the ability to engraft immunodeficient mice was always $CD34^+/CD38^-$ in another study [5]. In a third study analysis of the abilities of subsets defined by expression of CD34 and Thy-1 showed that the phenotype of AML cells with long-term abilities was $CD34^+/Thy1^-$ in five of six cases evaluated [10]. In one case, $CD34^+$ cells failed to initiate leukemia and only $CD34^+$ cells showed the ability to engraft. Thus, the $CD34^+/CD38^-$ subset of AML generally contains AML cells with long-term potential. However, such AML cells occur in a minority of cases [9]. AML stem cells may express variable immunophenotypes. Apparently, expression of the CD34 antigen is not strictly associated with long-term abilities of AML.

AML Progenitors More Immature Than CFU-AML

The AML progenitor cells identified as CFU-AML actively synthesize DNA. This has been shown in thymidine suicide studies [11]. In normal bone marrow, the antimetabolite chemotherapeutic agent 5-fluorouracil (5-FU) preferentially eliminates hematopoietic cells that are in S-phase or show active mRNA synthesis [12]. 5-FU resistance is a property of murine hematopoietic cells with long-term in vivo repopulating abilities and long-term abilities in vitro, indicating that these cells are mainly in a kinetically quiescent state (G_0-phase) [13-17]. Most early hematopoietic progenitors in humans show similar resistance to 5-FU [2, 18, 19]. Prolonged incubation of unseparated human hematopoietic cells with 5-FU in the presence of cytokines selects for pluripotent cells in G_0 phase with an immature phenotype [20]. Hence, incubation with 5-FU may be used as a strategy to select for stem cells. The technique has also been applied with the purpose to investigate whether the AML cell population contains AML cells more immature than the AML-CFU [4] . Exposure of AML cells to 5-FU in vitro eliminates up to 3 log of the AML-CFU subset. However, most AML cells initiating leukemia in SCID mice survived the 5-FU treatment. Similarly, a major fraction of primitive leukemia CAFCs (i.e., 31%-82% of CAFCs as assessed at week 6 in culture) retained their viability after exposure to 5-FU. Thus, apparently, the AML cell populations contains a 5-FU resistant fraction of cells with long-term abilities both in vivo and in vitro, a condition similar to normal hematopoiesis. Because growth of AML may be initiated with AML cell populations depleted of AML-CFU, AML-CFU do not appear representative of leukemic stem cells. As the week 2 CAFC express a sensitivity to 5-FU that is greater than that of week 6 CAFCs and less than that of AML-CFU [4], the maturation stage of week 2 CAFCs appears intermediate between CFU-AML and week 6 primitive CAFCs.

Hierarchy of the AML Cell Population

The data discussed above show that AML cells constitute a hierarchically ordered cell population. This hierarchy resembles that of normal hematopoiesis in many, although not all, respects. SCID mouse leukemia-initiating cells and week 6 CAFCs measure closely related AML cell populations. Immature precursors in AML may incidentally be CD34⁻, which is in contrast to normal hematopoiesis. This appears indicative of a maturation asynchrony in certain cases of leukemia. The question at which maturation stage more exactly the AML cells lose their long-term potential requires additional study.

Possible Application of Assays for Primitive AML Progenitors to the Development of AML Therapy

Several investigators have correlated the in vitro sensitivity of CFU-AML to cytostatic drugs with the clinical efficacy of these drugs. However, to date, these tests have unsatisfactory predictive value [21]. The deleterious effects of individual cytostatic drugs on transient and long-term growth of normal bone marrow could be predicted using results of the CAFC assay [22, 23]. The experiments with 5-FU showed minimal cell kill of primitive AML cell progenitors and considerable killing of more mature AML cell subsets. Thus, the quantification of cytotoxic effects specifically targeted at primitive versus less primitive subsets of AML may now be feasible. Primitive AML cells as an index of the repopulative potential of the neoplasm and to assess efficacy of AML stem cell kill may provide a convenient endpoint for the development of AML therapy.

REFERENCES

1 Lapidot T, Pflumio F, Doedens M et al. Cytokine stimulation of human hematopoiesis from immature cells transplanted into SCID mice. Science 1992;255:1137-1141.

2 Breems DA, Blokland EAW, Neben S et al. Frequency analysis of human primitive haematopoietic subsets using a cobblestone area forming cell assay. Leukemia 1994;8:1095-1104.

3 Terpstra W, Prins A, Ploemacher RE et al. Long term leukemia initiating capacity of a CD34 negative subpopulation of acute myeloid leukemia. Blood 1996;87:2187-2194.

4 Terpstra W, Ploemacher RE, Prins A et al. Fluorouracil selectively spares AML cells with long-term growth abilities in immunodeficient mice and in culture. Blood 1996;88:1944-1950.

5 Bonnett D, Dick JE. The CD34⁺⁺/CD38⁻ stem cell fraction is responsible for the initiation of human acute myeloid leukemia in NOD-SCID mice. Exp Hematol 1996;24:1126a.

6 Lapidot T, Sirard C, Vormoor J et al. A cell initiating human acute leukemia after transplantation into SCID mice. Nature 1994;367:645-648.

7 Namikawa R, Uedo R, Kyoizumi S. Growth of human myeloid leukemias in the human marrow environment of SCID-hy mice. Blood 1993;82:2526-2536.

8   Terstappen LWMM, Huang S, Safford M et al. Sequential generation of hematopoietic colonies from single non-lineage committed $CD34^+$ $CD38^-$ progenitor cells. Blood 1991;77:1218-1227.

9   Blair A, Ailles LE, Hogge DE et al. Phenotype of primitive AML cells which engraft NOD/SCID mice. Exp Hematol 1996;24:1126a.

10 Terstappen LWMM, Safford M, Unterhalt M et al. Flow cytometric characterization of acute myeloid leukemia: comparison to the differentiation pathway of normal hematopoietic progenitor cells. Leukemia 1992;6:993-1000.

11 Minden MD, McCulloch EA. Proliferative state of blast cell progenitors in acute myeloblastic leukemia. Blood 1978;52:592.

12 Lenz HJ, Manno DJ, Danenberg KD et al. Incorporation of 5-fluorouracil into U2 and U6 snRNA inhibits mRNA precursor splicing. J Biol Chem 1994;269:31962-31968.

13 Hodgson GS, Bradley TR. Properties of hematopoietic stem cells surviving 5-fluorouracil treatment. Evidence for a pre-CFU-S cell? Nature 1979;281:381.

14 Van Zant G. Studies of the hematopoietic stem cell spared by 5-fluorouracil. J Exp Med 1984;159:679.

15 Lerner C, Harrison DE. 5-fluorouracil spares hemopoietic stem cells responsible for long term repopulation. Exp Hematol 1990;18:114.

16 Stewart FM, Crittenden RB, Lowry PA et al. Long-term engraftment of normal and post-5-fluorouracil murine marrow into normal nonmyeloblated mice. Blood 1993;81:2566-2571.

17 Down JD, Ploemacher RE. Transient and permanent engraftment potential of murine hematopoietic stem cell subsets: differential effects of host conditioning with gamma-irradiation and cytostatic drugs. Exp Hematol 1993;21:913-921.

18 Brandt J, Baird N, Lu L et al. Characterization of a human hematopoietic progenitor cell capable of forming blast cell containing colonies in vitro. J Clin Invest 1988;82:1017-1027.

19 Stewart FM, Temeles D, Lowry PA et al. Post-5-fluorouracil human marrow: stem cell characteristics and renewal properties after autologous marrow transplantation. Blood 1993;81:2283-2289.

20 Berardi AC, Wang A, Levine JD et al. Functional isolation and characterization of human hematopoietic stem cells. Science 1995;267:104-108.

21 Griffin JD, Löwenberg B. Clonogenic cells in acute myeloblastic leukemia. Blood 1986;68:1185.

22 Down JD, Ploemacher RE. Transient and permanent engraftment potential of murine hematopoietic stem cell subsets: differential effects of host conditioning with gamma irradiation and cytostatic drugs. Exp Hematol 1993;21:913-921.

23 Down JD, Boudewijn A, Dillingh JH et al. Relationships between ablation of distinct hematopoietic cell subsets and the development of donor bone marrow engraftment following recipient pretreatment with different alkylating drugs. Br J Cancer 1994;70:611-616.

Definition of the Leukemic Stem Cell:
An Achievable Goal

P.J. QUESENBERRY,[a] **LUDWIKA KREJA**[b]

[a]Cancer Center, University of Massachusetts Medical Center,
Worcester, Massachusetts, USA; and [b]Department of Clinical Physiology,
Occupational and Social Medicine, University of Ulm, Ulm, Germany

The discussion of leukemic stem cells focused on the characterization and definition of this cell. *Dr. Robert Löwenberg* presented studies suggesting that leukemic cellular subsets could be characterized by assays involving growth in NOD-SCID mice, growth on stromal cell (cobblestone-forming area cell) or clonal colony growth in semisolid cultures. The cells were further characterized by expression of CD34. The meaning of these assays was extensively discussed. A critical issue was whether or not they truly represented stem cells for the leukemic process and, even, whether the concept of leukemic stem cells was valid.

The different assays might reflect different functional states of the same cell, possibly tied to the phase of cell cycle or other, separate parameter. Could leukemic cells which do not grow in any of the assays at a specific point in time express their ability to grow in NOD-SCID mice, on stroma or in culture at latter time points? Could the CFU become a NOD-SCID grower, etc., and could the function of these cells repeatedly fluctuate over time? It was generally acknowledged that the meaning of these assays was, as yet, unclear, and that their relationship to the many genetic changes and cytogenetic subtypes of leukemia not established.

Progressive genetic changes clearly occur in acute and chronic leukemias, apparently increasing the malignant nature of the leukemic cells. Do such changes occur in specific subtypes, and do such manipulations as autologous bone marrow transplantation select for cells with lesser genetic damage? Might cells with acquired genetic changes engraft less well, and thus transplantation select for a more benign form of the disease?

The studies presented by *Allen Eaves* could be viewed in the same light. Chronic myelogenous leukemic (CML) cells cultured under "Dexter"-like conditions may lose the leukemic stem/progenitor cell phenotype, and, when used for transplantation in support of high-dose approaches, can apparently give rise to prolonged survival, although usually in the presence of the leukemic clone. A major question here was whether the results using cultured CML cells are different from simply using CML marrow in an autologous transplant setting; this latter point appears not to have been settled.

Overall, from the viewpoint of the past 20 years, it appears that while we still do not have a reasonable characterization of the leukemic stem cell, the tremendous developments in molecular genetics, clonal assays, immunodeficient mouse models and cell separative approaches indicate that a true definition of this cell and validation of the stem cell concept should be forthcoming in the near future. At the present time, we have many intriguing questions awaiting answers.

Human Hematopoietic Progenitor in Bone Marrow and Peripheral Blood

H.A. Messner

Princess Margaret Hospital, Toronto, Ontario

Key Words. *Peripheral blood · Peripheral blood progenitor cell · Bone marrow transplants · Allografts · Autografts · CD34⁺ progenitors · Steady-state marrow*

ABSTRACT

The ability to enhance the frequency of progenitors in the peripheral circulation has resulted in peripheral blood progenitor cell collections being the preferred procurement method for autologous transplants and an accepted alternative for allografts. In autografts, peripheral blood-derived progenitor cells appear to have an advantage over conventional marrow transplants in the form of earlier engraftment without compromising sustained marrow function.

Studies were performed to evaluate the broad class of CD34⁺ progenitors and their subtypes in preparations of bone marrow and peripheral blood cells. As a result, peripheral blood appears to contain a larger quantity of more mature progenitors, which is the likely reason for a more rapid return of granulocytes and platelets. However, controveries continue to exist as to whether the measurements derived from these studies can be used to predict time to engraftnment and subsequent reestablishment of a marrow reserve. Some of these issues have been addressed in pilot studies where allografts using G-CSF-mobilized peripheral blood progenitor cells were compared to conventionally harvested bone marrow and bone marrow obtained from G-CSF-stimulated donors. The time to engraftment of neutrophils and platelets were shortened when G-CSF-mobilized peripheral blood or marrow progenitor cells were used compared to case-matched grafts of steady-state marrow. The significance of the suggested differences between steady-state bone marrow grafts and mobilized peripheral blood cells remains to be determined. However, preparations of cytokine-mobilized peripheral blood progenitor cell preparations are being used with increasing frequency to replace conventional marrow harvests. *Stem Cells 1998;16 (suppl 1):93-96*

INTRODUCTION

The presence of marrow-protecting cells in peripheral blood was first convincingly demonstrated by investigators using the elegant model of parabiotic animals that are surgically joined and share in their circulation. Radiation of one partner with dosages known to be lethal were survived through circulating blood cells from the healthy partner [1, 2]. The opportunity of using peripheral blood as a source of marrow repopulating cells was systematically explored in dogs [3-5] culminating in the successful clinical application of this technology [6]. Under steady-state conditions the method is limited by low yields achieved with individual collections. Pre-exposure to chemotherapy or cytokines enhances the content of early progenitors to facilitate engraftment by a small number of collections.

This observation supports the concept that the relevant cell populations are able to migrate freely under steady-state conditions and hemopoietic stress. It is now also understood that the actual number of progenitor cells found in the peripheral circulation are subject to diurnal variations [7, G. *Bjarnason,* personal communication]. The ability to enhance the frequency of progenitors in the peripheral circulation has resulted in peripheral blood progenitor cell collections as the preferred procurement method for autologous transplants and more recently as an accepted alternative for allografting. At least in autografts peripheral blood-derived progenitor cells appear to have advantages over conventional marrow transplants in the form of earlier engraftment without compromising sustained marrow function. This observation has prompted the question as to whether marrow-repopulating cells derived from alternative sources may differ in their quantity and/or biological properties. Studies to answer these questions became feasible after assays were established that permitted the quantitation of functionally determined progenitor populations. These techniques include the flow cytometric assessment of relevant surface markers that characterize progenitor cells, evaluation of their proliferative potential and ability to differentiate under defined culture conditions, and ultimately examination of their role to initiate and maintain hemopoiesis in vivo.

Characterization of Hemopoietic Progenitors

The most likely candidates for human marrow-repopulating cells express the CD34 antigen on their surface in the absence of HLA-DR or lineage-specific markers [8, 9]. In addition they are characterized by the expression of adhesion molecules and cytokine receptors. As demonstrated by embryonal stem cells, determinants such as CD34, *c-kit* and FLT2/FLK3 [10, 11] are expressed constitutively, although the level of expression may vary over time. As cells mature they acquire lineage-specific properties and/or markers of activation.

A number of studies were performed to evaluate the broad class of CD34$^+$ progenitors and their subtypes in preparations of bone marrow and peripheral blood cells. The proportion of CD34$^+$, HLA-DR⁻, Lin⁻ cells appears to be similar in both sources. Cells of this phenotype are able to initiate and sustain for some time the production of more mature pluripotent or lineage-restricted clonogenic progenitors in long-term cultures. In contrast CD34$^+$ cells with more mature phenotype (CD38$^+$, HLA-DR$^+$) are limited to colony formation in primary semisolid cultures or sustain liquid cultures for about two weeks [12, 13]. Peripheral blood appears to contain a larger quantity of more mature progenitors characterized by a CD34$^+$, CD38$^+$, Lin$^+$ phenotype. The presence of these more mature cells in peripheral blood-derived progenitor preparations is the likely reason for a more rapid return of granulocytes and platelets. Sustained engraftment in autologous peripheral blood transplants is usually observed, although it is not clear whether permanent hemopoiesis results from reinfused cells or endogeneous regeneration. The follow-up of peripheral blood-derived allografts is not as extensive. However, since late graft failures are not reported, it is likely that these allografts contain sufficient long-term marrow-repopulating cells.

Peripheral blood and marrow-derived CD34$^+$ cells differ in other aspects. The proportion of cycling cells as determined by CD71 expression is significantly higher in steady-state bone marrow compared to peripheral blood [14, 15]. In addition, bone marrow-derived CD34$^+$ cells contain higher proportions of cells expressing B cell markers but demonstrate lower levels of CD45 antigen [15].

Clinical Correlations

Extensive studies are available to evaluate bone marrow and peripheral blood-derived grafts using the above-mentioned parameters. While there is some understanding about the minimal number of progenitor cells as determined by flow cytometry or cell culture necessary for engraftment, controversies continue to exist about the notion that these measurements can be used to predict time to engraftment and subsequent re-establishment of a marrow reserve. The most optimistic data are presented for autografts where the engraftment process is less complicated through events related to prophylaxis for graft-versus-host-disease and treatment for viral complications.

We have addressed some of these issues in a series of pilot studies in which allografts using G-CSF-mobilized peripheral blood progenitor cells were compared to conventionally harvested bone marrow and bone marrow obtained from G-CSF-stimulated donors. The time to engraftment of neutrophils and platelets were shortened when G-CSF-mobilized peripheral blood or marrow progenitor cells were used compared to case-matched grafts of steady-state marrow. The median time to engraftment was 18 days for neutrophils from both sources, 21 days for platelets in peripheral blood grafts and 22 days for platelets from bone marrow grafts. The respective case-matched controls from steady-state conventionally harvested marrow showed neutrophil engraftment after 22.5 days and platelet engraftment after 27.5 days. It is of note that the time to engraftment was neither correlated with the number of CD34$^+$ cells nor with any one of the clonogenic cell populations which included colony-forming units (CFU)-blasts, CFU-granulocyte, erythroid, macrophage, megakaryocyte, CFU-granulocyte-macrophage, CFU-megakaryocyte and BFU-E.

These pilot studies are of interest. Whether the suggested differences between steady state bone marrow grafts and mobilized peripheral blood cells are of clinical significance remains to be evaluated by randomized studies. Besides the well-publicized study conducted by the European Bone Marrow Transplant Group, there are currently two studies under way to address this issue, one by the Canadian Bone Marrow Transplant Group and one by the Transplant Centre in Seattle.

CONCLUSIONS

Preparations of cytokine-mobilized peripheral blood progenitor cell preparations are being used with increasing frequency to replace conventional bone marrow harvests. While certain differences in the composition of CD34$^+$ subpopulations are detected, both sources are able to promote long-term engraftment. In autologous transplants the choice of peripheral blood cells appears to lead to a significant shortening of the time to engraftment, at least for some indications. While promising in pilot studies, the value and role of peripheral blood progenitor cells in allogeneic transplants remains to be determined.

REFERENCES

1 Woenckhaus, E. Beitrag zur Allgemeinwirkung der Roentgenstrahlen. Arch f Exp Path und Pharm 1930;150:182.

2 Brecher G, Cronkite EP. Post-radiation parabiosis and survival in rats. Proc Soc Exp Biol Med 1951;77:292-294.

3 Cavins JA, Scheer SC, Thomas ED et al. The recovery of lethally irradiated dogs given infusions of autologous leukocytes preserved at -80°C. Blood 1964;23:38-43.

4 Storb R, Epstein RB, Raçde H et al. Marrow engraftment by allogeneic leukocytes in lethally irradiated dogs. Blood 1967;30:805-811.

5 Fliedner TM, Flad HD, Bruch CH et al. Treatment of aplastic anemia by blood stem cell transfusion: a canine model. Haematologica 1967;61:141-148.

6 Körbling M, Dorken B, Ho AD et al. Autologous transplantation of blood-derived hemopoietic stem cells after myelablative therapy in a patient with Durkitt's lymphoma. Blood 1986;67:529-532.

7 Smaaland R, Laerum OD, Sothern RB et al. Colony-forming unit-granulocyte-macrophage and DNA synthesis of human bone marrow are circadian stage-dependent and show covariation. Blood 1992;79:2281-2287.

8 Berenson RJ, Andrews RG, Bensinger WI et al. Antigen CD34$^+$ marrow cells engraft lethally irradiated baboons. J Clin Invest 1988;81;951-955.

9 Sutherland HJ, Eaves HJ, Eaves CJ et al. Characterization and partial purification of human marrow cells capable of initiating long-term hematopoiesis in vitro. Blood 1989;74:1563-1570.

10 Yarden Y, Kuang W-J, Yang-Feng et al. Human proto-oncogene *c-kit*: a new cell surface receptor tyrosine kinase for an unidentified ligand. EMBO J 1987;6:3341-3351.

11 Rosent O, Schiff C, Pebusque J-J et al. Human FKT3/FLK2 gene; cDNA clone and expression in hematopoietic cells. Blood 1993;82:1110-1119.

12 Prosper F, Vanoverbeke K, Stroncek D et al. Primitive long-term culture initiating cells

(LTC-ICs) in granulocyte colony-stimulating factor mobilized peripheral blood progenitor cells have similar potential for ex vivo expansion as primitive LTC-ICs in steady state bone marrow. Blood 1997;89:3991-3997.

13 de Wynter EA, Nadali G, Coutinho LH et al. Extensive amplification of single cells from CD34[+] subpopulations in umbilical cord blood and identification of long-term culture-initiating cells is present in two subsets. STEM CELLS 1996;14:566-576.

14 Bender JG, Unverzagt KL, Walker DE et al. Identification and comparison of CD34-positive cells and their subpopulations from normal peripheral blood and bone marrow using multicolor flow cytometry. Blood 1991;77:2591-2596.

15 Rumi C, Rutella S, Teofili L et al. RhG-CSF-mobilized CD34[+] peripheral blood progenitors are myeloperoxidase-negative and noncycling irrespective of CD33 or CD13 coexpression. Exp Hematol 1997;25:246-251.

Hemopoietic Progenitor Cells in the Blood as Indicators of the Functional Status of the Bone Marrow after Total-Body and Partial-Body Irradiation: Experiences from Studies in Dogs

WILHELM NOTHDURFT,[a] LUDWIKA KREJA[b]

[a]Department of Radiotherapy and [b]Department of Clinical Physiology, Occupational and Social Medicine, University of Ulm, Ulm, Germany

Key Words. GM-CFC · Peripheral blood · Indicators · Bone marrow function · Dogs · Total-body irradiation · Partial-body irradiation

ABSTRACT

The granulocyte-macrophage colony-forming cells (GM-CFC) were studied in the blood of dogs to evaluate their relationship to the bone marrow GM-CFC under normal conditions and their involvement in hemopoietic regeneration after different types of exposure to ionizing radiation. The GM-CFC could be defined as regular blood elements showing characteristic levels of their concentration in individual dogs in the range from 20 to 300 cells per ml. In relative terms, the GM-CFC numbers present in the whole blood of normal dogs were found to be on the order of 0.1% of the GM-CFC numbers present in the bone marrow. A small fraction of the GM-CFC population in the bone marrow, i.e., about 1%, can be mobilized into the peripheral blood within three h by intravenous injection of dextran sulfate (DS). These cells are characterized by a small size and a low S-phase fraction similar to the GM-CFC that are normally present in the blood.

Total-body irradiation with single doses of 0.8 Gy and more caused a characteristic pattern of sequential changes in the blood GM-CFC concentration that were related to the recovery of the bone marrow GM-CFC population. The blood GM-CFC concentration showed an extreme depression within the first 15 days, a transient increase from day 17 to day 35 and remained at subnormal values for several weeks and months. The regeneration of the GM-CFC population in the bone marrow that could be mobilized into the blood by DS was similarly delayed as the recovery of the blood GM-CFC values.

In dogs which were kept under continuous radiation exposure (0.019 Gy/day) causing permanent damage to the hemopoietic system, the GM-CFC numbers in the blood remained permanently depressed. Partial-body irradiation of dogs with a myeloablative dose (11.7 Gy) given to the anterior part of their body was followed by sequential changes in the blood GM-CFC concentration specific for this type of exposure. The pattern of changes was determined by direct radiation effects, the compensatory responses in the protected bone marrow and the regeneration events in the irradiated bone marrow. On the other hand, it could be shown that the repopulation and the restoration of the hemopoietic tissue is initiated by the seeding of hemopoietic cells (including GM-CFC) from the protected marrow. *Stem Cells 1998;16(suppl 1):97-111*

INTRODUCTION

In the 1970s conclusive evidence had accumulated indicating that hemopoietic progenitor cells and stem cells are present in the blood not only of rodents, but of the mammalian organism in general. The role of these elements in hemopoiesis under normal as well as pathophysiological conditions has been studied with increasing interest in different experimental models and clinical situations. The various facets of this field of research and the progress achieved in the last decades are reviewed in this issue in considerable detail by *Fliedner* [1]. This review makes reference to some of our studies performed on dogs to examine the response of the hemopoietic system to exposures to ionizing radiation under different conditions.

The fact that the hemopoietic cell populations in the peripheral blood had to be understood as integrating elements of the hemopoietic system led us to suppose that these cell populations could be sensitive indicators of radiation-induced damage to the hemopoietic tissues for several reasons. Any damage to the active bone marrow, homogeneous or local nature, could be expected to interfere with the dynamic equilibrium between the hemopoietic cell populations in the bone marrow on the one hand and in the peripheral blood on the other. As a consequence the hemopoietic cell populations could be expected to respond to radiation exposures in a sensitive fashion.

This paper will give a review of the radiohematological research performed in dogs, in which special attention was paid to the response of the granulocyte-macrophage progenitor cells (GM-CFC) in the blood to total-body irradiation (TBI) and partial-body irradiation. The biology of this type of cell in dogs under normal conditions will be considered in the first section of this article.

RESULTS

Characterization of GM-CFC in Canine Blood

GM-CFC Concentration in Blood

Sequential determinations of the GM-CFC concentration in the blood over periods of several weeks to months until one year revealed characteristic levels of the average GM-CFC numbers per ml blood in individual dogs. Fluctuations of the actual daily values around this mean were remarkably small in several of the animals studied, but could amount by a factor of two or more in other dogs for unknown reasons. Typical numbers per 1 ml obtained for five dogs studied in initial experiments over a period of 80 days (three to six times a week) were (mean $\pm$ 1 SD): 27 ± 21, 181 ± 93, 205 ± 107, 313 ± 148 and 341 ± 117 [2].

GM-CFC Pools

Under steady-state conditions of hemopoiesis, the GM-CFC is distributed over three main organ systems. The number of GM-CFC in the whole blood volume is on the order of 0.1% of the total number present in the normal dog; 96% to 99% are found in the bone marrow and 1% to 4% are present in the spleen [3-6]. However, in five dogs studied in more detail, no correlation was found between the total numbers of GM-CFC in bone marrow on the one hand and in the blood on the other [3]. Comparative analyses of blood-derived GM-CFC and GM-CFC from bone marrow revealed that the GM-CFC in the blood constitute quite a homogenous population of small cells with a low proliferation rate (i.e., small S-phase fraction) in comparison to the bone marrow GM-CFC population, for which much broader cell-size distribution profiles with higher mean values of cell size and a larger S-phase fraction were obtained [7]. The GM-CFC in the spleen are characterized by an S-phase fraction of about 16%, i.e., as small as in the GM-CFC population in the blood, indicating that the GM-CFC residing in the spleen are a major fraction of the GM-CFC population in the blood [4].

Migratory GM-CFC in the Bone Marrow

Among the heterogeneous GM-CFC population in the bone marrow there is a small subpopulation of cells that is able to emigrate from the extravascular sites and to enter the blood (migratory GM-CFC), in contrast to the major fraction.

A rapid rise in the GM-CFC concentration in the blood is obtained after intravenous injections of the heparin-like compound dextran sulfate ([DS], mw=10,000) with the maximum values obtained after about three h after injection [8]. This increase was interpreted as a result of mobilization of the migratory GM-CFC, though the mechanisms leading to the transient accumulation remained unclear (Fig. 1). Based on the maximum increases obtained in the blood GM-CFC concentrations after DS injection, it was calculated that the size of the migratory GM-CFC population was on the order of 1% of the total bone marrow GM-CFC population [5]. These cells are characterized by a low proliferation rate and their small size similar to those present in the blood under normal conditions [7], indicating that both the migratory cells in the bone marrow and the GM-CFC present in the peripheral blood (and in the spleen) represent members of the same subpopulation distributed over different organs.

The mean transit time for GM-CFC in the blood as derived from the kinetics of DS-mobilized GM-CFC has been determined to be on the order of 1.4 h [5]. Another approach to study the kinetics of GM-CFC migration and to estimate the pool size of cells involved was the collection of GM-CFC from the blood by continuous leukapheresis [1].

The Role of the Spleen

A splenectomy did not influence the GM-CFC concentration in the blood of individual dogs long-term, i.e., after splenectomy the blood GM-CFC concentration remained within the same range as before [3]. The mobilization test with DS performed in splenectomized dogs revealed quantitative correlations between the GM-CFC in the blood and the DS-mobilizable population similar to those as obtained from dogs with their spleen present.

TBI

Short Single Exposures with Uniform Dose Distributions

The first experimental approach was to study the response of the blood GM-CFC to short single exposures to TBI. The dogs were exposed to an x-ray beam bilaterally receiving TBI with increasing doses in the range from 0.2 Gy to 0.8 Gy at homogeneous dose distributions [2].

The curves obtained for the blood granulocyte counts showed no clear changes in the dogs irradiated with 0.4 Gy, although characteristic marginal alterations were found after the higher dose of 0.8 Gy within the first 25 days after TBI. Similarly, the lymphocytes showed no radiation-associated changes after 0.2 and 0.4 Gy (Fig. 2). However, a significant depression and slow recovery took place in dogs receiving the largest dose of 0.8 Gy.

In contrast, the blood GM-CFC showed a slight but lasting depression in the dogs which had received a dose of 0.4 Gy (Fig. 3). The higher dose of 0.8 Gy was clearly followed by an immediate reduction of the GM-CFC numbers within 24 h to extremely low levels of about 5% of the average initial values. This effect was much

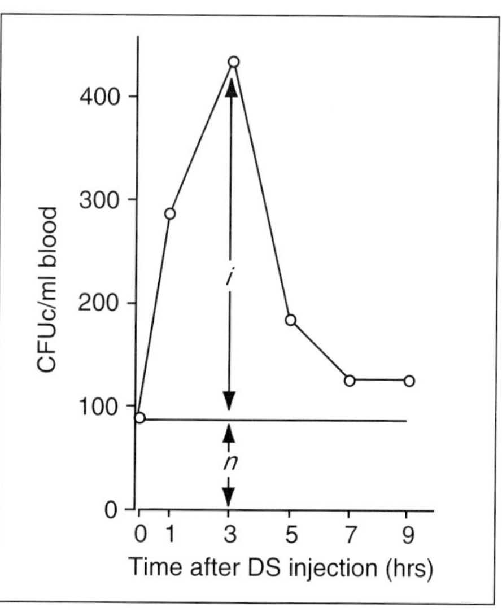

Figure 1. Typical curve of the time-dependent changes in the GM-CFC concentration in the blood of a normal dog after intravenous injection of DS. Parameter (i) is the maximum increase in the GM-CFC concentration over the normal value (n) just before the injection. Reprinted, with modifications, with permission from [5].

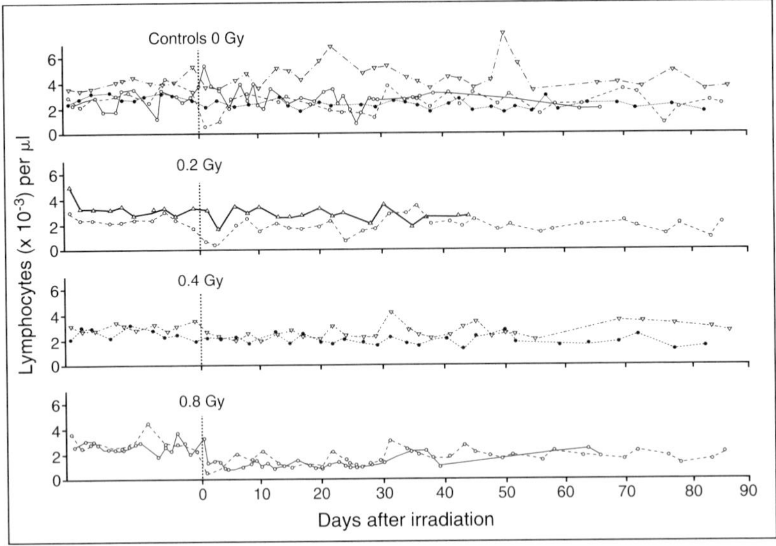

Figure 2. Sequential changes in the blood lymphocyte concentration of dogs after TBI with increasing radiation doses given in a single session. Reprinted with permission from [2].

stronger than the immediate response of the lymphocytes. Furthermore, the recovery of the GM-CFC population was extremely delayed for more than three months. There seemed to be a certain response pattern, characterized by an increase in GM-CFC numbers between day 17 and day 35 to 40, a certain decrease thereafter and a stabilization at subnormal levels in the later period.

Reduced Mobilizable GM-CFC Population

To get insight into mechanisms possibly involved in the radiation-induced progenitor cell reduction, another experiment was performed [9]. Two reasonable approaches were employed in this study to characterize both the bone marrow and the blood GM-CFC populations and their functional relationship to each other: A) The mobilization assay by means of DS that allows estimation of the pool size of migratory GM-CFC in the bone marrow and B) determinations of the cell-size distribution profiles for blood and bone marrow GM-CFC by means of velocity sedimentation separation [7].

In these experiments the dogs received TBI with radiation doses of 0.8 Gy or 1.6 Gy. The mobilization test with DS (standard dosage 15 mg/kg) was performed at regular intervals before and after irradiation.

Both radiation doses caused a strong and lasting depression of the blood GM-CFC numbers (Fig. 4).

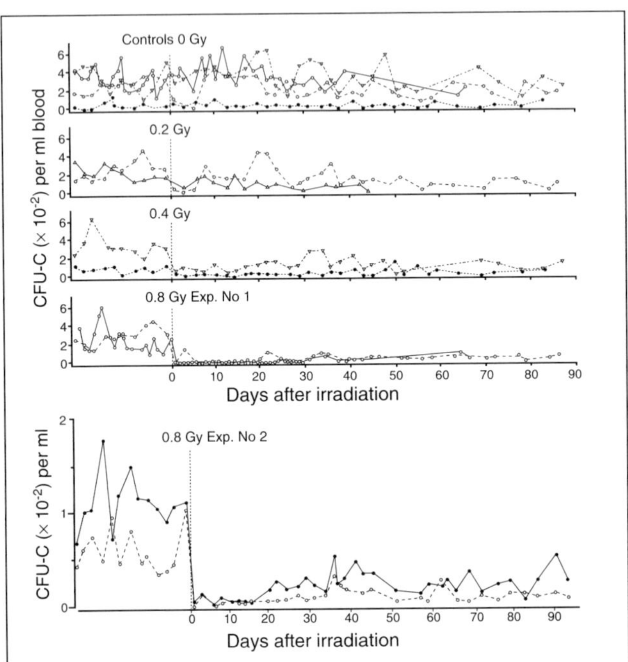

Figure 3. Sequential changes in the blood GM-CFC concentration of dogs after TBI with increasing radiation doses given in a single session. Reprinted with permission from [2].

The effect was independent of the initial normal GM-CFC concentration in that in the animals receiving 0.8 Gy, the concentration was higher than in those receiving the higher radiation dose. The pattern of changes was similar to that in the 0.8 Gy-irradiated dogs as shown before. In any case the GM-CFC numbers increased in the period up to day 40, but showed no further increase thereafter and remained at subnormal levels (50% to 60% of normal) until day 160 after TBI.

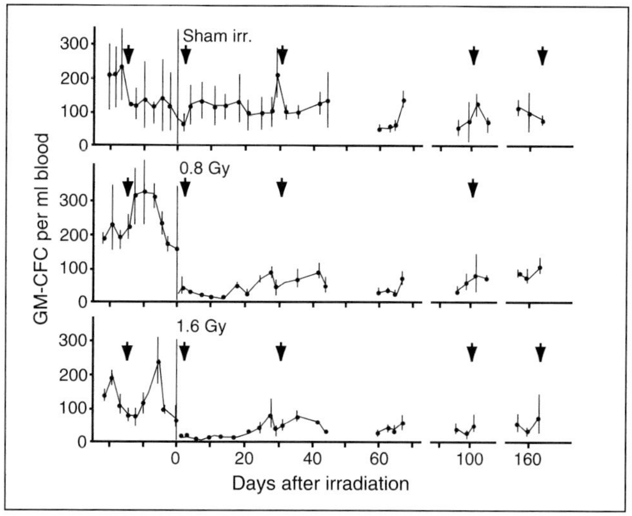

Figure 4. Sequential changes in the blood GM-CFC concentration of dogs after TBI with a radiation dose of 0.8 Gy or 1.6 Gy given in a single session. The arrows mark the days on which the mobilization test with dextran sulfate was performed. Reprinted with permission from [9].

For each mobilization test performed in all the animals before TBI or sham-irradiation, the maximum net increase in the blood GM-CFC concentration was plotted versus the individual initial GM-CFC concentration (Fig. 5A). A statistical correlation is observed; there is a quantitative relationship (within limits) between the GM-CFC numbers actually found in the peripheral blood and the size of a certain GM-CFC subpopulation in the bone marrow that could rapidly be mobilized into the blood by DS.

The DS mobilization test was performed in the irradiated animals at day 2, day 30, day 100 and day 160 after TBI. A correlation similar to that as shown for dogs with a normal hematological status was obtained for the irradiated animals (Fig. 5B). But in contrast, a large portion of all the values was within the lower left area of the graph compared to the values obtained for nonexposed animals. Thus, from these differences it can be concluded that in the course of regeneration until 160 days after TBI, the pool size of the mobilizable GM-CFC in the bone marrow was reduced in a fashion as indicated

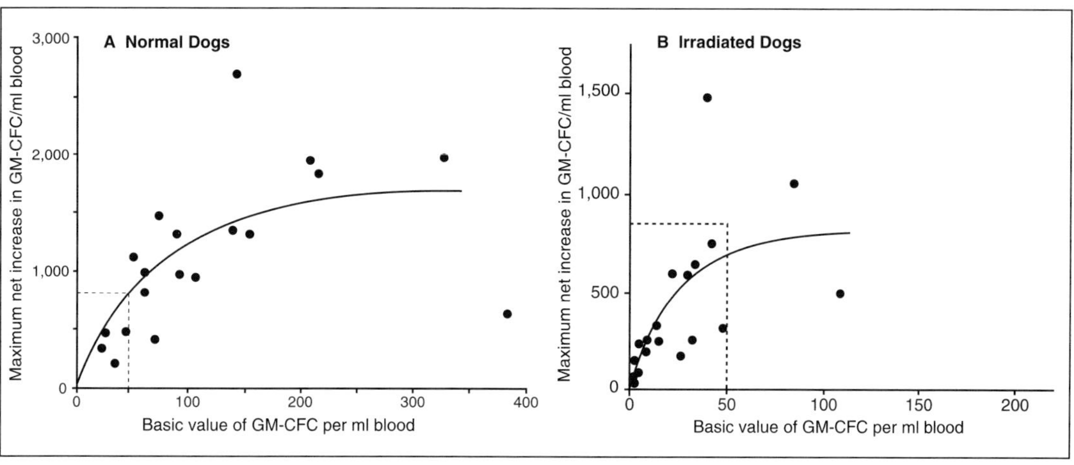

Figure 5. Correlations between the number of mobilizable GM-CFC and the basic value before the DS injection (A) in normal dogs and (B) in irradiated dogs at different times after TBI with a radiation dose of 0.8 Gy or 1.6 Gy (Fig. 4). Reprinted with permission from [9].

by the subnormal blood GM-CFC levels.

The findings obtained from the analyses of bone marrow GM-CFC by velocity sedimentation separation showed that in the irradiated dogs, the portion of GM-CFC with the smaller volume (constituting the migratory subpopulation [7]) was strongly reduced after TBI [10].

The Role of the Spleen

The impact of the spleen on the response of the blood GM-CFC was examined in dogs which underwent splenectomy and were exposed to TBI (radiation dose 0.8 Gy) 23 weeks after surgery. The radiation-induced alterations in the blood GM-CFC values in sham-operated animals were similar to those presented in Fig. 3, i.e., about day 90 after TBI the values had recovered to 30% of the preirradiation levels. In the splenectomized animals the regeneration of the blood GM-CFC was faster. There was a stronger increase between day 17 and 40, and at day 80 to 90 the GM-CFC values in the splenectomized animals had recovered to about 60% of the preirradiation levels. The DS mobilization test performed in splenectomized dogs after TBI (0.8 Gy) revealed quantitative correlations between the GM-CFC in the blood and the mobilizable population similar to those as obtained for irradiated dogs with their spleen present.

Repeated Exposures to Small Doses

In view of the strong response of the blood GM-CFC population to relatively small doses of TBI, it was of interest to study the alterations of the indicator system to repeated exposures to small radiation doses. Two dogs received four exposures to 0.2 Gy, each given at intervals of 10 or 11 days between each TBI (*Nothdurft et al.,* unpublished). No clear changes of the GM-CFC concentration could be detected within the 10 day intervals following the first or second irradiation. However, the third exposure (i.e., the cumulative dose of 0.6 Gy) was followed by a clear decrease of the GM-CFC concentration in the blood to about 20% of the initial values. The fourth exposure caused a further depression. The recovery process was extremely delayed and at day 120 after the last TBI, the GM-CFC had recovered to about 40% to 50% of their initial concentration. These numbers were slightly above the level of about 30% to 40% obtained for dogs, which had received the same total dose of 0.8 Gy, but in a single exposure.

Continuous TBI of Low-Dose Rate

In studies performed at the Argonne National Laboratory (USA), dogs were exposed to continuous TBI by γ-rays from a Co-60 source with daily doses of 0.019 Gy for indefinite times [11]. The counts of the blood lymphocytes, neutrophilic granulocytes and thrombocytes uniformly showed decreases within the first 200 to 500 days corresponding to cumulative doses in the range from 3.8 to 9 Gy, but remained stable at subnormal levels in the period of 1,700 days of exposure. The erythrocyte concentration showed minor changes only at cumulative doses in the range of 20 to 35 Gy. The GM-CFC numbers in bone marrow samples from the ribs showed a strong decrease within the first 150 days of exposure at cumulative doses of about 3 Gy, preceding the changes of the blood granulocyte concentration (Fig. 6A). A transient partial recovery of the GM-CFC was observed at later times followed by another decrease to extremely low values at cumulative doses in the range of 32 Gy. The blood GM-CFC showed a response pattern corresponding to the alterations in the GM-CFC numbers in the bone marrow (Fig. 6B): a strong initial decrease at doses in the range of up to 3 Gy was followed by a persistent depression of the GM-CFC numbers under cumulative doses to 32 Gy.

Inhomogeneous Dose Distribution

An experiment was performed to test the concept that exposures to TBI under conditions of different dose distributions should cause similar patterns of response of the blood GM-CFC if in either case the degree of overall systemic damage to the bone marrow would have been the same [12]. Three dogs received TBI by bilateral exposure resulting in a rather homogeneous dose distribution with bone marrow doses generated in different sites varying from 1.5 Gy to 2.0 Gy at most. In contrast, another six dogs were exposed to the beam of the x-ray machine from one side only, resulting in an inhomogeneous distribution with a gradient of bone marrow doses ranging from 0.9 Gy (iliac crest, right side) to 3.1 Gy (head of the humerus, left side) as the extremes. The total survival fractions of the bone marrow GM-CFC were in the range of 6.7% and 7.7%, respectively, i.e., rather similar for both exposure conditions.

The pattern of changes in the blood granulocyte and lymphocyte concentrations was similar in both groups of dogs until day 370 after exposure. The lymphocyte counts were nearly normal at this

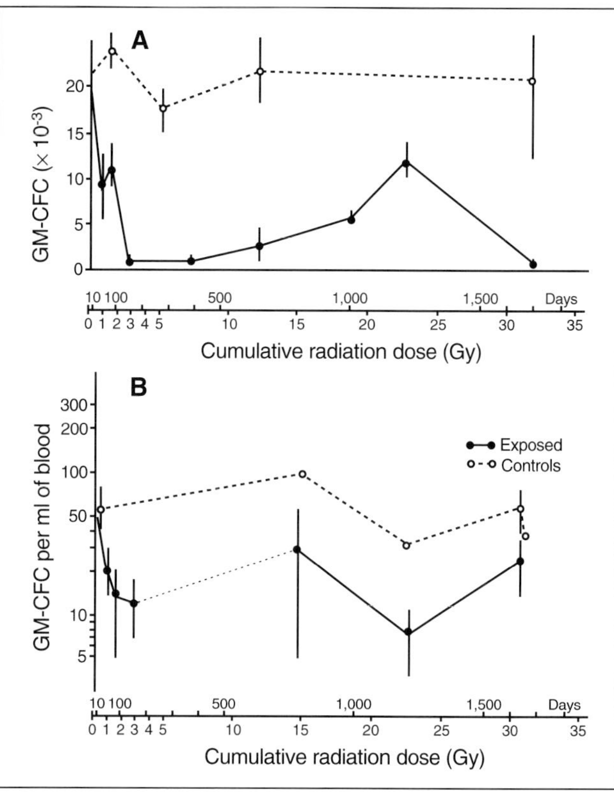

Figure 6. Sequential changes (A) in the total numbers of GM-CFC in the bone marrow from a piece of the rib and (B) in the GM-CFC concentration in the blood in dogs during continuous low-dose rate exposure to 0.019 Gy/day. Mean values obtained from irradiated animals (•) and nonexposed dogs (○). Reprinted, with modifications, with permission from [11].

latter time, in contrast to the granulocyte concentration that had recovered to 70% or 75% of the initial values, i.e., in either case they remained clearly subnormal. On the other hand, the thrombocyte concentration, also showing an extreme depression between day 10 and day 20 after TBI, was nearly normal or normal in the period from day 30 to one year after the exposure in both groups of dogs. Similarly, the parameters of the erythroid lineage after initial decreases between day 11 and 21 days after TBI showed complete recovery, i.e., no long-term residual defects [13].

The pattern of radiation-induced alterations in the blood GM-CFC concentration also was rather similar in both groups of dogs, indicating that a comparable degree of systemic damage to the bone marrow GM-CFC population indeed was expressed in corresponding changes in the migratory GM-CFC population (Fig. 7). Furthermore, the extremely reduced values from day 1 to day 20 in both curves do reflect the extreme damage to the bone marrow GM-CFC population. The characteristic increase in the blood GM-CFC concentration thereafter in the period until day 35 paralleled the strong rise in the bone marrow GM-CFC concentration within the same time interval. However, the blood GM-CFC remained clearly subnormal for at least one year, reflecting persistent residual damage to the granulocyte progenitor cell system as was also reflected in the blood granulocyte values.

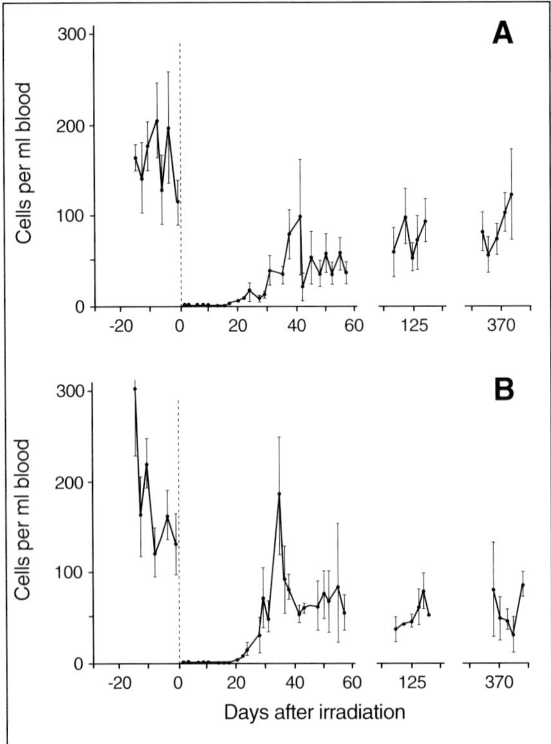

Figure 7. Sequential changes in the concentration of GM-CFC in the blood of dogs after TBI given by (A) a unilateral exposure (inhomogenous dose distribution) and (B) bilateral exposure (homogenous dose distribution). Reprinted with permission from [12].

Partial-Body Irradiation

General Aspects

Partial-body irradiation will reduce the numbers of proliferative cells in the irradiated volume in an exponential fashion, but leave certain fractions of the hemopoietic cell populations undamaged, depending on the amount of bone marrow protected. This is in contrast to TBI with homogeneous or inhomogeneous dose distributions.

Recent experiments were performed on dogs which were exposed with their anterior part to a single dose of 11.7 Gy. Under these conditions about 72% of the total bone marrow mass was included in the irradiated volume [14]. The experiments had two aims: A) to study in detail the involvement of the GM-CFC in the blood in bone marrow regeneration and B) to try to accelerate the reconstitution of the hemopoietic tissue in the aplastic sites by means of therapeutic treatment with growth factors. The essential findings are considered in the following paragraphs. For details see *Nothdurft et al.* [15].

GM-CFC in the Blood in Relation to Overall Hemopoietic Activity

The GM-CFC in the blood were extremely depressed within the first seven days after the exposure (Fig. 8). An increase associated with considerable fluctuations took place at about day 10 approaching the maximum about day 25. Thereafter, the GM-CFC decreased again and remained subnormal to at least day 70.

The GM-CFC in the irradiated bone marrow (humerus and sternum) were reduced (as expected) 24 h after the exposure by nearly five orders of magnitude of the initial values to extremely low numbers (Fig. 8). Similar depressions were observed for the BFU-E. Repopulation took place in an exponential fashion in the period to day 21, followed by a further modest increase in the period to day 35 when the GM-CFC had recovered to 40% of the initial value. Thereafter the GM-CFC numbers decreased again and remained reduced until at least day 70, but were back within the normal range at about day 170 after the exposure.

The absolute GM-CFC numbers in the protected marrow as represented by the iliac crest clearly showed an abscopal response to the eradication of the major fraction of the total bone marrow mass (Fig. 8). This was characterized by a decrease in the first seven days and a recovery in the period to day 21. Interestingly, the GM-CFC (and BFU-E) decreased thereafter similarly to those in the irradiated bone marrow and also remained subnormal in the interval to at least day 70.

It becomes evident that there is a close interrelationship between the pattern of the blood GM-CFC changes on the one hand and the radiation-induced alterations in both the irradiated as well as the protected bone marrow on the other (see **Discussion**).

Interestingly, the granulocyte counts in the blood showed a transient recovery (after the strong initial cytopenia) to normal values in the period from day 25 to day 35, but thereafter decreased again and showed subnormal values in the interval between day 40 to day 80. In contrast, the thrombocyte counts and erythrocyte counts, after having recovered from the initial reduction about 30 days after the exposure remained stable within the range of the preirradiation values.

Growth Factor-Stimulated Progenitor Cell Migration

The concept of the therapeutic approaches was as follows: an early expansion of the migratory cell populations in the protected bone marrow should increase the seeding rate to the irradiated sites and thus accelerate the repopulation [15].

Three dogs received treatment with recombinant human (rHu)G-CSF (Filgrastim) for seven days (daily dosage 2 × 15 µg/kg) after partial-body irradiation, starting with the subcutaneous injections 24 h after the exposure. The essential findings are presented in Figure 8. G-CSF clearly increased the GM-CFC concentration in the blood in comparison to the controls within two to three days of treatment and caused a strong transient rise between day 5 and day 15 after partial-body irradiation (Fig. 8, upper panel). However in the period from day 45 to day 70, the values were subnormal, similar to those in the controls.

As becomes evident from the curve in Figure 8 (middle panel), the expansion of the migratory GM-CFC population within the first 15 to 21 days clearly was associated with an accelerated regeneration of the GM-CFC (but also of the BFU-E and the absolute cell num-

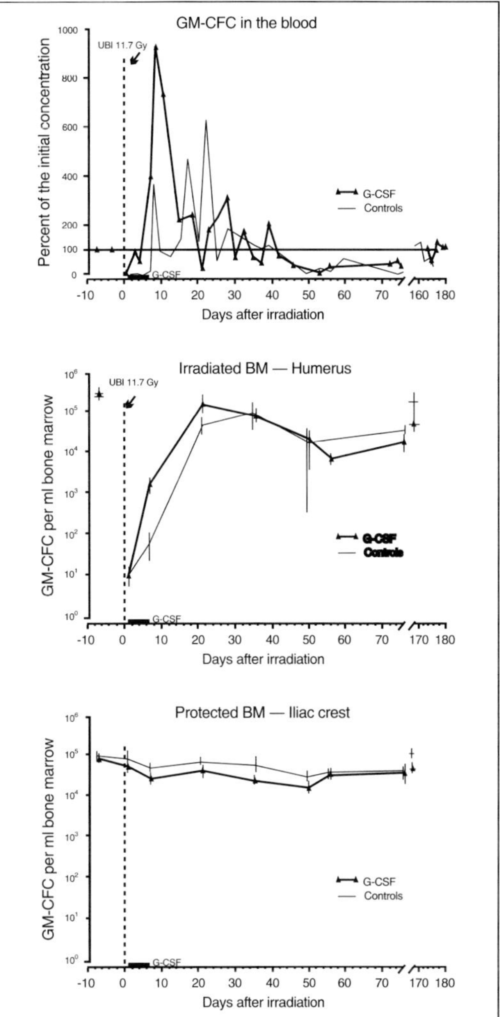

Figure 8. Sequential changes in the concentration of GM-CFC in the blood, in the irradiated bone marrow of the humerus and in the protected bone marrow of the iliac crest in dogs after irradiation with a dose of 11.7 Gy given to the anterior part of the body. Controls (—): *three dogs received injections of saline for seven days; G-CSF (▲–▲): three dogs received subcutaneous injections of rHuG-CSF (Filgrastim; 2 × 15 µg/kg/day) for seven days starting the day after the exposure. Reprinted, with modifications, with permission from [15].*

bers) in the irradiated bone marrow sites up to day 21, but no longer. On the other hand, no clear effect of the G-CSF treatment (when compared to the controls) could be detected in the protected bone marrow on the basis of the determinations of the GM-CFC numbers (Fig. 8, lower panel), the BFU-E and the cellularity.

It is of interest to notice that in the G-CSF-treated animals, the blood GM-CFC values between day 45 and day 70 showed a similar depression as established in the control animals, and that this depression also was associated with decreasing GM-CFC numbers in the irradiated as well as protected bone marrow.

Kinetics of Cells with DNA Damage

The assessment of cells with radiation-induced DNA damage in the peripheral blood and in samples from the irradiated as well as protected bone marrow was performed by means of the comet assay according to *Singh et al.* [16] with slight modifications [17]. In these studies a value of three for the tail-moment (TM) was applied as the minimum value for defining a significant amount of radiation-induced genomic damage. Since in the present studies no gross differences could be detected between the sequential findings obtained from the animals of the different treatment groups, the data obtained from five to eight dogs were processed and evaluated collectively.

The pattern of sequential changes in the frequency of cells in the bone marrow with TM>3 is shown in Figure 9. On day 1 after the exposure, cells with TM>3 clearly were more frequent in the protected bone marrow than in the irradiated sites (in which the absolute cell numbers were reduced to less than 10% of the initial value). At day 7 and in the following time up to one year after the exposure, the frequency of strongly damaged cells was statistically not different between the irradiated and protected marrow sites. There was an increasing trend in the proportion of cells with a TM>3 in the irradiated as well as the nonexposed marrow in the period until day 35 to 50 after irradiation and a decrease thereafter to the normal preirradiation range. In contrast, the peripheral blood cells with TM>3 were most frequent in the first hours after irradiation (Fig. 9). One week after the exposure the proportion of cells with TM>3 was in the range characteristic for normal animals and remained at that level at least up to one year after irradiation.

DISCUSSION

Normal Dogs

The findings obtained in normal dogs with different experimental approaches indicate that the GM-CFC in the peripheral blood represent a subgroup of cells from the whole GM-CFC compartment that are characterized by a relatively small size and a low S-phase fraction in comparison to the bone marrow. However, it has not definitely been shown whether these cells, including those present in the spleen and those in the bone marrow that can be mobilized into the blood by DS or leukapheresis, constitute an

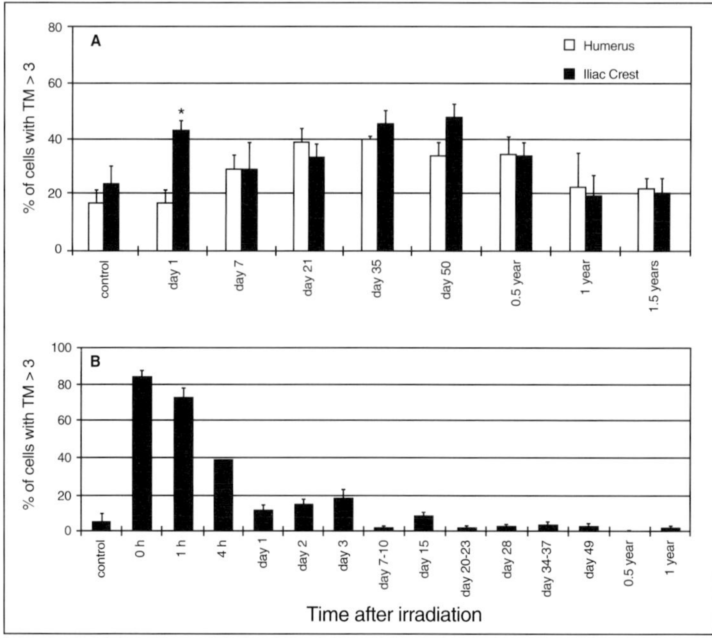

Figure 9. Relative numbers of cells with DNA damage as assessed by the comet assay (A) in the bone marrow of the irradiated humerus and the protected iliac crest and (B) in the blood of dogs after irradiation of the anterior part of the body with a dose of 11.7 Gy. Reprinted with permission from [32].

immature subpopulation of the heterogeneous GM-CFC compartment. Alternatively, these cells may be G_1 cells from subpopulations at different stages in the hierarchy of GM-CFC that preferentially are released from the marrow, in contrast to cells in the other phases of the cell cycle. The fact that the total number of migratory GM-CFC is small in comparison to the whole bone marrow GM-CFC population supports the first assumption. Eventually, both the mechanisms under consideration may be operative.

The close quantitative correlations between the GM-CFC number present in the blood of individual dogs at any time and the migratory GM-CFC population in the bone marrow as evidenced by the mobilization assay by means of DS indicates that there is indeed a quantitative relationship between both pools on the basis of a rapid exchange [5], i.e., the cells present in the blood are an indicator of that subpopulation of GM-CFC in the bone marrow that is able to migrate. On the other hand, the relationship between the blood GM-CFC and the bone marrow GM-CFC population as a whole seems to be more complex [3].

Progenitor cell migration in man shows similar characteristics as described for the dog. GM-CFC obtained from the peripheral blood are smaller than most of those present in the bone marrow and show an S-phase fraction smaller than the latter [18-20]. The latter also holds true for pluripotent hemopoietic progenitor cells [21]. Recent studies performed on $CD34^+$ cells from blood and bone marrow have confirmed these earlier results, showing that progenitor cells present in the blood under normal conditions and in the course of "mobilization" under the influence of G-CSF or GM-CSF are not in S/G_2-M, in contrast to the cells from the bone marrow [22-24].

Radiation-Induced Alterations—General Aspects

The results obtained from irradiated dogs—taken together—indicate that for any condition of radiation exposure tested, pronounced responses of the blood GM-CFC population could be established. In any case, among the different blood elements, the GM-CFC in the blood showed the strongest immediate reduction. Specifically, after TBI under different conditions as well as after extended-field partial-body irradiation, the GM-CFC number in the peripheral blood was reduced more strongly in the first week than the lymphocyte counts. The particularly sensitive response of the lymphocytes to any form of radiation exposure is well established [25-27].

After TBI or partial-body irradiation, the blood GM-CFC showed characteristic patterns of sequential changes each in association to the regeneration events in the bone marrow. In contrast, the lymphocyte counts showed a rather uniform pattern of response independent of the type of the exposure, i.e., the strongest reduction within the first three days after irradiation followed by a continuous increase in the weeks and months thereafter.

TBI

TBI was followed by a comparatively strong reduction of the blood GM-CFC concentration within at least 24 h. This effect can be related in part to the fact that during the exposure, major fractions of those cell populations were sterilized that actually were present in the circulation as well as those that were located in the bone marrow constituting the migratory GM-CFC. However, there must have been an additional mechanism interfering with the release of GM-CFC from marrow, probably the early initial events of hemopoietic regeneration. In fact, the typical pattern of the blood GM-CFC changes is a reflection of the radiation-induced alterations in the bone marrow GM-CFC and their recovery, as evidenced in several of the studies under consideration [2, 9, 10, 12].

The regeneration events in the bone marrow were characterized by low GM-CFC concentrations for about 14 days after irradiation associated with a strongly elevated S-phase fraction in the first 14 to 21 days (depending on the radiation dose), thus indicating that the GM-CFC were strongly proliferating but also differentiating. Just in this phase the blood GM-CFC showed their strongest depression, which is in accordance with the observation that under normal conditions, S-phase cells are rare within the blood GM-CFC population. In the interval from day 20 to 35, when the blood GM-CFC values showed their strongest increase, the bone marrow GM-CFC concentration also showed their strongest rise (indicating an increasing pool size) and a decreasing S-phase fraction tending to the normal value.

However, at the end of this transient recovery phase, the blood GM-CFC concentration remained at clearly subnormal levels after radiation doses of 0.8 Gy and more given in a single session (or in four fractions), and showed only minimum further recovery in the weeks and months thereafter signaling residual alterations in the bone marrow GM-CFC compartment.

The results obtained by the GM-CFC mobilization test by means of DS in dogs which had been exposed to TBI (0.8 and 1.6 Gy) are support for the assumption that the persisting subnormal blood GM-CFC values were due to a delayed reconstitution of the migratory GM-CFC population in the bone marrow [9], the mechanisms of which are not understood.

In view of the lasting depression of the GM-CFC concentration in the blood as a consequence of TBI with a single dose, it is not surprising that the blood GM-CFC values were found permanently depressed in dogs which were continuously exposed, due to the permanent damage to the granulocytic system, that in part was compensated by an increased proliferation rate [11].

To evaluate the significance of the findings obtained from dogs, attention should be paid to reports from some other experimental studies in which the radiation response of hemopoietic cells in the blood after TBI was examined. In mice TBI with doses of 3.5 Gy or 7 Gy caused a reduction of colony-forming units-spleen (CFU-S) in the blood to extremely low numbers in the first seven days [28]. Thereafter the CFU-S values per ml increased, and between day 10 to day 63 they were temporarily higher after the larger dose than after the lower one. On the other hand, the studies by *Micklem et al.* [29] show that after TBI, stem cell migration was significantly involved in hemopoietic regeneration only after a large dose, i.e., 6 Gy that caused an extreme depletion of the stem cell pool distributed over the whole skeleton, but not after smaller doses employed (1 Gy and 3.5 Gy).

The sequential alterations in the concentration of $CD34^+$ cells in the blood of monkeys were studied after TBI with a single dose of 5 Gy [30]. A slight increase in the numbers of $CD34^+$ cells per ml was already found on the first day after the exposure followed by elevated levels until at least day 28. It cannot be excluded that certain clonogenic subpopulations of this group of cells, e.g., GM-CFC, may show a somewhat different pattern of alterations due to specific mechanisms of cell migration during hemopoietic regeneration.

Partial-Body Irradiation

The response pattern of the blood GM-CFC after partial-body irradiation shows certain similarities to the alterations as observed after TBI, but also characteristics associated with this type of exposure. Generally, the mechanisms determining the GM-CFC concentration in the blood were more complex than after TBI, since a certain fraction of the bone marrow was completely ablated and the remaining part was protected.

The extreme reduction of the GM-CFC in the blood in the first seven days may be surprising, but is easy to explain. In the case of anterior body irradiation, the radiation dose of 11.7 Gy causes complete ablation of 70% of the total hemopoietic tissue including the GM-CFC with its migratory subpopulation. Furthermore, a major fraction of the GM-CFC present in the whole blood during the exposure (of three h) and passing the field was sterilized by appropriate transit doses. These effects were the main causes of the strong reduction of the blood GM-CFC numbers within the first 24 h after exposure.

Similarly to TBI the reduced GM-CFC concentration in the blood in the first few days after partial-body irradiation was due to the low number of migratory GM-CFC present in the protected marrow in the early phase of hemopoietic compensation characterized by a strong proliferation of GM-CFC and an associated differentiation [14, 31]. On the other hand, in the irradiated marrow some repopulation could already be detected seven days after the exposure. The seeding of hemopoietic cells in the irradiated sites (that were released from the protected marrow) could have significantly influenced the pattern of temporal changes in the blood GM-CFC concentration.

The transient increase in the blood GM-CFC concentration thereafter lasting from about day 10 to day 35 after the exposure of the anterior part of the body was related to the return of the GM-CFC pool in the protected marrow to a normal functional status, i.e., showing nearly normal numbers again and a normal proliferation rate [14, 31]. At later times progenitor cells could have been released from the irradiated marrow (when the hemopoietic tissue had attained a certain degree of recovery) and contributed to the transiently increased blood GM-CFC concentration. It is an interesting observation that, following this increase, the blood GM-CFC levels remained reduced for several weeks. Such a decrease was also found in dogs which had received irradiation of the lower part of their body, containing only 30% of the total active bone marrow, but this was of a much shorter duration than in the animals of which the anterior part was exposed [1]. This secondary decrease in the blood GM-CFC concentration resulted from and was indicative of an overall systemic decrease, for unknown reasons, in the GM-CFC number in the irradiated as well as protected bone marrow (as reflected by the curves in Fig. 8). Interestingly, the decreasing GM-CFC numbers were associated with corresponding changes in the blood granulocyte counts that, after a transient increase to normal levels, showed subnormal values again for several weeks [15].

The findings obtained by means of the comet assay may offer a possible explanation for the persisting subnormal GM-CFC values in the irradiated as well as protected bone marrow. Though fragmentary, the data show that surviving hemopoietic cells with DNA damage were distributed between different bones and persisted in the marrow of the irradiated as well as protected bones for more than 50 days [32]. Due to the DNA damage, such cells could have had limited proliferative potential and have been the basis of the reduced GM-CFC numbers and the reduced overall bone marrow cellularity for several weeks after the exposure. Such defects seem to be specifically related to the granulopoietic renewal system, since no such residual defects were observed in erythropoiesis and thrombopoiesis as reflected by the blood cell counts that, after their recovery, remained stable within the preirradiation range [15].

The findings obtained in partial-body-irradiated dogs clearly have shown that the restoration of the hemopoietic tissue in the bones exposed to a large single radiation dose is essentially dependent on the seeding of hemopoietic cells that originate in the protected marrow sites [33]. Consequently, the early expansion of the migratory GM-CFC population in the protected marrow, as achieved by the treatment with rHuG-CSF, caused an accelerated repopulation of the irradiated sites in comparison to untreated animals and in contrast to animals which were treated with rHuGM-CSF, but showed no early progenitor cell mobilization [15].

Experiences from Clinical Studies

Some reports from clinical studies indicate that therapeutic irradiations involving significant fractions of the active bone marrow are causing progenitor cell changes in the blood similar to those observed in the canine experiments. In patients treated for malignant lymphomas with protracted fractionated TBI (3 $\times$ 0.1 Gy per week) to a cumulative dose of 1.1 Gy, the concentration of the GM-CFC in the blood already decreased in the course of treatment and remained subnormal for at least six weeks [34]. A remarkably strong depression of GM-CFC mobilization by G-CSF was observed in a patient receiving fractionated irradiation (total dose 40.8 Gy) to the pelvis involving 40% of the active bone marrow when the mobilization was performed three weeks after irradiation, but not at six weeks after the exposure [35]. Generally, in patients the efficiency of different protocols of progenitor cell mobilization is significantly influenced by previous broad range radiotherapy, among others [36, 37].

ACKNOWLEDGMENT

The research work has been supported by the Bundesminister des Inneren (BMI) and the Bundesminister für Umwelt, Naturschutz und Reaktorsicherheit (BMU) of the Bundesrepublik Deutschland; the Deutsche Forschungsgemeinschaft (SFB 112) and the Commission of the European Communities. The authors gratefully acknowledge the excellent technical work performed by our technicians *H. Bauer, G. Baur, M. Buchenscheit, B. Burr, I. Fache, B. Lehner, B. Petras, E. Rüber, I. Sachse, K. Siebert, K. Steinhoff,* and *C. Wieland.*

REFERENCES

1 Fliedner TM. The role of blood stem cells in hemopoietic cell renewal. STEM CELLS 1998;16(suppl 1):13-29.

2 Nothdurft W, Fliedner TM. The response of the granulocytic progenitor cells (CFU-C) of blood and bone marrow in dogs exposed to low dose of X irradiation. Radiat Res 1982;89:38-52.

3 Nothdurft W. Die Reaktionen der granulozytär determinierten Stammzellen im Blut des Hundes nach Röntgenganzkörperbestrahlung und ihre Bedeutung als Indikatoren für Strahlenbelastungen. Thesis (Habilitationsschrift), University of Ulm, 1980:1-112.

4 Nothdurft W, Calvo W, Fliedner TM et al. Investigations on the pool size, proliferative state and differentiation pattern of splenic CFUc in normal dogs. Exp Hematol 1980;8:988-995.

5 Nothdurft W, Steinbach KH, Ross W et al. Quantitative aspects of granulocytic progenitor cell (CFUc) mobilization from extravascular sites in dogs using dextran sulphate (DS). Cell Tissue Kinet 1982;15:331-340.

6 Nothdurft W. Use of peripheral blood stem cells for transplantation. Experimental protocols performed by the Ulm group. In: Seidel HJ, ed. The Hemopoietic Stem Cell. Ulm: Universitätsverlag GmbH, 1990:73-92.

7 Gerhartz HH, Fliedner TM. Velocity sedimentation and cell cycle characteristics of granulopoietic progenitor cells (CFUc) in canine blood and bone marrow: influence of mobilization and CFUc depletion. Exp Hematol 1980;8:209-218.

8 Ross WM, Körbling M, Nothdurft W et al. The role of dextran sulfate in increasing the CFUc - concentration in dog blood. Proc Soc Exp Biol Med 1978;157:301-305.

9 Nothdurft W, Steinbach KH, Fliedner TM. Dose- and time-related quantitative and qualitative alterations in the granulocyte/macrophage progenitor cell (GM-CFC) compartment of dogs after total-body irradiation. Radiat Res 1984;98:332-344.

10 Gerhartz HH, Nothdurft W, Fliedner TM. Effect of low-dose whole-body irradiation on granulopoietic progenitor cell subpopulations: implications of CFUc release. Cell Tissue Kinetic 1982;15:371-379.

11 Nothdurft W, Fliedner TM, Fritz TE et al. Response of hemopoiesis in dogs to continuous low dose rate total body irradiation. STEM CELLS 1995;13(suppl 1):261-267.

12 Baltschukat K, Nothdurft W. Hematological effects of unilateral and bilateral exposures of dogs to 300 kVp X rays. Radiat Res 1990;123:7-16.

13 Kreja L, Weinsheimer W, Selig C et al. Effects of total-body irradiation on bone marrow erythroid burst-forming units (BFU-E) and hemopoietic regeneration in dogs. Radiat Res 1993;135:315-319.

14 Nothdurft W, Calvo W, Klinnert et al. Acute and long-term alterations in the granulocyte/macrophage progenitor cell (GM-CFC) compartment of dogs after partial-body irradiation: irradiation of the upper body with a single myeloablative dose. Int J Radiat Oncol Biol Phys 1986;112:949-957.

15 Nothdurft W, Kreja L, Selig C. Acceleration of hemopoietic recovery in dogs after extended-field partial - body irradiation by treatment with colony - stimulating factors: rhG-CSF and rhGM-CSF. Int J Radiat Oncol Biol Phys 1997;37:1145-1154.

16 Singh NP, McCoy MT, Tice RR et al. A simple technique for quantitation of low levels of DNA damage in individual cells. Exp Cell Res 1988;175:184-191.

17 Kreja L, Selig C, Nothdurft W. Assessment of DNA damage in canine peripheral blood and bone marrow after total body irradiation using single-cell gel electrophoresis technique. Mutat Res 1996;359:63-70.

18 Tebbi K, Rubin S, Cowan DH et al. A comparison of granulopoiesis in culture from blood and bone marrow cells of nonleukemic individuals and patients with acute leukemia. Blood 1976;48:235-243.

19 Wells JR, Opelz G, Cline MJ. Characterization of functional distinct lymphoid and myeloid cells from human blood and bone marrow. II. Separation by velocity sedimentation. J Immunol Methods 1977;18:79-93.

20 Liu YK, Stallard SS, Koo V et al. The proliferative states of circulating granulopoietic stem cells in man. Scand J Haematol 1979;22:258-262.

21 Lepine J, Messner HA. Pluripotent hemopoietic progenitors (CFU-GEMM) in chronic myelogenous leukemia. Int J Cell Cloning 1983;1:230-239.

22 Leitner A, Strobl H, Fischmeister G et al. Lack of DNA synthesis among CD34$^+$ cells in cord blood and in cytokine-mobilized blood. Br J Haematol 1996;92:255-262.

23 Lemoli RM, Tafuri A, Fortuna A et al. Cycling status of CD34$^+$ cells mobilized into peripheral blood of healthy donors by recombinant human granulocyte colony stimulating factor. Blood 1997;89:1189-1196.

24 Rumi C, Rutella S, Teofili L et al. RhG-CSF mobilized CD34$^+$ peripheral blood progenitors are myeloperoxidase-negative and noncycling irrespective of CD33 or CD13 coexpression. Exp Hematol 1997;25:246-251.

25 Bond VP, Fliedner TM, Archambeau JO. Mammalian Radiation Lethality. A Disturbance of Cellular Kinetics. New York: Academic Press, 1965.

26 Maruyama Y, Feola JM. Relative sensitivities of the thymus, spleen and lymphopoietic systems. In: Lett JT, Altman KI, eds. Relative Radiation Sensitivities of Human Organ Systems (Advances in Radiation Biology, Vol. 12). New York: Academic Press, 1987:1-82.

27 Grosse-Wilde H, Schaefer UW. Lymphatic system. In: Scherer E, Streffer C, Trott KR, eds. Radiopathology of Organs and Tissues. Berlin, Heidelberg, New York: Springer-Verlag, 1991:171-190.

28 Barnes DWH, Loutit JF. Effects of irradiation and antigenic stimulation on circulating hemopoietic stem cells of the mouse. Nature 1967;213:1142-1143.

29 Micklem HS, Ogden DA, Evans EP et al. Compartments and cell flows within the mouse haemopoietic system. II. Estimated rates of interchange. Cell Tissue Kinet 1975;8:233-248.

30 Wagemaker G, Neelis KJ, Wognum AW. Surface markers and growth factor receptors of immature hemopoietic stem cell subsets. STEM CELLS 1995;13(suppl 1):165-171.

31 Baltschukat K, Fliedner TM, Nothdurft W. Hematological effects in dogs after irradiation of the lower part of the body with a single myeloablative dose. Radiother Oncol 1989;14:239-246.

32 Nothdurft W, Kreja L, Selig C. Untersuchungenüber die Wirkung hämopoetischer Wachstumsfaktoren auf die Strahlenempfindlichkeit der Hämopoese und ihr Regenerationsvermögen. In: Der Bundesminister für Umwelt, Naturschutz und Reaktorsicherheit, Hrsg. Schriftenreihe Reaktorsicherheit und Strahlenschutz BMU - 1996-472,1996.

33 Nothdurft W. Bone Marrow. In: Scherer E, Streffer C, Trott KR, eds. Radiopathology of Organs and Tissues. Berlin, Heidelberg, New York: Springer-Verlag, 1991:113-169.

34 Labedzki L, Schmidt RE, Hartlapp JH et al. Ganzkörperbestrahlungen bei malignen Lymphomen niedriger Malignität. Strahlentherapie 1982;158:195-201.

35 Braun MP, Masiarz RT. Abscopal depression of G-CSF mobilized peripheral stem cells. Bone Marrow Transplant 1994;14:1005-1007.

36 Demirer T, Bensinger WI. Optimalization of peripheral blood stem cell collection. Curr Opin Hematol 1995;2:219-226.

37 To LB, Haylock DN, Simmons Pj et al. The biology and clinical uses of blood stem cells. Blood 1997;89;2233-2258.

Role of the CD34$^+$38$^-$ Cells in Posttransplant Hematopoietic Recovery

PH. HÉNON,[a,b] H. SOVALAT,[a] D. BOURDERONT,[c] M. OJEDA-URIBE,[b]
Y. ARKAM,[b] E. WUNDER,[a] J.P. RAIDOT,[d] F. HUSSEINI,[d] B. AUDHUY[d]

[a]Institut de Recherche en Hématologie et Transfusion, [b]Department of Hematology,
[c]Bio Statistical Unit, Hôpitaux de Mulhouse and [d]Department of Onco-Hematology,
Hôpital Pasteur, Colmar, France

Key Words. *Autologous blood cell transplantation · CD34$^+$ cells · CD34$^+$38$^-$ cells · Hematopoietic recovery
· Engraftment kinetics · Hematopoietic growth factors*

ABSTRACT

Using three different statistical tests in parallel, we showed in a preliminary study that neither mononuclear cells, CD34$^+$33$^+$ or 33$^-$ cells, nor CD34$^+$38$^+$ cells significantly correlated with engraftment kinetics following autologous blood cell transplantation (ABCT). We additionally demonstrated here, in a series of patients suffering from malignant diseases, that the graft content in CD34$^+$38$^-$ cells is individually a more sensitive indicator of the earliest, as well as the latest post-ABCT trilineage hematopoietic recovery than the colony-forming units-granulocyte-macrophage and even the total CD34$^+$ cell content. This suggests that the CD34$^+$38$^-$ cell population is itself subdivided into two more subsets, one being already lineage-committed and responsible for short-term engraftment, the other containing only very primitive hematopoietic cells responsible for sustained engraftment. Strong arguments favor the probability that these subsets correspond to HLA-DR$^+$ and DR$^-$ cells, respectively. We also defined an optimal threshold value of 0.05 $\times$ 10^6 CD34$^+$38$^-$ cells/kg of the patient's body weight (b.w.) above which a rapid and sustained trilineage engraftment safely occurs. In fact, infusion of lower numbers of cells seems to have a more significant impact on long-term compared to short-term neutrophil recovery and on platelet kinetics engraftment. We additionally looked for the eventual influence on engraftment time of the type of disease, and of post-ABCT administration of hematopoietic growth factors (HGF). When the type of disease appeared to have no influence on the engraftment time, posttransplant HGF administration significantly reduced the time to trilineage engraftment in patients transplanted with < 0.05 $\times$ 10^6 CD34$^+$38$^-$ cells, thus justifying it in case of reinfusion of low numbers of CD34$^+$38$^-$ cells. On the other hand, the administration of HGF after infusion of more than 0.05 $\times$ 10^6 CD34$^+$38$^-$ cells/kg b.w. did not hasten more, or only very little, the engraftment time, thus becoming not only unprofitable for the patients but costly as well. *Stem Cells 1998;16(suppl 1):113-122*

INTRODUCTION

Blood is now commonly used as source of hematopoietic stem cells for autografting as well as allografting [1, 2]. Numerous studies have attempted to define which blood cell (BC) subpopulation could predict at best the kinetics of a further engraftment. However, their results are somewhat contradictory

[3-6]. Colony-forming units-granulocyte-macrophage (CFU-GM) and/or total CD34$^+$ cell assessments are the most widely applied tools, but their correlation with hematopoietic recovery does not seem to be linear and suffers from a huge variability [7-10].

We have shown in a preliminary study [11] using three different statistical tests in parallel that, whatever the statistical test, there was no significant correlation between the infused number of mononuclear cells (MNC), CD34$^+$33$^+$ cells, CD34$^+$33$^-$ cells, CD34$^+$38$^+$ cells and trilineage engraftment kinetics. On the other hand, the number of infused CFU-GM, total CD34$^+$ cells and overall CD34$^+$38$^-$ cells seemed to better correlate with engraftment kinetics. As a consequence, we have subsequently focused our attention on these cell subvarieties in an attempt to better define which of them would actually reflect the quality of the blood graft products and therefore predict the rapidity of engraftment.

PATIENTS AND METHODS

Patients

Eighteen patients with malignant lymphoma, 11 patients with multiple myeloma, 8 patients with solid tumors (ST) and 6 patients with acute lymphoblastic leukemia (ALL) were consecutively enrolled in this study. Their median age was 42 years (range 18-67 years), with a male/female ratio of 23/20.

Prior to blood hematopoietic progenitor cell mobilization, all patients had received various chemotherapy courses in accordance with the type and stage of their disease. The mobilization regimen always comprised a chemotherapy adapted to the type of disease. In addition, all the patients except two with lymphoma and those with ALL, were subcutaneously administered hematopoietic growth factor(s) (HGF), either G-CSF alone (31 patients) or interleukin 3 + G-CSF (four patients), from the day after chemotherapy until completion of leukaphereses (LKs), at a daily dosage of 5 μg/kg.

LK Procedure and BC Cryopreservation

BC collection was performed with a Baxter-Fenwal CS 3000, set to a modified "programme 1," using a small volume chamber. LKs were started when at least the peripheral blood (PB) CD34$^+$ cell baseline count (previously determined in our laboratory as being 2×10^3/ml) was reached. On average 10 l of blood were processed during each LK session at a flow-rate of 50-60 ml/min, with a final leukapheresis product (LKP) volume of 50 ml of MNC suspension. MNCs were subsequently counted and adjusted to a concentration of 2×10^7/ml, then mixed volume to volume in a 20% dimethylsulfoxide-albumin solution. The final cell suspension was transferred into Gambro DF700 freezing bags (Dialysatoren GmBH; Hechingen, Germany) and progressively frozen to 140°C with a Nicool 416 controlled-cryopreservation device (Compagnie des Produits Oxygénés; Paris, France). The frozen cells were finally stored at -196°C into the liquid phase of nitrogen.

Evaluation of the Graft Content in CD34$^+$ Cells and Subsets

CD34$^+$ cells were identified and quantified using the double-staining method and flow cytometry assay we previously described [12].

For detection of CD34$^+$CD38 subsets, cell aliquots were stained with 8G12 monoclonal antibody (mAb) using the same method, then incubated with 20 μl of fluoroscein isothiocyanate (FITC)-conjugated anti-CD38 mAb (Immunotech; Marseille, France). In parallel, both unstained cells and cells stained with a control isotype, applied as a combination of nonspecific FITC-IgG1 with phycoerythrin (PE)-IgG1 (Simultest Control, Becton Dickinson; Mountain View, CA), were used as negative controls. After a 30-min incubation, the cells were mixed with 4 ml of lysing reagent (Ortho; Raritan, NJ) and washed twice in Dulbecco's phosphate buffer saline ([D-PBS], Gibco; Cergy-Pontoise, France) with 2% fetal calf serum (FCS). They were then immediately analyzed by flow cytometry with a FACStar (Becton Dickinson) equipped with a 5 W argon laser. Fifty thousand cells were acquired in a list mode file, and the data were analyzed with the Consort 30 program. Cell aggregates and debris were excluded by gating in acquisition. CD34[+] cells were obtained by side-scatter cytogram (SSC) versus red fluorescence (PE). 530 nm and 570 nm filters were used for selection of green and red fluorescence attributable to FITC and PE-labeled antibodies (Ab). Compensation levels were set to limit the superposition of fluorochrome emission spectrum. CD34[+] cell subpopulations were determined by electronic gating on the CD34[+] population identified in a two-color display of PE-8G12 versus side scatter. These gated CD34[+] events were studied with FITC-labeled Ab. Subpopulations of CD34[+] cells were identified on the cytogram of PE versus FITC fluorescence. The limit between negative and positive expression of the CD38 markers was set according to negative control-Ab (PE versus FITC fluorescence) on the lymphocyte region as shown in Figure 1.

Finally, absolute quantification per ml of CD34[+] cells and their subsets was evaluated in LKP samples by multiplying the MNC count determined with a STKS Cell Counter Coulter (Coultronics; Margency, France) with the percentage of CD34[+] cells determined by flow cytometry. Results were finally expressed as the number of total CD34[+] cells or subsets per kg of the patient's body weight (b.w.).

CFU-GM Colony Assay

Fresh MNCs from each LKP sample were adjusted and plated at a concentration of 2×10^5 viable cells n duplicate in a culture medium consisting of 0.8% methylcellulose supplemented with 20% human placental-conditioned medium (standardized against Medium H431; Stem Cell Technologies; Vancouver, Canada) and 20% FCS. Plates were incubated at 37°C and 5% CO_2 in humidified atmosphere. Colonies containing more than 50 cells were scored on day 12, using an inverted microscope.

Myeloablative Conditioning Therapy and Autologous Blood Cell Transplantation (ABCT)

Pretransplant conditioning regimens depended on the disease. Fractionated total body irradiation (TBI = 10-12 Gy delivered in five to six fractions) was combined with high-dose chemotherapy (HDCT) in 23 patients while the 20 others underwent HDCT only. Twenty-four hours after completion of high-dose therapy, cryopreserved blood cells were thawed at the patient's bedside and immediately reinfused. Fourteen out of 43 patients (all patients with ST and several other patients reinfused with low number of cells) received G-CSF posttransplant (5 μg/kg/day) from day +2 until achievement of ANC $\geq 0.5 \times 10^9$. The kinetics of engraftment were defined as the number of days from graft infusion to reach ANC of 0.5, 1 and 2×10^9/l, platelet counts of 20 and 50×10^9/l without transfusion support and absolute reticulocyte counts of 30 and 50 $\times 10^9$/l, on two consecutive days.

Statistical Analyses

The nonparametric Spearman rank correlation test was used for examining the relationships

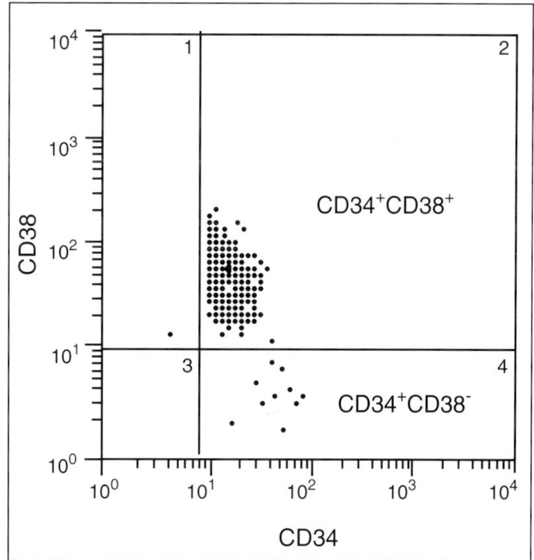

Figure 1. CD34[+]CD38[+] and CD38[-] subpopulations in peripheral blood of a patient having received a mobilizing regimen combining high-dose chemotherapy plus G-CSF. All cells being considered CD34[+] are shown. The majority shows intermediate to high CD38 expression and forms a cluster in the upper right quadrant; simultaneously, these cells express the CD34 surface antigen at a lower level than the CD34[+]CD38[-] subpopulation, as shown in the lower right quadrant.

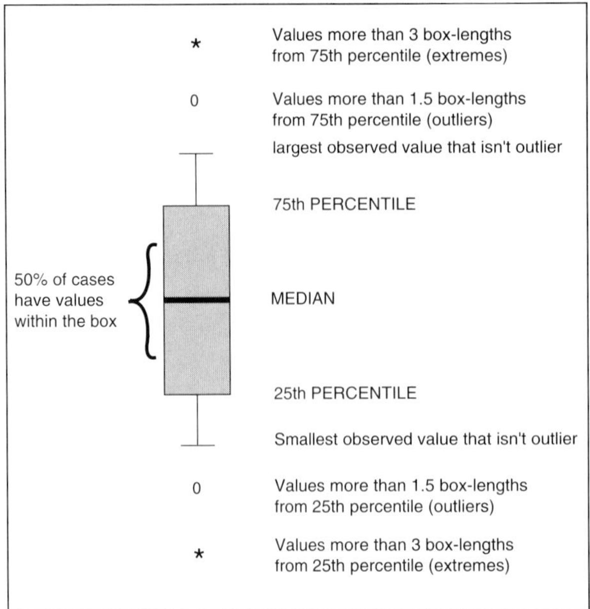

Figure 2. The box-plot model is particularly useful for comparing the distribution of values in several groups.

between the individual amounts of different subvarieties of cells reinfused and the number of days required for hematopoietic recovery after ABCT for each patient. When dependent and predictive variables were related, the parameters of a linear regression model ($Y = b_o + b_1 \times$ cells) and a log-inverse model ($Y = e[b_o + b_1 \times$ cells]) were estimated and the goodness-of-fit of the models was evaluated with the coefficient of determination (R^2). Patients who died before engraftment of either lineage were censored at the date of death.

The possible influence of the type of disease and of posttransplant administration of growth factors on the average number of days required for trilineage engraftment was estimated with the "box-plot" graphic procedure, particularly useful for comparing the distribution of data among several groups (Fig. 2). A set of a priori contrasts, according to the different subgroups of patients, was tested with the Mann-Whitney or Kruskal-Wallis nonparametric tests.

Data analyses were performed with SPSS$^®$ 6.1.2. for Windows^{TM} software. Results were considered as significant for p value < 0.05.

RESULTS

Posttransplant Hematopoietic Recovery

Average numbers of each reinfused PB cell subvariety are detailed in Table 1. The average times to reach ANC of 0.5, 1, and 2 $\times$ 10^9/l were 11, 12 and 20 days, respectively. The average times to reach 20 and 50 $\times$ 10^9/l platelets were 17 and 25 days. However, four patients never reached 50 $\times$ 10^9 platelets/l before they respectively died on day 14, 35, 120 and 550. Absolute reticulocyte counts reached 30 and 50 $\times$ 10^9/l within an average of 17 and 22 days, respectively.

Correlation Analysis between the Number of Infused Cells and the Kinetics of Engraftment

The individual amounts of the different cell subvarieties reinfused for transplant were plotted against the number of days to reach the different ANC, platelet and reticulocyte counts defining the trilineage engraftment kinetics for each patient. The infused number of CFU-GM satisfactorily correlated with the time to ANC $\geq$ 0.5 $\times$ 10^9/l whatever the statistical test, but not at all with the later stages of neutrophil recovery; furthermore, they only weakly correlated with platelet and erythroid engraftment in the sole Spearman's test. On the other hand, the number of total CD34$^+$ cells

Table 1. Average numbers of different subvarieties of blood cells contained in reinfused graft products

Blood cell subtype	n of reinfused cells (range)
CFU-GM ($\times$ 10^4/kg)	14.9 (2.8–57.7)
Total CD34$^+$ ($\times$ 10^6/kg)	2.94 (0.3–10.42)
CD34$^+$38$^-$ ($\times$ 10^6/kg)	0.15 (0.011–1.62)

Table 2. Summary of relationships between each subvariety of infused cells and each parameter of engraftment kinetics depending on the statistical model: 1) Spearman's test, 2) Linear regression model (L), 3) Log-inverse model (S)

Type of reinfused cells		ANC ($\times 10^9$/l)			Platelets ($\times 10^9$/l)		Reticulocytes ($\times 10^9$/l)	
		≥ 0.5	≥ 1	≥ 2	≥ 20	≥ 50	≥ 30	≥ 50
	1)	+	-	-	++	++	+	+
CFU-GM	2)	++	-	-	-	-	-	-
	3)	+	-	-	-	-	-	-
	1)	++	+++	+++	+++	+++	+++	+++
CD34$^+$	2)	++	++	++	+++	++	+	+
	3)	-	-	++	+++	+++	++	++
	1)	++	++	++	++	++	++	++
CD34$^+$38$^-$	2)	++	++	++	++	++	+	+
	3)	++	++	++	+++	+++	++	++

The *p*-value relationships between the three statistical models are expressed as follows:

Spearman's correlation coefficient	R square (L and S models)	*p* values	Relationship expression
$r \geq -0.50$	R2 ≥ 0.30	≤ 0.001	+++
$r \geq -0.40$	R2 ≥ 0.20	≤ 0.01	++
$r \geq -0.30$	R2 ≥ 0.15	≤ 0.05	+
$r < -0.30$	R2 < 0.15	> 0.05	—

correlated well with most of the engraftment kinetics parameters in the three statistical tests, except with the two first stages of ANC recovery in the log-inverse model. However, the more constant correlations within the three statistical models were significantly and surprisingly observed between the number of infused CD38$^-$ cells and each of the trilineage engraftment parameters. All correlative values are summarized in Table 2.

Moreover, the log-inverse model interestingly allowed determination of a plateau of the CD38$^-$ engraftment kinetics correlation curves, similarly starting from an infused dose of 0.05×10^6 CD34$^+$38$^-$ cells/kg for the three cell lineages. Under this cell dose, the correlation values were extremely scattered and unpredictable, when, on the other hand, infusion of higher cell amounts seemed not to further shorten the time of trilineage recovery (Fig. 3A, B, C). Although less convincing because of the lack of correlation with the earliest ANC recovery parameters, a "cut-off" value of 2×10^6 total CD34$^+$ cells could also be determined from the log-inverse curves for all the other engraftment parameters (curves not shown).

In an attempt to confirm these two "cut-off" values as clinically useful threshold cell doses, we further compared trilineage engraftment kinetics in the subgroups of patients determined in function of those. It clearly appeared in Table 3 that patients receiving more than 2×10^6 CD34$^+$ and 0.05×10^6 CD34$^+$38$^-$ cells/kg globally experienced a faster average trilineage engraftment than those receiving less. However, when examining in detail each patient's data, discrepancies in the influence of the two cell subvarieties on hematopoietic recovery sometimes appeared. For example, seven patients who were transplanted with less than 2×10^6 total CD34$^+$ cells/kg, but more than 0.05×10^6 cells of the CD38$^-$ subset, all achieved a prompt and sustained trilineage engraftment. On the other hand, for two patients who received more than 2×10^6 total CD34$^+$ cells, but only a few cells of the CD38$^-$ subset, the return to normal platelet counts and hemoglobin levels was very slow or not even reached after six months posttransplant. Therefore, individual assessment of the graft content in CD34$^+$38$^-$ cells seems to be a more reliable predictive parameter of posttransplant hematopoietic recovery than that of the total CD34$^+$ cell content.

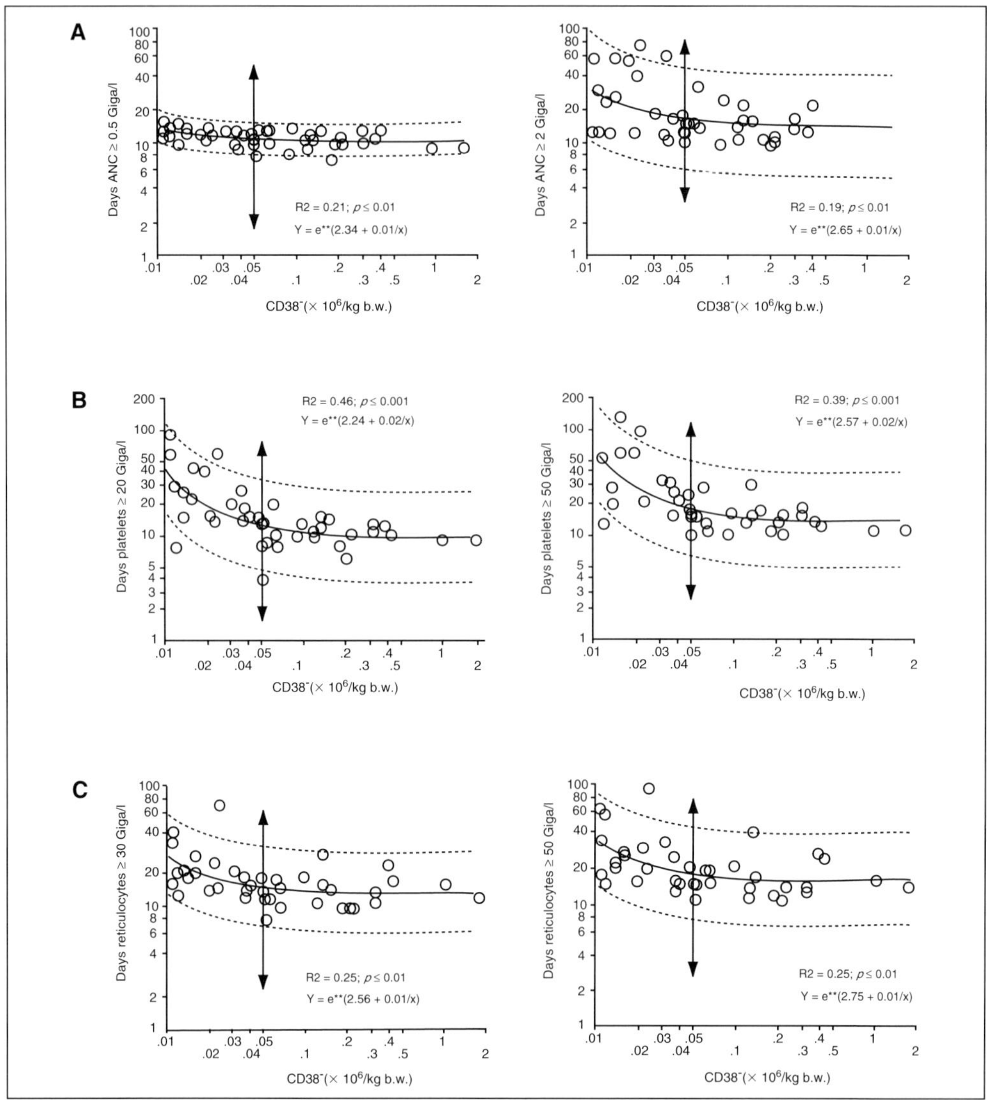

Figure 3. The inversion of the slope of the CD38$^-$ engraftment correlation curves in the log-inverse model similarly started from infused doses of 0.05 $\times$ 10^6 CD34$^+$38$^-$ cells/kg for (A) the granulocytic, (B) the platelet, and (C) the reticulocyte lineages.

Analysis of the Potential Influence of the Type of Disease and of HGF Posttransplant Administration on Engraftment Kinetics

Using the box-plot model, the type of disease did not appear to have any significant influence on posttransplant hematopoietic recovery, whichever the engraftment kinetics parameter considered (data not shown).

On the contrary, posttransplant HGF administration seemed to play a variable role in hematopoietic reconstitution, depending on the cell dose reinfused to the patients. Patients who were transplanted with more than 0.05 $\times$ 10^6 CD34$^+$38$^-$ cells/kg and underwent posttransplant HGF administration did not improve or improved very little, in terms of rapidity of trilineage engraftment, over those who did not receive HGF. On the contrary, patients who were transplanted with amounts of CD34$^+$38$^-$ cells < 0.05 $\times$ 10^6/kg clearly benefited from posttransplant HGF administration. Their hematopoietic reconstitution was, indeed, as fast

Table 3. Comparison of trilineage engraftment kinetics depending on the total $CD34^+$ or the $CD34^+38^-$ cell dose reinfused. p values were determined by the Mann-Whitney nonparametric test

Number of patients	Number of reinfused cells	ANC ($\times 10^9/l$)			Platelets ($\times 10^9/l$)		Reticulocytes ($\times 10^9/l$)	
		≥ 0.5	≥ 1.0	≥ 2.0	≥ 20	≥ 50	≥ 30	≥ 50
27	$<2 \times 10^6$/kg	12.9	14.8	28.0	24.0	34.2	21.6	29.6
	(extremes)	(8–16)	(9–22)	(9–100)	(10–90)	(13–130)	(10–71)	(12–90)
CD34⁺								
16	$\geq 2 \times 10^6$/kg	9.0	11.5	12.3	12.0	15.7	14	17.8
	(extremes)	(7–12)	(8–14)	(10–22)	(4–15)	(10–24)	(10–18)	(11–26)
	Mean difference	3.9	3.3	15.7	12.0	18.5	7.6	11.8
	(p value)	(< 0.05)	(< 0.05)	(< 0.01)	($p < 0.01$)	($p < 0.01$)	($p < 0.01$)	($p < 0.001$)
20	$< 0.05 \times 10^6$/kg	12.2	14.8	29.3	27.7	38.5	22.2	28.9
	(extremes)	(8–18)	(9–22)	(13–100)	(10–90)	(12–130)	(11–71)	(13–90)
CD38⁻								
23	$\geq 0.05 \times 10^6$/kg	10.8	12.6	15.4	10.9	14.5	13.8	17.2
	(extremes)	(7–12)	(8–15)	(10–33)	(4–13)	(10–17)	(8–22)	(10–26)
	Mean difference	1.4	2.2	13.9	17.2	24	8.4	11.7
	(p value)	(< 0.05)	(< 0.05)	(< 0.01)	($p < 0.001$)	($p < 0.001$)	($p < 0.001$)	($p < 0.001$)

as that of patients having received more than 0.05×10^6 $CD34^+38^-$ cells, i.e., significantly more rapid than that of patients having also received low cell doses but who were not administered HGF (Fig. 4 A, B, C).

DISCUSSION

Despite the intensive development of ABCT within recent years, the cell subpopulation which could predict at best the kinetics of posttransplant hematopoietic engraftment remains to be defined. CFU-GM assessment finally appears not to be a reliable predictive engraftment indicator. While some reported its significant, but usually weak, correlation with granulocytic and even platelet recovery kinetics [3, 7, 8], others disclaimed its predictive interest [4, 5, 9]. Our present results are not more convincing. We only found a weak correlation of graft CFU-GM with the three statistical tests in the earliest phase of granulocytic recovery, and with the Spearman's test alone for platelets and erythroid engraftment.

Most investigators now insist on the powerful predictive role of the graft content in $CD34^+$ cells in optimally predicting the rapidity of the further engraftment kinetics [4, 5, 10, 13]. However, many investigators did not find any linear correlation between the number of infused $CD34^+$ cells and neutrophil engraftment, and had instead attempted to define $CD34^+$ cell threshold values above those where prompt engraftment occurs with increasing confidence. Threshold $CD34^+$ cell values varying from 2 to 5 $\times$ 10^6/kg have been suggested to be necessary to achieve rapid neutrophil and platelet recovery from BC infusion [5, 10, 13-15]. In fact, our present study found a linear correlation between the time to recovery of PB cell counts postautograft and the absolute number of $CD34^+$ cells in the graft. It also brought an additional confirmation that the $CD34^+$ "cut-off" of 2 $\times$ 10^6/kg may be a valuable clinical indicator under which hematopoiesis is significantly delayed in most, if not all, patients.

However, as both immature stem cells and committed progenitors express the $CD34^+$ antigen as well, it might be clinically interesting to better refine stem cell measurement by evaluating $CD34^+$ subsets, which could avoid overestimating the true stem cell content of the graft. Despite the conjunction of high cell enrichment usually obtained in LKP and recent advances in flow cytometry methodology, which altogether allows minor $CD34^+$ cell subpopulations to become visible in the fluorescence-activated cell sorter analysis, only very few investigators have clinically applied such measurements to

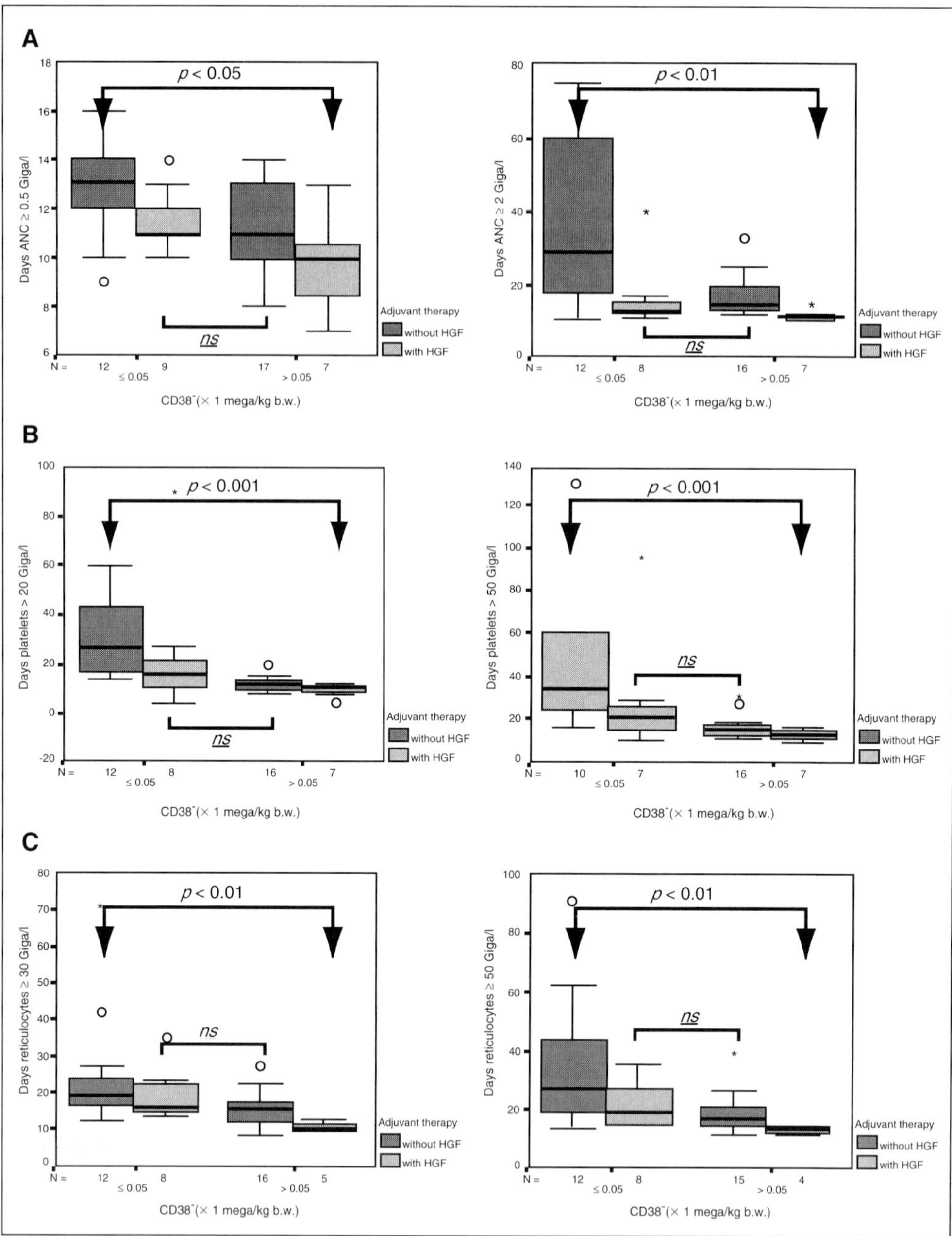

Figure 4. Box-plot model: analysis of the influence of HGF posttransplant administration on trilineage engraftment kinetics: (A) ANC, (B) platelets, (C) reticulocytes. Giga/l: $\times 10^9/l$ - Mega/kg: $10^6/kg$.

study posttransplant hematopoietic recovery.

Our results concerning the strong correlations in the three statistical tests we used in parallel between the number of transplanted CD34⁺CD38⁻ cells and all stages of trilineage engraftment, including the earliest, were somewhat surprising. They seem to suggest a functional heterogeneity of the CD38⁻ subpopulation, initially supposed to be only very immature and to solely participate in late, complete hematopoietic reconstitution. It surprisingly appears to also have a correlation with early trilineage engraftment, sufficient to suggest its involvement in such a way, and could indicate at least a partial lineage-commitment of the CD38⁻ subpopulation. Recent studies have suggested that this small CD38⁻ subpopulation was itself divided into two more subsets: HLA-DR⁺ and HLA-DR⁻. Double-negative (CD38⁻ DR⁻) cells would constitute approximatively 14% of the CD34⁺CD38⁻ subset in the bone marrow (BM) [16]. In adults, very primitive stem cells seem to be essentially contained within the CD34⁺CD38⁻ DR⁻ subset, capable of increasing progeny of all hematopoietic lineages in vitro, although it might also contain few committed hematopoietic progenitors [16, 17]. On the other hand, in fetal BM, the hematopoietic stem cells seem to reside within the CD34⁺, CD38⁻, HLA-DR⁺ cell subpopulation [18].

Buscemi et al. reported data almost similar to ours, in a short study enrolling seven patients transplanted with BC [19]. They also found, using a linear regression analysis, that the total number of grafted CD34⁺ cells correlated with platelet, but not with early neutrophil recovery. They did not find any correlation between hematopoietic recovery, and neither the CD34⁺CD33⁺ and CD34⁺CD38⁺ subsets, nor MNC and CFU-GM-infused numbers. But overall they found a very strong correlation between platelet recovery and the CD34⁺CD38⁻ subset. Interestingly, using three-color flow cytometry analysis, they showed that the grafted CD34⁺CD38⁻ cells were either HLA-DR⁺ or HLA-DR⁻. Therefore, they suggested a lineage commitment, implying that CD34⁺ cells negative for CD38 also comprise committed progenitors and, more specifically, megakaryocytic ones. *Sandhaus et al.* have analyzed LKP samples from 36 sequential patients, also using a three-color flow cytometry assay [20]. Two hundred fifty thousand ungated events were acquired from each sample into a list mode file. Spearman's correlation of CD34⁺38⁻ cells with early marrow engraftment of neutrophils was highly significant here. Still more recently, *Waller et al.* studied the contribution of CFU-GM, CFU-megakaryocyte, total CD34⁺ cells and CD34⁺38⁻ cells in BM graft products on the kinetics of platelet engraftment in a series of 24 patients with breast cancer or lymphoma, undergoing autologous bone marrow transplantation (ABMT) [21]. From all of these cell parameters, the content of CD34⁺38⁻ cells (with an average of 0.07×10^6/kg) was the sole significant predictor of the time to achieve a platelet count of $> 20 \times 10^9$/l posttransplant.

Thus, although more fragmentarily, the results of these recent studies are along the same lines as ours. They all tend to confirm that assessment of the CD34⁺38⁻ cell graft content yields clinically relevant data that would help to predict engraftment following autologous PB or BM transplant. Therefore, it would be of the greatest interest now to propose a CD34⁺38⁻ threshold dose clinically applicable. In our hands, the "cut-off" of 0.05×10^6 (=5×10^4) CD34⁺38⁻ cells/kg seems to be reliable, regardless of the type of disease. Under this value, even if the time to achieve 0.5×10^9 neutrophil/l never exceeded 18 days, which in short is not longer than that observed after ABMT [9, 22], achievement of higher neutrophil counts and, overall, platelet kinetics recovery was significantly delayed, or never even reached. Therefore, it may be suggested that infusion of a low CD34⁺38⁻ cell dose has a consistently more significant impact on long-term than short-term neutrophil recovery and on platelet and reticulocyte kinetics recovery. However, posttransplant HGF administration seems to significantly correct this delay, thus justifying its use in this situation. On the other hand, when more than 5×10^4 CD34⁺38⁻ cells/kg are reinfused to the patient, the benefit, in terms of hematopoietic recovery, of additional HGF administration is too small (or even null) to be clinically profitable and to justify its important overcost.

Because of the difficulty in standardizing the measurement of CD34⁺ cells and subsets [23], the "cut-off" value we propose will, however, require further validation before its widespread clinical use.

Acknowledgment

We thank *Mrs. Jeanne Bachorz, Michèle Baerenzung, Paulette Fuchs, Huguette Lewandowski* and *Valérie Chabouté* for their excellent technical assistance, and *Mrs. Francine Morgenthaler* and *Colette Sparks* for typing the manuscript.

REFERENCES

1 Hénon Ph. Peripheral blood stem cell transplantation: past, present and future. STEM CELLS 1993;11:154-172.

2 Körbling M, Przepiorka D, Huh YO et al. Allogeneic blood stem cell transplantation for refractory leukemia and lymphoma: potential advantage of blood over marrow allografts. Blood 1995;85:1659-1665.

3 Takamatsu Y, Harada M, Teshima T et al. Relationship of infused CFU-GM and CFU-MK mobilized with chemotherapy with or without G-CSF to platelet recovery after autologous blood stem cell transplantation. Exp Hematol 1995;23:8-13.

4 Bensinger WI, Longin K, Appelbaum F et al. Peripheral blood stem cells (PBSCs) collected after recombinant granulocyte colony stimulating factor (rhG-CSF): an analysis of factors correlating with the tempo of engraftment after transplantation. Br J Haematol 1994;87:825-831.

5 Urashima M, Ohkawara J, Hoshi Y et al. Peripheral blood progenitor cell transplantation estimated by three-colour (CD34, HLA-DR, CD 33) flow cytometry. Acta Haematol 1994;92:23-28.

6 Smith RJ, Sweetenham JW. A mononuclear cell dose of 3 × 10^8/kg predicts early multilineage recovery in patients with malignant lymphoma treated with carmustine, etoposide, Ara-C and melphalan (BEAM) and peripheral blood progenitor cell transplantation. Exp Hematol 1995;23:1581-1588.

7 Pierelli L, Iacone A, Quaglietta AM et al. Haematopoietic reconstitution after autologous blood stem cell transplantation in patients with malignancies: a multicentre retrospective study. Br J Haematol 1994;86:70-75.

8 Van der Walle E, Richel DJ, Holtkamp MJ et al. Bone marrow reconstitution after high-dose chemotherapy and autologous peripheral blood progenitor cell transplantation: effect of graft size. Ann Oncol 1994;5:795-802.

9 Hénon Ph, Liang H, Beck-Wirth G et al. Comparison of hematopoietic and immune recovery after autologous bone marrow or blood stem cell transplants. Bone Marrow Transplant 1992;9:285-291.

10 Bender JG, Lum L, Unverzagt KL et al. Correlation of colony-forming cells, long-term culture initiating cells and CD34$^+$ cells in apheresis products from patients mobilized for peripheral blood progenitors with different regimens. Bone Marrow Transplant 1994;13:479-485.

11 Hénon Ph, Sovalat A, Becker M et al. Assessment of the CD34$^+$38$^-$ content in autologous blood graft products as predictive factor of posttransplant trilineage engraftment. Exp Hematol 1996;9:1049a.

12 Herbein G, Sovalat H, Wunder E et al. Isolation and identification of two CD34$^+$ cell subpopulations from normal human peripheral blood. STEM CELLS 1994;12:187-197.

13 Tricot G, Jagannath S, Vesole D et al. Peripheral blood stem cell transplants for MM: identification of favorable variables for rapid engraftment in 225 patients. Blood 1995;85:588-596.

14 Bensinger W, Appelbaum F, Rowley S et al. Factors that influence collection and engraftment of autologous peripheral blood stem cells. J Clin Oncol 1995;13:2547-2555.

15 Haynes A, Hunter A, McQuaker G et al. Engraftment characteristics of peripheral blood stem cell mobilised with cyclophosphamide and the delayed addition of G-CSF. Bone Marrow Transplant 1995;16:359-363.

16 Rusten LS, Jacobsen SEW, Kaalhus O et al. Functional differences between CD38$^-$ and DR-subfractions of CD34$^+$ bone marrow cells. Blood 1994;84:1473-1481.

17 Terstappen L, Huang S, Safford M et al. Sequential generation of hematopoietic colonies derived from single nonlineage-committed CD34$^+$CD38$^-$ progenitor cells. Blood 1991;77:1218-1227.

18 Huang S, Terstappen L. Lymphoid and myeloid differentiation of single human CD34$^+$, HLA DR$^+$, CD38$^-$ hematopoietic stem cells. Blood 1994;83:1515-1526.

19 Buscemi F, Indovina A, Scimè R et al. CD34$^+$ cell subsets and platelet recovery after PBSC autograft. Bone Marrow Transplant 1995;16:855-856 (correspondence).

20 Sandhaus L, Tubbs R, Edinger M et al. CD34$^+$ cell determination for peripheral blood progenitor cell transplantation: how many is enough? Exp Hematol 1996;24:1024a.

21 Waller EK, Worford LJ, Lynn M et al. Platelet recovery following autologous bone marrow transplantation correlates with the content of CD34$^+$38$^-$ cells in the marrow graft. Exp Hematol 1997;25:899a.

22 To LB, Roberts MM, Haylock DN et al. Comparison of hematological recovery times and supportive care requirements of recovery phase following autologous peripheral blood stem cell transplants, autologous bone marrow transplants, and allogeneic bone marrow transplants. Bone Marrow Transplant 1992;9:277-284.

23 Sutherland DR, Anderson L, Keeney M et al. Response to letter to the Editor: Toward a worldwide standard for CD34$^+$ enumeration. J Hematother 1997:85-89.

Hematopoietic Progenitor Cells in the Blood and Bone Marrow in Various Hematologic Disorders

SURAPOL ISSARAGRISIL, YAOWALAK U-PRATYA, MANEENOP YIMYAM, KRIANGSAK PAKDEESUWAN, ARCHROB KHUHAPINANT, WANNA MUANGSUP, KOVIT PATTANAPANYASAT

Division of Hematology, Department of Medicine, Faculty of Medicine, Siriraj Hospital, Mahidol University, Bangkok, Thailand

Key Words. *Hematopoietic progenitor cells · Aplastic anemia · Paroxysmal nocturnal hemoglobinuria · Thalassemia*

ABSTRACT

Hematopoietic progenitor cells are present in the blood and the bone marrow. Changes in the numbers of hematopoietic progenitor cells reflect alteration of pluripotent stem cells. We discuss such changes in common hematologic diseases including aplastic anemia, paroxysmal nocturnal hemoglobinuria (PNH) and thalassemia. In aplastic anemia, the numbers of burst forming units-erythroid (BFU-E) and colony-forming units-granulocyte-macrophage (CFU-GM) are much decreased; the decrease still exists after recovery from therapy. In PNH, the numbers of progenitor cells are low, even in the presence of marrow hypercellularity. In thalassemia, the numbers of progenitor cells are much increased; more pronounced in splenectomized patients. *Stem Cells 1998;16(suppl 1):123-128*

INTRODUCTION

Hematopoietic progenitor cells, both erythroid and myeloid, are present in the bone marrow and blood. The number of progenitor cells in the blood is high prior to birth and decreases rapidly after birth. Only a small number of progenitor cells has been demonstrated in adult blood. In various conditions and diseases with the involvement of hematopoietic stem cells, either physiologic or pathologic as well as abnormal cytokine production, the progenitor cells can be affected. In this communication, we discuss the changes in the number of progenitor cells in three common hematologic diseases including aplastic anemia, paroxysmal nocturnal hemoglobinuria (PNH) and thalassemia.

Aplastic Anemia

Aplastic anemia, characterized by pancytopenia with a fatty bone marrow, was first described by *Paul Ehrlich* in 1888 [1]. It is a rare but severe disease of unknown etiology. Its incidence is known to vary throughout the world [2-4]. A long-standing impression of the local hematologists and visitors from the West is that aplastic anemia is more common in the Far East [2, 3]. This belief is based on the relatively higher number of patients seen annually in the Far East compared to western hospitals. In Thailand, there are at least 60 new cases seen annually at Siriraj Hospital and more than 1,500 cases have been documented in our hematological clinic. However, the number of cases may not represent the true incidence but rather reflect selective referral from other hospitals in Bangkok and the rural areas.

Since 1989, a population-based case-control study has been conducted in Thailand in order to verify the high incidence of aplastic anemia in Thailand and to investigate the possible risk factors. The annual incidence was 3.9 per million in Bangkok [5, and *Issaragrisil, Leaverton, Chansung et al.,* submitted for publication], two times higher than the rate in Europe and Israel as reported by the International Agranulocytosis and Aplastic Anemia Study [4]. The incidence was somewhat higher, at five per million in Khonkaen in the Northeast and lower, at three per million in Songkla in the South [*Issaragrisil, Leaverton, Chansung et al.,* submitted for publication]. This is higher than any recently published rate in western countries. The differences among the three geographic regions studied may result from different environmental and occupational patterns in these areas. With regard to age incidence, there are two peaks at 15-24 years and at 60 years and over in Bangkok. In Khonkaen and Songkla the pattern is more conventional, with a consistent increase in incidence with increasing age.

Aplastic anemia has many clinical associations including a wide variety of drug and chemical exposures, some viral infections and pregnancy; however, most cases are considered idiopathic and without clinical associations [1]. The results of the case-control study in Thailand, the largest epidemiologic study of aplastic anemia conducted to date, suggest that only a small proportion of Thai cases can be accounted for by drugs and there is no association with chloramphenicol [6]. The environmental and occupational exposures may be the important etiologic factors. We have documented an inverse association between aplastic anemia and socioeconomic status [7], increased risk among rice farmers [8] and an association with past exposure to hepatitis A virus [9]. It is not clear that any of these factors are relevant to the association. Their occurrence may constitute indirect evidence of the effect of water- or soil-born infectious agents.

Progenitor Cells in Aplastic Anemia

Hematopoiesis is greatly impaired in aplastic anemia. The most consistent finding in all laboratories is the very low numbers of blood and bone marrow hematopoietic progenitor cells including CFU-GM, BFU-E, CFU-erythroid (CFU-E) and CFU-granulocyte, erythroid, macrophage, megakaryocyte (CFU-GEMM) [1]. Our study indicates that the numbers of BFU-E and CFU-GM are very low in the blood and bone marrow and there are no colonies observed in about one-third of the patients studied [10]. It is of interest to note that the presence of colonies is related to a good clinical response to therapy with anabolic steroids. Of 37 patients studied, 11 had no colonies at all and the remaining 26 patients had a small number of colonies. In those with no colonies, five patients died, one failed to respond to therapy, two recovered and three were lost to follow-up. Of 26 patients with the presence of colonies, 11 patients responded, four failed to respond, four died and seven were lost to follow-up [10].

In patients who recover after therapy with anabolic steroids, the numbers of BFU-E and CFU-GM are still low (10% and 20% of the normal controls) although they are higher compared to those with active disease [11]. Those patients who respond to ATG/ALG treatment have lower numbers of BFU-E and CFU-GM in the blood and bone marrow as well [12].

Primitive progenitor and stem cells can be identified by CD34 expression. The number of CD34 cells is much reduced in aplastic anemia [13, 14]. Recently, it has been shown that there is a profound defect in long-term initiating cells which have the frequency, phenotype and kinetic properties of true stem cells [15, 16].

PNH

PNH is an acquired disorder, characterized by chronic intravascular hemolysis resulting from an increased sensitivity of erythrocytes to activated complements [17]. Absence of red cell surfaces of complement regulatory proteins such as CD59 and decay-accelerating factor (DAF) is responsible for the hypersensitivity to complement of the red cells [18, 19]. DAF, CD59 and some other membrane proteins are inserted to the red cell surface via a glycosylphosphatidylinositol (GPI) moiety. Impaired synthesis of GPI anchor results in the deficiency of such proteins from the red cell membrane. Studies with abnormal lymphoid cell lines established from PNH patients indicate that the first step of GPI anchor synthesis is defective [20, 21]. The genes responsible for this particular step, called PIG-A, PIG-C and PIG-H, have been cloned and characterized [22, 23]. Somatic mutation of only X-linked PIG-A has been shown to be responsible in over 100 patients studied [24].

PNH is relatively more common in Thailand [25]. There are 5-10 new cases seen annually at Siriraj Hospital; more than 100 patients are collected in our series [25]. PNH is common in the younger age group of 21-30 years [25]. The association between PNH and aplastic anemia has been described; PNH occurs in approximately 9% of aplastic anemia patients [26]. During the course of PNH, one-third of the patients die of bone marrow failure. It has been reported that PNH, aplastic anemia and acute leukemia occurred in a single patient [27]. PNH as well as aplastic anemia are more frequent in Thailand.

Progenitor Cells in PNH

Defective hematopoiesis is observed in PNH. There are markedly decreased numbers of BFU-E and CFU-GM in the blood and bone marrow [28]. The numbers of progenitor cells, both BFU-E and CFU-GM, in the blood are only 20% of normal whereas the number of BFU-E in the bone marrow is about 10% and CFU-GM is approximately one-half of normal. The decrease is observed even in the presence of marrow hypercellularity. However, those patients with marrow hypocellularity have a lower number of BFU-E and CFU-GM. The finding of decreased numbers of progenitor cells suggests the involvement of hematopoietic stem cells; however, the degree of depletion is not as great as that in aplastic anemia. Quantitative analysis of CD34 cells shows a lower number in PNH compared to normal individuals. The mean percentage is about one-third of normal (0.03% versus 0.08%), and the absolute number is about one-half of the normal (2.5×10^6/l versus 4.9×10^6/l). In those with aplastic/PNH syndrome, the number of CD34 cells is lower, about one-third of normal. Lower numbers of blood progenitor cells in PNH is partly due to complement-mediated cytolysis since increased sensitivity to complement of BFU-E, CFU-GM and CFU-megakaryocyte has been demonstrated [29, 30].

Corticosteroid therapy in PNH can produce an improvement in 60% of the patients [31]. A prolonged interval from diagnosis to treatment decreases the chance of a favorable hematologic response to therapy. Those with a higher number of progenitor cells in the blood and bone marrow have a higher rate of response.

Thalassemia

Thalassemia is widespread throughout the world; Southeast Asia in particular has high frequencies [32, 33]. The most common abnormal genes are α-thalassemia, β-thalassemia, hemoglobin (Hb) E and Hb Constant Spring (CS). The severe form of α-thalassemia, α-thalassemia 1, is most common in this region and Hb E is the hallmark of Southeast Asia. α-thalassemia is very common, attaining frequencies of 20%-40% in the northeastern corner of Southeast Asia. Hb E is mostly found at the junction of Cambodia, Laos and Thailand, the so-called Hb E triangle, where the frequency of Hb E reaches 50%-60%. β-thalassemia and Hb CS are scattered throughout the region at a low percentage (3%-9% for β-thalassemia and 1%-8% for Hb CS). Abnormal genes in various combinations lead to more than 60 thalassemic syndromes. Of these there are four common syndromes including Hb Bart's hydrop fetalis, Hb H disease, homozygous β-thalassemia and β-thalassemia/Hb E disease. In Thailand, about 500,000 people are afflicted with this disease and 18-24 million people are heterozygous for these abnormal genes. The annual numbers of birth are 625 for homozygous β-thalassemia, 3,250 for β-thalassemia/Hb E disease, 1,250 for Hb Bart's hydrop fetalis and 7,000 for Hb H disease. The high number of people afflicted with these syndromes makes thalassemia one of the major socioeconomic burdens on Southeast Asia. Migrations of the people have rapidly brought the Southeast Asian thalassemic genes to the West.

Progenitor Cells in Thalassemia

The numbers of BFU-E and CFU-GM in the blood of thalassemic patients are higher than normal individuals (six to eight times for BFU-E and two to three times for CFU-GM) [34]. There is a positive correlation between the number of colonies and the absolute number of nucleated red cells. Thalassemic patients have a higher number of progenitor cells after splenectomy. In thalassemia, the spleen acts as a filter site for migrating immature cells and a pool of hematopoietic progenitors, as well as represents a site of extramedullary erythropoiesis. After splenectomy, the filter function is abolished; however, hematopoietic stimulation in the bone marrow still persists. The numbers of progenitor cells as well as nucleated red cells are therefore increased postsplenectomy.

The number of CD34 cells is increased in thalassemia compared to normal individuals. Those with splenectomy have a higher number of CD34 cells than nonsplenectomized patients. The mean percentage of CD34 cells was 0.33% and 0.25% for those with and without splenectomy, respectively, whereas it was 0.08% ± 0.02% in normal individuals. The absolute number of CD34 cells was 44.9 $\times$ 10^6/l and 18.3 $\times$ 10^6/l for splenectomized and nonsplenectomized patients, respectively; the value in normal controls was 5.3 ± 1.3 $\times$ 10^6/l.

The developmental stages of erythroid precursors in thalassemia were studied by using a two-phase liquid culture [35]. The first phase was cultured in 10% conditioned media from the 5637 bladder cancer cell line which contained various growth factors excluding erythropoietin. After six days of culture, the nonadherent cells were harvested and recultured in media containing erythropoietin. The cultured cells were studied for cell count, morphology and flow cytometry at various time intervals. In normal persons, during the beginning of the second phase, the cell number decreased together with the appearence of many blast-like cells. The pronormoblast first appeared on day 3 after reculture. The erythroid precursors were rapidly proliferating and differentiating thereafter and reached the peak around the middle of the third week to the beginning of the fourth week. Then the cell number declined and the erythroid precursors started to disintegrate.

In thalassemia, there was more proliferation than normal controls, splenectomized more than nonsplenectomized patients, indicating that there are considerable numbers of erythroid progenitors in the blood of thalassemic patients. The rate of disintegration of erythroid precursors seems to be more accelerated in nonsplenectomized patients at the beginning of the fourth week while a small number of some erythroid precursors in splenectomized patients were still in their early stages and began to proliferate and differentiate further. At six weeks, early erythroid precursors were still observed in splenectomized patients although none were found in culture of normal or nonsplenectomized cases. This finding indicates that there are still some immature precursors at the sixth week of the culture in splenectomized patients. In nonsplenectomized patients the erythroid precursors seem to disintegrate more rapidly than controls, in contrast to the flow cytometry result of a high percentage of double-positive cells at week 5 and 6, and the confocal image result of the small cells whose stages could not be recognized visually. These small cells in thalassemia may be destroyed erythroid precursors in which the size of dying cells is reduced and the expression of surface markers is less affected. Such accelerated cell destruction is partly responsible for the ineffective erythropoiesis in thalassemia. The mechanism of cell death in thalassemia has been proposed to be apoptosis [36].

ACKNOWLEDGMENT

This work was supported by grants from Mahidol University, Prince Chainat-Narainthorn Foundation, The Wellcome Trust and Public Health Service (Grant HL 35068), and the National Heart, Lung, and Blood Institute, National Institutes of Health.

REFERENCES

1 Young NS, Alter BP. Aplastic anemia: acquired and inherited. Philadelphia: W.B. Saunders, 1994:1-11.

2 Gordon-Smith EC, Issaragrisil S. Epidemiology of aplastic anemia. Baillieres Clin Haematol 1992;5:475-491.

3 Young NS, Issaragrisil S, Chieh CW et al. Aplastic anaemia in the Orient. Br J Haematol 1986;62:1-6.

4 Kaufman DW, Kelly JP, Levy M et al. The Drug Etiology of Agranulocytosis and Aplastic Anemia. New York: Oxford University Press, 1991:1-404

5 Issaragrisil S, Sriratanasatavorn C, Piankijagum A et al. Incidence of aplastic anemia in Bangkok. Blood 1991;77:2166-2168.

6 Issaragrisil S, Kaufman DW, Anderson T et al. Low drug attributability of aplastic anemia in Thailand. Blood 1997;89:4034-4039.

7 Issaragrisil S, Kaufman DW, Anderson TE et al. An association of aplastic anemia in Thailand with low socioeconomic status. Br J Haematol 1995;91:80-84.

8 Issaragrisil S, Chansung K, Kaufman DW et al. Association of aplastic anemia in rural Thailand with grain farming and agricultural pesticide exposure. Am J Public Health 1997;87:1551-1554.

9 Issaragrisil S, Kaufman D, Thongput A et al. Association of seropositivity for hepatitis viruses and aplastic anemia in Thailand. Hepatology 1997;25:1255-1257.

10 Issaragrisil S, Tangnaitrisorana Y, Chinprasertsuk S et al. Studies on the pathogenesis of aplastic anemia in Thailand: evidence of immune mediated mechanism. Asian Pac J Allergy Immunol 1988;6:33-37.

11 Issaragrisil S, Piankijagum A, Tangnaitrisorana Y. Abnormalities of hematopoietic progenitor cells in patients with aplastic anemia after hematologic recovery. J Med Assoc Thai 1989;72:643-648.

12 U-pratya Y, Yimyam M. The hematopoietic committed progenitor cells studied in aplastic anemia treated with antilymphocyte globulin. Mahidol Univ J 1996;4:105-108.

13 Maciejewski JP, Anderson S, Katevas P et al. Phenotypic and functional analysis of bone marrow progenitor cell compartment in bone marrow failure. Br J Haematol 1994;87:227-234.

14 Scopes J, Bagnara M, Gordon-Smith EC et al. Haemopoietic progenitor cells are reduced in aplastic anaemia. Br J Haematol 1994;86:427-430.

15 Maciejewski JP, Selleri C, Sato T et al. A severe and consistent defecit in marrow and circulating primitive hematopoietic cells (long-term culture-initiating cells) in acquired aplastic anemia. Blood 1996;88:1983-1991.

16 Schrezenmeier H, Jenal M, Herrmann F et al. Quantitative analysis of cobblestone area-forming cells in bone marrow of patients with aplastic anemia by limiting dilution assay. Blood 1996;88:4474-4480.

17 Ross WF, Dacie JV. Immune lysis of normal human and PNH red blood cells. I. The sensitivity of PNH red cells to lysis by complement and specific antibody. J Clin Invest 1966;45:736-748.

18 Kinoshita T, Medof ME, Silber R et al. Distribution of decay-accelerating factor in the peripheral blood of normal individuals and patients with paroxysmal nocturnal hemoglobinuria. J Exp Med 1985;162:75-92.

19 Fujioka S, Yamada T. Varying populations of CD59-negative, partly positive and normally positive blood cells in different cell lineages in peripheral blood of paroxysmal nocturnal hemoglobinuria patients. Am J Hematol 1994;45:1150-1161.

20 Mahoney JF, Urakaze M, Hall S et al. Defective glycosylphosphatidyl inositol anchor synthesis in paroxysmal nocturnal hemoglobinuria granulocytes. Blood 1992;79:1400-1403.

21 Takahashi M, Takeda J, Hirose S et al. Deficient biosynthesis of N-acetyl-glucosaminyl-phosphatidylinositol, the first intermediate of glycosyl phosphatidyl-inosital anchor biosynthesis, in cell lines established from patients with paroxysmal nocturnal hemoglobinuria. J Exp Med 1993;177:517-521.

22 Miyata T, Takeda J, Iida Y et al. The cloning of PIG-A, a component in the early step of GPI-anchor biosynthesis. Science 1993;259:1318-1320.

23 Inoue N, Watanabe R, Takeda J et al. PIG-C, one of the three human genes involved in the first step of glycosylphosphatidylinositol biosynthesis is a homologue of saccharomyces cerevisiae GP12. Biochem Biophys Res Commun 1996;226:193-199.

24 Pramoonjago P, Wannchiwanawin W, Chinprasertsuk S et al. Somatic mutations of PIG-A in Thai patients with paroxysmal nocturnal hemoglobinuria. Blood 1995;86:1736-1739.

25 Kruatachue M, Wasi P, Na-Nakorn S. Paroxysmal nocturnal haemoglobinuria in Thailand with special reference to an association with aplastic anaemia. Br J Haematol 1978;39:267-276.

26 de Planque MM, Bacigalupo A, Wursch A et al. Long-term follow up of severe aplastic anaemia patients treated with antithymocyte globulin. Br J Haematol 1989;73:121-126.

27 Wasi P, Kruatrachue M, Na-Nakorn S. Aplastic anemia-paroxysmal nocturnal hemoglobinuria

syndrome-acute leukemia in the same patient. J Med Assoc Thai 1970;53:656-661.

28 Issaragrisil S, Piankijagum A, Chinprasertsuk S et al. Growth of mixed erythroid-granulocytic colonies in culture derived from bone marrow of patients with paroxysmal nocturnal hemoglobinuria without addition of exogenous stimulator. Exp Hematol 1986;14:861-866.

29 Dessypris EN, Clark DA, McKee LC et al. Increased sensitivity to complement of erythroid and myeloid progenitors in paroxysmal nocturnal hemoglobinuria. N Engl J Med 1983;309:690-693.

30 Dessypris EN, Gleaton JH, Clark DA. Increased sensitivity to complement of megakaryocyte progenitors in paroxysmal nocturnal haemoglobinuria. Br J Haematol 1988;69:305-309.

31 Issaragrisil S, Piankijagum Aj, Tangnaitrisorana Y. Corticosteroids therapy in paroxysmal nocturnal hemoglobinuria. Am J Haematol 1987;25:77-83.

32 Wasi P. Haemoglobinopathies including thalassaemia. Clin Haematol 1981;10:707-729.

33 Wasi P, Pootrakul S, Pootrakul P et al. Thalassemia in Thailand. Ann NY Acad Sci 1980;344:352-363.

34 Issaragrisil S, Tangnaitrisorana Y, Piankijagum A et al. Study of hematopoietic progenitors in patients with thalassemia: the effect of splenectomy. Birth Defects 1988;23:323-329.

35 Khuhapinant A, Bunyaratvej A, Sahaphong S et al. An in vitro study on thalassemic erythroid precursors in liquid culture. Southeast Asian J Trop Med Public Health 1997 (in press).

36 Yuan J, Angelucci E, Lucarelli G et al. Accelerated programmed cell death (apoptosis) in erythroid precursors of patients with severe β-thlassemia (Cooley's anemia). Blood 1993;82:344-377.

Chapter V

Mobilization of Blood Stem Cells

In Vivo Expansion of the Circulating Stem Cell Pool
Martin Körbling

Mobilization of Blood Stem Cells
Anne Kessinger, J. Graham Sharp

Mobilization and Transplantation of Peripheral Blood Stem Cells
Richard K. Shadduck, Zella R. Zeigler, D. Frank Andrews III, Gary L. Gilmore, John Lister

The Role of Endothelium in the Regulation of Hematopoietic Stem Cell Migration
Robert Möhle, Shahin Rafii, Malcolm A.S. Moore

Rapidly Mobilizable Stem Cells. Do They Belong to a Special Subpopulation?
Julia Gidáli, I. Fehér

In Vivo Expansion of the Circulating Stem Cell Pool

MARTIN KÖRBLING

University of Texas, M.D. Anderson Cancer Center, Houston, Texas, USA

Key Words. *CD34⁺ cells · Stem cell mobilization · G-CSF · Thrombopoietin · Anti-VLA₄ monoclonal antibody*

ABSTRACT

Stem cell trafficking between extravascular marrow sites and circulating blood is an essential part of the blood stem cell transplantation technology. Recombinant human G-CSF (rHuG-CSF) is widely used for stem cell peripheralization alone or together with chemopriming mobilizing early and pluripotent CD34⁺ cell subsets. New cytokine/chemokine mobilization regimens are under investigation such as combined rHuG-CSF and rHu thrombopoietin, rHuG-CSF and interleukin 3, rHuG-CSF and rHu stem cell factor, rHuG-CSF and Flt-3 ligand, human macrophage inflammatory protein, interleukin 1, and interleukin 8. Modifying the adherence of CD34⁺ cells to extracellular matrix molecules is a new mechanism by which hematopoietic progenitor cells are released into the circulating blood. Blocking the $\alpha_4\beta_1$ integrin receptor on CD34⁺ progenitor cells by using monoclonal antibodies specific for the heterodimeric complex $\alpha_4\beta_1$ has been shown to further increase the circulating stem cell concentration when given following rHuG-CSF priming.

The current clinical research is primarily focused on improving stem cell mobilization efficiency in heavily pretreated and poorly mobilizing patients, and to decrease adverse effects of cytokine treatment. *Stem Cells 1998;16(suppl 1):131-138*

INTRODUCTION

The circulating stem cell pool has almost entirely replaced bone marrow (BM) as a stem cell source for autologous support after myeloablative or near-myeloablative chemotherapy. Allogeneic blood stem cell transplantation is now emerging as a new transplantation modality with potential advantages over allogeneic BM transplantation.

Transient shifting of hematopoietic progenitor cells including stem cells is a precondition for sufficient stem cell collection from both patients and normal stem cell donors. In the following, we describe mechanisms that increase the circulating stem cell concentration as part of stem cell trafficking between extravascular sites and circulating blood.

Circulating Hematopoietic Progenitor Cells

BM and blood stem cell pools are in dynamic equilibrium to each other allowing hematopoietic progenitor cells migrating from extravascular marrow sites or marginal pools into circulation and vice versa [1]. In the unperturbed peripheral blood (PB) from normal subjects, the percentage of hematopoietic progenitor cells, phenotypically characterized as CD34⁺, among circulating nucleated cells is, on the average, 0.06% [2] compared to 1.1% in a BM aspirate (Table 1). The absolute number of circulating CD34⁺ cells in normal individuals has been reported to be 3.8 ($\pm$ 0.8 SD) $\times$ 10^3/ml PB (n = 14) [2] or 3.8 ($\pm$ 3.2 SD) $\times$ 10^3/ml PB (n = 10) [3]. The more primitive circulating CD34$^+$ subset concentrations such as CD34$^+$ Thy-1^{dim} and CD34$^+$ Thy-1^{dim} CD38$^-$ encompassing 30% and 2.5%, respectively, of the unperturbed circulating CD34$^+$ cell pool are 1.1 $\times$ 10^3/ml and 0.095 $\times$ 10^3/ml, respectively [2] (Table 1).

Mobilization of Hematopoietic Progenitor Cells from Extravascular Marrow Sites or Marginal Pools into the Circulation of Normal Donors

For complete and sustained hematopoietic engraftment after myeloablative chemo- or chemo/radiotherapy, patients must receive a sufficient number of early and pluripotent hematopoietic progenitor cells with indefinite self-renewal potential. The stem cell concentration in steady-state PB is considered insufficient to provide a CD34$^+$ cell engraftment dose by single or multiple apheresis in a reasonable time period. A temporary peripheralization of CD34$^+$ cells and subsets into the circulating blood is therefore a necessity to significantly increase the yield of blood stem cells, thus minimizing the number of aphereses needed to achieve a CD34$^+$ cell engraftment dose.

Successful temporary shifting of hemopoietic progenitor cells from extravascular marrow sites into circulation by chemotherapy-induced rebounding of peripheral blood progenitor cell (PBPC) concentration has first been reported in man by *Richman et al.* [4]. Such "chemopriming" treatment combined with cytokine application is still considered standard treatment for stem cell mobilization in cancer patients. For obvious ethical reasons, mobilization of stem cells from normal donors for allogeneic transplantation cannot rely on chemotherapy as shown to be effective in the autologous transplant setting, when combined with cytokine treatment [5]. Cytokine priming alone, however, has emerged as an acceptable and efficient treatment alternative in normal donors for stem cell mobilization. As shown by *Dexter's* group [6] in a sex-mismatched mouse model, the transplantation of 10 µl recombinant human (rHu)G-CSF-treated PB was equivalent to 3,000 µl unperturbed PB in rescuing $\geq$ 98% of lethally irradiated mice.

Optimal Cytokine for Stem Cell Mobilization in Normal Donors

rHuG-CSF has emerged so far as the preferred cytokine for stem cell mobilization in normal donors partly based on the positive experience and toxicity profile reported with its administration to granulocyte donors [7, 8]. rHuGM-CSF appears to be less effective in mobilizing CD34$^+$ progenitors in normal stem cell donors [9, 10] although comparative data are scarce. In a recent study a combined rHuG-CSF and rHuGM-CSF mobilization treatment was similarly well-tolerated in normal individuals. The combined treatment did not, however, translate into a higher mobilization of CD34$^+$ progenitors when compared to rHuG-CSF alone, but resulted in a significantly greater peripheralization of CD34$^+$ cells with the early CD34$^+$CD38$^-$ subtype [10]. These findings suggest that rHuGM-CSF in combination with other cytokines deserves further investigation as a mobilizing agent in normal individuals.

Table 1. CD34$^+$ cells and subsets in the peripheral blood of normal subjects at steady state and at the fourth day of rHuG-CSF treatment

	CD34$^+$ cells $\times$ 10^3/ml	% CD34$^+$ cells among TNC	CD34$^+$ Thy-1^{dim} cells $\times$ 10^3/ml	% CD34$^+$ Thy-1^{dim} cells among TNC	CD34$^+$ Thy-1^{dim} CD38$^-$ cells $\times$ 10^3/ml	% CD34$^+$ Thy-1^{dim} CD38$^-$ cells among TNC
Steady-state PB	3.8	0.06	1.1	0.017	0.095	0.0015
PB at the fourth day of rHuG-CSF treatment	61.9	0.93	26.6	0.4	2.2	0.03

PB: peripheral blood; TNC: total nucleated cells.

Effect of rHuG-CSF Treatment on the Peripheralization of WBC, Polymorphonuclear (PMN) Cells, Lymphocytes, and CD34$^+$ Cells and Subsets in Normal Subjects

To assess the effects of rHuG-CSF (12 μg/kg/day) on the peripheralization of hematopoietic progenitor cells and lymphoid subsets, we studied a cohort of 41 normal blood stem cell donors. After three days of rHuG-CSF treatment, the WBC, PMN and lymphocyte concentrations in the donor's PB exceeded baseline by 6.4-, 8.0- and 2.2-fold, respectively [2]. A similar increase of T lymphocytes by day 3 of 16 μg/kg/day rHuG-CSF has been reported by *Weaver et al.* [11], namely 1.5 to 2.0 times over baseline. On the other hand, PB CD34$^+$ cells and primitive subsets such as CD34$^+$ Thy-1^{dim}, and CD34$^+$ Thy-1^{dim} CD38$^-$ cells increased by 16.3-fold, 24.2-fold and 23.2-fold, respectively, suggesting a selective peripheraiization effect of rHuG-CSF on hematopoietic progenitor cells and, in particular, on their more primitive stem cell subsets [2, 12]. The percentage of CD34$^+$ cells among total nucleated cells increases up to almost 1% at the fourth day of rHuG-CSF treatment (Table 1).

The clonogenic potential of rHuG-CSF-mobilized PBSC is also reported to be significantly higher: in a study on PBSC obtained from G-CSF-treated normal individuals, the replating capacity of primary colonies from five-week-old long-term culture (LTC) systems was found to be significantly higher than the five-week-old LTC initiated in a steady state [13]. In normal donors, a five-day course of G-CSF increased the frequency of LTC-initiating cells among CD34$^+$ cells by ninefold over baseline [12].

Kinetics of CD34$^+$ Cells and Subsets under rHuG-CSF Mobilization Treatment

The kinetics of WBC and progenitor cell subsets under rHuG-CSF treatment are quite uniform in an unperturbed, normal hematopoietic system, although a remarkable interindividual variability in the degree of progenitor cell mobilization has become evident [3, 14, 15]. When monitored over six days on a daily basis under rHuG-CSF treatment (12 μg/kg/day), the kinetics of circulating CD34$^+$ cells and subsets paralleled each other reaching a plateau from day 4 on (day 1 = first day of cytokine treatment). Based on that data and data reported by others [3, 14-17], the most favorable day for stem cell collection (15- to 35-fold increase of circulating CD34$^+$ cells at peak level over baseline values) would appear to be day 4 or day 5 of cytokine treatment. Continuation of rHuG-CSF administration beyond a five-day course leads to a progressive decline in the mobilization efficiency of CD34$^+$ progenitors [15, 18].

Dose-Dependent Mobilization of CD34$^+$ Progenitor Cells

It has been shown that, at least for rHuG-CSF doses between 5 and 10 μg/kg/day, a dose-response relationship exists between rHuG-CSF dose and degree of mobilization of CD34$^+$ progenitor cells [18, 19, 20]. Although rHuG-CSF doses up to 24 μg/kg/day have been employed [21, 22], experience with such a dose range remains limited. rHuhG-CSF given to normal donors at a dose of 10 - 12 μg/kg twice daily resulted in a higher yield of CD34$^+$ cells compared to 10 μg/kg given once a day [22]. Nevertheless, bone pain and headache were more severe in the high-dose rHuG-CSF donor cohort, but still tolerable.

Even low (2.5 μg/kg/day) daily doses of rHuG-CSF consistently induce a significant increase in circulating colony-forming units granulocyte/macrophage (CFU-GM) and BFU-E, which is paralleled by an increase in the circulating level of CD34$^+$ cells [23].

Factors Affecting Mobilization of CD34$^+$ Progenitor Cells

In an effort to elucidate factors affecting mobilization in normal donors and stem cell yield by apheresis, the CD34$^+$ cell yield from the first day of apheresis in 119 donors who underwent apheresis on days 4-6 of rHuG-CSF treatment (12 μg/kg/day) was analyzed. The CD34$^+$ cell yield was significantly lower in donors > 55 years of age, or who underwent apheresis on day 4 of rHuG-CSF treatment. There was also a correlation between CD34$^+$ cell yield and baseline WBC, pre-apheresis WBC and pre-apheresis mononuclear cell (MNC) count. Twenty-one (18%) donors were considered "poor mobilizers" yielding less than 20 $\times$ 10^6 CD34$^+$ cells/l donor blood processed. In the multivariate analysis, the only significant risk factor for inferior mobilization was age > 55 years, which conferred a 3.8-fold increased risk ($p = 0.04$). As poor mobilizers occurred in all age groups, the predictive value (and clinical usefulness) of the model was limited [24].

New Stem Cell Mobilization Regimens Including Cytokines/Chemokines and Anti-VLA₄ Monoclonal Antibody

The heparinoid dextran sulfate, a synthetic low molecular weight polyanion of strong negative charge, has been successfully used as a first stem cell mobilization agent in a canine transplantation model [25, 26]. rHuG-CSF is, at the present time, considered the mobilization treatment of choice for normal donors. Clinical experience with other cytokines alone or in combination with rHuG-CSF is limited.

Combined rHuG-CSF and rHu Thrombopoietin (TPO)

rHuTPO is a growth factor that stimulates the proliferation and differentiation of megakaryocytic progenitor cells, inducing the full maturation of megakaryocytes and release of platelets [27]. *Molineux et al.* [28] reported that irradiated mice that received PBSC mobilized by PEGylated recombinant human megakaryocyte growth and development factor (PEG-rHuMGDF) showed a significantly reduced period (four or five days) of thrombocytopenia ($<10^{11}$/l) compared to those that received unmobilized PBSC transplantation (nine days). In this model, rHuMGDF also modestly stimulates the mobilization of myeloid progenitor cells, and rHuMGDF-mobilized PBSC accelerate platelet recovery in transplant recipients.

As shown in an ongoing phase I clinical trial [29], combined mobilization treatment with rHuG-CSF and rHuTPO in patients with stage II/III breast cancer results in a higher CD34⁺ cell apheresis yield compared to rHuG-CSF treatment alone (34.5×10^6/kg versus 15.3×10^6/kg CD34⁺ cells in the apheresis product). A possible effect of rHuTPO treatment on circulating megakaryocytic progenitor cells (CD34⁺ CD41a⁺) and a possible shortening of the post-transplant period of cytopenia including thrombocytopenia, remains to be shown in this and further clinical trials.

Combined rHuG-CSF and Interleukin 3 (IL-3)

Combined treatment with rHuG-CSF and IL-3 has been reported to further increase circulating progenitor cells in patients with Hodgkin's disease and non-Hodgkin's lymphoma compared to rHuG-CSF alone. rHuG-CSF alone (5 μg/kg/day over five days) increased the number of circulating CFU-GM over baseline by 21-fold, whereas combined treatment with IL-3 (5 mg/kg/day for seven days) followed by rHuG-CSF at the same dose level for five days further increased the circulating CFU-GM level by 56-fold over baseline [30]. When rHuG-CSF (5 μg/kg/day) was administered for seven consecutive days either alone or preceded by rHuIL-3 (5 μg/kg/day) for four consecutive days in sequential or partially overlapping schedules, the mean circulating CD34⁺ cell counts on day 3 of cytokine treatment were significantly higher in the sequential treatment group [31].

Human Macrophage Inflammatory Protein (MIP-1a)

MIP-1α is considered a potential myeloprotective cytokine based on its myelosuppressive and cycle inhibitory functions [32]. As reported by *Lord et al.* [33], MIP-1α also induces a rapid mobilization effect on early progenitor cells into circulation in mice. In a phase I clinical trial the administration of BB10010, a genetically engineered and stable variant of MIP-1α, at 5 or 10 μg/kg significantly reduced cycling rates of BM progenitor cells, as well as its concentration, but increased the number of circulating progenitor cells between 2.6- and 4.1-fold over baseline [34].

IL-1 and IL-8

IL-1 is a newly studied compound for potential stem cell mobilization. In studies in mice, IL-1 administration (1 μg) increases the number of circulating CFU-GM by 30-fold over baseline.

Transplantation of IL-1-mobilized blood progenitor cells resulted in long-term donor chimerism [35]. IL-8, a chemotactic cytokine, has been shown to induce rapid (15 - 30 min) mobilization of hematopoietic progenitor cells [36]. Fifteen minutes after single intraperitoneal injection of 30 μg IL-8 into mice, circulating CFU-GM increased by 17-fold over baseline, and returned to almost pretreatment values after 60 min. Sex-mismatched transplantation of IL-8-mobilized hematopoietic progenitor cells resulted in complete and permanent hematopoietic reconstitution.

Combined rHuG-CSF and recombinant methionyl Human Stem Cell Factor (r-metHuSCF)

While r-metHuSCF alone exerts little effect on in vitro colony formation of normal BM progenitor cells, the combination of r-metHuSCF with rHuGM-CSF, rHuG-CSF or IL-3 synergistically increases colony formation [37]. As shown by *Andrews et al.* in nonhuman primates [38], low-dose rHuSCF treatment in combination with rHuG-CSF resulted in a 14-fold higher yield of progenitor cells contained in the apheresis product compared to rHuG-CSF administration alone. WBC, PMN and platelets engrafted significantly faster when using the rHuSCF and rHuG-CSF-treated blood stem cell autograft. Several clinical phase I/II trials have been reported to assess the ability of r-metHuSCF in combination with rHuG-CSF to mobilize stem cells in patients with solid tumors or malignant hematologic disorders. In patients with advanced stage breast cancer, a combined rHuSCF (10 μg/kg/day) and rHuG-CSF (10 μg/kg/day) resulted in a fourfold increase in the percentage of $CD34^+$ cells in the apheresis product compared to rHuG-CSF treatment (10 μg/kg/day) alone [39]. Another multicenter phase I/II trial in non-Hodgkin's lymphoma patients using escalating doses of subcutaneously administered r-metHuSCF (0 - 20 μg/kg/day) combined with 10 μg/kg/day rHuG-CSF for seven days has recently been reported [40]. r-metHuSCF was well-tolerated in conjunction with a multiagent premedication regimen. In patients with prior extensive chemopriming and combined cytokine treatment, the $CD34^+$ cell apheresis yield was 1.76×10^6/kg versus 0.28×10^6/kg, and the time to an untransfused platelet count of 20×10^9/l was 10.5 days shorter.

Combined Flt-3 Ligand and rHuG-CSF

Flt-3 ligand is believed to have similar biologic activities on the hematopoietic system as is known for SCF. *Molineux et al.* [41] studied the effect of a combined Flt-3 ligand and rHuG-CSF treatment on circulating CFU-GM in mice. Whereas Flt-3 ligand alone was a relatively modest mobilizer of CFU-GM (2.3-fold increase over baseline), combined Flt-3 ligand and rHuG-CSF treatment resulted in a 645-fold increase of circulating CFU-GM. Based on those data and data reported for a combined rHuSCF and rHuG-CSF treatment, a synergistic effect of rHuG-CSF with either rHuSCF or Flt-3 ligand on the peripheralization of hematopoietic progenitor cells seems to exist. Flt-3 ligand is also known to increase the number of circulating dendritic cells that might, together with increased numbers of natural killer cells, mediate a nonspecific tumoricidal effect in the transplant recipient [42].

Since Flt-3 ligand primarily acts through lymphoid proliferation compared to the mast cell degranulation effect of rHuSCF, Flt-3 ligand might also have a different toxicity profile.

Combined rHuG-CSF and Anti-VLA₄ Monoclonal Antibody (mAb)

Hematopoietic progenitor cells predominantly interact with the extracellular matrix molecule fibronectin through expression of cell-surface receptors belonging to the integrin family. The $\alpha_4\beta_1$ integrin (= very late activation antigen-4; VLA₄) and the $\alpha_5\beta_1$ integrin (= very late activation antigen-5; VLA₅) receptors are the principle ones through which hematopoietic progenitor cells adhere to fibronectin [43, 44].

Papayannopoulou and *Nakamoto* [45] reported a preclinical study in primates using anti-VLA₄ mAb (anti-CD49d) to peripheralize hematopoietic progenitor cells. Daily injections of anti-VLA₄ for four days resulted in an increase of PB CFU-GM concentration by 8- to 100-fold over baseline 24 h after injection, and an 18- to > 200-fold increase of PB BFU-E concentration. When pretreated with rHuG-CSF for five days, anti-VLA_4 treatment, however, additively augmented peripheralization of progenitors in animals. The five-day rHuG-CSF treatment increased the PB CFU-GM from a baseline concentration of 89 per ml up to 2,000 per ml PB. After two additional injections of anti-VLA_4 on days 6 and 7, there was a significant increase in CFU-GM beyond the level observed at day 5 of rHuG-CSF, from 2,000 per ml to 13,000 per ml PB. This increase was maintained for about three days after the last anti-VLA_4 treatment and occurred while the WBC concentration was decreasing. In contrast to rHuG-CSF alone, there was a significant increase in BFU-E, circulating CFU-E and nucleated red blood cells.

It is believed that some cytokines, including rHuG-CSF, also interfere with the adhesive properties of $\beta 1$ integrins on hematopoietic progenitor cells [35] thus providing a potentially additive effect to anti-VLA_4 mAb treatment.

Transient Post-Donation Cytopenias in Normal Donors

Stem cell apheresis and, in particular, large-volume stem cell apheresis has been reported to cause a transient decrease in the donor's platelet count [46, 47]. A causative direct role of rHuG-CSF mobilization treatment has also been discussed [48]. Clinically asymptomatic, transient drops in PB lymphocyte and granulocyte concentrations below baseline occasionally resulting in lymphocytopenia and/or granulocytopenia have also been reported following rHuG-CSF mobilization and stem cell collection [48-51]. $CD34^+$ cells and subsets as well as lymphoid subsets (CD3, CD4, CD8, $CD3^-16^+56^+$, CD19) bottom out by day 7 to regain baseline values by day 30 to 100 after rHuG-CSF treatment and apheresis [50]. A reactive lymphocytopenia by day 7 was also reported by *Martinez et al.* [51] regaining baseline values 30-90 days after apheresis. From the data reported so far, there is, up to now, no evidence of a possible clinical relevance of these findings.

CONCLUSIONS

Stem cell trafficking between extravascular marrow sites and circulating blood is an essential part of the blood stem cell transplantation technology. We are now in the early stage of understanding the marrow microenvironment which regulates adherence and release of hematopoietic progenitor cells and immunocompetent cells. Data accumulated so far from clinical studies show by no doubt a preferential mobilization of hematopoietic progenitor cells over lymphoid cells when using rHuG-CSF treatment. It is foreseeable that proper use of cell release mechanisms through the marrow-blood barrier, including blocking cell adherence, might enable us to construct in vivo a stem cell graft that fulfills clinical needs by minimizing the donor's risk and discomfort.

REFERENCES

1 Fliedner TM, Steinbach KH. Repopulating potential of hematopoietic precursor cells. Blood Cells 1988;14:393-410.

2 Körbling M, Huh YO, Durett A et al. Allogeneic blood stem cell transplantation: peripheralization and yield of donor-derived primitive hematopoietic progenitor cells ($CD34^+$ $Thy-1^{dim}$) and lymphoid subsets, and possible predictors of engraftment and GVHD. Blood 1995;86:2842-2848.

3 Link H, Arseniev L, Bähre O et al. Combined transplantation of allogeneic bone marrow and $CD34^+$ blood cells. Blood 1995;86:2500-2508.

4 Richman C, Weiner RS, Yankee RA. Incerase in circulating stem cells following chemotherapy in man. Blood 1976;47:1031-1034.

5 Socinski MA, Cannistra SA, Elias A et al. Granulocyte macrophage colony stimulating factor expands the circulating hematopoietic progenitor cell compartment in man. Lancet 1988;28:1194-1198.

6 Molineux G, Pojda Z, Hampson IN et al. Transplantation potential of peripheral blood stem cells induced by granulocyte colony-stimulating factor. Blood 1990;76:2153-2158.

7 Bensinger WI, Price TH, Dale DC et al. The effects of daily recombinant human granulocyte colony-stimulating factor administration on normal granulocyte donors undergoing leukapheresis. Blood 1993;81:1883-1888.

8 Caspar CB, Seger RA, Burger J et al. Effective stimulation of donors for granulocyte transfusions with recombinant methionyl granulocyte colony-stimulating factor. Blood 1993;81:2866-2871.

9 Peters WP, Rosner G, Ross M et al. Comparative effects of granulocyte-macrophage colony-stimulating factor (GM-CSF) and granulocyte colony-stimulating factor (G-CSF) on priming peripheral blood progenitor cells for use with autologous bone marrow after high-dose chemotherapy. Blood 1993;81:1709-1719.

10 Lane TA, Law P, Maruyama M et al. Harvesting and enrichment of hematopoietic progenitor cells mobilized into the peripheral blood of normal donors by granulocyte-macrophage colony-stimulating factor or G-CSF: potential role in allogeneic marrow transplantation. Blood 1995;85:275-282.

11 Weaver CH, Longin K, Buckner CD et al. Lymphocyte content in peripheral blood mononuclear cells collected after administration of recombinant human granulocyte colony-stimulating factor. Bone Marrow Transplant 1994;13:411-415.

12 Prosper F, Stroncek D, Verfaillie CM. Mobilization of LTC-IC in normal donors treated with G-CSF: phenotypic analysis of mobilized PBSC. Blood 1995;86:464a.

13 Fujisaki T, Otsuka T, Harada M et al. Granulocyte colony-stimulating factor mobilizes primitive hematopoietic stem cells in normal individuals. Bone Marrow Transplant 1995;16:57-62.

14 Tjonnfjord GE, Steen R, Evensen SA et al. Characterization of CD34$^+$ peripheral blood cells from healthy adults mobilized by recombinant human granulocyte-stimulating factor. Blood 1994;84:2795-2801.

15 Grigg AP, Roberts AW, Raunow H et al. Optimizing dose and scheduling of filgrastim (granulocyte colony-stimulating factor) for mobilization and collection of peripheral blood progenitor cells in normal volunteers. Blood 1995;86:4437-4445.

16 Tanaka R, Matsudaira T, Tanaka I et al. Kinetics and characteristics of peripheral blood progenitor cells mobilized by G-CSF in normal healthy volunteers. Blood 1994;84(suppl 1):541a.

17 Dreger P, Haferlach T, Eckstein V et al. G-CSF-mobilized peripheral blood progenitor cells for allogeneic transplantation: safety, kinetics and mobilization, and composition of the graft. Br J Haematol 1994;87:609-613.

18 Stroncek D, Clay M, Jaszcz W et al. Longer than 5 days of G-CSF mobilization of normal individuals results in lower CD34$^+$ cell counts. Blood 1994;84:541a.

19 Höglund M, Smedmyr B, Simonsson B et al. Dose-dependent mobilisation of haematopoietic progenitor cells in healthy volunteers receiving glycosylated rHuG-CSF. Bone Marrow Transplant 1996;18:19-27.

20 Stroncek D, Clay M, Lennon S et al. Collection of two blood progenitor cell components from healthy donors. Blood 1996;88:396a.

21 Bensinger WI, Weaver CH, Appelbaum FR et al. Transplantation of allogeneic peripheral blood stem cells mobilized by recombinant human granulocyte colony-stimulating factor. Blood 1995;85:1655-1658.

22 Waller CF, Bertz H, Wenger MK et al. Mobilization of peripheral blood progenitor cells for allogeneic transplantation: efficacy and toxicity of a high-dose rhG-CSF regimen. Bone Marrow Transplant 1996;18:279-283.

23 Matsunaga T, Sakamaki S, Kohgo Y et al. Recombinant human granulocyte colony-stimulating factor can mobilize sufficient amounts of peripheral blood stem cells in healthy volunteers for allogeneic transplantation. Bone Marrow Transplant 1993;11:103-108.

24 Anderlini P, Przepiorka D, Seong D et al. Factors affecting mobilization of CD34$^+$ cells in normal donors treated with filgrastim. Transfusion 1997;37:507-512.

25 Körbling M, Fliedner TM, Calvo W et al. Albumin density gradient purification of canine hemopoietic blood stem cells (HBSC): long-term allogeneic engraftment without GVH-reaction. Exp Hematol 1979;7:277-288.

26 Ross WM, Körbling M, Nothdurft W et al. The role of dextran sulfate in increasing the CFUc - concentration in dog blood. Proc Soc Exp Biol Med 1978;157:301-305.

27 Kaushansky K. Thrombopoietin: the primary regulator of platelet production. Blood 1995;86:419-431.

28 Molineux G, Hartley C, McElroy P et al. Megakaryocyte growth and development factor accelerates platelet recovery in peripheral blood progenitor cell transplant recipients. Blood 1996;88:366-376.

29 Champlin R, Körbling M, Donato M et al. Recombinant human thrombopoietin (rhTPO) for mobilization of peripheral blood progenitor cells (PBPC) for autologous transplantation in breast cancer: preliminary results of a phase I trial. Proc Am Soc Clin Oncol 1997;16:100a.

30 Geissler K, Peschel C, Niederwieser D et al. Potentiation of granulocyte colony-stimulating

factor-induced mobilization of circulating progenitor cells by seven-day pretreatment with interleukin-3. Blood 1996;87:2732-2739.

31 Huhn RD, Yurkow EJ, Tushinski R et al. Recombinant human interleukin-3 (rhIL-3) enhances the mobilization of peripheral blood progenitor cells by recombinant human granulocyte colony-stimulating factor (rhG-CSF) in normal volunteers. Exp Hematol 1996;24:839-847.

32 Hunter MG, Bawden L, Brotherton D et al. BB-10010: an active variant of human macrophage inflammatory protein-1α with improved pharmaceutical properties. Blood 1995;86:4400-4408.

33 Lord BI, Woolford LB, Wood LM et al. Mobilization of early hematopoietic progenitor cells with BB-10010: a genetically engineered variant of human macrophage inflammatory protein -1α. Blood 1995;85:3412-3415.

34 Broxmeyer HE, Hague NL, Sledge GW et al. Suppression of marrow and mobilization of blood myeloid progenitors in vivo by BB10010, a genetically engineered variant of human macrophage inflammatory protein (MIP-1a), in a phase I clinical trial in patients with relapsed/refractory breast cancer. Blood 1995;86(suppl 1):12a.

35 Levesque JP, Leavesley DI, Niutta S et al. Cytokines increase human hemopoietic cell adhesiveness by activation of very late antigen (VLA)-4 and VLA-5 integrins. J Exp Med 1995;181:1805-1815.

36 Laterveer L, Lindley IJD, Hamilton MS et al. Interleukin-8 induces rapid mobilization of hematopoietic stem cells with radioprotective capacity and long-term myelolymphoid repopulating ability. Blood 1995;85:2269-2275.

37 McNiece IK, Langley KE, Zsebo KM et al. Recombinant human stem cell factor synergizes with GM-CSF, G-CSF, Il-3 and EPO to stimulate human progenitor cells of the myeloid and erythroid lineages. Exp Hematol 1991;19:226-231.

38 Andrews RG, Briddell RA, Knitter GH et al. Rapid engraftment by peripheral blood progenitor cells mobilized by recombinant human stem cell factor and recombinant human granulocyte colony-stimulating factor in nonhuman primates. Blood 1995;85:15-20.

39 McNiece I, Glaspy J, LeMaistre F et al. Effects of recombinant methionyl human stem cell factor (rhSCF) and filgrastim (rhG-CSF) on mobilization of peripheral blood progenitor cells: preliminary laboratory results from a phase I/II study. Blood 1993;82(suppl 1):84a.

40 Moskowitz CH, Stiff P, Gordon MS et al. Recombinant methionyl human stem cell factor and filgrastim for peripheral blood progenitor cell mobilization and transplantation in non-Hodgkin's lymphoma patients - results of a phase I/II trial. Blood 1997;89:3136-3147.

41 Molineux G, McCrea C, Yan XQ et al. Flt-3 ligand synergizes with granulocyte colony-stimulating factor to increase neutrophil numbers and to mobilize peripheral blood stem cells with long-term repopulating potential. Blood 1997;89:3998-4004.

42 Lynch DH, Andreasen A, Maraskovsky E et al. Flt3 ligand induces tumor regression and antitumor responses in vivo. Nat Med 1997;3:625-631.

43 Verfaillie C, Hurley R, Bhatia R et al. Role of bone marrow matrix in normal and abnormal hematopoiesis. Crit Rev Oncol Hematol 1994;16:201-224.

44 Simmons PJ, Masinovsky B, Longenecker BM et al. Vascular cell adhesion molecule-1 expressed by bone marrow stromal cells mediates the binding of hematopoietic progenitor cells. Blood 1992;80:388-395.

45 Papayannopoulou T, Nakamoto B. Peripheralization of hematopoietic progenitors in primates treated with anti-VLA$_4$ integrin. Proc Natl Acad Sci USA 1993;90:9374-9378.

46 Malachowski ME, Comenzo RL, Hillyer CD et al. Large-volume leukapheresis for peripheral blood stem cell collection in patients with hematologic malignancies. Transfusion 1992;32:732-735.

47 Hillyer CD, Tiegerman KO, Berkman EM. Increase in circulating colony-forming units-granulocyte-macrophage during large-volume leukapheresis: evaluation of a new cell separator. Transfusion 1991;31:327-332.

48 Stroncek D, Clay M, Lennon S et al. Neutropenia following the collection of granulocyte colony-stimulating factor mobilized blood progenitor cell components is due to the collection of progenitor cells. Blood 1996;88:396a.

49 Anderlini P, Przepiorka D, Seong D et al. Transient neutropenia in normal donors after G-CSF mobilization and stem cell apheresis. Br J Haematol 1996;94:155-158.

50 Körbling M, Anderlini P, Durett A et al. Delayed effects of rhG-CSF mobilization treatment and apheresis on circulating CD34$^+$ and CD34$^+$Thy-1^{dim} CD38$^-$ progenitor cells, and lymphoid subsets in normal stem cell donors for allogeneic transplantation. Bone Marrow Transplant 1996;18:1073-1079.

51 Martinez C, Urbano-Ispizua A, Rozman C et al. Effects of G-CSF administration and peripheral blood progenitor cell collection in 20 healthy donors. Ann Hematol 1996;72:269-272.

Mobilization of Blood Stem Cells

Anne Kessinger, J. Graham Sharp

University of Nebraska Medical Center, Omaha, Nebraska, USA

Key Words. *Blood stem cells · Transplantation · Mobilization inhibition · Hematopoietic recovery*

Abstract

Deliberately increasing the number of hematopoietic stem and progenitor cells in the circulation allows faster and more efficient collection of sufficient cells for transplantation in both the allogeneic and autologous settings. These mobilized stem cells, when transplanted, provide quicker hematopoietic recovery for the patient than do nonmobilized blood stem cells or steady-state marrow-derived stem cells. Currently used clinical procedures to produce stem cell mobilization include administration of G-CSF or GM-CSF, either as single agents or in combination with myelosuppressive chemotherapy. Some autologous blood stem cell donors exhibit indifference to currently applied mobilization therapies. This failure to mobilize has been associated with prior stem cell toxic therapy, e.g., radiation therapy and chemotherapy, but the association is incomplete. The observation that occasional normal donors have failed to respond to mobilization therapy indicates that factors other than stem cell damage could also be involved. Recently, a murine model has provided evidence that a circulating factor inhibits mobilization in some settings. Preliminary investigations have suggested that a circulating factor may inhibit mobilization of human hematopoietic progenitor cells in some instances. Studies to identify this factor(s) are underway. The mechanisms of blood stem cell mobilization are still poorly understood and there continues to be the potential to improve this process. *Stem Cells 1998;16(suppl 1):139-143*

Introduction

Manipulations designed to increase the number of human hematopoietic stem and progenitor cells in the circulation of potential peripheral blood stem/progenitor cell donors have not only made collection of these cells with apheresis a more efficient process, but also produced a graft product which restores hematopoiesis more rapidly than steady-state marrow cell grafts [1]. Mobilization techniques currently considered standard for clinical use include administration of myelosuppressive chemotherapy and a growth factor which affects the granulocyte lineage (sargramostim [2] or filgrastim [3]) or administration of either of these growth factors alone [1, 4]. Occasionally, autologous donors fail to respond to mobilization-inducing therapies. Factors which sometimes predict for failure to mobilize have included prior chemotherapy and radiation therapy [5]. Although some patients previously treated with chemotherapy and/or radiation therapy exhibit vigorous mobilization in response to growth factors and/or myelosuppressive chemotherapy, these associations have led to the understandable assumption that failure to mobilize is in some way related to a damaged stem cell pool. However, the recent advent of allogeneic peripheral blood stem cell transplantation has revealed that an occasional normal donor fails to mobilize following growth factor administration [6], suggesting that factors other than, or in addition to, stem cell damage may be involved when indifference to mobilization occurs. Because a murine mobilization study suggested that a circulating factor could play a role in the etiology of failure to respond to mobilizing therapy [7], a study was undertaken to determine if a circulating factor(s) might influence the magnitude of response to clinical mobilization attempts.

MATERIALS AND METHODS

Murine Assay Model

A murine model of mobilization inhibition induced by partial body irradiation was developed [7], whereby injection of mobilizing growth factors failed to result in a large increase of circulating progenitors if 2 Gy of partial body irradiation (lower limbs, upper hemibody or lower hemibody) was administered on the same days as the growth factors. Table 1 shows the significant degree of mobilization of colony-forming cells (CFU) in the blood and spleen and the slight increase in femoral marrow CFU in recipients of growth factors only. Upper hemibody radiation (XRT) greatly inhibited mobilization of CFU into the blood and spleen as did lower limb XRT. Both lower limb and lower hemibody XRT completely inhibited mobilization of CFU into the blood.

Since the effect occurred regardless of the site irradiated, the inhibition was suspected to be systemic. To test this premise, plasma from hemibody irradiated mice was injected i.v. into untreated mice 10 min before receiving the mobilizing growth factors. The effect on mobilization of CFU to the spleen 24 h later was assessed compared to recipients of either saline or normal donor plasma. Plasma from part-body irradiated mice inhibited blood stem cell mobilization [7] to a level of 16% of that observed in the control. The hypothesis was formulated that radiation therapy released or activated a circulating inhibitor of blood stem cell mobilization. This murine inhibition model was then adapted for the current study to demonstrate proof of principal that a circulating mobilization-inhibiting factor could be functioning in autologous and normal donors who failed to mobilize well.

Human Subjects

Five individuals, three autologous donors undergoing mobilizing growth factor administration for blood stem cell collection with poor mobilization responses and two normal volunteers, were identified. Following administration of filgrastim 10 μg/kg s.c. for mobilization for five days, and for one patient erythropoietin (EPO) 300 U/kg for five days along with the filgrastim, these patients required 9, 10 and 4 apheresis procedures to collect 0.59, 1.12, and 0.37 $\times$ 10^6 CD34$^+$ cells/kg, respectively. After informed consent was given by the participants, heparinized plasma was obtained from a blood sample of each person. This study was approved by the University of Nebraska Institutional Review Board.

Table 1. Impact of lower limb (LL), upper hemibody (UHB) or lower hemibody (LHB) irradiation (XRT) on growth factor-induced mobilization in murine blood, femoral marrow and spleen

	Peak mobilization (fold increases over nonmobilized) for each treatment[a]			
	Growth factor only[b]	Growth factor plus LL-XRT	UHB-XRT	LHB-XRT
Blood	$\times$20	none	$\times$4	none
Spleen	$\times$36	$\times$10	$\times$5	irradiated[c]
Femoral marrow	$\times$3	irradiated[c]	$\times$3	irradiated[c]

[a]Colony-forming cells (CFU-GM, CFU-mix, HPP-CFC) were assayed before and after treatment. The average peak-fold increase is presented. Growth factor was administered daily each morning, and a 2 Gy fraction of XRT each afternoon for five days. Peak mobilization occurred after three to five days of treatment.
[b]500 U/kg EPO plus 15 μg/kg filgrastim.
[c]This tissue was included in this irradiation field; therefore, CFC numbers were decreased from the control value.

Mice

The study employed young adult female Balb/c mice purchased from Charles River (Wilmington, MA). The mice were maintained on a 12-h light, 6:00 a.m. to 6:00 p.m., 12-h dark cycle and provided both sterilized food and acidified (pH2) sterile water ad libitum. They were maintained in filter-top cages in laminar airflow cabinets.

Growth Factors

Recombinant EPO 500 U/kg (Ortho Biotech; Raritan, NJ) and filgrastim 15 μg/kg (Amgen; Thousand Oaks, CA) were used as the mobilizing regimen for the murine mouse model.

Hematopoietic Colony Assay

Mobilization of stem cells was assessed by in vitro hematopoietic colony-forming assay; high proliferative potential-colony-forming cells (HPP-CFC). Briefly, at necropsy, spleens were removed aseptically and cells were gently teased from the spleens with 25 gauge needles into Hank's balanced salt solution (HBSS) without calcium and magnesium. Clumps were dispersed by repeated aspiration with a 1 cc syringe without a needle. Cells were washed once and resuspended in Tris-buffered ammonium chloride (ACT) for five min to lyse mature red blood cells. After five min, an equal volume of complete medium containing serum was added to halt the action of the ACT. The cells were washed once and resuspended in HBSS without calcium and magnesium. These cells were then enumerated and employed in the colony assay detailed below.

HPP-CFC Assay

Spleen (1×10^5) cells were plated in 60 mm dishes containing Iscove's modified Dulbecco's medium, 0.3% agar, 15% fetal bovine serum, 100 units penicillin, 100 μg streptomycin, 50 μM 2-mercaptoethaol and 10 ng interleukin 3 (IL-3) with 10% L cell conditioned medium (or recombinant M-CSF) as sources of colony-stimulating activity. Dishes were incubated for 11 days at 37°C in a humidified atmosphere containing 5% CO_2 in air. The colonies were enumerated using an inverted microscope. Microscopic colonies containing 50 cells and less and greater than 2 mm diameter were counted.

Data Analysis

Means and standard deviations were calculated when possible. One tailed Student's t test was employed to determine significant differences.

Experimental Design

Plasma, 0.2 ml, from either autologous donors receiving filgrastim for mobilization and identified as poor mobilizers or from normal volunteers or 0.2 ml plasma harvested from mice after receiving hemibody irradiation as described above was injected into nonirradiated control BALB/c mice 10 min prior to injection of EPO, 500 U/kg and filgrastim, 15 μg/kg. The mobilization response was determined in the murine assay system by measuring HPP-CFC in the spleen of the animals using methods described above.

RESULTS

The effect of the plasma collected from the various sources listed above on mobilization in the mouse treated with EPO and filgrastim is listed in Table 2. Using the one-tailed Student's t test, the difference between the mobilization observed in the mice treated with plasma from poorly mobilizing patients and the growth factor-treated control mice showed a statistically significant difference ($p \leq .005$). The mice treated with plasma from normal volunteers also had significantly different mobilization than the mice injected with plasma from the poorly mobilizing patients ($p \leq .025$). The difference in mobilization between the control mice and the mice pretreated with plasma from previously irradiated mice was significant ($p \leq .01$), but mobilization in the mice treated with plasma from normal volunteers was not significantly different from that observed in the control mice.

Table 2. Impact of plasma from normal volunteers, partial-body irradiated mice and poorly mobilizing cancer patients on growth factor mobilization in the mouse

Plasma source[a]	Mobilization (% of saline control)[b]
None, growth factor + saline only	100 ± 14
Plasma from partial-body irradiated mice[c]	29 ± 13
Plasma from normal volunteers	72 ± 13
Plasma from poorly mobilizing patients	22 ± 12

[a]0.2 ml heparinized plasma injected i.v. Plasma was injected at mid-morning 10 min prior to growth factor (500 μ/kg EPO plus 15 μg/kg G-CSF) injection.
[b]Mobilization was assessed as HPP-CFC per 1×10^5 spleen cells, 24 h following growth factor only or growth factor and plasma injection. Mean values ± standard deviations are presented.
[c]Partial body irradiation of mice inhibits blood stem cell mobilization via a circulating inhibitor. This was employed as a control for positive inhibition.

DISCUSSION

Some patients undergoing growth factor-mobilized autologous blood stem harvests do not mobilize well and require more than the minimum anticipated number of leukaphereses to collect a suitable graft product. Patients with prior exposure to chemotherapy and/or radiation therapy were more likely to be poor mobilizers, and damaged stem cells were believed to play a role in poor mobilization. However, some normal donors with no history of stem cell toxic prior therapy have also exhibited poor mobilization. Given that a circulating inhibitor of blood stem mobilization had been detected in partial-body irradiated mice, the mouse assay of inhibition of blood stem cell mobilization was adapted to assay plasma from normal donors, poorly mobilizing normal donors and cancer patients. The preliminary results of these assays (Table 2) suggested that plasma from normal donors caused some inhibition (to 72% of the control). Inhibition resulting from injection of plasma collected from normal poorly mobilizing donors was noted, as mobilization in the animal model was 76% of the control value. The plasma from the poorly mobilizing cancer patients was even more inhibitory (to 22% of the control) at a level comparable to that of plasma from partial-body irradiated mice. These results lead to the suggestion that an inhibitor of blood stem cell mobilization may be found in the plasma of some cancer patients and normal donors. Whether this is the same inhibitor or similar to that found in the circulation of mice following radiation therapy remains to be defined.

A recent study of different wild-type murine strains [8] revealed that genetic influences may play a role in the response to growth factor-induced mobilization attempts. The patterns of mobilization observed included rapid vigorous response, intermediate response and indifference to growth factor administration (e.g., inhibition) depending upon the genetic strain being examined.

The nature of the inhibition is obviously of considerable interest, as is the mechanism of action. Recently, inhibitors of growth factor signaling have been described [9-11]. Some of these inhibitors are growth factor-induced, suggesting that a negative feedback loop may be operational. Potentially, endogenous cytokines induced by irradiation of mice, induced by cytotoxic chemotherapy, radiation therapy or the presence of malignancy in cancer patients and induced by virtue of genetic constitution in response to an underlying relatively benign event, such as a recent infection in some normal donors, may be responsible for this inhibition of blood stem cell mobilization. Obviously, the ability to detect patient donors and/or normal donors with the active circulating inhibitor and the ability to neutralize this inhibitor would increase the efficiency and cost-effectiveness of blood stem cell collection for these donors.

Currently, new combinations of growth factors which potentially tailor the cellular content of the harvest for therapeutic purposes, e.g., IL-2-responsive cells, dendritic cells, are being pursued. These developments, as well as a better understanding of the mechanisms of blood stem cell mobilization, offer the potential for further improvements in the application of this procedure.

ACKNOWLEDGMENT

It is a pleasure to thank *Sally Mann, Barbara O'Kane-Murphy* and *Kim Schmit-Pokorny* for excellent technical support and *Roxann Pierce* who typed the manuscript.

REFERENCES

1 Hartmann O, LeCorroller AG, Blaise D et al. Peripheral blood stem cell and bone marrow transplantation for solid tumors and lymphomas: hematologic recovery and costs. A randomized, controlled trial. Ann Intern Med 1997;126:600-607.

2 Tarella C, Boccadoro M, Omded P et al. Role of chemotherapy and GM-CSF on hemopoietic progenitor cell mobilization in multiple myeloma. Bone Marrow Transplant 1993;11:271-277.

3 Schwartzberg LS, Birch R, Hazelton B et al. Peripheral blood stem cell mobilization by chemotherapy with and without recombinant human granulocyte colony-stimulating factor. J Hematother 1992;1:317-327.

4 Bishop MR, Anderson JR, Jackson JD et al. High-dose therapy and peripheral blood progenitor cell transplantation: effects of recombinant human granulocyte-macrophage colony-stimulating factor on the autograft. Blood 1994;83:610-616.

5 Brugger W, Bross K, Frisch J et al. Mobilization of peripheral blood progenitor cells by sequential administration of interleukin-3 and granulocyte-macrophage colony-stimulating factor following polychemotherapy with etoposide, ifosfamide, and cisplatin. Blood 1992;79:1193-1200.

6 Bensinger WI, Clift RA, Anasetti C et al. Transplantation of allogeneic peripheral blood stem cells mobilized by recombinant human granulocyte colony stimulating factor. STEM CELLS 1996;14:90-105.

7 Kessinger A, Clausen S, Mann S et al. Indifference to blood stem cell mobilization attempts: prior stem cell damage is not the only causal factor. Blood 1996;88(suppl 1):225b.

8 Roberts AW, Foote S, Alexander WS et al. Genetic influences determining progenitor cell mobilization and luekocytosis induced by granulocyte colony-stimulating factor. Blood 1997;89:2736-2744.

9 Starr R, Willson TA, Viney EM et al. A family of growth factor-inducible inhibitors of signaling. Nature 1997;387:917-921.

10 Endo TA, Masuhara M, Yokouchi M et al. A new protein containing an SH2 domain that inhibits JAK kinases. Nature 1997;387:921-924.

11 Naka T, Narazaki M, Hirata M et al. Structure and function of a new STAT-induced STAT inhibitor. Nature 1997;387:924-929.

Mobilization and Transplantation of Peripheral Blood Stem Cells

RICHARD K. SHADDUCK, ZELLA R. ZEIGLER, D. FRANK ANDREWS III,
GARY L. GILMORE, JOHN LISTER

Western Pennsylvania Cancer Institute, The Western Pennsylvania Hospital,
Pittsburgh, Pennsylvania, USA

Key Words. *CD34 · Chemotherapy · Hematopoietic growth factors · Leukapheresis · Mobilization
· Peripheral blood stem cells · Stem cell transplantation*

ABSTRACT

Two hundred nineteen patients underwent peripheral blood stem cell (PBSC) transplantation from 1990 to 1997. Stem cells were mobilized with cyclophosphamide (CY), or with CY plus Taxol or etoposide, followed by cytokines, and collected when leukocyte counts $\geq 1,000/\mu l$, or when CD34$^+$ counts $\geq 20/\mu l$. On average, four to five collections were needed to obtain sufficient PBSC for engraftment. When CD34$^+$ counts were used, the average number of collections decreased from 5.4 to 4.2. A discrepancy was noted in the extraction ratios and number of collections that depended on the optical density (I/O) setting of the leukapheresis machine. Patients collected at a setting of 100 had higher extraction ratios and required fewer collections (mean = 2.7) than those collected at 150 (mean = 4.4). This result was unexpected, because the entire mononuclear cell layer is collected at the higher I/O setting. Further analysis revealed that a larger volume of red cells was collected at 150 than at 100. These procedures used a small-volume collection chamber, so the chamber was apparently overloaded by RBC at the higher setting.

More rapid recovery of neutrophil counts and platelet counts was seen in PBSC transplants than in autologous marrow transplants; moreover, PBSC transplant patients required fewer RBC and platelet transfusions.

Sixteen out of 21 normal donors for allogeneic PBSC transplants gave adequate collections ($> 2.5 \times 10^6$ CD34$^+$ cells/kg), but three donors failed to yield $\geq 1.5 \times 10^6$ CD34 cells/kg. This suggests an inherent difference among certain normal donors that may make PBSC mobilization difficult. *Stem Cells 1998;16(suppl 1):145-158*

INTRODUCTION

High-dose chemoradiotherapy with allogeneic or autologous bone marrow rescue has been successful in the treatment of many hematologic malignancies. Although such transplants are potentially curative, they are also associated with considerable morbidity and mortality. Donors require bone marrow harvest in the operating room and replacement of red cell volume by transfusions and have several days of discomfort afterwards.

A number of observations suggested that circulating stem cells were also capable of restoring hematopoiesis after marrow-lethal chemoradiotherapy. The recovery of an irradiated parabiotic animal after shielding of the "donor" animal [1, 2] and recovery of individual animals after split dose hemibody irradiation [3] amply demonstrated the existence of circulating hematopoietic stem cells. Subsequently, transfused blood leukocytes were shown to restore blood cell production in lethally irradiated dogs [4, 5].

Despite these observations, there was still concern that there were insufficient stem cells in the circulation for clinical transplantation. In a series of experiments *Fliedner* and colleagues showed that both autologous and allogeneic blood mononuclear cells were sufficient for engraftment in the canine model [6-8]. Moreover, the concept of stem cell mobilization was defined by infusing dextran sulfate and increasing the number of circulating clonogenic progenitor cells [9].

The availability of cell separation machines permitted large volume leukapheresis, then provided the technology for developing blood stem cell transplantation. Using large-volume blood leukocyte collections, *Korbling* [10], *Juttner* [11], *Kessinger* [12], *Reiffers* [13], and others, initiated peripheral blood stem cell transplants in the mid 1980s. Recovery rates paralleled those of marrow transplants until mobilized stem cells were employed. Initial studies showed that treatment with cyclophosphamide and adriamycin was associated with a rebound in the number of circulating colony-forming cells [14]. Subsequently, *Gianni* [15] extended these observations to show that addition of GM-CSF led to further augmentation in the number of circulating progenitor cells. Using such suitably mobilized stem cells, it has become apparent that recovery from marrow ablative therapy is much faster after peripheral blood stem cells than after autologous bone marrow transplants (ABMT). This has led to a revolution in the approach to marrow transplantation with a rapid shift from bone marrow to peripheral blood stem cell transplants.

The Western Pennsylvania Cancer Institute Bone Marrow Transplant Program began peripheral blood stem cell transplants in December 1990, and has transplanted 219 patients with carcinoma of the breast, ovary, lymphoma, Hodgkin's disease, myeloma, acute myelogenous leukemia, chronic myelogenous leukemia, and acute lymphocytic leukemia. In this paper, we have examined the different mobilization regimens and collection methods for obtaining stem cells, and have compared these findings to the recovery rates observed after ABMT.

METHODS

The records from 275 patients who had undergone autologous bone marrow or stem cell transplantation from September 1990 through May 1997 were reviewed. An initial series of 56 patients had autologous bone marrow transplants; those with carcinoma of the breast and non-Hodgkin's lymphoma were analyzed with respect to recovery times and utilization of blood and platelet transfusions post-transplantation. Twenty-six patients were transplanted in 1991 with both bone marrow and peripheral blood stem cells; since then, an additional 193 patients received only peripheral blood stem cell transplants. As recovery times were similar, these latter two groups have been combined for a total of 219 patients undergoing blood stem cell transplants. Diagnoses included carcinoma of the breast (98), carcinoma of the ovary (5), non-Hodgkin's lymphoma (70), Hodgkin's disease (10), multiple myeloma (20), acute myelogenous leukemia (10), chronic myelogenous leukemia (1), and acute lymphocytic leukemia (5).

Mobilization protocols have evolved from chemotherapy or growth factors alone to a combined approach. The initial 35 patients with lymphoid malignancies were given 4 gm/M^2 cyclophosphamide (CY) (16 patients), CY followed by 250 μg/M^2 GM-CSF (13 patients), or CY followed by 600 μg G-CSF (6 patients) [16].

Twenty-two patients were entered onto interleukin 3 (IL-3) studies, in which they received IL-3 alone, G-CSF alone, or IL-3 in combination with or followed by GM-CSF or G-CSF [17]. Further groups of patients were treated with growth factors alone or growth factors following 4 gm/M^2 CY. In January 1995, mobilization protocols were modified to include additional chemotherapy. Patients with carcinoma of the breast or ovary were given 4 gm/M^2 CY and 170 mg/M^2 Taxol [18]. Patients with lymphoid malignancies such as Hodgkin's disease, non-Hodgkin's lymphoma, myeloma or with acute myelogenous or acute lymphocytic leukemia were given 4 gm/M^2 CY and 600 mg/M^2 etoposide [19].

The mobilization chemotherapy was administered during a 24-h hospital admission. All patients had indwelling triple lumen Foley catheters. They underwent continuous 24-h bladder irrigation with 300 ml/h of a 3% sterile sorbitol solution to prevent hemorrhagic cystitis [20]. A single dose of 500 mg of ciprofloxacin was given orally at the time of catheter removal. Starting five days after mobilization, patients were given 500 mg ciprofloxacin every 12 h. Patients were given 5 μg/kg G-CSF s.c. every 12 h, (CY-Taxol) or 8 μg/kg G-CSF s.c. every 12 h (Cy-VP16) starting 24 h after mobilization chemotherapy. All received 1 mg folic acid daily.

Complete blood counts were started five days after mobilization and obtained daily. Patients were transfused with red cells for symptomatic anemia or hemoglobin values below 8 gm/dl and received single donor platelets for a bleeding diathesis or for a platelet count below 15,000/μl. All blood products were irradiated with 2,500 cGy. Those patients who developed a temperature of 38.5 °C were admitted to the hospital and treated with intravenous antibiotics.

Stem cell collections were initiated when the leukocyte count reached 1,000 and continued until 6-8 $\times$ 10^8 MNC/kg were collected. CFU-GM assays were performed; however, results were not known prior to completion of the cell collections. The technique was modified in April 1995 so that each daily collection was tested for CD34 positive cells; phereses were continued until 4 $\times$ 10^6 CD34 cells/kg were obtained. In order to improve the efficiency of stem cell collections in February 1996, the number of circulating CD34 cells was tested as soon as the leukocyte count reached 1,000/μl. Collection procedures were delayed until a minimum of 20 CD34 cells/μl was achieved.

Most patients required an indwelling catheter for stem cell collections. A double lumen apheresis catheter (Mahurkar catheter; Quinton Instrument Company; Seattle, WA) was inserted under local anesthesia. Apheresis was performed with the CS3000 Plus Blood Cell Separator (Fenwal Division; Baxter-Biotech; Deerfield, IL) as described previously [21]. Whole blood flow rates were adjusted from 40 to 85 ml/min, depending on patient tolerance. Anticoagulation was accomplished with ACD-A, with a whole blood to ACD-A ratio of 10:1. The granulocyte chamber was used as a separation chamber, and a small-volume chamber (50 ml) was used as the collection chamber. For most collections, the optical density (I/O) was set at 150 to optimize collection of the entire mononuclear cell layer, as described previously [22]. Patients who were entered onto a protocol for CD34 selection on the Isolex 300i (Baxter Biotech) were collected with an I/O setting of 100.

Heparin (10 units/ml of pheresis product) was added to the collected cells. The cells were then added to a cryopreservation solution containing pentastarch, normosol R, and DMSO, as described previously [21]. An equal volume of cryopreservative was added to the cell suspension to bring the final concentrations to 5% DSMO, 6% pentastarch, and 4% albumin. The blood freezing bags were placed in aluminum cassettes and held in a minus 70°C freezer until transplant. The cryopreserved cells were thawed in a sterile 37°C water bath, and the contents pooled for infusion. All peripheral blood stem cells were infused within one hour of thawing.

The number of granulocyte-macrophage colony-forming cells was assessed by the in vitro myeloid colony assay [21]. 3 $\times$ 10^5 cells/ml were suspended in methylcellulose tissue culture medium. Colony-stimulating activity was provided by 2.5 ng of recombinant human GM-CSF (Immunex; Seattle, WA). Culture plates were incubated in a humidified 5% CO_2, 5% O_2 atmosphere at 37° for 14 days. Colonies containing more than 50 cells were assessed with the aid of an inverted microscope.

CD34$^+$ cells were determined by adding a fluorescein-conjugated anti-CD34$^+$ monoclonal antibody (anti-HPCA-2; Becton & Dickinson; Mountain View, CA), and subsequently the cells were treated with FACS lysing solution (Becton & Dickinson). After several washes, the cells were fixed in 0.5% paraformaldehyde in phosphate-buffered saline. Flow cytometry was performed on a FACS scan flow cytometer with LYSIS II software. Cells were gated on the entire nucleated population and the lymphocyte population using "back-gating" with CD14 and CD45.

Percoll (Pharmacia Biotech; Uppsala, Sweden) was diluted 90% v/v with 10% v/v 1.5 M NaCl to make stock isotonic percoll (SIP). Six gradients (1.070, 1.068, 1.066, 1.064, 1.062, and 1.050 g/ml) were made by diluting the SIP with 0.15 M NaCl. The discontinuous gradient was made by carefully layering

1 ml of each density gradient on top of the other in a 15 ml conical polypropylene tube. Cells from heparinized blood collected from patients prior to apheresis were lysed using the water lysis method and were washed once in PBS. They were resuspended in 5 ml SIP. The 5 ml cell suspension was underlaid in the prepared Percoll discontinuous gradient tube and centrifuged at $400 \times g$ for 20 min in a Beckman tabletop swinging bucket centrifuge. After centrifugation, each layer of cells was carefully removed using a Pasteur pipette, enumerated and assayed for CD34 cells.

RESULTS

The initial 35 patients with lymphoid malignancies were treated with 4 gm/M^2 (high-dose) CY or CY followed by GM-CSF or G-CSF. Of those patients given chemotherapy alone, 73% developed neutropenic fevers and required hospital admission for intravenous antibiotics. This decreased to 32% in patients receiving growth factor support. The high rate of readmission was most likely due to the fact that these patients were not receiving prophylactic antibiotics. There was one fatality with sudden death at home 10 days after mobilization, in a 51-year-old patient who had been well several hours previously when evaluated by a health care professional.

Most patients required an indwelling Mahurkar catheter for their large-volume pheresis. Stem cells were collected by a daily 12-l leukapheresis using the Baxter CS3000. The machine settings were modified from the manufacturer's recommendation to an I/O of 150 as described by *Rosenfeld et al.* [22]. This allowed the machine to collect further into the buffy coat layer, thus improving the mononuclear cell collection, which was thought to increase the recovery of hematopoietic stem cells. The numbers of cells collected from the three groups of patients are shown in Table 1. Mononuclear cells ranged from 5.9 to 8.7 $\times$ 10^8/kg. CFU-GM and CD34 positive cells (the latter assayed on thawed pooled collections) all exceeded the concentrations believed necessary for rapid engraftment.

In order to assess the recovery rates from PBSC, the initial 35 patients did not receive growth factors post-transplant. An absolute neutrophil count of 500 was achieved 14.5 days after PBSCT. This compared favorably with our similar data, indicating a 21-day recovery after autologous bone marrow transplant. Platelet recovery was prompt with achievement of 50,000 platelets/μl at day 20 after transplant.

Following these initial transplants, various studies were conducted to determine whether there were better techniques for enhancing stem cell mobilization. Patients received CY alone, growth factors alone (including IL-3 in conjunction with or followed by GM-CSF or G-CSF) in 22 patients or combinations of chemotherapy and growth factors. Since January 1995, patients with carcinoma of the breast or ovary received CY plus Taxol, whereas those with lymphoma, Hodgkin's disease, myeloma, or acute leukemia were given CY plus VP16. Twenty-four h after chemotherapy, G-CSF was administered in a dose of 5 μg/kg every 12 h (CY-Taxol). This dose was increased to 8 μg/kg s.c. every 12 h for patients receiving

Table 1. Cell collections

Mobilization regimen	n of patients	MNC (10^8/kg)	CFU-GM ($\times$ 10^4/kg)	CD34** (10^6/kg)
CY	15	5.9* (4.6-7.2)	15.4* (7.5-33.2)	8.7 (5.4-14.6)
CY + GM-CSF	13	8.1 (7.4-8.7)	60.4 (40.5-86.6)	5.9 (3.3-15.9)
CY + G-CSF	6	8.7 (7.4-11.0)	35.1 (7.7-94.2)	13.8 (1.0-35.7)

*Values represent medians.
**CD34 assays were done on thawed samples.
Reprinted with permission from [16].

Table 2. Autologous stem cell collections

Diagnosis	Chemo	HGF	Chemo + HGF	Total
Breast CA	3.0 (1)	3.3 (16)	4.3 (51)	4.1 (68)
Lymphoma	8.5 (2)	5.9 (6)	5.0 (31)	5.5 (39)

Values represent the mean numbers of daily pheresis procedures necessary to collect 4×10^6 CD34 cells/kg. Values in parentheses represent the number of patients in each treatment group. Patients were given chemotherapy (Chemo), hematopoietic growth factor (HGF), or a combination of agents for mobilization.

CY-VP16 in January 1995; the G-CSF was continued until completion of apheresis with no dose reductions for side effects or marked leukocytosis.

The average number of pheresis procedures to obtain sufficient cells for engraftment in patients with breast cancer or lymphoma is shown in Table 2. In general, fewer procedures were required to obtain an adequate stem cell product with carcinoma of the breast than with lymphoma, irrespective of the method of mobilization.

In February 1996, the criteria for stem cell collections were changed from a white count >

Table 3. Autologous stem cell collections

	Mean # collections	# Patients
CD34 (product)	5.4 ± 0.4	90
CD34 (blood)	4.2 ± 0.4	59
	$p = 0.03$	

Values represent the number of daily pheresis procedures necessary to collect 4×10^6 CD34 cells/kg. CD34 assays were done either on the collected product or were measured prospectively from the blood prior to stem cell collection.

1,000 per µL to a CD34 count $\geq 20/\mu L$. In many patients, this delayed the initiation of the leukapheresis for several days but seemed to shorten the process of stem cell collections (Table 3). A mean of 4.2 collections was employed with prospective CD34 assays of the blood as compared with 5.4 collections when CD34 cells were only assessed in the stem cell product. Moreover, the collections were more efficient with higher numbers of CD34 cells and CFU-GM collected, while requiring only half the number of mononuclear cells in the product (Fig. 1).

To determine whether the number of circulating CD34 cells correlated with those collected in the product, values were plotted from all collections in which circulating CD34 cells were analyzed in a prospective fashion. As shown in Figure 2, there was a considerable increase in collected CD34 positive cells in those patients with higher numbers of circulating CD34 cells at the time of pheresis. It was of concern, however, that with values at 20-25/µL, the anticipated recovery of CD34 positive cells from a 12-l pheresis was on the

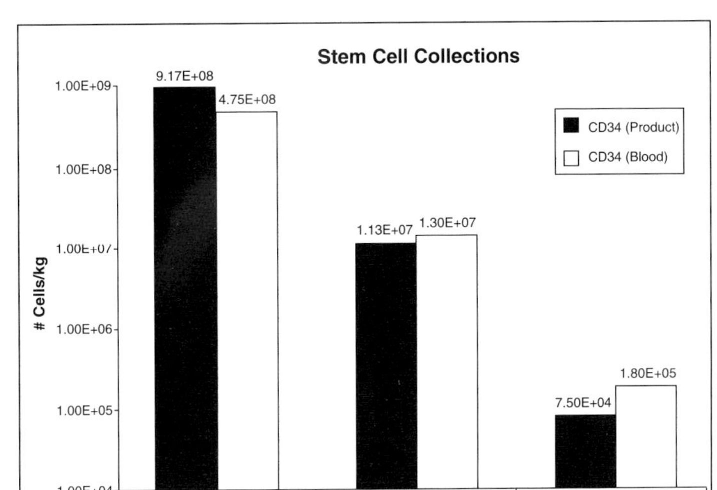

Figure 1. Stem cell collections: values represent the total number of mononuclear cells/kg, CD34 cells/kg or CFU-GM (granulocyte-macrophage colony-forming cells/kg). CD34 cells were assessed after collection in the product or were assayed prospectively in the blood prior to pheresis.

Table 7. Red cell volume in CD34 collections

Machine settings	RBC (ml)
I/O 100	16.7 ± 0.6
I/O 150	21.1 ± 0.2
	$p < 0.00005$

Values represent the volume of red cells in the stem cell collections using two different optical density settings for the pheresis.

Table 8. Neutrophil and platelet recovery

	Days	
	ANC > 500	Plt > 50,000
Total (48)	11.2 ± 0.4	17.9 ± 1.4
Lymphoma (14)	11.9 ± 0.5	20.0 ± 3.1
Breast (25)	10.7 ± 0.4	14.6 ± 1.0
		$p = 0.047$

Values represent the number of days to achieve a neutrophil count (ANC) of 500 or platelet count of 50,000/μl after transplantation.

sumably by egress from the chamber and return to the patient during the procedure.

All patients undergoing autologous peripheral blood stem cell transplant since January 1993 have received hematopoietic growth factors post-transplant. Depending on current studies, either GM-CSF or G-CSF was administered in doses of 250-400 μg by daily s.c. injections.

The rates of blood cell recovery of patients transplanted in the last year are shown in Table 8. Neutrophil and platelet recovery times were shorter in patients with breast cancer than with lymphoma. When compared with recoveries in our earlier patients with lymphoma, it appears neutrophil recovery was accelerated by growth factor treatment from 14.5 days to 11.9 days, but as anticipated, there was no change in platelet recovery, with a mean time of 20 days to achieve a platelet count of 50,000. The dose of CD34 positive cells administered seemed to have no effect on neutrophil or platelet recovery times (Figs. 5A and 5B); however, it should be noted that most patients received more than 4×10^6 CD34 positive cells/kg, which appears to be above the dose necessary to achieve the shortest engraftment time.

The numbers of red cell and platelet transfusions used after autologous BMT and autologous PBSCT are shown in Figures 6A and 6B. In addition to enjoying more rapid neutrophil recovery, patients undergoing peripheral blood stem cell transplants required fewer red cell and platelet transfusions. This resulted in shorter hospital stays and a decrease in costs associated with the transplant procedure.

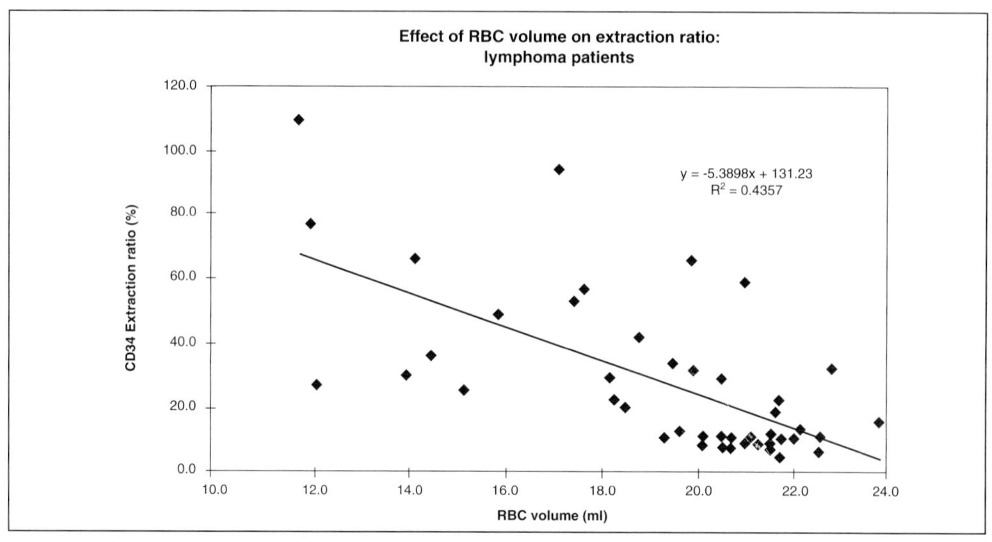

Figure 4. Effect of RBC volume in stem cell collections on extraction ratio. *Observations were obtained from patients with lymphoma.*

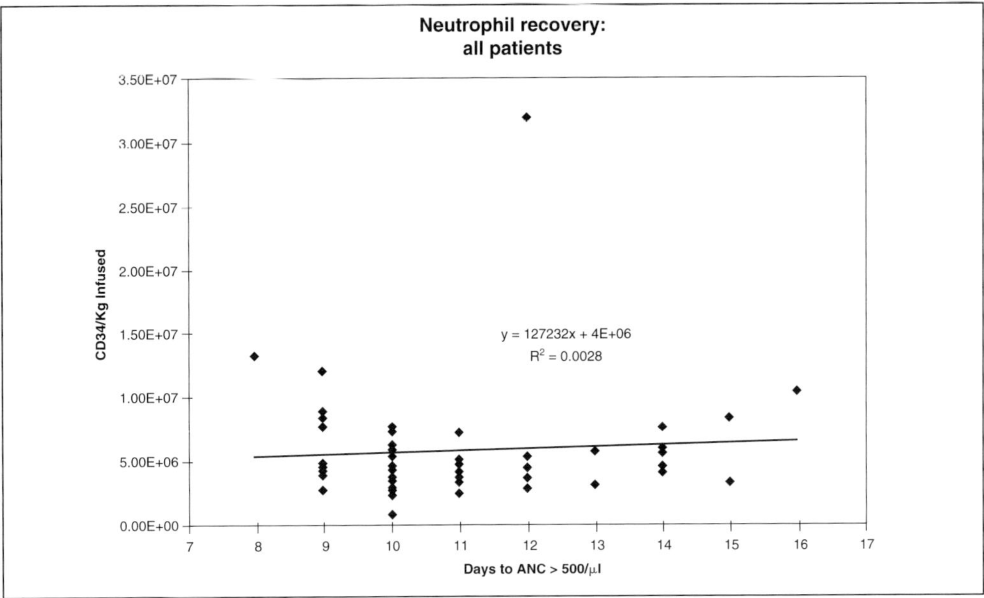

Figure 5A. Neutrophil recovery to greater than 500 cells/μl. *Values were obtained from all patients with carcinoma of the breast and lymphoma.*

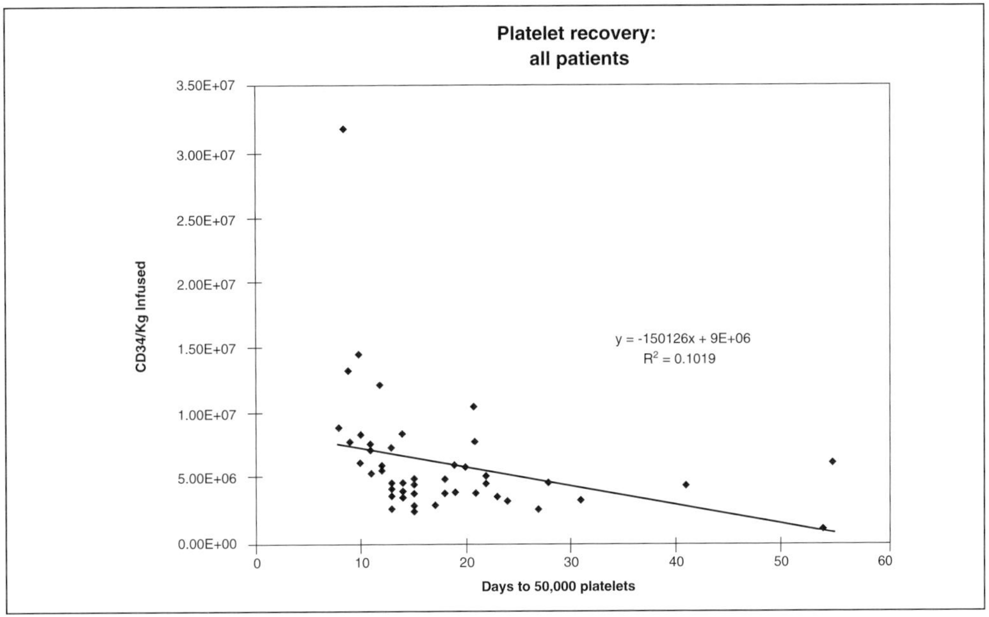

Figure 5B. Platelet recovery to > 50,000 platelets/μl. *Values were obtained from all patients with carcinoma of the breast and lymphoma.*

Mobilization of allogeneic blood stem cells was attempted from 21 normal donors using G-CSF 5 μg/kg s.c. every 12 h for four days. Leukapheresis was initiated on the fifth day of growth factor therapy. As shown in Table 9, only half the normal donors yielded > than 4×10^6 CD34/kg with either one or several collections. Sixteen of 21 donors had collections of greater than 2.5×10^6/kg, yet three donors failed to yield sufficient cells and subsequently had a bone marrow harvest performed. Those donors with

13-21 CD34 cells/µl proved to have poor collections, whereas adequate numbers of cells were obtained for the 18 donors with 35-135 CD34 positive cells/µl.

DISCUSSION

Over the last 5-7 years, there has been a dramatic change in the approach to high-dose chemoradiotherapy with stem cell rescue. Virtually all patients are receiving peripheral blood stem cells rather than bone marrow transplants owing to: A) the relative ease of cell collections; B) the ability to obtain cells when conditions preclude marrow harvests, and C) the more rapid recovery seen after peripheral blood stem cell transplants. Despite this rapid shift in the approach to transplantation, optimal conditions for mobilization and cell collection have not been fully defined.

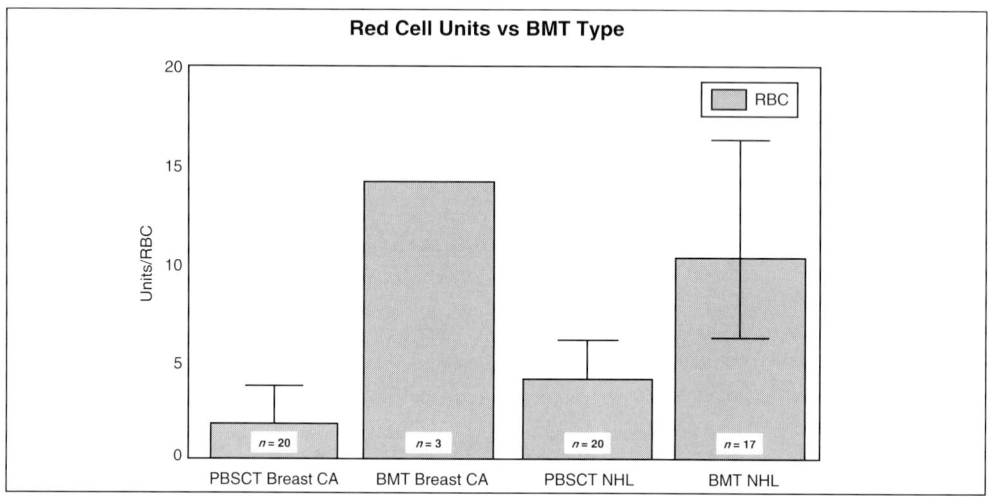

Figure 6A. Red cell transfusion requirements with autologous peripheral blood stem cell and bone marrow transplants.

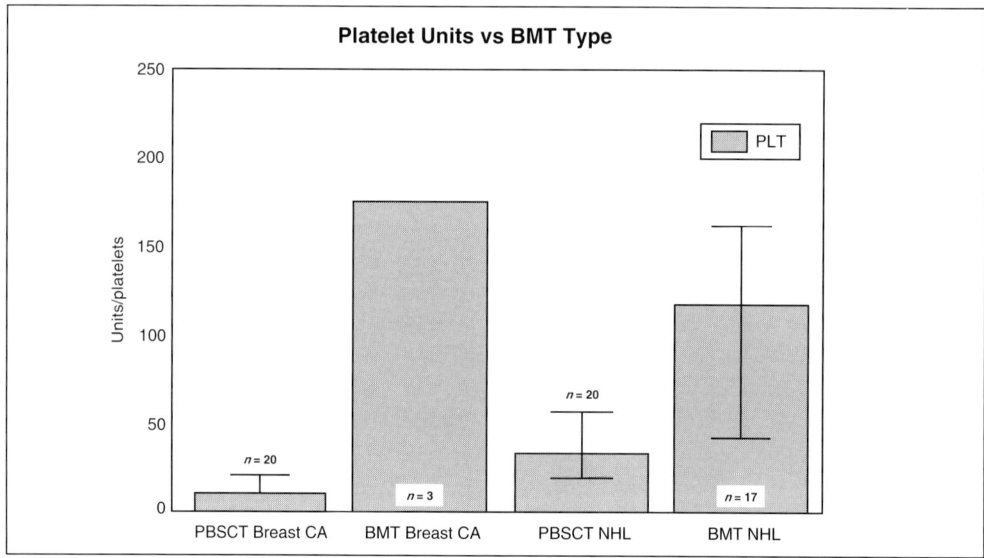

Figure 6B. Platelet transfusion requirements with autologous peripheral blood stem cell and bone marrow transplants. A single donor platelet pheresis was counted as 10 units of random donor platelets (PLT).

It seems clear that stem cell mobilization with high-dose chemotherapy and growth factor support is reasonably safe and well tolerated. The one fatality in our series of 219 patients was most likely due to a cardiovascular event rather than an infectious cause. With the use of prophylactic antibiotics, the readmission rate for neutropenic fever is now below 15%-20%. Moreover, neutrophil recovery frequently ensues within two to three days of the febrile episode. The average time to a leukocyte count greater than $1,000/\mu l$ is 8-12 days from chemotherapy. Since the leukocyte count does not fall for at least five days following chemotherapy, the total duration of neutropenia is less than a week in most patients.

Table 9. Allogeneic stem cell collections

CD34/kg		
$> 4 \times 10^6$	1 collection	9/21
	all collections	11/21
$> 2.5 \times 10^6$	1 collection	11/21
	all collections	16/21
$< 1.5 \times 10^6$	all collections	3/21
(G-CSF 5 μg/kg q 12 hr $\times$ 4 days)		

Values represent the number of patients with sufficient stem cell collections as judged by the number of CD34 positive cells obtained.

All patients in our series since January 1995 received combination chemotherapy with high-dose CY plus either Taxol or VP16. As reported by others [17, 18, 23, 24], we have found this to be a safe approach with no increase in toxicity as compared with CY alone. In our studies, we have largely abandoned the use of growth factors alone for stem cell mobilization except in patients with cardiac dysfunction and a low ejection fraction. In addition to improving CD34 yields, high-dose chemotherapy causes further cytoreduction of the tumor and serves as a predictor for response to transplantation.

In the past, the timing of pheresis procedures was largely dictated by a rise in leukocyte count to $1,000/\mu l$. This frequently meant obtaining a product with less than 1×10^6 CD34 cells/kg. Using the peripheral CD34 count as a guideline [25, 26], we are now delaying collections until there are > 20 CD34 cells/μl. This usually occurs on days 10-12 after mobilization and may be dependent on the amount of previous chemotherapy or radiotherapy. Although prospective analysis of the blood CD34 levels delays the onset of collections, it permits a greater recovery of CD34 cells and reduces the total number of phereses necessary for an adequate stem cell product.

Previous studies have shown that marrow involvement, diagnoses other than carcinoma of the breast, large numbers of chemotherapy cycles, and previous irradiation all reduce the mobilization of CD34 positive cells [27-29]. Our studies show that additional phereses were required for patients with non-Hodgkin's lymphoma as compared to carcinoma of the breast. In part, this may reflect prior treatment, however, the data indicated a much lower extraction ratio in patients with lymphoma, as compared to carcinoma of the breast. One possible explanation could be stem cell exhaustion during the collection. As shown in Figure 3, most patients had approximately 50% of the baseline CD34 cells still remaining in the circulation after the 12-liter exchange. Alternatively, the poor collection may have resulted from poor extraction during the pheresis procedure. *Hayloc et al.* [30] found that the instantaneous collection efficiency (extraction ratio) of the Baxter CS3000 machine was 95% for mononuclear cells and CFU-GM as judged by assays on the inlet and outlet lines during pheresis. However, the overall collection efficiency ratings during the procedure were 64% and 56% for the mononuclear cell and CFU-GM recoveries, respectively. This discrepancy between the single-pass removal and the overall removal of cells was due to a fall in mononuclear cells during the collection, dilution by ACD-A and the operational dead space of the machine. When these factors were considered, the overall collection efficiency or extraction ratio approached 95%. However, these authors used a larger-volume collection chamber and a different program for cell collection.

As shown in Table 4, there appears to be heterogeneity in the density profile of circulating CD34 positive cells. Thus, it would seem the collection of the entire mononuclear cell layer would most likely optimize the CD34 recovery. Studies from our institution suggested optimal recovery of mononuclear cells using an OD setting that would remove and collect the majority of blood mononuclear cells [22]. The I/O setting of 150 was shown to collect a higher proportion of mononuclear cells, as well as 1%-2% neutrophils, thus suggesting maximal removal of the mononuclear cell layer. *Stroncek et al.* [31] have used a similar approach with an I/O setting of 140 for over 100 allogeneic stem cell collections. In their studies, only 7 to 8 l of blood have been processed, as compared with 12 l in our studies. Based on the volume of red cells in each pheresis product, it would appear that the small-volume collection chamber has become overloaded during the 12-l collection, thus returning CD34 cells to the patient during the latter part of the procedure. Several approaches may be taken to correct this technical problem. Cells may be collected using a large-volume collection chamber; however, this also removes a large number of platelets, thus increasing the need for platelet transfusions during the recovery phase from chemotherapy. Alternatively, a machine setting of 100 would seem more appropriate for large-volume (12-l) pheresis procedures. Another approach would be to manually empty the collection chamber into the collection bag halfway through the procedure. These possibilities are now under study with kinetic analysis of CD34 removal at periodic intervals during the large-volume pheresis.

Despite problems with collection, most patients in this series received more than 4×10^6 CD34 cells/kg. Recoveries were prompt, with neutrophil counts greater than 500 by day 10-11 when growth factors were administered post-transplant. This represented a 3-4 day reduction in the duration of neutropenia as compared to the first 35 patients who did not receive growth factors post-transplant. Platelet recoveries were also prompt and more rapid in patients with carcinoma of the breast than with those having lymphoma. This may again reflect more exposures to chemotherapy prior to the peripheral blood stem cell transplant in the lymphoma group.

Mobilization and collection of allogeneic stem cells also appeared suboptimal; only one-half of the donors had a satisfactory collection with a single pheresis procedure. In part, this may have reflected use of the 150 I/O setting; however, three donors failed to mobilize sufficient cells for collections as judged by low levels of circulating CD34 positive cells. This finding has been noted by other groups [31-33] and may reflect genetic variations in expression of adhesive proteins that respond to high levels of G-CSF.

SUMMARY

Autologous PBSC transplantation offers several advantages over autologous bone marrow transplantation; patients receiving PBSC transplants typically have faster neutrophil and platelet recoveries and need fewer red cell and platelet transfusions. Optimizing PBSC collections remains a clinical goal; as this study shows, collecting PBSC when peripheral $CD34^+$ counts are $> 20/\mu l$ permits adequate numbers of stem cells to be harvested in fewer collections, thereby reducing the costs and physiological stresses of the procedure. PBSC collections are also useful for allogeneic transplants, where adequate numbers of stem cells for transplantation are often collected with a single leukapheresis.

ACKNOWLEDGMENTS

The authors gratefully acknowledge the excellent assistance of *Margo Steinsdoerfer* in preparation of the manuscript, and *Connie Domenick* and *John Weimerskirch* in compiling much of the data. We also thank *Charlene Briedenbaugh*, *Tammy Tarosky* and *Gale Kennedy* for excellent technical assistance with the stem cell collections and transplantation.

REFERENCES

1 Woenckhaus E. Beitrag zur Allgemeinwirkung der Roentgenstrahlen. Arch f Exp Path und Pharm 1931;160:19-28.

2 Brecher G, Cronkite EP. Post-radiation parabiosis and survival in rats. Proc Soc Exp Biol and Med 1951;77:292-294.

3 Swift MN, Taketa FT, Bond VP. Regionally fractionated-x-irradiation equivalent in dose to total body exposure. Radiat Res 1954;1:241-252.

4 Cavins JA, Scheer SC, Thomas ED. The recovery of lethally irradiated dogs given infusions of autologous leukocytes preserved at -80°C. Blood 1964;23:38-42.

5 Storb R, Epstein RB, Ragde H et al. Marrow engraftment by allogeneic leukocytes in lethally irradiated dogs. Blood 1967;30:805-811.

6 Fliedner TM, Flad HD, Bruch C et al. Treatment of aplastic anemia by blood stem cell transfusion: a canine model. Haematologica 1976;61:141-156.

7 Calvo W, Fliedner TM, Herbst EW et al. Regeneration of blood forming organs after autologous leukocyte transfusion in lethally irradiated dogs. Distribution and cellularity of the marrow in irradiated and transfused animals. Blood 1976;47:593-601.

8 Körbling M, Fliedner TM, Calvo W et al. Albumin density gradient purification of canine hemopoietic blood stem cells (HBSC): long-term allogeneic engraftment without GVH reaction. Exp Hematol 1979;7:277-288.

9 Ross WM, Körbling M. Role of dextran sulfate in increasing CFU-C concentration in dog blood. Proc Soc Exp Biol Med 1978;157:301-305.

10 Körbling M, Dorken B, Ho AD et al. Autologous transplantation of blood-derived hemopoietic stem cells after myeloablative therapy in a patient with Burkitt's lymphoma. Blood 1986;67:529-532.

11 Juttner CA, To LB, Haylock DN et al. Circulating autologous stem cells collected in very early remission from acute non-lymphoblastic leukaemia produce prompt but incomplete haemopoietic reconstitution after high dose melphalan or supralethal chemoradiotherapy. Br J Haematol 1985;61:739-745.

12 Kessinger A, Armitage JO, Landmark JD et al. Reconstitution of human hematopoietic function with autologous cryopreserved circulating stem cells. Exp Hematol 1986;14:192-196.

13 Reiffers J, Bernard P, David B et al. Successful autologous transplantation with peripheral blood hemopoietic cells in a patient with acute leukemia. Exp Hematol 1986;14:312-315.

14 Richman CM, Weiner RS, Yankee RA. Increase in circulating stem cells following chemotherapy in man. Blood 1976;47:1031-1039.

15 Gianni AM, Siena S, Bregni M et al. Granulocyte-macrophage colony-stimulating factor to harvest circulating haemopoietic stem cells for autotransplantation. Lancet 1989;2:580-585.

16 Rosenfeld CS, Shadduck RK, Zeigler ZR et al. Cyclophosphamide-mobilized peripheral blood stem cells in patients with lymphoid malignancies. Bone Marrow Transplant 1995;15:433-438.

17 Rosenfeld CS, Bolwell B, LeFever A et al. Comparison of four cytokine regimens for mobilization of peripheral blood stem cells: IL-3 alone and combined with GM-CSF or G-CSF. Bone Marrow Transplant 1996;17:179-183.

18 Demirer T, Buckner CD, Bensinger WI et al. Peripheral-blood stem-cell collections after paclitaxel, cyclophosphamide and recombinant human granulocyte colony-stimulating factor in patients with breast and ovarian cancer. J Clin Oncol 1995;13:1714-1719.

19 Schwartzberg R, Birch R, Blanco R et al. Rapid and sustained hematopoietic reconstitution by peripheral blood stem cell infusion alone following high-dose chemotherapy. Bone Marrow Transplant 1993;11:369-374.

20 Rosenzweig MQ, Schaefer PM, Rosenfeld CS. Prevention of transplant-related hemorrhagic cystitis using bladder irrigation with sorbitol. Bone Marrow Transplant 1994;14:491-492.

21 Rosenfeld CS, Gremba C, Shadduck RK et al. Engraftment with peripheral blood stem cells using noncontrolled-rate cryopreservation: comparison with autologous bone marrow transplantation. Exp Hematol 1994;22:290-294.

22 Rosenfeld CS, Cullis H, Tarosky T et al. Peripheral blood stem cell collection using the small volume collection chamber in the Fenwal CS-3000 Plus blood cell separator. Bone Marrow Transplant 1994;13:131-134.

23 Demirer T, Buckner CD, Bensinger WI. Optimization of peripheral blood stem cell mobilization. STEM CELLS 1996;14:106-116.

24 Bensinger W, Appelbaum F, Rowley S et al. Factors that influence collection and engraftment of autologous peripheral blood stem cells. J Clin Oncol 1995;13:2547-2555.

25 Siena S, Bregni M, Brando B et al. Circulation of $CD34^+$ hematopoietic stem cells in the peripheral blood of high dose cyclophosphamide-treated patients: enhancement by intravenous recombinant human granulocyte-macrophage colony-stimulating factor. Blood 1989;74:1905-1914.

26 Siena S, Bregni M, Brando B et al. Flow cytometry for clinical estimation of circulating hematopoietic progenitors for autologous transplantation in cancer patients. Blood 1991;77:400-409.

27 Kotasek D, Shepherd KM, Sage RE et al. Factors affecting blood stem cell collections following high-dose cyclophosphamide mobilization in lymphoma, myeloma and solid tumors. Bone Marrow Transplant 1992;9:11-17.

28 Haas R, Mohle R, Fruhauf S et al. Patient characteristics associated with successful mobilizing and autografting of peripheral blood progenitor cells in malignant lymphoma. Blood 1994;83:3787-3794.

29 Bensinger WI, Longin K, Appelbaum F et al. Peripheral blood stem cells (PBSCs) collected after recombinant granulocyte colony stimulating factor (rhG-CSF): an analysis of factors correlating with the tempo of engraftment after transplantation. Br J. Haematol 1994;87:825-831.

30 Haylock DN, Canty A, Thorp D et al. A discrepancy between the instantaneous and the overall collection efficiency of the Fenwal CS3000 for peripheral blood stem cell apheresis. J Clin Apheresis 1992;7:6-11.

31 Stroncek DF, Clay ME, Petzoldt ML et al. Treatment of normal individuals with granulocyte-colony-stimulating factor: donor experiences and the effects on peripheral blood CD34[+] cell counts and on the collection of peripheral blood stem cells. Transfusion 1996;36:601-610.

32 Roberts AW, DeLuca E, Begley CG et al. Broad inter-individual variations in circulating progenitor cell numbers induced by granulocyte colony-stimulating factor therapy. STEM CELLS 1995;13:512-516.

33 Bensinger WI, Clift RA, Anasetti C et al. Transplantation of allogeneic peripheral blood stem cells mobilized by recombinant human granulocyte colony stimulating factor. STEM CELLS 1996;14:90-105.

The Role of Endothelium in the Regulation of Hematopoietic Stem Cell Migration

Robert Möhle,[a,b] Shahin Rafii,[c] Malcolm A.S. Moore[a]

[a]Laboratory of Developmental Hematopoiesis, Sloan-Kettering Institute, New York, NY, USA;
[b]Department of Medicine II, University of Tübingen, Tübingen, Germany; [c]Cornell University
Medical College, Division of Hematology & Oncology, New York, NY, USA

Key Words. *Endothelium · Hematopoietic stem cells · Migration · Mobilization · Homing · Adhesion molecules
· Cytokines · Chemokines*

Abstract

Mobilization of hematopoietic progenitor cells appears to be a multifactorial process which is at least partially regulated at the level of bone marrow microvascular endothelium (BMEC). In order to study the regulation of progenitor cell migration by endothelium in vitro, methods have been developed to isolate BMEC from bone marrow aspirates. In addition, immortalized BMEC cell lines have been generated. Using an in vitro model of migration across bone marrow endothelium, we demonstrate that only a small number of more mature, committed progenitors migrate spontaneously. In this model, adhesion molecules of the β2-integrin family and the corresponding endothelial ligands are involved. The low spontaneous migratory capacity suggests that, in addition to adhesion molecules which mediate direct cellular contacts, paracrine cytokines and chemokines may play a role in progenitor migration across endothelium. Growth-factor-stimulated hematopoietic cells can produce cytokines which act on endothelial cells (e.g., vascular endothelial growth factor, VEGF), modifying their motility, growth, permeability, and fenestration. Therefore, VEGF might be involved in the mobilization and homing of hematopoietic progenitor cells. Furthermore, transendothelial migration of progenitors in vitro is substantially enhanced by the chemokine stromal-cell-derived factor-1 (SDF-1), which is produced by bone marrow stromal cells. More primitive progenitors, which do not migrate spontaneously, also respond to this chemokine. We conclude that transendothelial progenitor cell migration is regulated by adhesion molecules, paracrine cytokines, and chemokines. Mobilizing hematopoietic growth factors stimulate proliferation of hematopoietic cells, which may indirectly result in changes of the local cytokine and chemokine milieu, adhesion molecule expression, and eventually the mobilization of hematopoietic progenitor cells. *Stem Cells 1998;16(suppl 1):159-165*

Possible Role of Endothelium in Progenitor Cell Mobilization

In contrast to the well-established clinical use of mobilized peripheral blood hematopoietic progenitor cells for autologous or allogeneic transplantation, the mechanisms of mobilization and homing of hematopoietic stem cells have still remained elusive. Since endothelium separates the resting (bone marrow stroma) from the circulating progenitor cell compartment (peripheral blood) [1], it is conceivable that hematopoietic progenitor cell trafficking is at least partially regulated at the level of the sinusoidal bone marrow endothelium. In

Characteristics and Potentials of Blood Stem Cells
Stem Cells 1998;16(suppl 1):159-165 ©AlphaMed Press. All rights reserved.

vivo and in vitro studies suggest that progenitor cell mobilization is a multifactorial process, determined by the reciprocal interactions of the hematopoietic, endothelial, and stromal cells. Regulation of these interactions most likely involves adhesion molecules, paracrine cytokines, and chemokines.

During steady-state hematopoiesis (without administration of exogenous cytokines), only low numbers of circulating progenitor cells can be found in the peripheral blood. Mobilization with hematopoietic growth factors or regeneration of hematopoiesis post-chemotherapy induces a shift of the progenitor cell equilibrium from the resting to the circulating pool [2-4]. Increasing numbers of progenitors in the peripheral blood could be due to either an active release from the bone marrow or a reduced ability of the progenitor cells to leave the circulation and home to the bone marrow. The latter could indirectly increase the number of peripheral blood progenitor cells as a result of the longer time progenitors stay in the circulation. Thus, presentation of adhesion molecules by bone marrow endothelium which are recognized by circulating progenitors during the process of homing might also play an indirect role for the mobilization.

Bone Marrow Endothelial Cells In Vitro

To investigate mechanisms involved in the regulation of hematopoietic progenitor cell trafficking in vitro, we and other groups have developed techniques for the isolation and cultivation of bone marrow endothelial cells [5, 6]. Microvascular endothelium can be separated from bone marrow spicules after collagenase digestion followed by immunomagnetic isolation (Fig. 1). Virtually pure cultures (as assessed by immunocytological analysis) may require repeated isolation steps. Fluorescence-activated cell sorting (FACS) has also been used to isolate endothelium from the bone marrow [6]. However, endothelial cells can be obtained more efficiently from isolated microvessels and might represent microvascular endothelium more appropriately than sorting of single cells from the mononuclear cell fraction. Early passages of bone marrow endothelial cells have successfully been immortalized, which allows study of the interaction of hematopoietic cells with a more homogeneous endothelial cell population [7, 8]. These cells retain the phenotype of bone marrow microvascular endothelium (BMEC) more closely and stably than primary BMEC after several passages in vitro. For in vitro analysis of transendothelial progenitor cell migration, we have used the immortalized cell line BMEC-1 [8]. Similar to early passages of primary BMEC, this cell line is positive for characteristic endothelial markers, such as CD34 and factor VIII/von Willebrand factor (vWF). Low levels of adhesion molecules of the immunoglobulin superfamily (ICAM-1) are constitutively expressed and can be upregulated by inflammatory cytokines.

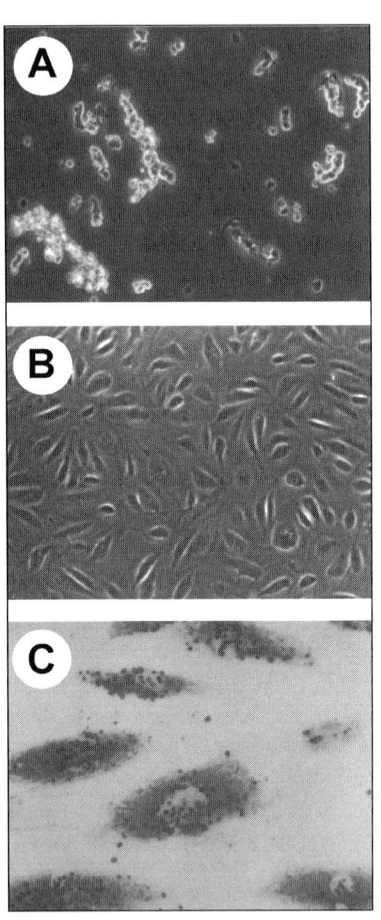

Figure 1. Isolation of bone marrow endothelial cells. (A) After digestion of spicules from bone marrow aspirates with collagenase, microvessel fragments were obtained (original magnification × 100). (B) After separation using antibodies or lectins recognizing endothelial antigens, virtually pure confluent layers of BMEC grown on gelatin-coated dishes were established (× 100). (C) The purity of the cell population can be assessed by immunocytology for factor VIII/von Willebrand factor (× 400).

Factors Involved in the Regulation of Progenitor Cell Mobilization by Endothelial Adhesion Molecules

Phenotypic analysis of hematopoietic progenitor cells has shown that bone marrow and mobilized peripheral blood progenitors express a variety of adhesion molecules such as selectins, selectin ligands, integrins, and PECAM [9-12]. The repertoire of adhesion molecules expressed on hematopoietic progenitor cells is sufficient for the consecutive steps of leukocyte extravasation. This process involves reversible ("rolling," mediated by selectins) and firm adhesion (mediated by integrins), followed by migration across the endothelial layer (mediated by integrins, PECAM, and other adhesion molecules), and requires sequential action of these adhesion molecules [13]. However, most studies of leukocyte migration refer to extravasation at sites of inflammation. It is unknown whether these mechanisms of leukocyte migration play a role in hematopoietic progenitor cell mobilization and homing, which are obviously not inflammation-related processes. However, bone marrow microvascular endothelium in vitro may constitutively express adhesion molecules such as VCAM and E-selectin [14, 15], which are usually only found after stimulation with inflammatory cytokines.

The fact that the level of the β1-integrin, very late activation-antigen-4 (VLA-4), and β2-integrin LFA-1 (leukocyte function antigen-1) is lower on circulating progenitors indicates that downmodulation of adhesion molecules may contribute to the release of progenitors from the bone marrow [16, 17]. Bone marrow stromal and endothelial cells express VCAM-1 and ICAM-1, the ligands for these adhesion molecules [14, 18]. Disrupting the β1-integrin-mediated adhesion by administration of antibodies to VLA-4 mobilizes progenitors in vivo [19]. Furthermore, antibodies to VLA-4 and VCAM inhibit homing of stem cells to the bone marrow, which further supports the idea that adhesion via integrins is involved in stem cell migration [20].

To analyze the contribution of adhesion molecules to transendothelial progenitor cell migration, we have developed an in vitro model using primary bone marrow endothelial cells or BMEC-1 cells grown on 3 μm microporous transwell membranes, separating an upper and lower chamber in a six-well tissue culture plate [8]. After addition of hematopoietic progenitor cells to the upper chamber of the transmigration system and incubation for several hours, transmigrated cells can be quantified and characterized (Fig. 2). The contribution of adhesion molecules to the transendothelial migration can be assessed by blocking antibodies which are also added to the upper chamber.

Without addition of cytokines or chemokines, only a small number (1.6 ± 0.3% within 24 h) of CD34$^+$ mobilized peripheral blood hematopoietic progenitor cells migrates across bone marrow endothelium in vitro [8]. These cells display the phenotype of committed progenitors (CD34$^+$/CD38^{++}), while CD34$^+$/CD38$^-$ cells, which comprise more primitive progenitors, are not found among the transmigrated cells. Transmigration can be partially inhibited with blocking antibodies to the β2-integrin LFA-1, which is expressed on hematopoietic progenitor cells, while blocking antibodies to the β1-integrin VLA-4 and L-selectin showed no effect. These results suggest that, in contrast to mature leukocytes (e.g., monocytes), which can spontaneously migrate across endothelium [21], efficient migration, particularly of more primitive progenitors requires additional factors, such as paracrine cytokines or chemokines.

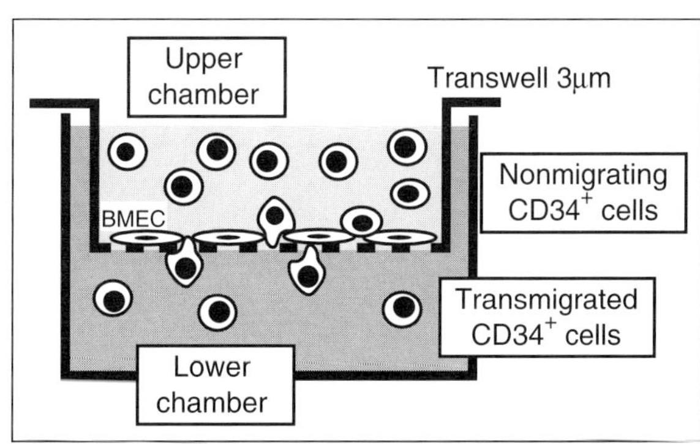

Figure 2. Transendothelial migration of hematopoietic progenitor cells in vitro. Primary bone marrow endothelial cells or cell lines were grown to confluence on 3 μm microporous transwell membrane inserts, separating an upper from a lower chamber in a six-well tissue culture plate. Hematopoietic progenitor cells were added to the upper chamber of the transmigration system. Transmigrated progenitors could be recovered from the lower chamber after incubation for 10 h or 24 h at 37°C/5% CO₂.

Cytokines

If present in a membrane-bound form, cytokines can also act as adhesion molecules. For example, stem cell factor ([SCF], c-kit ligand) is expressed on the cell surface of bone marrow stromal and endothelial cells [22, 23]. The low level of c-kit on circulating, mobilized progenitors may indicate that loss of the SCF receptor facilitates the egress of progenitor cells from the bone marrow [24].

Recent studies also suggest that proliferating hematopoietic cells produce cytokines that act on endothelial cells and may support the release of hematopoietic progenitor cells from the bone marrow. Vascular endothelial growth factor (VEGF) is a cytokine which specifically acts on endothelial cells, induces endothelial proliferation and vascular remodeling, and increases endothelial fenestration [25-27]. We have demonstrated that hematopoietic growth factors such as interleukin 3 (IL-3) and thrombopoietin induce VEGF secretion in proliferating hematopoietic precursor and mature cells, which may also contribute to the release of progenitors [28]. In reverse, VEGF induces production of hematopoietic cytokines in endothelial cells without inflammatory endothelial activation, resulting in a paracrine loop (Fig. 3). Locally secreted VEGF could allow transit of hematopoietic cells by increasing the vascular permeability and endothelial fenestration. VEGF supports proliferation of endothelial cells and angiogenesis, which is associated with a unique pattern of cell surface molecules, including expression of E-selectin [29]. Indeed, this endothelial adhesion molecule seems to be constitutively expressed on bone marrow endothelium in vivo, and might therefore play a role in stem cell homing [15]. Both, establishment of hematopoiesis and development of vasculature is absent in VEGF deficient mice, further supporting the idea that VEGF is an important cytokine involved in the reciprocal interaction between hematopoietic and endothelial cells [30].

Chemokines

Chemokines represent a group of cytokines with chemotactic effect on hematopoietic cells. While the majority of chemokines act on mature cells (e.g., IL-8 on granulocytes), recent studies have revealed that the chemokine stromal-cell-derived factor-1 (SDF-1), which is produced by bone marrow stromal cells (but also by stromal cells of other tissues), is chemotactic also for hematopoietic progenitor cells [31, 32]. SDF-1 is a member of the CXC chemokine family which is characterized by an intervening residue separating the first two cysteine residues within a conserved motif [33]. In vivo, constitutive production of SDF-1 by bone marrow stromal cells could result in a transendothelial gradient supporting migration of circulating hematopoietic progenitors into the bone marrow

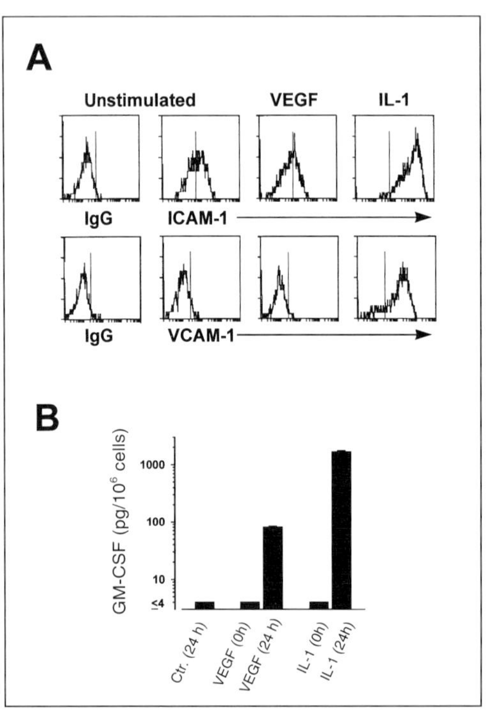

Figure 3. VEGF induces secretion of hematopoietic growth factors in bone marrow endothelial cells without activation. (A) Incubation of bone marrow endothelial cells with VEGF (50 ng/ml for 12 h) did not induce expression of the adhesion molecules ICAM-1 or VCAM-1, as assessed by flow cytometry. In contrast, upregulation of these endothelial adhesion molecules was observed after activation with IL-1β (10 ng/ml). Fluorescence histograms are shown; IgG = isotype specific IgG control. (B) After incubation for 24 h, significant production of GM-CSF was observed when BMEC were incubated with VEGF (50 ng/ml) using a sensitive immunoassay (ELISA). As a positive control, IL-1β-induced production of GM-CSF is shown. Incubation without cytokines (Ctr. 24 h), and VEGF or IL-1β-supplemented medium without incubation (VEGF 0 h, IL-1 0 h) served as negative controls.

stroma. In our transmigration system, addition of SDF-1 containing conditioned medium from the stromal cell line MS-5 or recombinant SDF-1 dramatically increases the number of CD34$^+$ peripheral blood progenitor cells migrating across bone marrow endothelium (Fig. 4). Indeed, peripheral blood progenitor cells express the receptor for SDF-1, the CXC chemokine receptor-4 (CXCR-4), and respond to the chemokine with a rapid intracellular calcium mobilization (Fig. 5). Similar to lymphocytes [34], the SDF-1 effect can be partially blocked by CXCR-4 antibodies demonstrating that this receptor is responsible for the SDF-1 effect also in hematopoietic progenitor cells. SDF-1-induced transendothelial migration in vitro is also controlled by bone marrow endothelium, as suggested by the blocking effect of β2-integrin antibodies (39% reduction of the transmigrated CD34$^+$ progenitor cells when the LFA-1β antibody TS 1/18 is added at 5 mg/ml to the upper chamber of the transmigration system). However, the blocking effect of this antibody on spontaneous migration is greater (61% reduction).

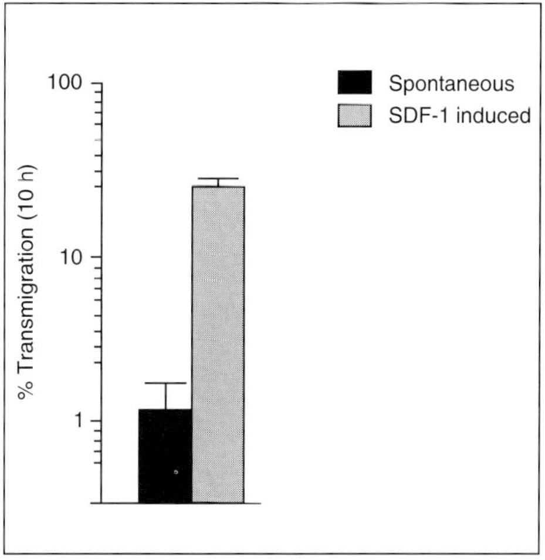

Figure 4. SDF-1 enhances transendothelial migration of hematopoietic progenitors. *Conditioned medium from the cell line MS-5, which contains large amounts of SDF-1, was added to the lower chamber of the transmigration system shown in Figure 2. As a control for spontaneous migration, unconditioned medium was used. Transmigrated cells were recovered from the lower chamber after 10 h and enumerated.*

The fact that circulating progenitors migrate less avidly in response to SDF-1 than bone-marrow-derived CD34$^+$ cells [32] and that bone marrow hematopoiesis is reduced in SDF-1-deficient mice [35] suggests that SDF-1-mediated transendothelial migration plays a role in stem cell mobilization and homing. However, it is not clear how migration in response to SDF-1 is regulated. Both reduced production of SDF-1 and downmodulation of the SDF-1 receptor on hematopoietic progenitor cells could be mechanisms involved in progenitor mobilization.

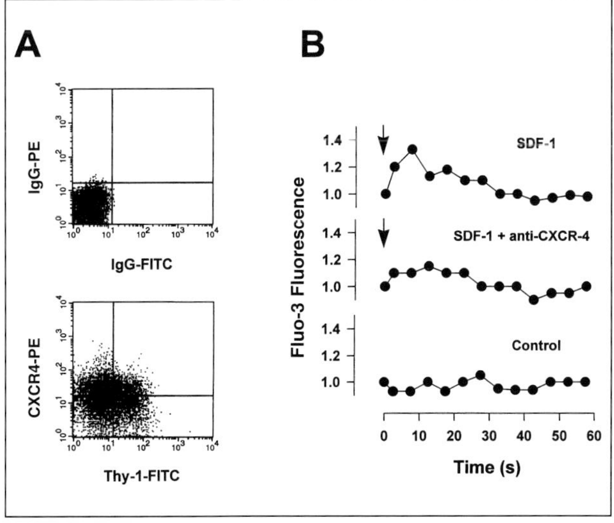

Figure 5. The functionally active SDF-1 receptor (CXCR-4) is expressed on hematopoietic progenitors. *(A) Mobilized CD34$^+$ cells from the peripheral blood were stained with Thy-1-FITC, CXCR-4 PE, and CD34-PerCP, and analyzed with flow cytometry. CD34$^+$ cells were gated and further analyzed for Thy-1 and CXCR-4 coexpression (dot plots are shown; IgG = isotype specific IgG control). CD34$^+$ cells expressed CXCR-4 at a moderate fluorescence intensity. The proportion of CXCR-4-expressing cells in the CD34$^+$/Thy-1$^+$ subpopulation was at least as great as in the CD34$^+$/Thy-1$^-$ subset, indicating that more primitive progenitors also express the SDF-1 receptor. (B) To determine whether CXCR-4 is functionally active in CD34$^+$ progenitor cells, SDF-1 (300 ng/ml) was added [9] to CD34$^+$ cells that had been loaded with the calcium-dependent fluorescence dye Fluo-3. Within seconds, intracellular calcium was mobilized by SDF-1, resulting in an increased Fluo-3 fluorescence. The effect was reduced by the partially blocking CXCR-4 antibody 12G5.*

CONCLUSIONS

The results of our studies and those from other investigators suggest that regulation of hematopoietic progenitor mobilization by endothelium is a multifactorial process which involves adhesion molecules (e.g., integrins and their receptors), cytokines (e.g., SCF, VEGF), and chemokines (e.g., SDF-1). Since addition of a single cytokine does not alter adhesion molecule expression or migratory behavior of hematopoietic progenitor cells [36], the mobilizing effect of hematopoietic growth factors such as G-CSF is most likely indirectly mediated. These cytokines induce proliferation of hematopoietic progenitor and precursor cells which modulates the local cytokine and chemokine milieu, and change the expression and avidity of adhesion molecules on hematopoietic, endothelial, and stromal cells. Eventually, mobilization of hematopoietic progenitor cells occurs as an indirect result of the altered hematopoietic microenvironment.

ACKNOWLEDGMENTS

We thank *Barbara Ferris* and *Michael Querijero* for excellent technical assistance.

This work was supported by the Gar Reichman Fund of the Cancer Research Institute (*M.A.S.M.*), by NIH grant KO8-HL-02926, Dorothy Rodbell Cohen Foundation for Sarcoma Research, and The Rich Foundation (*S.R.*). *R.M.* was recipient of a fellowship from the Dr. Mildred Scheel Stiftung für Krebsforschung (Germany).

REFERENCES

1 Weiss L. The hematopoietic microenvironment of the bone marrow: an ultrastructural study of the stroma in rats. Anat Rec 1976;186:161-184.

2 Demuynck H, Pettengell R, deCampos E et al. The capacity of peripheral blood stem cells mobilised with chemotherapy plus G-CSF to repopulate irradiated marrow stroma in vitro is similar to that of bone marrow. Eur J Cancer 1992;28:381-386.

3 Dührsen U, Villeval JL, Boyd J et al. Effects of recombinant human granulocyte colony-stimulating factor on hematopoietic progenitor cells in cancer patients. Blood 1988;72:2074-2081.

4 Richman CM, Weiner R, Yankee RA. Increase in circulating stem cells following chemotherapy in man. Blood 1976;47:1031-1039.

5 Rafii S, Shapiro F, Rimarachin J et al. Isolation and characterization of human bone marrow microvascular endothelial cells: hematopoietic progenitor cell adhesion. Blood 1994;84:10-19.

6 Schweitzer CM, van der Schoot CE, Dräger AM et al. Isolation and culture of human bone marrow endothelial cells. Exp Hematol 1995;23:31-48.

7 Candal FJ, Rafii S, Parker JT et al. BMEC-1: a human bone marrow microvascular endothelial cell with primary cell characteristics. Microvasc Res 1996;52:221-234.

8 Möhle R, Moore MAS, Nachman RL et al. Transendothelial migration of CD34$^+$ and mature hematopoietic cells: an in vitro study using a human bone marrow endothelial cell line. Blood 1997;89:72-80.

9 Lund-Johansen F, Terstappen LWMM. Differential surface expression of cell adhesion molecules during granulocyte maturation. J Leukoc Biol 1993;54:47-55.

10 Saeland S, Duvert V, Caux C et al. Distribution of surface-membrane molecules on bone-marrow and cord blood CD34$^+$ hematopoietic cells. Exp Hematol 1992;20:24-33.

11 Zannettino ACW, Berndt MC, Butcher C et al. Primitive human hematopoietic progenitors adhere to P-selectin (CD62P). Blood 1995;85:3466-3477.

12 Watt SM, Williamson J, Genevier H et al. The heparin binding PCAM-1 adhesion molecule is expressed by CD34$^+$ hematopoietic precursor cells with early myeloid and B-lymphoid phenotypes. Blood 1993;82:2649-2663.

13 Carlos TM, Harlan JM. Leukocyte-endothelial adhesion molecules. Blood 1994;84:2068-2101.

14 Jacobsen K, Kravitz J, Kincade PW et al. Adhesion receptors on bone marrow stromal cells: in vivo expression of vascular cell adhesion molecule-1 by reticular cells and sinusoidal endothelium in normal and gamma-irradiated mice. Blood 1996;87:73-82.

15 Schweitzer KM, Drager AM, van der Valk P et al. Constitutive expression of E-selectin and vascular cell adhesion molecule-1 on endothelial cells of hematopoietic tissues. Am J Pathol 1996;148:165-175.

16 Möhle R, Murea S, Kirsch M et al. Differential expression of L-selectin, VLA-4, and LFA-1 on CD34$^+$ progenitor cells from bone marrow and peripheral blood during G-CSF enhanced recovery. Exp Hematol 1995;23:1535-1542.

17 Dercksen MW, Gerritsen WR, Rodenhuis S et al. Expression of adhesion molecules on CD34[+] cells: L-selectin[+] cells predict a rapid platelet recovery after peripheral blood stem cell transplantation. Blood 1995;85:3313-3319.

18 Teixido J, Hemler ME, Greenberger JS et al. Role of $\beta 1$ and $\beta 2$ integrins in the adhesion of human CD34[hi] stem cells to bone marrow stroma. J Clin Invest 1992;90:358-367.

19 Papayannopoulou T, Nakamoto B. Peripheralization of hemopoietic progenitors in primates treated with anti-VLA4 integrin. Proc Natl Acad Sci USA 1993;90:9374-9378.

20 Papayannopoulou T, Craddock C, Nakamoto B et al. The VLA4/VCAM-1 adhesion pathway defines contrasting mechanisms of lodgement of transplanted murine hemopoietic progenitors between bone marrow and spleen. Proc Nat Acad Sci USA 1995;92:9647-9651.

21 Muller WA, Weigl SA. Monocyte-selective transendothelial migration: dissection of the binding and transmigration phases by an in vitro assay. J Exp Med 1992;176:819-828.

22 Flanagan JG, Chan DC, Leder P. Transmembrane form of kit ligand growth factor is determined by alternative splicing and is missing in the Sld mutant. Cell 1991;64:1025-1035.

23 Fleischman RA, Simpson F, Gallardo T et al. Isolation of endothelial-like stromal cells that express kit ligand and support in vitro hematopoiesis. Exp Hematol 1995;23:1407-1416.

24 Möhle R, Haas R, Hunstein W. Expression of adhesion molecules and c-kit on CD34[+] hematopoietic progenitor cells: comparison of cytokine-mobilized blood stem cells with normal bone marrow and peripheral blood. J Hematother 1993;2:483-489.

25 Connolly DT, Heuvelman DM, Nelson R et al. Tumor vascular permeability factor stimulates endothelial growth and angiogenesis. J Clin Invest 1989;84:1470-1478.

26 Dvorak HF, Brown LF, Detmar M et al. Vascular permeability factor/vascular endothelial growth factor, microvascular hyperpermeability, and angiogenesis. Am J Pathol 1995;146:1029-1039.

27 Roberts WG, Palade GE. Increased microvascular permeability and endothelial fenestration induced by vascular endothelial growth factor. J Cell Sci 1995;108:2369-2379.

28 Möhle R, Green D, Moore MAS et al. Constitutive production and thrombin-induced release of vascular endothelial growth factor by human megakaryocytes and platelets. Proc Natl Acad Sci USA 1997;94:663-668.

29 Bischoff J, Brasel C, Kraling B et al. E-selectin is upregulated in proliferating endothelial cell in vitro. Microcirculation 1997;4:279-287.

30 Ferrara N, Carver-Moore K, Chen H et al. Heterozygous embryonic lethality induced by targeted inactivation of the VEGF gene. Nature 1996;380:439-442.

31 Nagasawa T, Kikutani H, Kishimoto T. Molecular cloning and structure of a pre-B-cell growth-stimulating factor. Proc Natl Acad Sci USA 1994;91:2305-2309.

32 Aiuti A, Webb IJ, Bleul C et al. The chemokine SDF-1 is a chemoattractant for human hematopoietic progenitor cells and provides a new mechanism to explain the mobilization of CD34[+] progenitors to peripheral blood. J Exp Med 1997;185:111-120.

33 Wells TN, Power CA, Lusti-Narasimhan M et al. Selectivity and antagonism of chemokine receptors. J Leukoc Biol 1996;59:53-60.

34 Bleul CC, Wu L, Hoxie JA et al. The HIV coreceptors CXCR4 and CCR5 are differently expressed and regulated on human lymphocytes. Proc Natl Acad Sci USA 1997;94:1925-1930.

35 Nagasawa T, Hirota S, Tachibana K et al. Defects of B-cell lymphopoiesis and bone marrow myelopoiesis in mice lacking the CXC chemokine PBSF/SDF-1. Nature 1996;382:635-638.

36 Yong KL, Watts MJ, Thomas NSB et al. Transendothelial migration of CD34[+] cells requires prior activation by growth factors and is mediated by PECAM-1. Blood 1996;88:475a

Rapidly Mobilizable Stem Cells.
Do They Belong to a Special Subpopulation?

JULIA GIDÁLI, I. FEHÉR

National Institute of Haematolgy and Immunology Budapest, Budapest, Hungary

Key Words. *Rapidly mobilized CFU-S · Self-renewal capacity · Anchorage of stem cells*

ABSTRACT

Some characteristics of rapidly mobilized stem cells as a possible distinct subset of the murine bone marrow stem cell population are overviewed. Some of the agents that rapidly mobilize stem cells are toxic and possibly act through disrupting anchorage to the microenvironment. The mobilization occurring days after cytostatics and/or colony-stimulating factors (CSF), however, is a consequence of increased production or differentiation. While stem cells (colony-forming units-spleen; CFU-S) circulating normally in blood have low self-renewal capacity (SRC), SRC of rapidly mobilized CFU-S is closer to that of bone marrow stem cells and is similar to that of the late mobilized stem cells. The survival rate of mice after transplantation of rapidly mobilized stem cells did not differ from that of bone marrow stem cells. One year after transplantation of rapidly mobilized stem cells, the SRC value of bone marrow did not differ from those transplanted with bone marrow cells. Replacement of a rapidly mobilizable stem cell pool requires 48 h under physiological conditions and a longer time after damage to hemopoiesis (irradiation, hydroxyurea injection). Possible physiological mechanisms in the anchorage of stem cells are discussed. *Stem Cells 1998;16 (suppl 1):167-174*

INTRODUCTION

The presence of primitive hemopoietic cells in peripheral blood was proven three decades ago [1-4]. By applying various mobilizing agents, the transplantation of peripheral blood progenitors has become an alternative technique for bone marrow transplantation first in animals [5] and then in humans [6-8].

On one hand there is ample evidence that normal blood stem cells have poor self-renewal ability [9]; on the other hand mobilizable stem cells can adequately reconstitute the hemopoiesis after myeloablative chemotherapy in humans [6-8]. This virtual contradiction can be well explained by comparing self-maintaining features of the spontaneously circulating blood stem cells to mobilized stem cells in mice. In our previous experiments the rapidly mobilized stem cells seemed to represent a special subset of the pluripotent bone marrow stem cell pool [10], therefore the overview of the characteristics of these rapidly mobilizable stem cells may offer some insight into the physiology of circulating stem cells, too. Recent elaboration of new techniques for determining primitive and late stem cells from human leukapheresis products [11, 12] may help to extrapolate these data for clinical practice.

MATERIALS AND METHODS

Experimental Animals

12-14-week-old BDF1 mice were used.

Colony-Forming Unit-Spleen (CFU-S) Assay and Bone Marrow and Peripheral Stem Cell Transplantation

Recipients were irradiated with 9.0 Gy from a ^{60}Co γ source. Cells were injected from isologous donors. If not otherwise stated, spleen colonies were counted on day 9. Sixty-day survival was followed in groups receiving bone marrow or peripheral blood stem cells.

Mobilization of Stem Cells

1.5 mg trypsin (Bacto trypsin, Difco Laboratories; Detroit, MI), 1 mg zymosan (Sigma-Aldrich; Milwaukee, WI) and 150 µg endotoxin (Difco Laboratories) were injected i.v. for rapid mobilization, and 200 mg/kg cyclophosphamide (CY) (Endoxan; Asta AG; Frankfurt, Germany) i.p. or 250 µg/kg/day G-CSF (Neupogen, filgastrim, recombinant human (rHu)G-CSF, Hoffman-La Roche; Switzerland), divided into two equal doses s.c. were injected for late mobilization. Mice were bled from the axillary vessels 30 min after i.p. injection of 100 IU heparin.

Self-Renewal Capacity (SRC)

SRC was studied by transplanting single cell suspensions corresponding to 1/10 of whole spleen of primary recipients of blood and bone marrow CFU-S 10 days after transplantation into secondary 9 Gy irradiated recipients. Index of SRC was calculated from the ratio of day 9 CFU-S recovered from secondary recipients per CFU-S injected into primary recipients [13].

RESULTS

When the effect of various CFU-S mobilizing agents was compared, we found that some of the agents induce rapid stem cell mobilization while others induce release of stem cells into the circulation some days after the mobilization. Some of the agents that were found to induce rapid mobilization (i.e., within 60 min) are toxic. The chemokine interleukin 8 (IL-8), that was reported recently as a potent rapid mobilizer, has no toxic effect [14] (Table 1).

Mobilization kinetics can best be studied after trypsin injection. A single i.v. injection of 1.5 mg/mouse trypsin induced a significant increase of blood day 9 CFU-S level (from 22.4 ± 1.6/ml blood to 310 ± 41.7/ml blood). Then the blood CFU-S level gradually decreased to the control level (Fig. 1). Ratios of day 12 to day 8 colony-forming cells from normal bone marrow and rapidly mobilized stem cells were found to be identical. (Table 2).

One of the most characteristic features of a stem cell population is the SRC. Therefore, SRCs of

Table 1. Stem cell mobilizing agents in mice

Group of agents	Agent	Peak of mobilization	Increase in blood CFU-S	Reference
Enzymes	trypsin	minutes	20 ×	[10]
	zymosan		10 ×	[10]
Toxic agents	endotoxin	biphasic	15 ×	[10]
	WR 2721*	1-2 h	10 ×	
Others	IL-8	15 min	20 ×	[14]
Hormones	depersolone	1 h	5 ×	[10]
Cytostatics	CY	5-6 days	20 ×	[17]
CSFs	G-CSF	4-6 days	50 ×	[15, 17]
	SCF			
	IL-3			
	GM-CSF			

*Aminofostine, a chemical radioproetctive agent 200 mg/kg i.p.

rapidly mobilized and late mobilized stem cells were compared. As expected, SRC of normal blood stem cells proved to be significantly lower than that of bone marrow, while self-renewal of rapidly mobilized stem cells was closer to that of bone marrow than of blood. Although after rapid mobilization the increase in the blood CFU-S level has never reached that achieved after CY injection or G-CSF treatment, SRCs

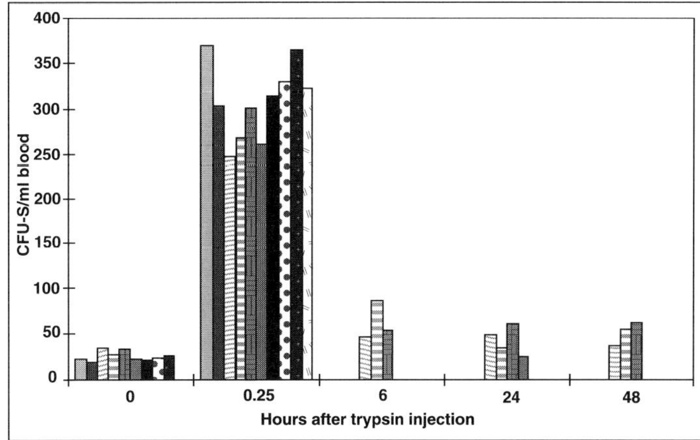

Figure 1. Blood CFU-S level after the i.v. injection of trypsin (1.5 mg/mouse). Each column is the mean of 10 recipients. Based on experiments originally published in [10].

of stem cells mobilized by CY or G-CSF were close to that of rapidly mobilized stem cells. This means that the quality of mobilized stem cells did not differ whether they were obtained from regenerating (CY-treated) mice, G-CSF-treated mice or after rapid mobilization (Table 3).

Up to a certain amount of mobilized stem cells, a close correlation could be observed between SRC of circulating stem cells and quantity of stem cells in the circulation (Fig. 2). Over 300 CFU-S/ml blood, however, SRC value oscillated around a plateau and this correlation could not be observed any more.

When injecting a comparable graft size into lethally irradiated mice, the repopulating ability of rapidly and late mobilized stem cells did not differ significantly (Table 4).

One year after transplantation bone marrow CFU-S concentration and SRC were studied in lethally irradiated female BDF$_1$ mice transplanted with bone marrow cells or rapidly mobilized blood stem cells from male mice. If comparable graft sizes were used, SRC of the chimeras of rapidly mobilized stem cells did not significantly differ from the bone marrow-transplanted group or of normal bone marrow (Table 5).

If rapidly mobilized stem cells represent a transient stem cell population, the rapidly mobilizable pool has to be exhausted by a certain mobilizer and there has to be a definite time interval for the replacement of the pool during which no mobilization can be induced [10]. After rapid mobilization (i.e., after the injection of 1.5 mg trypsin) a significant increase in circulating CFU-S was found and 24 h after trypsin injection, the blood CFU-S level approached the control level. Then, however, with a second trypsin injection, no CFU-S mobilization could be induced. Forty-eight h after the first injection, however, a second shot induced the same rapid mobilization as the first (Table 6).

Table 2. The amount of day 8 and day 12 CFU-S from normal BDF1 bone marrow or rapidly mobilized peripheral cells

Source of cells	Injected cell count or injected blood volume	d-8 CFU-S[*]	d-12 CFU-S*	d-12 /d-8 CFU-S
Bone marrow	6×10^4	16.5 ± 2.3	13.1 ± 2.8	0.79
Bone marrow	6×10^4	8.3 ± 1.7	6.0 ± 1.9	0.72
Mobilized peripheral cells[*]	0.05 ml	23.7 ± 3.3	16.9 ± 2.3	0.71
Mobilized peripheral cells[**]	0.05 ml	14.6 ± 1.9	12.0 ± 2.7	0.82

[*] Mean ± SD of 12 recipients
[**] Obtained 15 min after 1.5 mg trypsin

Table 3. Self-renewal capacity of rapidly and late mobilized stem cells

Source of stem cells	CFU-S/ml blood	SRC[*]	Reference[**]
Bone marrow		27.8 [spl]	[10]
		36.2 [spl]	[10]
		28.6 [spl]	[10]
		33.3 [spl]	[15]
		23.2 [bm]	[17]
Normal blood	22 ± 2	0.7 [spl]	[10]
	32 ± 4	0.9 [spl]	[10]
		2.9 [bm]	[17]
Blood after rapid mobilization			
trypsin	314 ± 25	11.6 [spl]	[10]
endotoxin	282 ± 26	4.6 [spl]	[10]
zymosan	309 ± 42	9.9 [spl]	[10]
Blood after CY mobilization	900 ± 95	5.2 [spl]	
		2.3 [bm]	[17]
Blood after G-CSF mobilization		8.0 [bm]	[17]
Blood after CY+ G-CSF mobilization	2000	N.T.	
		5.3 [bm]	[17]

[*] [bm]= bone marrow, [spl]= spleen.
[**]Reference number. No reference: present data.
SRC: self-renewal capacity.

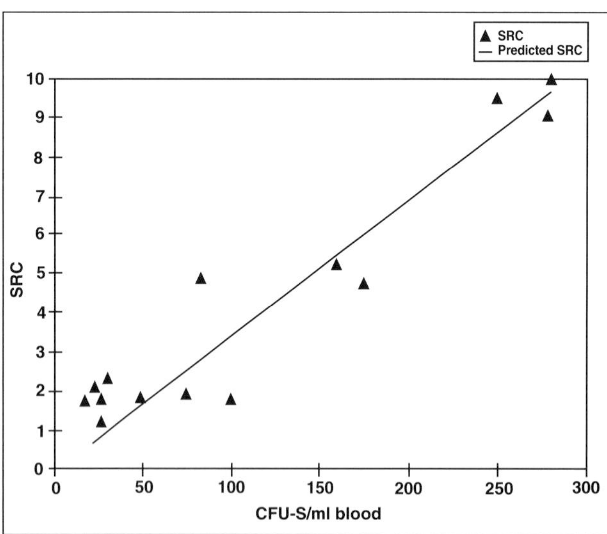

Figure 2. Correlation between SRC and level of circulating CFU-S level (CFU-S: 20 to 300/ml blood) SRC was calculated as described in Materials and Methods. Curve was fitted to a linear regression (r= 0.8835) Based on experiments originally published in [20].

Next we studied the amount of rapidly mobilizable CFU-S after damage to hemopoiesis. Twenty-four h after the injection of 500 mg/kg hydroxyurea (HU) or four days after 3.5 Co Gy γ irradiation, no mobilization could be observed. On the other hand, during regeneration of hemopoiesis (10 days after 3.5 Gy irradiation) a low blood CFU-S level was observed and CFU-S could not be mobilized by trypsin. Trypsin did not induce further mobilization when the blood CFU-S level was high (five days after endotoxin injection). After severe blood loss, however, when the circulating CFU-S level was not high, rapid mobilization was even higher than in the control groups. After a serious cycling wave induced by prostaglandin E_1, rapid mobilization of CFU-S could be induced. No correlation between femoral CFU-S level and mobilizable CFU-S or S phase CFU-S and mobilizable cells was found (Table 7).

Table 4. Repopulation of lethally irradiated BDF1 mice after transplantation of mobilized peripheral blood stem cells

Source of cells	Time of cell harvest	Injected d-9 CFU-S[*]	60-day survival N/N_0[**]
Normal bone marrow		188 ± 27	12/12
		155 ± 63	12/12
Blood after endotoxin	30 min	83.3 ± 5.7	12/12
	30 min	70.0 ± 11.5	12/12
Blood after CY	6 days	35.0 ± 6.5	10/12
Blood after CY+ G-CSF	6 days	20.0 ± 2.5	10/12
	6 days	100.0 ± 10.0	11/12

[*] Mean ± SD of 12 mice.
[**] 9.0 Gy irradiated recipients.

Table 5. Bone marrow CFU-S level and SRC one year after transplantation of rapidly mobilized blood stem cells

Source of graft	Injected d-9 CFU-S	CFU-S/10^6 bone marrow cells[*]	SRC[**]
Bone marrow	220 ± 36	253 ± 21.2	11.9
	155 ± 64	192 ± 44.9	17.3
	188 ± 27	183 ± 47	NT
Blood	83.3 ± 5.7	167 ± 35	17.2
	210 ± 34.5	140 ± 14.9	24.5
Control bone marrow		235 ± 25.4	28.6
		214.7 ± 47.5	19.2

[*] Mean ± SD of 12 recipients.
[**] SRC: Self-renewal capacity.

Table 6. Replacement of a mobilizable CFU-S pool after rapid release of stem cells into the circulation

Time after mobilization*	CFU-S/ml blood[**]	CFU-S/ml blood after the second mobilization[**]	Calculated mobilization[***]
15 min	626 ± 186		581
24 h	67 ± 17	83 ± 47	16
48 h	133 ± 59	633 ± 266	500
None	45 ± 15		

[*]1.5 mg trypsin/mouse i.v.
[**]Mean ± SD of three experiments four donor and 12 recipient mice per group.
[***]Difference between second and third column.

DISCUSSION

Although the presence of repopulating stem cells in blood has been accepted for a long time, they were proven to have limited transplantation potential [9] and were therefore not recommended for transplantation purposes. Animal experiments and clinical data, however, proved that structure of circulating stem cells can be manipulated: following the administration of CY and/or G-CSF, stem cell factor (SCF), IL-3, etc., the number of circulating stem cells increase and their self-reproducing quality (i.e., ratio of primitive to late stem cells) approaches that of bone marrow stem cells [15-17].

Long-term mobilization of stem cells may be the result of the production of new stem cells [18]. Rapid mobilization of stem cells, however, is not preceded by increased proliferation. This suggests that upon the effect of some agents, only a preformed subset of bone marrow stem cells (characterized by

Table 7. Rapidly mobilizable CFU-S after perturbation of stem cell pool

Perturbation	CFU-S per femur[*]	% of cells in S phase[**]	CFU-S/ml blood	Mobilizable CFU-S[***]
none (control)	5497 ± 725	6	30 ± 7	329 ± 61
bleeding (48 h)	4735 ± 321	25	41 ± 10	385 ± 78
endotoxin (5 days)	5274 ± 251	39	453 ± 52	41 ± 11
HU (24 h)[a]	760 ± 150	NT	5 ± 3	4 ± 1
3.5 Gy ^{60}Co γ (4 days)	360 ± 220	NT	1 ± 0.8	0
3.5 Gy ^{60}Co γ (10 days)	2358 ± 209	NT	6.0 ± 0.3	11 ± 2
prostaglandin E$_1$ (24 h)[b]	5700 ± 423	38.1	NT	332 ± 16
prostaglandin E$_1$ (48 h)[b]	5473 ± 368	10	24 ± 2	394 ± 57

NT = Not tested.
[*] Mean ± SD of three donors and 12 recipients.
[**] % of CFU-S loss after 30 min incubation with ^{3}HTdR.
[***] 15 min after trypsin injection.
[a] HU = 500 mg/kg i.v.
[b] PGE$_1$ = 10^{-1} µg/g body weight s.c.

their mobility) is released into the blood. Recently the complete clonal repertoire of CFU-S originating from bone marrow or peripheral blood was found to be identical [19], therefore the mobilizable stem cells belong to the standard constituents of the bone marrow stem cell population. As a working hypothesis we assumed that these rapidly mobilizable stem cells represent a more mature, transient subpopulation of the heterogeneous bone marrow stem cell population [10]. In the present paper properties of these easily mobilizable stem cells are summarized in comparison to the features of murine stem cells mobilized days after CY or G-CSF administration (that may serve as a model for human peripheral blood stem cell transplantation).

Assessed by their self-renewal or cobblestone-forming cell profile, early and late mobilized murine stem cells are as heterogeneous as the bone marrow stem cell population [10, 15, 17].

SRC or ratio of day 8 to day 12 CFU-S of stem cells mobilized by trypsin, endotoxin, zymosan (Tables 2, 3) or IL-8 [14] did not differ from those mobilized by CY or G-CSF [15, 17], suggesting that mobilized stem cells share similar properties irrespective of the mode of mobilization. This idea was supported by the close correlation between the SRC level of circulating CFU-S up to a certain blood CFU-S level [20] (Fig. 2). At more than 300 CFU-S/ml blood, a plateau level of SRC is reached, but the SRC of mobilized stem cells did not reach that of bone marrow.

The repopulating ability of rapidly mobilized stem cells did not differ from those mobilized by CY and CSFs (Table 4) [15, 17]. One year after transplantation mice reconstituted with rapidly mobilized stem cells showed a similar concentration of bone marrow CFU-S. The SRC of bone marrow stem cells was similar from bone marrow of rapidly mobilized stem cell chimeras.

Since within 48 h a second trypsin injection could not induce mobilization, upon the effect of trypsin the total amount of a preformed mobilizable pool seemed to be released into the circulation. These data contradict those reported by the Ulm group who found a continuous migration of CFU-GM during leukapheresis in dogs [21, 22]. If one assumes that leukapheresis does not mobilize the total mobilizable progenitor pool within an hour, a slow replenishment may be responsible for this phenomenon. This has already been proved after the administration of rHu IL-7 alone or in combination with rHu G-CSF in mice. The increases in the blood CFU-S and blood progenitor level were followed by a significant increase in the cycling rate of circulating and bone marrow stem cells, and the percentage of progenitors in bone marrow was maintained in spite of mobilization of pluripotent stem cells to the periphery [18]. Our finding that, after HU injection or sublethal irradiation, no CFU-S mobilization can be provoked fits well into this hypothesis [23]. On the other hand, increased cycling rate of CFU-S per se did not induce an increased mobilizable pool.

Relatively little is known about the physiology of mobilization. Although the mechanism by which stem cells are released from the bone marrow is not completely understood, data published during the last few years proved the expression of a wide range of adhesion molecules (e.g., very late-acting antigen-4 [VLA-4], VLA-5, leukocyte function-associated antigen-1 [LFA-1], LFA-3, L-selectin) on $CD34^+$ progenitors, suggesting their role in anchorage of stem cells in the bone marrow [24].

β_1 integrin was found to be expressed on day 12 CFU that was adhered to fibronectin [25], and 70% of day 28 cobblestone area-forming cells also adhere to fibronectin [26].

When the study of adhesion molecules expressed on $CD34^+$ progenitors mobilized by G-CSF after chemotherapy was compared to that on bone marrow $CD34^+$ cells, it gave inconsistent results. Some found decreased VLA-4 expression and increased LFA-1 expression [27], while others reported decreased LFA-1 expression and no change in VLA-4 expression [28]. A recent paper using $CD34^+$ enriched GM-CSF-mobilized progenitors strongly suggested that decreased expression of adhesion molecules (VLA-4, LFA-1, ICAM-1, LFA-3) on progenitor cells plays a role in their selective mobilization [29].

These data may support our earlier hypothesis that upon the effect of a mobilizing agent, a subset of the heterogeneous bone marrow stem cell population is released into the circulation.

ACKNOWLEDGMENT

This work was supported by the National Research Foundation of the Hungarian Academy of Sciences (OTKA 017737) and the Scientific Research Council of the Ministry of Welfare, Hungary 221/1996).

REFERENCES

1 Goodman JW, Hodgson GS. Evidence of stem cells in the peripheral blood of mice. Blood 1962;19:702-705.

2 Trobaugh FE, Lewis JP. Repopulating potential of blood and marrow. J Clin Invest 1964;43:1306-1309.

3 Storb R, Epstein RB, Thomas ED. Marrow repopulating ability of peripheral blood cells compared to thoracic duct cells. Blood 1968;32:662-667.

4 McCredie KB, Freireich EJ, Hersch EM et al. Early bone marrow recovery after chemotherapy following the transfusion of peripheral blood leukocytes in identical twins. Proc Am Assoc Cancer Res 1970;11:54-61.

5 Fliedner TM, Flad DH, Bruch C. Treatment of aplastic anaemia by blood stem cell transfusion. A canine model. Haematologica 1976;61:141-148.

6 Körbling M, Dörken B, Ho AD et al. Autologous transplantation of blood derived haemopoietic stem cells after myeloablative therapy in a patient with Burkitt lymphoma. Blood 1986;67:529-532.

7 Kessinger A, Armitage JO, Landmark JD et al. Reconstitution of human haemopoietic function with autologous cyropreserved circulating stem cells. Exp Hematol 1986;14:192-196.

8 Bender JG, Williams SF, Myers S et al. Characterization of chemotherapy mobilized peripheral blood progenitor cells for use in autologous stem cell transplantation. Bone Marrow Transplant 1992;10:281-285.

9 Micklem HS, Anderson N, Ross E. Limited potential of circulating haemopoietic stem cells. Nature 1975;256:41-43.

10 Fehér I, Gidáli J. Mobilizable stem cells: characteristics and replacement of the pool after exhaustion. Exp Hematol 1982;10:661-667.

11 Breems DA, van Hennik PB, Kusadasi N et al. Individual stem cell quality in leukapheresis products is related to the number of mobilized stem cells. Blood 1996;87:5370-5378.

12 Pettengell R, Luft T, Henschler R et al. Direct comparison by limiting dilution analysis of long term culture initiating cells in human bone marrow, umbilical cord blood and blood stem cells. Blood 1994;84:2653-2659.

13 Hodgson GS. Properties of haemopoietic stem cells in phenylhydrazine treated mice. Cell Tissue Kinet 1973;6:199-205.

14 Laterveer L, Lindley IJ, Hamilton MS et al. Interleukin-8 induces rapid mobilization of hematopoietic stem cells with radioprotective

capacity and long-term myelolymphoid repopulating ability. Blood 1995;85:2269-2275.

15 Molineux G, Pojda Z, Hampson IN et al. Transplantation potential of peripheral blood stem cells induced by granulocyte colony-stimulating factor. Blood 1990;76:2153-2158.

16 Drize N, Gan O, Zander A. Effect of recombinant human granulocyte colony stimulating factor treatment of mice on spleen colony forming unit number and self-renewal capacity. Exp Hematol 1993;21:1289-1293.

17 Neben S, Marcus K, Mauch P. Mobilization of hematopoietic stem and progenitor cell subpopulations from the marrow to the blood of mice following cyclophosphamide and/or granulocyte colony-stimulating factor. Blood 1993;81:1960-1967.

18 Grzegorzewski KJ, Komschlies KL, Franco JL et al. Quantitative and cell-cycle differences in progenitor cells mobilized by recombinant human interleukin-7 and recombinant human granulocyte colony-stimulating factor. Blood 1996;88:4139-4148.

19 Varas F, Bernad A, Bueren JA. Granulocyte colony-stimulating factor mobilizes into peripheral blood the complete clonal repertoire of hematopoietic precursors residing in the bone marrow of mice. Blood 1996;88:2495-2501.

20 Fehér I, Gidáli J. Self-renewal capacity of mobilized murine haemopoietic stem cells. Haematologica 1987;20;15-23.

21 Kovács P, Bruch C, Herbst EW et al. Collection of in vitro colony forming units from dogs by repeated continuous flow leukapheresis. Acta Haemat 1978;60:172-181.

22 Fliedner TM, Calvo W, Körbling M et al. Collection, storage and transfusion of blood stem cells for the treatment of hemopoietic failure. Blood Cells 1979;5:313-326.

23 Gidáli J, Fehér I. The amount of mobilizable stem cells in perturbed hemopoiesis. Int J Cell Cloning 1985;3:149-155.

24 Coulombel L, Auffray I, Gaugler MH et al. Expression and function of integrins on hematopoietic progenitor cells, Acta Haematol 1997;97:13-21.

25 Williams DA, Rios M, Stephens C et al. Fibronectin and VLA-4 in haematopoietic stem cell-microenvironment interactions. Nature 1991;352:438-441.

26 Van der Sluijs JP, Baert MR, Ploemacher RE. Differential adherence of murine hematopoietic stem cells subsets to fibronectin. Exp Hematol 1994;22:1236-1243.

27 Dercksen MW, Gerritsen WR, Rodenhuis et al. Expression of adhesion molecules on CD34[+] cells: CD34[+] L selectin[+] cells predict a rapid platelet recovery after peripheral blood stem cell transplantation. Blood 1995;85:3313-3319.

28 Mohle R, Murea S, Kirsch M et al. Differential expression of L-selectin, VLA-4 and LFA-1 on CD34[+] progenitor cells from bone marrow and peripheral blood during G-CSF-enhanced recovery. Exp Hematol 1995;23:1535-1542.

29 Watanabe T, Dave B, Heimann DG et al. GM-CSF-mobilized peripheral blood CD-34[+] cells differ from steady-state bone marrow CD-34[+] cells in adhesion molecule expression. Bone Marrow Transplant 1997;19:1175-1181.

CHAPTER VI

IN VITRO SELECTION AND EXPANSION OF BLOOD STEM CELLS

Changes in the Cytokine Regulation of Stem Cell Self-Renewal During Ontogeny

C. Eaves,[a,b,c] P. Zandstra,[d,e] E. Conneally,[a,c] C. Miller,[a,f]
J. Cashman,[a,b] A. Petzer,[a] J. Piret[d,e]

[a]Terry Fox Laboratory, British Columbia Cancer Agency and [b]Departments of Medical Genetics, [c]Pathology and Laboratory Medicine, [d]Chemical and Bio-Resource Engineering and [e]Biotechnology Laboratory, University of British Columbia, British Columbia, Canada; and [f]StemCell Technologies, Inc., Vancouver, British Columbia, Canada

Key Words. *Stem cells · Cytokines · Ontogeny · Cord blood · Long-term culture-initiating cell (LTC-IC)*

Abstract

The last 10 years have seen the development of a quantitative assay that is specific for transplantable totipotent murine hematopoietic cells with durable in vivo blood-forming ability. Recently, this assay has been successfully adapted to allow the detection and enumeration of an analogous population of human hematopoietic stem cells using myelosuppressed immunodeficient (nonobese diabetic/severe-combined immunodefiency) mice as recipients. Characterization of the cells detected by this assay indicates their close relationship in both mice and humans with cells detected in vitro as long-term culture-initiating cells (LTC-IC). Culture conditions have now been identified that support a significant net expansion of these cells from both species. More detailed analyses of the cytokine requirements for this response indicate that the viability, mitogenesis and maintenance of LTC-IC function by human $CD34^+CD38^-$ cells can be independently regulated by exogenous factors. Superimposed on this uncoupling of hematopoietic stem cell "self-renewal" and proliferation control is a change during ontogeny in the particular cytokines that regulate their responses. These findings unite stochastic and deterministic models of hematopoietic stem cell control through the concept of a molecular mechanism that actively blocks stem cell differentiation and must be maintained when these cells are stimulated to divide by exposure to certain types and concentrations of cytokines. *Stem Cells 1998;16(suppl 1):177-184*

Introduction

The field of hematopoietic stem cell biology stands at a new crossroad in biomedicine where cellular behavior and disease processes are beginning to be described in molecular terms. At such an exciting time in the rapid evolution of this field, it is particularly inspiring to join with those individuals who have helped shape its history over the last several decades and pay tribute to the ground-breaking concepts they helped to establish. *Ted Fliedner* is one of these individuals who, in spite of this celebration of his past, maintains that youthful and unrelenting joy in exploring the unknown, thus creating a permanent bond between the past and the future. As a friend and colleague for many years, it is a pleasure to summarize our recent data for this Workshop in his honor.

Characteristics and Potentials of Blood Stem Cells

THE POWER OF A QUANTITATIVE ASSAY WITH SPECIFICITY FOR HEMATOPOIETIC STEM CELLS

Nobody can agree on a precise definition of a hematopoietic stem cell and this is probably telling us something either about our lack of knowledge of the issue or that we are looking for a unifying molecular description where there may not be one. However, there are many practical opportunities for exploiting knowledge about primitive hematopoietic cells and these have spurred a particular interest in the biology of those cells that have been known for decades to be able as single entities to permanently reconstitute the entire hematopoietic system, either endogenously, or after transplantation into another individual. The realization in the early 1980s that the spleen-colony assay detects many cells that do not have long-term reconstituting ability [1, 2] highlighted the need for alternative ways of quantitating such cells with greater specificity, in particular to allow investigation of conditions that would support their proliferation and self-renewal in vitro.

Much of our efforts in the last 15 years has focused on the development and validation of assays that have proved useful for this purpose. The competitive repopulating unit (CRU) assay allows murine cells with long-term in vivo lympho-myeloid repopulating activity to be enumerated through the use of a limiting dilution analysis approach [3]. It is thus rigorously quantitative and allows CRU frequencies to be determined independent of their absolute lympho-myeloid cell outputs (above a threshold required for their detection which is ~1% of the normal circulating leukocyte population of 10^5 cells/mouse/day for $\geq$ 4 months [4]). This is not an issue for CRU of comparable outputs, but is when CRU outputs change as, for example, occurs during ontogeny and can thus be seen when CRU from fetal and adult murine sources are compared [5]. In addition, the CRU assay allows frequency measurements to be derived from limiting numbers of CRU. This becomes an important practical issue for many types of experiments, particularly those involving in vitro manipulations of highly purified cell populations.

A few years ago it was discovered that human hematopoietic cells with lympho-myeloid differentiation potential can reproducibly and at useful efficiency engraft the bone marrow of irradiated, intravenously transplanted, immunocompromised (nonobese diabetic/severe-combined immunodeficiency) mice for several months [6, 7]. We have taken advantage of this finding to adapt the principles of the murine CRU assay for the detection and quantitation of a similar type of human lympho-myeloid stem cell [8, 9]. The greater frequency of such cells in human cord blood than in adult marrow [10, 11] has focused initial attention on their characterization in cord blood samples. The second assay for primitive hematopoietic cells that has proven useful is the long-term culture-initiating cell (or LTC-IC) assay. This assay relies on an ability of primitive hematopoietic cells to generate differentiating progeny for many weeks in response to signals they receive when cocultured with certain types of fibroblasts [12-14]. Although it is not yet clear what the molecular nature of these signals may be, it has been shown that simply prolonging the interval allowed to elapse before the cultures are assessed allows an input cell that is separable from most in vitro colony-forming cells (CFC) and, in the mouse from most colony-forming units-spleen (CFU-S), to be discriminated (Table 1). When conditions for detecting LTC-IC are optimized, CFC outputs can be shown to be linearly related to LTC-IC

Table 1. Evidence that murine LTC-IC are stem cells (CRU)

Property	LTC-IC	CRU	Day-12 CFU-S	CFC
Number per femur	640	1,100	3,200	68,000
Enrichment in Sca-1$^+$Lin$^-$ wheat germ agglutinin$^+$ fraction	690×	500×	—	24×
Rh uptake	dull	dull	mixed	bright
Decrease after 5-fluorouracil in vivo	3×	4×	80×	120×
Proliferation in LTC	+	+	+	+

Data drawn from [12, 14, 20, 31].

> **Table 2.** Evidence that human CRU and LTC-IC are overlapping populations (and are different from CFC)
>
> 1. Similar prevalence of CRU and LTC-IC in the CD38$^-$ subpopulation of CD34$^+$ cord blood cells, whereas most CFC are in the CD38$^+$ subpopulation.
>
> 2. CRU and LTC-IC numbers are similarly amplified in cultures of CD34$^+$CD38$^-$ cord blood cells but to a lesser extent than CFC, and by different cytokines.
>
> 3. Retroviral-mediated gene transfer efficiencies to CRU and LTC-IC correlate, but between CRU and CFC, no correlation is seen.
>
> Based on results published in [8, 30, 32].

inputs over a wide range, thus allowing LTC-IC frequencies to be determined from bulk assays (rather than by limiting dilution analysis) if the average immediate (five to six weeks) CFC output per LTC-IC is already known. Assessment of this value for different sources of LTC-IC and different LTC-IC assay conditions has shown that significant variations are encountered for LTC-IC present at different stages of ontogeny. Moreover, these may be further influenced by the presence of additional cytokines in the LTC-IC assay itself [15]. However, marked changes have not yet been seen to accompany the maintenance or even amplification in vitro of a given source of LTC-IC [16-18].

Comparisons of CRU and LTC-IC of murine and human origin have indicated that even as originally defined, the cells detected by these two assays are likely to represent closely related, if not overlapping, populations in normal hematopoietic tissues (Tables 1 and 2). More recent studies have suggested that the original five-week human LTC-IC assay may not necessarily detect cells with CRU function, although it may be possible to recapture this correlation using a more prolonged culture period and/or the provision of cytokines that selectively enhance primitive LTC-IC plating efficiency and their average CFC output in the assay [14, 15, 17, 19].

AMPLIFICATION OF LTC-IC AND CRU IN VITRO

The identification of conditions that allow hematopoietic stem cell populations to be amplified in vitro has been a longstanding goal of many investigators. Our initial studies focused on attempts to expand LTC-IC populations. They involved a variety of strategies to manipulate conditions operative in the LTC system, based on the knowledge that most LTC-IC and some CRU could be shown to divide over the course of four to six weeks when maintained under "LTC" conditions [13, 17, 20]. A number of modifications of the LTC system were made which resulted in an increased production of various cytokines and accompanying increases in LTC-IC-derived CFC output, LTC-IC detection and LTC-IC maintenance [15, 16]. However, none of these changes were sufficient to cause a significant net increase over time in the size of the input LTC-IC population until the cells were placed in spinner cultures. This prevented the close-range interactions that occur between hematopoietic cells and adherent cells (fibroblasts and macrophages) in standard, static LTC and allowed significant amplifications of the LTC-IC population to be reproducibly obtained for the first time in our center [21].

This finding was confirmed independently by *Verfaillie's* group [22] and coincided with initial reports of the discovery and isolation of Flt3-ligand (FL) [23-25]. Preliminary experiments provided evidence of the ability of this "new" cytokine to stimulate human LTC-IC proliferation [26] and these findings prompted us to undertake a further study of the possibility that human LTC-IC expansion might be achieved under completely defined cytokine conditions [17]. Because we did not anticipate how successful this approach would eventually prove to be, these first experiments were designed to evaluate the extent of LTC-IC expansion that might occur within individual clones stimulated to develop from CD34$^+$CD38 cells isolated from normal adult human bone marrow. The results were overwhelming. Not only was the original objective achieved, the cocktail used, FL + steel factor (SF) + interleukin 3 (IL-3)

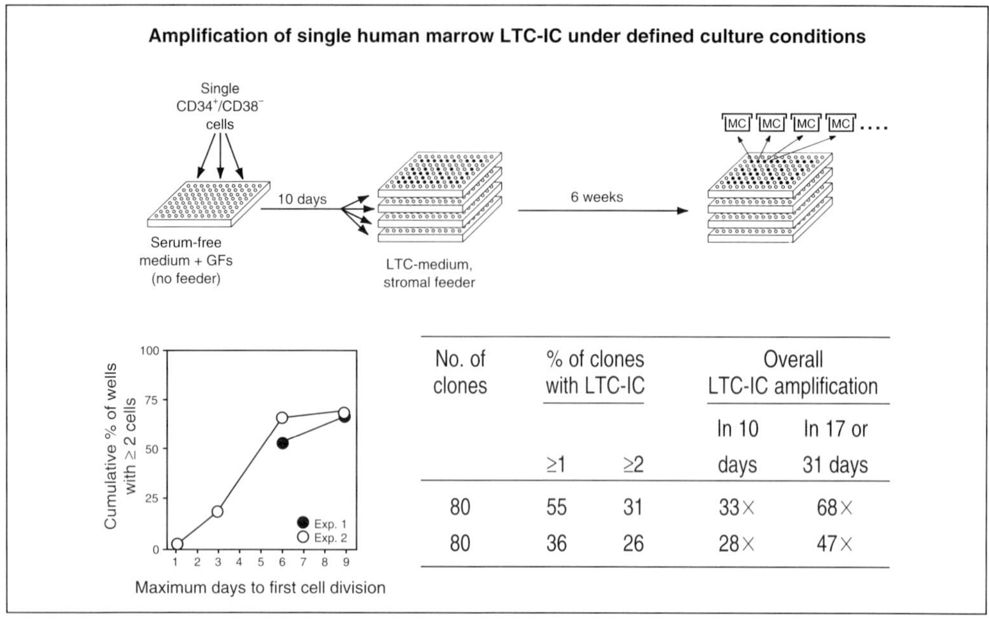

No. of clones	% of clones with LTC-IC		Overall LTC-IC amplification	
			In 10 days	In 17 or 31 days
	≥1	≥2		
80	55	31	33×	68×
80	36	26	28×	47×

Figure 1. Diagram illustrating the experimental design used to follow the recruitment into cycle of individual CD34+CD38− cells isolated from normal adult human bone marrow and cultured for 10 days in a defined medium containing 100 ng/ml FL and SF, 20 ng/ml of IL-3, IL-6, G-CSF and 5 ng/ml β-NGF. (Data for two independent experiments are plotted in the graph shown in the bottom left corner.) The LTC-IC content of all of the clones generated was measured on each at the end of the initial 10 days of culture. (Data for the same two experiments, in each of which 80 clones were analyzed, are tabulated in the bottom right corner of this figure.) Results are from [17].

+ IL-6 + G-CSF + β nerve growth factor (β-NGF), was found to stimulate the division within 10 days of every CD34+CD38− cell that remained viable, and approximately half of the clones thus produced had detectable LTC-IC among the progeny generated (Fig. 1). Moreover, when the total extent of LTC-IC amplification in these experiments was calculated, greater LTC-IC expansions than had ever previously been documented were noted.

This launched a new phase of hematopoietic stem cell expansion experiments in which the emphasis was redirected towards the use of highly purified starting populations and the identification of which cytokines were needed to support net increases in LTC-IC (and CRU). Multifactorial analysis of the roles of the cytokines used in the first experiments, in addition to an extensive survey of other types and concentrations of cytokines, revealed high concentrations of FL, SF and IL-3 to be necessary and sufficient to maximize the amplification of LTC-IC (>50-fold over input values within the first 10 days in culture) from starting populations of CD34+CD38− human bone marrow cells [18]. The addition of a fourth cytokine (either G-CSF, IL-6 or β-NGF) is, however, required to maximally enhance the accompanying expansion of cells detectable as CFC [27].

Extension of these studies to human cord blood CD34+CD38− cells provided the first definitive evidence that transplantable human stem cell populations can also be expanded in vitro with full retention of the functional properties of the original input stem cells. However, numerically, the expansions obtained for both the CRU and LTC-IC populations in these cord blood experiments were much more modest (net increases of two- and fourfold, respectively) [8]. Nevertheless, the developmental potential of the amplified CRU did not appear adversely affected by the amplification process. At about the same time, we were able to identify a slightly different cytokine cocktail that could support a similarly modest, but significant, expansion of transplantable murine stem cells of adult marrow origin [4].

Again, careful examination of the developmental potential of these expanded murine CRU demonstrated no decline in their subsequent regenerative potential and the extent to which both CRU and LTC-IC populations were expanded was similar.

EVIDENCE OF ONTOLOGICAL AS WELL AS CYTOKINE-MEDIATED REGULATION OF STEM CELL SELF-RENEWAL

Comparison of the cytokine dose response relationship for CFC and LTC-IC amplification in suspension cultures of $CD34^+CD38^-$ human bone marrow cells provided the first clue that the regulation of LTC-IC amplification by cytokines might involve specific pathways distinct from those responsible for blocking apoptosis and stimulating S-phase entry. The key finding in this regard came from the observation that to maximize LTC-IC expansion, it is necessary not only to stimulate the cells with particular cytokines, but also to ensure that these are present at very high concentrations, in fact >10-fold higher than the concentrations of the same cytokines that are sufficient to maximize expansion of CFC numbers in the same cultures [18]. We then performed experiments with single $CD34^+CD38^-$ cells to determine whether the reduced LTC-IC production obtained when suboptimal concentrations of cytokines are used is simply due to a failure of these conditions to stimulate a subset of $CD34^+CD38^-$ cells with high LTC-IC-generating potential. The results obtained did not support such a model. There was no difference in the number of cells initially stimulated to divide (clone frequency) nor in the total number of progeny they were stimulated to generate (clone size distribution) under the two cytokine conditions, in spite of the expected difference in the number of progeny with LTC-IC activity (Table 3).

A second series of experiments was then undertaken to investigate whether the ability to retain (or lose) LTC-IC function might be influenced by the relative concentration of cytokines present in the mixture (i.e., FL + SF + IL-3) that had been found to be effective [18]. The important results from these studies are summarized in Table 4. In this case additional single-cell experiments suggested that the presence of a high concentration of IL-3 and a reduced concentration of FL and SF (which had a strongly negative effect on the number of LTC-IC recoverable from 10-day cultures of $CD34^+CD38^-$ human bone marrow cells) was associated with some reduction in the viability and proliferative response of the input cells, even though there was no significant effect on the total output of CFC.

Taken together, these results provide strong evidence in favor of a deterministic effect of different cytokine treatments on the ability of mitogenically activated $CD34^+CD38^-$ human hematopoietic cells to maintain their state as LTC-IC. We therefore suggest that these cells depend on certain types of cytokine-induced signaling events to block the initiation of mechanisms that would begin to irreversibly restrict their ability to differentiate along more than a single lineage.

The finding that LTC-IC numbers are not as effectively amplified in cultures of $CD34^+CD38^-$ human cord blood cells as is seen when $CD34^+CD38^-$ adult human bone marrow cells are cultured under the

Table 3. Clone formation and progenitor expansion from single cell cultures of $CD34^+CD38^-$ adult human bone marrow cells

Cytokine concentration (ng/ml)		% of cells forming clones	Progenitor expansion	
FL/SF	IL-3/IL-6/G-CSF		LTC-IC	CFC
300	60	52 ± 7	57 ± 18	570 ± 50
30	6	61 ± 9	1.2 ± 0.5	430 ± 90

$CD34^+CD38^-$ cells were isolated and cultured as single cells in serum-free medium in the two cytokine cocktails shown. At the end of 10 days, the number of clones (± 2 cells/well) was assessed and then all cells from all clones generated under the same condition were pooled and assayed for LTC-IC and CFC to allow a comparison to the frequency of these two types of progenitors measured in the original input populations. Results are from [18].

Table 4. Positive and negative effects on LTC-IC amplification of changes in the concentration of individual components of an active cytokine cocktail in 10-day cultures initiated with CD34$^+$CD38$^-$ adult human bone marrow cells

Cytokine concentration (ng/ml)			Progenitor expansion	
FL	**SF**	**IL-3**	**LTC-IC**	**CFC**
300	300	60	45×	76×
300	300	2	22×	76×
300	10	60	33×	31×
300	10	2	18×	41×
10	300	60	4×	62×
10	300	2	4×	28×
10	10	2	4×	39×
10	10	60	0.3×	68×

CD34$^+$CD38$^-$ cells were isolated and cultured for 10 days under the eight different cytokine conditions shown and the suspensions then each assayed separately for their LTC-IC and CFC contents. Expansion values were calculated by comparison of these 10-day yields with the frequency of LTC-IC and CFC measured independently on the original input suspension. Data are from [18].

same conditions raised another question about the cytokine-mediated regulation of primitive hematopoietic cell properties. Indeed, at first glance this observation would seem to contravene the concept of a greater self-renewal potential (and hence an ultimately greater potential for primitive cell output) by ontologically "earlier" cells, suggested by previous comparisons of fetal liver, cord blood and adult marrow progenitors [5, 28, 29]. However, this decreased LTC-IC output by cord blood CD34$^+$CD38$^-$ cells could be shown to be accompanied by an increased output of both CFC and total cells for several weeks [30], consistent with previous reports. To explore the possibility that cord blood LTC-IC expansion may be optimized by exposure of the cells to different cytokines than are required by their adult counterparts, we carried out another large series of multifactorial design experiments. A different mixture of cytokines proved to be important not only for LTC-IC expansion from CD34$^+$CD38$^-$ cord blood cells but also for the concomitant generation of granulopoietic or erythroid and pluripotent CFC from CD34$^+$CD38$^-$ cord blood cells [30]. In light of the model described above, these findings would suggest that the signaling events responsible for blocking stem cell differentiation (promoting self-renewal divisions) may require the activation of different receptors on cells at different stages of ontogeny due to ontological changes in the number, distribution or types of intracytoplasmic mediators with which they may be associated. Alternatively, other downstream targets may change (or both possibilities may apply). Regardless of where the molecular mechanisms regulating hematopoietic stem cell behavior converge, these studies provide new evidence of heterogeneity in the molecular responses that can be elicited by different cytokine treatments which may or may not differentially regulate the ability of these cells to remain alive, proliferate and differentiate.

Acknowledgment

The authors thank Amgen, Cangene, Genetics Institute, Immunex, and Novartis and staff of the Terry Fox Laboratory for contributing many critical reagents and expertise, without which the work reviewed in this paper would not have been possible. The expert assistance of *Bernadine Fox* in preparing the manuscript is also acknowledged.

This work was supported by grants from the National Cancer Institute of Canada (NCIC) with funds from the Terry Fox Run, the E. Schrödinger Foundation (to *A. Petzer*), the USA National Institutes of Health (HL - 55435), the British Columbia Science Council and Novartis. *P. Zandstra* held Studentships from the Natural Sciences and Engineering Research Council of Canada and the British Columbia

Science Council; *E. Conneally,* a Terry Fox Physician-Scientist Fellowship; *C. Miller,* an Alberta Heritage Postdoctoral Fellowship and *C. Eaves,* a Terry Fox Cancer Research Scientist Award of the NCIC.

REFERENCES

1 Magli MC, Iscove NN, Odartchenko N. Transient nature of early haematopoietic spleen colonies. Nature 1982;295:527-529.

2 Jones RJ, Wagner JE, Celano P et al. Separation of pluripotent haematopoietic stem cells from spleen colony-forming cells. Nature 1990;347:188-189.

3 Szilvassy SJ, Humphries RK, Lansdorp PM et al. Quantitative assay for totipotent reconstituting hematopoietic stem cells by a competitive repopulation strategy. Proc Natl Acad Sci USA 1990;87:8736-8740.

4 Miller CL, Eaves CJ. Expansion in vitro of adult murine hematopoietic stem cells with transplantable lympho-myeloid reconstituting ability. Proc Natl Acad Sci USA 1997;94:13648-13653.

5 Rebel VI, Miller CL, Eaves CJ et al. The repopulation potential of fetal liver hematopoietic stem cells in mice exceeds that of their adult bone marrow counterparts. Blood 1996;87:3500-3507.

6 Pflumio F, Izac B, Katz A et al. Phenotype and function of human hematopoietic cells engrafting immune-deficient CB17-severe combined immunodeficiency mice and nonobese diabetic-severe combined immunodeficiency mice after transplantation of human cord blood mononuclear cells. Blood 1996;88:3731-3740.

7 Cashman JD, Lapidot T, Wang JCY et al. Kinetic evidence of the regeneration of multilineage hematopoiesis from primitive cells in normal human bone marrow transplanted into immunodeficient mice. Blood 1997;89:4307-4316.

8 Conneally E, Cashman J, Petzer A et al. Expansion in vitro of transplantable human cord blood stem cells demonstrated using a quantitative assay of their lympho-myeloid repopulating activity in nonobese diabetic-scid/scid mice. Proc Natl Acad Sci USA 1997;94:9836-9841.

9 Cashman J, Bockhold K, Hogge DE et al. Sustained proliferation, multi-lineage differentiation and maintenance of primitive human haematopoietic cells in NOD/SCID mice transplanted with human cord blood. Br J Haematol 1997;98:1026-1036.

10 Wang JCY, Doedens M, Dick JE. Primitive human hematopoietic cells are enriched in cord blood compared with adult bone marrow or mobilized peripheral blood as measured by the quantitative in vivo SCID-repopulating cell assay. Blood 1997;89:3919-3924.

11 Holyoake TL, Nicolini F, Cashman J et al. Development and validation of an improved in vivo assay for quantitating human hematopoietic stem cells. Blood 1997;90:(suppl 1):159a.

12 Ploemacher RE, Van Der Sluijs JP, Voerman JSA et al. An in vitro limiting-dilution assay of long-term repopulating hematopoietic stem cells in the mouse. Blood 1989;74:2755-2763.

13 Sutherland HJ, Lansdorp PM, Henkelman DH et al. Functional characterization of individual human hematopoietic stem cells cultured at limiting dilution on supportive marrow stromal layers. Proc Natl Acad Sci USA 1990;87:3584-3588.

14 Lemieux ME, Rebel VI, Lansdorp PM et al. Characterization and purification of a primitive hematopoietic cell type in adult mouse marrow capable of lympho-myeloid differentiation in long-term marrow "switch" cultures. Blood 1995;86:1339-1347.

15 Hogge DE, Lansdorp PM, Reid D et al. Enhanced detection, maintenance and differentiation of primitive human hematopoietic cells in cultures containing murine fibroblasts engineered to produce human Steel factor, interleukin-3 and granulocyte colony-stimulating factor. Blood 1996;88:3765-3773.

16 Sutherland HJ, Eaves CJ, Lansdorp PM et al. Differential regulation of primitive human hematopoietic cells in long-term cultures maintained on genetically engineered murine stromal cells. Blood 1991;78:666-672.

17 Petzer AL, Hogge DE, Lansdorp PM et al. Self-renewal of primitive human hematopoietic cells (long-term-culture-initiating cells) in vitro and their expansion in defined medium. Proc Natl Acad Sci USA 1996;93:1470-1474.

18 Zandstra PW, Conneally E, Petzer AL et al. Cytokine manipulation of primitive human hematopoietic cell self-renewal. Proc Natl Acad Sci USA 1997;94:4698-4703.

19 Hao QL, Thiemann FT, Petersen D et al. Extended long-term culture reveals a highly quiescent and primitive human hematopoietic progentior population. Blood 1996;88:3306-3313.

20 Fraser CC, Szilvassy SJ, Eaves CJ et al. Proliferation of totipotent hematopoietic stem cells in vitro with retention of long-term competitive in vivo reconstituting ability. Proc Natl Acad Sci USA 1992;89:1968-1972.

21 Zandstra PW, Eaves CJ, Piret JM. Expansion of hematopoietic progenitor cell populations in stirred

suspension bioreactors of normal human bone marrow cells. Biotechnology 1994;12:909-914.

22 Verfaillie CM. Direct contact between human primitive hematopoietic progenitors and bone marrow stroma is not required for long-term in vitro hematopoiesis. Blood 1992;79:2821-2826.

23 Lyman SD, James L, Vanden Bos T et al. Molecular cloning of a ligand for the flt3/flk-2 tyrosine kinase receptor: a proliferative factor for primitive hematopoietic cells. Cell 1993;75:1157-1167.

24 Hannum C, Culpepper J, Campbell D et al. Ligand for FLT3/FLK2 receptor tyrosine kinase regulates growth of haematopoietic stem cells and is encoded by variant RNAs. Nature 1994;368:643-648.

25 Mackarehtschian K, Hardin JD, Moore KA et al. Targeted disruption of the flk2/flt3 gene leads to deficiencies in primitive hematopoietic progenitors. Immunity 1995;3:147-161.

26 Ponchio L, Eaves C. Steel factor and Flk-2/Flt-3 ligand alone trigger quiescent human LTC-IC into S-phase more effectively than primitive quiescent clonogenic progenitor cells. J Hematother 1995;4:(suppl 3):217.

27 Petzer AL, Zandstra PW, Piret JM et al. Differential cytokine effects on primitive (CD34$^+$CD38$^-$) human hematopoietic cells: novel responses to flt3-ligand and thrombopoietin. J Exp Med 1996;183:2551-2558.

28 Lansdorp PM, Dragowska W, Mayani H. Ontogeny-related changes in proliferative potential of human hematopoietic cells. J Exp Med 1993;178:787-791.

29 Pawliuk R, Eaves C, Humphries RK. Evidence of both ontogeny and transplant dose-regulated expansion of hematopoietic stem cells in vivo. Blood 1996;88:2852-2858.

30 Zandstra PW, Conneally E, Piret JM et al. Changes during ontogeny in the cytokine responsiveness of human erythroid, myeloid and LTC-IC progenitors. Exp Hematol 1997;25:877.

31 Dexter TM, Spooncer E, Toksoz D et al. The role of cells and their products in the regulation of in vitro stem cell proliferation and granulocyte development. J Supramol Struc 1980;13:513-524.

32 Conneally E, Eaves CJ, Humphries RK. Efficient retroviral-mediated gene transfer to human cord blood stem cells with in vivo repopulating potential. Blood 1998 (in press).

In Vivo Expansion of Hemopoietic Stem Cells

GERARD WAGEMAKER, SIMONE C.C. HARTONG, KAREN J. NEELIS,
TORSTEIN EGELAND,[a] ALBERTUS W. WOGNUM

Institute of Hematology, Erasmus Universiteit Rotterdam, The Netherlands
and [a]Institute of Transplantation Immunology, Oslo, Norway

Key Words. *Stem cells · In vivo expansion of stem cells · Mobilization of stem cells · Thrombopoietin · CD34$^+$ cells
· Circulating CD34$^+$ cells · Rhesus monkeys · Hemopoietic growth factors*

ABSTRACT

Under conditions of steady-state hemo-poiesis, a small fraction of immature hemopoi-etic cells, including stem cells, circulates in peripheral blood (PB). In rhesus monkeys, a median number of 1.2×10^7/l CD34$^+$ cells was observed as opposed to a median number of 1.5×10^9/l in aspirated bone marrow (BM). The concentration of circulating CD34$^+$ cells is therefore approximately two logs less than that in BM. Since a 4-kg rhesus monkey has an estimated number of 3×10^{10} BM cells and approximately 300 ml of blood, the fraction of CD34$^+$ cells that circulates can be estimated at approximately 0.4% of the total pool of CD34$^+$ cells. During hemopoietic reconstitution following a cytotoxic insult such as results from a midlethal dose of TBI, PB CD34$^+$ cell numbers appeared to be correlated to those of BM, suggesting that PB CD34$^+$ cells may reflect reconstitution of BM CD34$^+$ cells. Reconstitution of BM immature cells can be accelerated by treatment with pharmacologi-cal doses of growth factors, resulting in large-ly expanded immature cell populations within a few weeks after TBI. Growth factors observed to exert such an effect included, notably, thrombopoietin. Such an acceleration can be monitored by daily assessment of cir-culating CD34$^+$ cells. Expansion of immature circulating cells indicates expansion of similar cells in the bone marrow rather than growth factor-induced selective mobilization of immature cells. *Stem Cells 1998;16(suppl 1):185-191*

INTRODUCTION

It is long known that a small fraction of hemopoietic stem cells circulates [1, 2], probably as part of homeostatic mechanisms required to control blood cell production from the scattered bone marrow (BM) sites. The fraction of circulating immature hemopoietic cells characterized by the CD34 sur-face antigen may be expanded by administration of pharmacological doses of growth factors such as G-CSF [3] and GM-CSF [4], Kit-ligand [5], Flt-3 ligand [6] and interleukin 8 (IL-8) [7], indicating that either their BM numbers or their mobilization into the peripheral blood (PB), or both, are under growth factor control. More recently, advantage has been taken from circulating stem cells in that these cells provide an alternative to BM to harvest large numbers of stem cells for either autologous or allogeneic transplantation [8, 9].

We have earlier advocated that these cells may also be used as an early marker for residual stem cell numbers and a monitor for immature cell reconstitution after TBI and/or hemopoietic cell transplantation [10], or during hemopoietic growth factor therapy. However, the relation of

Characteristics and Potentials of Blood Stem Cells
STEM CELLS 1998;16(suppl 1):185-191

PB to BM immature hemopoietic cells appeared to be complex [10], in part because of fluctuations and genetic influences [11] which determine circulating cell numbers. We approached these issues from experience in a preclinical model for radiation-induced myelosuppression in rhesus monkeys, with special reference to normal levels and expansion of immature BM and PB CD34$^+$ cells by thrombopoietin (TPO) [12-15] therapy. As described previously, TPO treatment accelerates the reconstitution of immature BM CD34$^+$ cells [16, 17], an effect that is augmented by coadministration of GM-CSF [18]. This feature is in accordance with the presence of the TPO receptor, c-Mpl, on immature BM cells and with stimulatory effects of TPO on immature hemopoietic cells in vitro [18-20].

MATERIALS AND METHODS

Animals

Purpose-bred male rhesus monkeys (*Macaca Mulatta*) weighing 2.5-4.0 kilograms and aged two to three years were used. The monkeys were housed in groups of four to six monkeys in stainless steel cages in rooms equipped with reverse-filtered air barrier, normal day light rhythm and conditioned to 20°C with a relative humidity of 70%. Animals were fed ad libitum with commercial primate chow and fresh fruits, and received acidified drinking water. All animals were free of intestinal parasites and seronegative for herpes B, simian T-lymphotropic viruses and simian immunodeficiency virus. Housing, experiments and all other conditions were approved by an ethical committee in conformity with legal regulations in the Netherlands.

TBI

Monkeys were irradiated with a single dose of 5 Gy TBI delivered by two opposing x-ray generators, operating at a tube voltage of 300 kV and a current of 10 mA. The half-layer thickness was 3mm^3. The focus skin distance was 0.8 m and the average dose rate 0.20-0.22 Gy/min. During TBI, the animals were placed in a cylindrical polycarbonate cage which rotated slowly (three times per min) around its vertical axis.

Supportive Care

Two weeks before TBI, the monkeys were placed in a laminar flow cabinet and the gastrointestinal tract was selectively decontaminated by giving orally Ciprofloxacin (Bayer; Mijdrecht, The Netherlands), Nystatin (Sanofi BV; Maassluis, The Netherlands) and Polymyxin B (Pfizer; New York, NY). This regimen was supplemented with systemic antibiotics, in most cases ticarcillin (Beecham Pharma; Amstelveen, The Netherlands) and cefuroxim (Glaxo; Zeist, The Netherlands), when leukocyte counts dropped below 10^9/l. Guided by fecal bacteriograms, the antibiotics were continued until leukocyte counts rose to levels >10^9/l. Dehydration and electrolyte disturbances were treated by appropriate fluid and electrolyte administration s.c. The monkeys received irradiated (15 Gy γ irradiation) platelet transfusions whenever thrombocyte counts reached values below 40 × 10^9/l, packed red cells whenever hematocrits were lower than 20% and occasionally, whole blood transfusions in case of coincidence of both transfusion criteria.

Test Drug

Recombinant full-length human TPO produced by Chinese hamster ovary cells was supplied by Genentech Inc. (South San Francisco, CA). The daily dose of 10 μg/kg was administered s.c. for 21 consecutive days after TBI. The dose was diluted to a volume of 1 ml with phosphate-buffered saline/0.01% Tween 20 prior to administration. The diluent was used as placebo. Each treatment group consisted of four consecutive monkeys.

BM Aspirates

BM was aspirated under neurolept anesthesia using Ketalar (Apharmo; Arnhem, The Netherlands) and Vetranquil (Sanofi; Maassluis, The Netherlands). Small BM aspirates for analytical purposes were taken from the shafts of the humeri using pediatric spinal needles and collected in bottles containing 2 ml Hank's buffered Hepes solution (HHBS) with 200 IU sodium heparin/ml (Leo Pharmaceutical Products; Weesp, The Netherlands). Low density cells were isolated using a Ficoll (density 1.077) (Nycomed Pharma AS; Oslo, Norway) separation.

Hematological Examinations

Complete blood cell counts were measured daily using a Sysmex F-800 hematology analyzer (Toa Medical Electronics Co., LTD.; Kobe, Japan).

Measurements of Surface Antigens

Once weekly, a fluorescence-activated cell sorter (FACS) scan analysis was done on PB and BM samples for a variety of surface antigens, including CD34, by use of a human CD34 monoclonal antibody (mAb 566) that had been fluoresceinated with fluorescein isothiocyanate (Sigma; St Louis, MO) according to standard procedures. For PB CD34$^+$ cells this analysis was done daily. 0.5 mL of whole blood or BM was lysed in 10 ml lysing solution (8.26 g ammonium chloride/1.0 g potassium bicarbonate and 0.037 g EDTA per l) for 10 min at 4°C. After lysing the cells were washed twice with HHBS containing 2% fetal calf serum and 0.05% (wt/vol) sodium azide (HFN). The cells were resuspended in 100 µl HFN containing 2% normal monkey serum to prevent a specific binding of the mAbs. mAbs were added in a volume of 5 µl and incubated for 30 min on ice. After two washes, the cells were measured on the flow cytometer. Ungated list mode data were collected for 10,000 events and analyzed using the Lysis II software (Becton-Dickinson; San Jose, CA).

Statistics

Standard deviations were calculated and are given in the text and in the figures on the assumption of a normal distribution. The significance of a difference was calculated by Fisher's exact test for categorical data, and for continuous data by a one-way analysis of variance followed by a nonpaired Student's *t*-test.

RESULTS

Normal Levels of BM Aspirate and PB CD34$^+$ Cells

Figure 1 shows the absolute numbers of CD34$^+$ cells in BM aspirates and PB of 50 consecutive

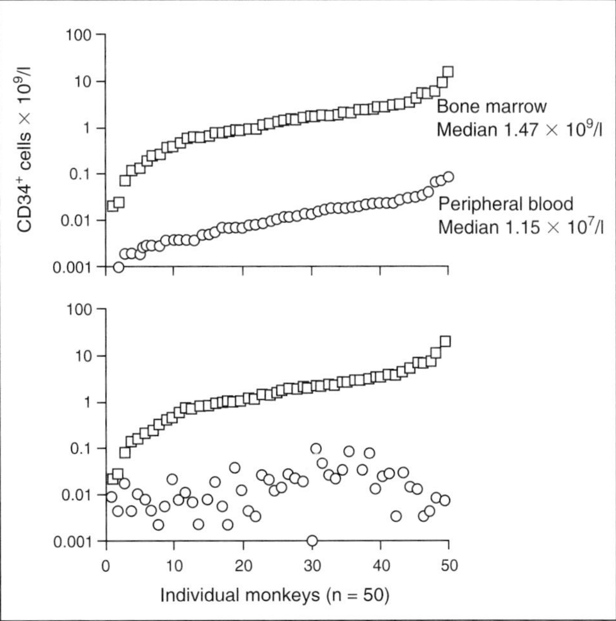

Figure 1. BM aspirate and PB CD34$^+$ cells in 50 consecutive normal rhesus monkeys, representing baseline data collected just before TBI. PB is presented by circles and BM by squares. Upper panel: BM and PB data of individual monkeys dissociated and ranked in ascending order. Lower panel: BM and PB data of individual monkeys associated, BM data ranked in ascending order.

Table 1. Distribution parameters of BM aspirate and PB CD34[+] cells of 50 normal rhesus monkeys

	BM CD34[+] cells	PB CD34[+] cells
Frequency (%)		
Mean ± SD	3.2 ± 3.5	0.2 ± 0.2
Median	2.2	0.1
Range	0.2 - 17.5	ND - 1.1
Absolute number ($\times 10^9$/l)		
Mean ± SD	2.2 ± 2.8	0.02 ± 0.02
Median	1.5	0.01
Range	0.02 - 16.5	ND - 0.09

ND: Not detectable.

Table 2. Approximation of the fraction of CD34[+] cells that circulates, based on median levels

Number of BM CD34[+] cells/monkey[a]	6.6×10^8
Number of PB CD34[+] cells/monkey[b]	0.3×10^7
Fraction of circulating CD34[+] cells	0.4%

[a]Calculated on the assumption that a 4-kg monkey has 3×10^{10} BM cells of which 2.2% are CD34[+].

[b]Calculated on the assumption that a 4-kg monkey has approximately 300 ml blood containing 10^7/l CD34[+] cells.

rhesus monkeys, sampled to obtain baseline data just before TBI. In the upper panel, the individual monkey BM and PB values are dissociated and both ranked in ascending order, displaying a median value of 10^7/l CD34[+] cells in PB and of 1.5×10^9/l in aspirated BM, and a variance which spans for both BM and PB approximately two logs in magnitude. In the lower panel, the PB CD34[+] cell numbers of individual monkeys are reassociated with those of the BM, which clearly shows that a direct relationship between BM and PB CD34[+] is not evident. The distribution parameters of the BM and PB CD34[+] cells are given in Table 1 and the calculation of the fraction of circulating CD34[+] cells is shown in Table 2, on which basis it is concluded that approximately 0.4% of the total pool of CD34[+] cells circulates.

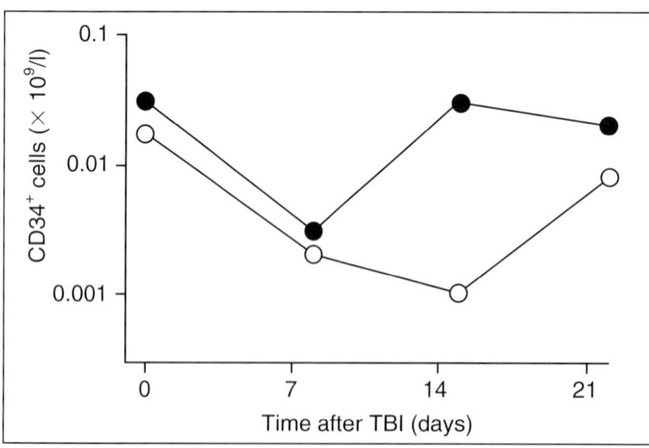

Figure 2. Circulating CD34[+] cells of TPO (closed circles) and placebo-treated (open circles) rhesus monkeys, revealing acceleration of CD34[+] cell reconstitution by TPO and consequently more than one-log expansion of those cells compared to placebo controls two weeks after TBI. Mean values of four individual monkeys in each group. The difference at two weeks is highly significant (p<0.01).

Effect of TPO on Circulating CD34[+] Cells during Hemopoietic Reconstitution Following 5 Gy TBI

Figure 2 demonstrates the PB levels of CD34[+] cells in monkeys treated with TPO for 21 consecutive days. The two-log expanded numbers of CD34[+] cells in the TPO-treated monkeys in the second week after TBI compared to

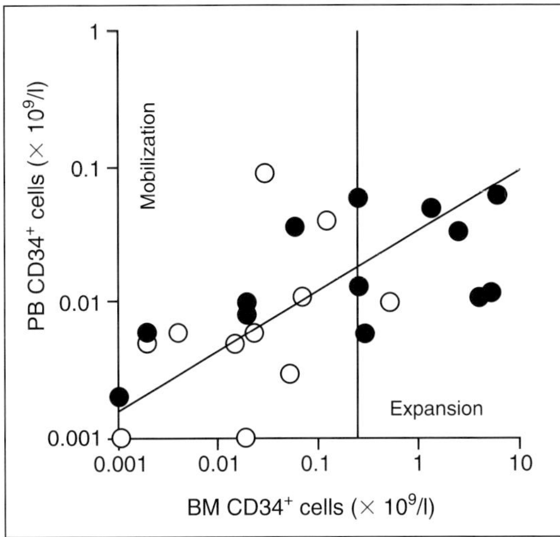

Figure 3. Correlation of BM and PB CD34⁺ cells during the first three weeks after TBI for TPO (closed circles) and placebo (open circles)-treated monkeys. The regression line for the placebo controls is shown and the vertical line presents the median BM CD34⁺ level of the TPO-treated monkeys. The shift to the right for the TPO BM CD34⁺ levels relative to those of the placebo controls is statistically significant (p = 0.01, Fisher's exact test), reflecting TPO-induced BM expansion. The regression line for the CD34⁺ cells of the TPO-treated monkeys (not shown) does not differ significantly from that of the placebo controls, direct evidence that TPO treatment does not result in a selective additional mobilization of CD34⁺ cells into the PB, but rather is a reflection of TPO-stimulated expansion in BM.

the placebo controls is evident. These data supplement our earlier reports on the hemopoietic effects [16, 21] and on expansion of BM CD34⁺ cells and clonogenic progenitors [21] in the same monkeys. The data were further processed to demonstrate the relation of BM and PB CD34⁺ cells during the first three weeks after TBI, shown in Figure 3, which also demonstrates that the increased levels of PB CD34⁺ cells are attributable to BM expansion rather than to selective mobilization of CD34⁺ cells.

DISCUSSION

In normal rhesus monkeys, an average of 0.4%, with a wide variation, of the total pool of immature CD34⁺ cells circulates in the PB. There appeared to be no direct relationship with the numbers of BM CD34⁺ cells, which is readily understandable from the fluctuating nature of the immature circulating cell number and genetic variation [11] of stem cell mobilization, as well as from variations in the quality of BM aspirates due to inevitable admixture with PB and in BM composition at the puncture site. Nevertheless, the median concentration of PB CD34⁺ being 1/100 of that in BM is in magnitude consistent with observations in other species, taking into account that BM stem cell concentrations tend to decrease with increasing species' body weight. It might be useful to dissect the CD34⁺ cells to reveal more immature circulating cells, e.g., the DR^{dull} fraction [10].

We further demonstrated that daily measurement of PB CD34⁺ cells can be used advantageously to monitor reconstitution of immature hemopoietic cells following myelosuppressive treatment and its acceleration by growth factor therapy using results obtained with preclinical evaluation of TPO treatment as an example. TPO appeared to be able to accelerate reconstitution of CD34⁺ BM cells, including the clonogenic progenitor cells [16], resulting in a two-log advantage two weeks after TBI over placebo-treated monkeys. This expansion was directly reflected by a one to two-log increase in PB CD34⁺ cells two weeks after TBI, a feature that was further analyzed by a simple correlation test which demonstrated that indeed the increased numbers of PB CD34 in TPO-treated monkeys should be explained by BM expansion rather than selective mobilization.

TPO is not unique in accelerating BM CD34⁺ cell expansion, but the magnitude of its effect is equivalent to that of coadministration of IL-3 and IL-6 (unpublished observations), whereas GM-CSF is less effective [17] and G-CSF even less [18] in an identical animal model. Consistent with the presence of Mpl on immature cells, TPO belongs with IL-3, IL-6 and IL-11 to a group of growth factors with the potential to expand immature multilineage reconstituting cells in vivo, which results in expansion of progenitor cells along myeloid and erythroid directions in addition to those of the megakaryocyte lineage and in multilineage efficacy [16, 19, 22]. In contrast to the latter growth factors, adverse effects of TPO treatment have not been observed, which makes TPO a key candidate growth factor to expand immature hemopoietic cells following myelosuppressive treatment or exposure to ionizing radiation in conjunction with other growth factors. The results also imply that growth factors that expand immature cells following myelosuppressive treatment and as a consequence increased numbers of circulating cells, such as TPO, should be distinguished from those that are highly effective mobilizers in normal individuals, such as G-CSF.

Growth factor-supported in vivo expansion of immature BM cells might be both an alternative and adjuvant to ex vivo expansion, and might be advantageously used in gene transfer protocols. However, there may be limitations in that, for instance, accelerated reconstitution of multilineage progenitors induced by TPO treatment after TBI of mice appeared to be accompanied by a proportional depletion of more immature cells (*Neelis et al.,* manuscript submitted for publication) be it not necessarily long-term repopulating cells. Also, TPO (and all other growth factors tested so far) proved to be ineffective under conditions of limited stem cell numbers, as occurs when small numbers of autologous BM cells or highly purified stem cells are transplanted after high-dose TBI [23]. In that condition, hemopoietic reconstitution appeared to be difficult to influence beneficially by exogenous growth factors although full hemopoietic reconstitution was reached in approximately four weeks, an indication that endogenous regulatory mechanisms may not always be inferior to administration of pharmacological doses of growth factors.

ACKNOWLEDGMENT

The authors wish to acknowledge the significant contributions of *Drs. G. Roger Thomas* and *Dan L. Eaton,* Genentech Inc., South San Francisco, CA, during the preclinical evaluation of TPO, the technical assistance of *Trudy P. Visser, Wati Dimjati, Hannie Busking-van der Lelie* and *Dorinde Kieboom-Pluimes,* and the animal care provided by *Albert Kloosterman* and *Ron Briegoos.* This work has been partly supported by the Netherlands Cancer Foundation Koningin Wilhemina Fonds, the Dutch Organization for Scientific Research NWO, the Royal Netherlands Academy of Arts and Sciences and Contracts of the Commission of the European Communities.

REFERENCES

1 Micklem HS, Anderson N, Ross E. Limited potential of circulating haemopoietic stem cells. Nature 1975;256:41-43.

2 Micklem HS, Ogden DA, Evans EP et al. Compartments and cell flows within the mouse haemopoietic system. II. Estimated rates of interchange. Cell Tissue Kinet 1975;8:233-248.

3 Briddell RA, Hartley CA, Smith KA et al. Recombinant human granulocyte colony-stimulating factor in vivo in mice to mobilize peripheral blood progenitor cells that have enhanced repopulating potential. Blood 1993;82:1720-1723.

4 Elias AD, Ayash L, Anderson KC et al. Mobilization of peripheral blood progenitor cells by chemotherapy and granulocyte-macrophage colony-stimulating factor of hematologic support after high-dose intensification for breast cancer. Blood 1992;79:3036-3044.

5 Mauch P, Lamont C, Neben TY et al. Hematopoietic stem cells in the blood after stem cell factor and interleukin-11 administration: evidence for different mechanisms of mobilization. Blood 1995;86:4674-4680.

6 Sudo Y, Shimazaki C, Ashihara E et al. Synergistic effect of Flt-3 ligand on the granulocyte colony-stimulating factor-induced mobilization of hematopoietic stem cells and progenitor cells into blood in mice. Blood 1997;89:3186-3191.

7 Laterveer L, Lindley IJ, Heemskerk DP et al. Rapid mobilization of hemopoietic progenitor cells in rhesus monkeys by a single intravenous injection of interleukin-8. Blood 1996;87:781-788.

8 Körbling M, Dorken B, Ho AD et al. Autologous transplantation of blood-derived hemopoietic stem cells after myeloablative therapy in a patient with Burkitt's lymphoma. Blood 1986;67:529-532.

9 Körbling M, Przepiorka D, Huh YO et al. Allogeneic blood stem cell transplantation for refractory leukemia and lymphoma: potential advantage of blood over marrow allografts. Blood 1995;85:1659-1665.

10 Wagemaker G, Neelis KJ, Wognum AW. Surface markers and growth factor receptors of immature hemopoietic stem cell subsets. STEM CELLS 1995;13(suppl 1)165-171.

11 Roberts AW, Foote S, Alexander WS et al. Genetic influences determining progenitor cell mobilization and leukocytosis induced by granulocyte colony-stimulating factor. Blood 1997;89:2736-2744.

12 De Sauvage FJ, Hass PE, Spencer SD et al. Stimulation of megakaryocytopoiesis and thrombopoiesis by the c-Mpl ligand. Nature 1994;369:533.

13 Lok S, Kaushansky K, Holly RD et al. Cloning and expression of murine thrombopoietin cDNA and stimulation of platelet production in vivo. Nature 1994;369:565-568.

14 Wendling F, Maraskovsky E, Debili N et al. cMpl ligand is a humoral regulator of megakaryocytopoiesis. Nature 1994;369:571-574.

15 Kaushansky K, Lok S, Holly RD et al. Promotion of megakaryocyte progenitor expansion and differentiation by the c-Mpl ligand thrombopoietin. Nature 1994;369:568-571.

16 Neelis KJ, Dubbelman YD, Qingliang L et al. Simultaneous TPO and G-CSF treatment of rhesus monkeys prevents thrombopenia, accelerates platelet and red cell reconstitution, alleviates neutropenia and promotes the recovery of immature bone marrow cells. Exp Hematol 1997;25:1084-1093.

17 Neelis SCC, Hartong T, Egeland GR et al. The efficacy of single-dose administration of thrombopoietin with coadministration of either granulocyte/macrophage or granulocyte colony-stimulating factor in myelosuppressed rhesus monkeys. Blood 1997;90:2555-2564.

18 Methia N, Louache F, Vainchenker W et al. Oligodeoxynucleotides antisense to the proto-oncogene c-mpl specifically inhibit in vitro megakaryocytopoiesis. Blood 1993;82:1395-1401.

19 Sitnicka E, Lin N, Priestley GV et al. The effect of thrombopoietin on the proliferation and differentiation of murine hematopoietic stem cells. Blood 1996;87:4998-5005.

20 Ku H, Yonemura Y, Kaushansky K et al. Thrombopoietin, the ligand for the Mpl receptor, synergizes with steel factor and other early acting cytokines in supporting proliferation of primitive hematopoietic progenitors of mice. Blood 1996;87:4544-4551.

21 Neelis KJ, Qingliang L, Thomas GR et al. Prevention of thrombocytopenia by thrombopoietin in myelosuppressed rhesus monkeys accompanied by prominent erythropoietic stimulation and iron depletion. Blood 1997;90:58-63.

22 Farese AM, Hunt P, Grab LB et al. Combined administration of recombinant human megakaryocyte growth and development factor and granulocyte colony-stimulating factor enhances multilineage hematopoietic reconstitution in nonhuman primates after radiation-induced marrow aplasia. J Clin Invest 1996;97:2145.

23 Neelis KJ, Dubbelman YD, Wognum AW et al. Lack of efficacy of thrombopoietin and granulocyte colony-stimulating factor after high dose total body irradiation and autologous stem cell or bone marrow transplantation in rhesus monkeys. Exp Hematol 1997;25:1094-1103.

Development of Natural Killer Cells from Lymphohematopoietic Progenitors of Murine Fetal Liver

YUICHI AIBA, MAKIO OGAWA

Ralph H. Johnson Department of Veterans Affairs Medical Center, Department of Medicine, Medical University of South Carolina, Charleston, South Carolina, USA

Key Words. *Natural killer cells · Lymphohematopoietic cells · Interleukins · Growth factors*

ABSTRACT

We established a clonal culture system which supports the growth of murine immature natural killer (NK) cells. When we plated day 14 fetal thymocytes in methylcellulose media containing interleukin 2 (IL-2), IL-7 and steel factor (SF), we observed diffuse colonies which could not be classified into known colony types. Cells in the colonies were blast-like and expressed Thy-1 and CD25 but not lineage-specific markers. Cells in the colonies developed into NK1.1$^+$ cells in fetal thymus organ culture indicating that the colonies consist of immature NK cells. We then examined the colony-forming ability of fetal liver cells. The combination of IL-2, IL-7 and SF with or without IL-11 supported formation of few immature NK cell colonies from purified progenitors. Interestingly, addition of IL-11 to the culture stimulated formation of mixed colonies consisting of immature NK cells, B cells, macrophages and/or mast cells. The clonal origin of the mixed NK cell colonies was confirmed by micromanipulation of the colony-forming cells. This culture assay should facilitate the analysis of the pathway and cytokine regulation of NK cell development. *Stem Cells 1998;16(suppl 1):193-198*

INTRODUCTION

Natural killer (NK) cells comprise a small subset of lymphocytes and are thought to play important roles in various immune responses [1, 2]. Although the functions of NK cells are being extensively studied, their ontogeny and regulation of development are largely unknown. It was reported that NK cells are closely related to T lymphocytes in their developmental pathways [3]. *Sánchez et al.* [4] have shown that NK/T common progenitors are present in human fetal thymus. However, it still remains to be clarified how NK or NK/T common progenitors develop from multipotential hematopoietic progenitors, and how and when NK/T common progenitors diverge to form separate NK and T cell lineages. The lineage relationship of NK cells with B and myeloid cells should also be clarified.

To investigate the pathway of NK cell development, it is necessary to establish a clonal culture system which supports the development of NK cells from multipotential hematopoietic progenitors. Here, we report that murine fetal thymocytes and liver cells plated in methylcellulose culture form immature NK cell colonies. We also found that mixed colonies consisting of NK, B and myeloid cells

Characteristics and Potentials of Blood Stem Cells

can develop from purified hematopoietic progenitors of fetal liver cells in the presence of interleukin 2 (IL-2), IL-7, steel factor (SF) and IL-11. We believe that this quantitative clonal culture is useful for analyzing the developmental pathway and cytokine regulation of NK cell progenitors.

MATERIALS AND METHODS

Mice and Cell Preparation

Female C57BL/6-Ly5.2 and male DBA/2 mice were purchased from Charles River (Raleigh, NC). Male C57BL/6-Ly5.1 mice were purchased from Jackson Laboratories (Bar Harbor, ME). Mice were allowed to mate for 18 h. The day of vaginal plugging was designated as day 0 of gestation. On day 14 of gestation, the mice were sacrificed and cell suspensions of fetal thymus and liver were prepared by gently pressing these organs between two slide glasses and by repeated pipetting. Purification of fetal liver progenitors had been described previously [5].

Cytokines

Purified murine recombinant IL-2 was purchased from R&D Systems (Minneapolis, MN). Recombinant human IL-7 was provided by Sanofi Winthrop, Inc. (Malvern, PA). Recombinant murine SF was a gift from Immunex (Seattle, WA). Recombinant human IL-11 was provided by Genetics Institute (Cambridge, MA). Concentrations of cytokines used were as follows: IL-2, 20 ng/ml; IL-7, SF, 100 ng/ml; 200 U/ml (20ng/ml); IL-11, 100 ng/ml.

Flow Cytometry and Cell Sorting

The following monoclonal antibodies were used for flow cytometric analysis and cell sorting: biotin-conjugated-anti-CD3 (clone;145-2C11) (Pharmingen; San Diego, CA); fluorescein isothio-cyanate (FITC) conjugated-anti-CD4 (YTS 191.1) (Caltag Laboratories; South San Francisco, CA); phycoerythrin (PE) conjugated-anti-CD8 (YTS 169.4) (Caltag); PE-conjugated-anti-CD25 (PC61.5.3) (Caltag); FITC-conjugated-anti-Thy1.2 (30-H12) (Pharmingen); biotin-conjugated-anti-NK1.1 (PK136) (Pharmingen); PE-conjugated-anti-B220 (RA3-6B2) (Pharmingen); biotin-conjugated-anti-c-kit (ACK4), biotin-conjugated-anti-Mac-1 (M1/70), biotin-conjugated-anti-Gr-1 (RB6-8C5) (Pharmingen); biotin-conjugated-anti-TER (TER119) (Pharmingen); FITC-conjugated-anti-Ly5.1 (A20-1.7, kindly provided by *Dr. H. Fleming* of Emory University, Atlanta, GA), and FITC-conjugated-anti-Ly5 (30F11.1). Basic techniques of cell staining had been described previously [6]. In all experiments, cells stained with appropriate isotype-matched control immunoglobulins were prepared as negative controls. After staining, cells were analyzed and/or sorted by using FACS Vantage (Becton Dickinson; Mountain View, CA).

Clonal Culture for Immature NK Cell Colonies

Methylcellulose culture was carried out by using 35mm Falcon suspension culture dishes (Becton Dickinson Labware; Lincoln Park, NJ). Fetal thymocytes or purified progenitor cells of fetal liver were cultured in the medium consisting of α-medium (Flow Laboratories; Rockville, MD), 1.2% 1,500-centipoise methylcellulose (Shinetsu Chemical; Tokyo, Japan), 5% fetal bovine serum, 1% deionized fraction-V bovine serum albium and 0.1mM 2-mercaptoethanol and cytokines. Dishes were incubated at 37°C in a humidified atmosphere flushed with 5% CO_2 for 14 or 18 days. Single-cell manipulation of colony-forming cells was carried out as described previously [7].

Fetal Thymus Organ Culture

Fetal thymus organ culture was performed as described previously [8]. Briefly, fetal thymi were first incubated with 4×10^4 test cells in a hanging drop culture for 20 h. Samples were then transferred onto filter membranes (Costar; Cambridge, MA; pore size, 8mm) and cultured for 11 days. Cells were recovered from the thymic lobes, stained with antibodies and analyzed by flow cytometry.

RESULTS

Immature NK Cell Colony Formation from Fetal Thymocytes

We chose day 14 murine fetal thymocytes as the material for growing candidate NK cell colonies because relatively high percentages of the cells had been shown to have the potential of developing into NK cells [9]. After testing several cytokine combinations, we found that fetal thymocytes cultured in the methylcellulose media containing IL-2, IL-7 and SF form diffuse colonies which cannot be classified into known colony types (Fig. 1). May-Grünwald Giemsa staining of the colonies revealed that the cells in the colonies are blast-like, showing no signs of cytoplasmic differentiation. Colony-forming frequency of the fetal thymocytes was about 1%. We then examined expression of surface molecules of the cells in the colonies by flow cytometry. As shown in Figure 2, the cells expressed Thy-1 and CD25 but not Mac-1, Gr-1, TER, CD3 or B220. Because the cells in the colonies expressed Thy-1 and CD25, it was likely that these cells are immature NK or T cells. Therefore, we next examined the NK and T cell potentials by culturing these cells in fetal thymus organ culture. Fetal thymocytes of C57BL/6-Ly5.1/Ly5.2 F1 mice were cultured in the methylcellulose media in the presence of IL-2, IL-7 and SF. After incubation for 14 days, candidate NK cell colonies were individually picked, pooled and plated in culture with fetal thymic lobes of C57BL/6-Ly5.2 mice. Ten days later cells recovered from the thymic lobes were analyzed for the expression of Ly5.1, CD3, NK1.1 and B220. As shown in Figure 3, most of test Ly5.1$^+$ cells expressed NK1.1 but neither CD3 nor B220. This result indicated that the diffuse colonies derived from the fetal thymocytes are immature NK cell colonies.

Mixed NK Cell Colony Formation from Fetal Liver Progenitors

We next examined the colony-forming ability of purified hematopoietic progenitors of fetal

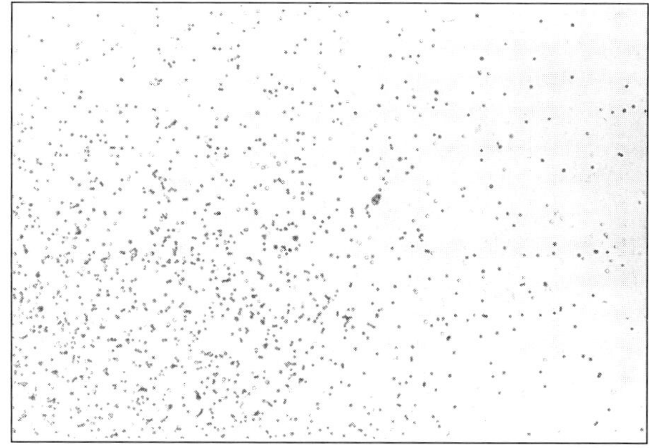

Figure 1. A photomicrograph of an immature NK cell colony. *One quarter of a representative immature NK cell colony seen on an inverted microscope.*

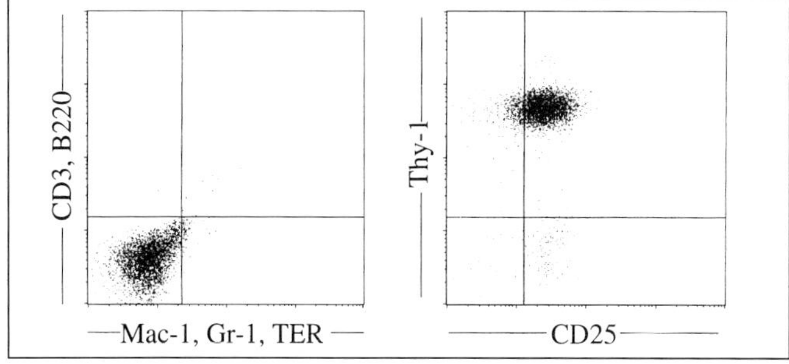

Figure 2. Surface phenotypes of the cells in the immature NK cell colonies. *Fetal thymocytes were cultured in methylcellulose media with IL-2, IL-7 and SF. After 14 days of culture, immature NK cell colonies were individually picked, pooled and stained with monoclonal antibodies specific for molecules indicated in each FACS profile.*

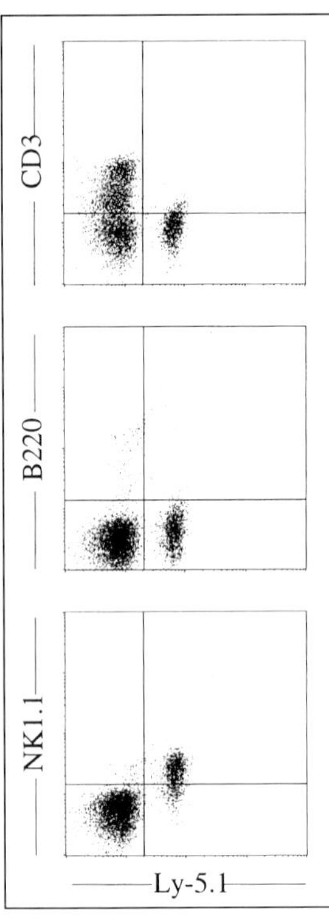

Figure 3. Surface phenotypes of the cells developing in fetal thymus organ culture. Fetal thymocytes from C57BL/6-Ly5.1/C57BL/-6-Ly5.2 F1 mice (Ly5.1/Ly5.2) were plated in methylcellulose culture with IL-2, IL-7 and SF. After 14 days of culture, immature NK cell colonies were individually picked, pooled and incubated in a hanging drop culture for 20 h with fetal thymus lobes from BDF1 (Ly5.2) mice. The lobes were then cultured on filter membranes for 10 days. Cells harvested from the lobes were stained with monoclonal antibodies specific for molecules indicated in each FACS profile.

liver cells. Low density (<1.0770), lineage marker-negative, c-kit$^+$Sca-1$^+$ cells were prepared from day 14 murine fetal liver. We have previously shown that colony-forming cells can be enriched by this method [5]. The cells were plated in methylcellulose media with IL-2, IL-7 and SF. As shown in Table 1, immature NK cell colonies developed although their frequencies were low. In an effort to increase the frequency of the colonies, we found that addition of IL-11 to the culture increases the frequency of colony-forming cells (Table 1). More interestingly, mixed colonies consisting of diffuse round cells characteristic of immature NK cells and other types of cells were also detected (Fig. 4). Table 1 shows the results of a representative study. In the same table, colony-forming ability of the fetal thymocytes is also shown.

To confirm the clonality of the mixed colonies, we next plated the c-kit$^+$Sca-1$^+$ cells individually by micromanipulation into methylcellulose media containing IL-2, IL-7, IL-11 and SF. From 100 individually plated cells, 12 mixed NK cell colonies developed after 18 days of culture. This study established the clonal origin of the mixed NK cell colonies. To characterize the cells in the mixed colonies in more detail, each colony was lifted individually from the culture and divided into two aliquots. Cells in one aliquot were examined for the expression of B220 and Thy-1 by flow cytometry. All colonies contained Thy-1$^+$ B220$^-$ cells. Eleven out of the 12 colonies contained B220$^+$ cells, suggesting that most of the colonies have B lineage cells. Representative fluorescence-activated cell sort profiles were shown in Figure 5. Cells in the other aliquot of the colonies were subjected to May-Grünwald Giemsa staining for examination of myeloid lineage cells. All mixed colonies contained macrophages; two out of the 12 contained mast cells. These results indicated that most of the mixed

Table 1. Colony formation from fetal liver and fetal thymus cells

Cells plated			# of Colonies					
Type	#/Dish	Cytokines	Mixed NK	Pure NK	Pre-B	M	Mast	M-mast
Sca-1$^+$c-kit$^+$FL	50	IL-2, IL-7, SF	0	1 ± 1	3 ± 1	7 ± 2	1 ± 1	2 ± 1
		IL-2, IL-7, IL-11, SF	7 ± 1	2 ± 1	4 ± 1	7 ± 1	1 ± 1	2 ± 1
FT	1,000	IL-2, IL-7, SF	0	11 ± 1	0	0	2 ± 1	0
		IL-2, IL-7, IL-11, SF	0	13 ± 1	0	0	3 ± 2	0

Sca-1$^+$c-kit$^+$ FL cells were prepared as described in **Materials and Methods.** Cells were cultured for 18 days in methylcellulose media in the presence of designated cytokines. Data represent mean ± SD of quadruplicate cultures. Abbreviations: Mixed NK: mixed NK colonies; Pure NK: NK cell colonies; Pre-B: Pre-B cell colonies; M: macrophage colony; mast: mast cell colony; M-mast: macrophage-mast cell mixed colony; FL: fetal liver; FT: fetal thymus.

NK cell colonies contain immature K, B and myeloid cells and suggested that the colonies are derived from lymphohematopoietic progenitors.

DISCUSSION

Although much effort has been made to clarify the pathway and regulation of NK cell development, there are still questions to be resolved in NK cell ontogeny. This is mainly because of the lack of a clonal culture system which supports the growth and development of NK cells from uncommitted progenitors. Here, we report the establishment of a clonal culture which supports the growth of immature NK cells, B cells, macrophages and/or mast cells from single hematopoietic progenitors of murine fetal liver.

Recently, several reports suggested that NK, T and B cells arise from common lymphoid progenitors [10-14]. However, because of the lack of a clonal culture which supports the growth of multiple lymphoid lineage cells simultaneously, the concept of common lymphoid progenitors was not established unequivocally. The culture system reported here will greatly facilitate identification of the common lymphoid progenitors. Our study revealed that fetal thymocytes cannot form mixed colonies containing NK and B lineage cells. This appears to indicate that fetal thymi contain committed NK and B cell progenitors but not common NK/B progenitors. Alternatively, very few thymocytes have the potential to develop to both NK and B cells and our culture is not sensitive enough to detect the few common progenitors. Regardless, our culture system will now allow direct study of the mechanisms regulating commitment of multipotent progenitors to NK cell lineage.

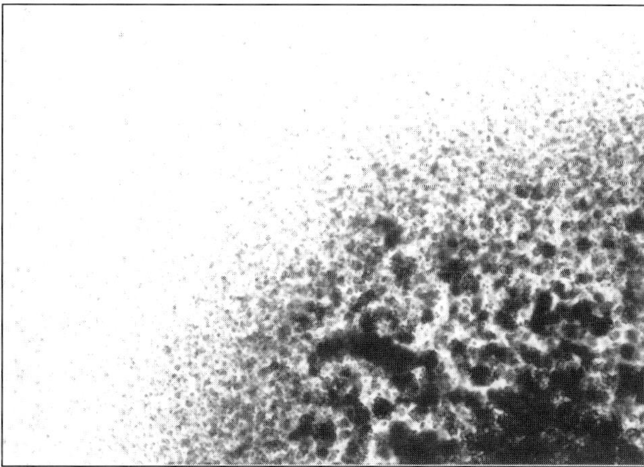

Figure 4. A photomicropraph of a mixed NK cell colony. One quarter of a representative mixed NK cell colony seen on an inverted microscope is shown.

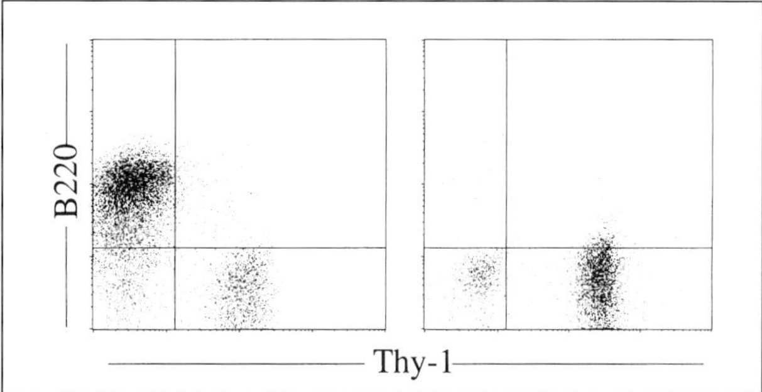

Figure 5. Representative FACS profiles of colonies derived from single cells. Sca-1$^+$c-kit$^+$ cells were prepared from fetal liver and were plated individually by micromanipulation into methylcellulose media containing IL-2, IL-7, IL-11 and SF. After 18 days of culture, colonies were identified in situ and picked individually. Cells from each colony were stained with PE-anti-B220 and FITC-anti-Thy-1 and analyzed by FACS Vantage. Left: a mixed NK colony with B lineage cells. Right: a mixed NK colony without B lineage cells.

ACKNOWLEDGMENT

We thank *Dr. Haiqun Zeng* for assistance in cell sorting and *Dr. Pamela N. Pharr* and *Mrs. Anne G. Leary* in preparation of this manuscript.

REFERENCES

1 Trinchieri G. Biology of natural killer cells. Adv Immunol 1989;47:187-376.

2 Herberman RB, Reynolds CW, Ortaldo JR. Mechanism of cytotoxicity by natural killer (NK) cells. Annu Rev Immunol 1986;4:651-680.

3 Lanier LL, Spits H, Phillips JH. The developmental relationship between NK cells and T cells. Immunol Today 1992;13:392-395.

4 Sánchez MJ, Muench MO, Roncarolo MG et al. Identification of a common T/natural killer cell progenitor in human fetal thymus. J Exp Med 1994;180:569-576.

5 Fujimoto K, Lyman SD, Hirayama F et al. Isolation and characterization of primitive hematopoietic progenitors of murine fetal liver. Exp Hematol 1996;24:285-290.

6 Hirayama, F, Shih J-P, Awgulewitsch A et al. Clonal proliferation of murine lymphohemopoietic progenitors in culture. Proc Natl Acad Sci USA 1992;89:5907-5911.

7 Suda T, Suda J, Ogawa M. Single-cell origin of mouse hemopoietic colonies expressing multiple lineages in variable combinations. Proc Natl Acad Sci USA 1983;80:6689-6693.

8 Aiba Y, Hirayama F, Ogawa M. Clonal proliferation and cytokine requirement of murine progenitors for natural killer cells. Blood 1997;89:4005-4012.

9 Rodewald H-R, Moingeon P, Lucich JL et al. A population of early fetal thymocytes expressing FcgRII/III contains precursors of T lymphocytes and natural killer cells. Cell 1992;69:139-150.

10 Galy A, Travis M, Cen D et al. Human T, B, natural killer, and dendritic cells arise from a common bone marrow progenitor cell subset. Immunity 1995;3:459-473.

11 Georgopoulos K, Bigby M, Wang J-H et al. The ikaros gene is required for the development of all lymphoid lineages. Cell 1994;79:143-156.

12 Matsuzaki Y, Gyotoku J-I, Ogawa M et al. Characterization of c-kit positive intrathymic stem cells that are restricted to lymphoid differentiation. J Exp Med 1993;178:1283-1292.

13 Wu L, Antica M, Johnson GR et al. Developmental potential of the earliest precursor cells from the adult mouse thymus. J Exp Med 1991;174:1617-1627.

14 Zúñiga-Pflücker JC, Jiang D, Lenardo MJ. Requirement for TNF-α and IL-1α in fetal thymocyte commitment and differentiation. Science 1995;268:1906-1909.

Ex Vivo Manipulation of Hematopoietic Stem and Progenitor Cells

LOTHAR KANZ, WOLFRAM BRUGGER, STEFAN SCHEDING

University of Tübingen, Medical Center, Department of Hematology, Oncology, and Immunology, Tübingen, Germany

Key Words. *Peripheral blood progenitor cells · Hematopoietic growth factor · High-dose chemotherapy · Myeloablative conditioning · Post-progenitor cells · Dendritic cells*

ABSTRACT

Approaches to manipulate peripheral blood progenitor cells (PBPC) ex vivo currently include the selection of CD34$^+$ cells as a means to purge contaminating tumor cells from leukapheresis preparations or to provide a homogeneous starting population for the expansion of hematopoietic progenitor cells as well as the induction of postprogenitor cells of either the myeloid or megakaryocytic lineage. The latter cell populations might be used for an additional transplantation together with PBPC to possibly shorten the period of aplasia. In addition, ex vivo expansion of CD34$^+$ cells can be used to generate autologous tumor-antigen-presenting dendritic cells for immunotherapeutic approaches aiming to treat minimal residual disease following high-dose chemotherapy. *Stem Cells 1998;16(suppl 1):199-204*

RATIONALE FOR THE EX VIVO EXPANSION OF STEM AND PROGENITOR CELLS

The potential uses of ex vivo-expanded CD34$^+$ peripheral blood progenitor cells (PBPC) are summarized in Table 1. There is increasing interest to supply sufficient numbers of progenitor cells for repetitive transplantation, particularly for sequential and double high-dose chemotherapy approaches, such as in breast cancer. Moreover, ex vivo expansion might enable an increase in progenitor cells in the case of patients with insufficient recruitment of CD34$^+$ cells, thus allowing high-dose chemotherapy to be administered in those "poor mobilizers." However, our own experience indicates that CD34-selected progenitor cells of "poor mobilizers" have only a very low expansion potential (unpublished observations). An increase of stem cells for allogeneic transplants, particularly in a

Table 1. Rationale for the ex-vivo expansion of stem and progenitor cells

▲ Use for repetitive high-dose chemotherapy (e.g., breast cancer, germ cell tumors).

▲ Potential for high-dose chemotherapy in patients with insufficient mobilization of PBPC ("poor mobilizers").

▲ Use of "high stem cell doses" in a mismatched, T cell-depleted allograft setting.

▲ Tumor cell purging (i.e., aim to amplify normal progenitors utilizing culture conditions which inhibit the survival of contaminating malignant cells).

mismatched, T cell-depleted setting has been shown to reduce the incidence of graft rejection [1-3]. In addition, effective ex vivo expansion procedures allow reduction of the sample volume that has to be collected from a patient to provide a suitable graft, thus reducing the overall tumor cell load in the final preparation and possibly avoiding leukapheresis [4]. Finally, ex vivo culture conditions might favor maintenance and/or expansion of normal stem/progenitor cells and restrict survival of malignant precursor cells, as already shown for Ph$^+$ chronic myelogenous leukemia and acute myeloid leukemia [5-7].

Ex Vivo Expansion of Stem and Progenitor Cells: Preclinical and Clinical Data

The optimal choice of hematopoietic growth factors for the ex vivo expansion of CD34$^+$ cells has not yet been defined. We have shown that a combination of stem cell factor (SCF), interleukin 1 (IL-1), IL-3, IL-6 and erythropoietin (EPO) is very potent in increasing the number of committed hematopoietic progenitor cells [8]. Long-term culture-initiating cells (LTC-IC), representing very early hematopoietic cells, are not lost during this procedure; however, no expansion of these cells was observed using this combination of hematopoietic growth factors [9].

Based on these in vitro experiments, we have performed a clinical phase I/II study of 10 patients using ex vivo-expanded CD34$^+$ cells [4]. Starting only with about 1/10 of a two-h leukapheresis preparation, we were able to generate a sufficient number of hematopoietic progenitor cells ex vivo that mediated rapid hematopoietic engraftment of both neutrophils and platelets in patients receiving high-dose chemotherapy. Interestingly, correlation analysis between the time to hematopoietic recovery and number of transplanted colony-forming cells indicated that a threshold dose of ex vivo-generated committed progenitor cells exists as a surrogate marker to ensure rapid engraftment. None of the patients studied had a secondary nadir of peripheral blood counts during follow-up. However, the capability of those ex vivo-generated cells to induce long-term hematopoiesis cannot be deduced by this study because autologous stem cells are likely to contribute to long-term hematopoiesis after nonmyeloablative high-dose chemotherapy as applied in this study (VIC-E high-dose chemotherapy) [4].

Besides our trial only one other recent report described the transplantation of ex vivo-expanded cells without other cellular support, such as unmanipulated PBPC or bone marrow. In their study *Holyoake et al.* demonstrated ex vivo-generated progenitor-mediated short-term hematopoietic recovery for neutrophils after TBI in the case of three out of four patients [10]. These observations confirm our data on the short-term capabilities of ex vivo-expanded cells. The one patient who did not engraft by day 14 furthermore received the lowest colony-forming units-granulocyte, macrophage dose; however, two of the three patients failed to sustain hematopoietic engraftment following this myeloablative conditioning regimen. Although TBI probably might have decreased vascular adhesion and transit of expanded progenitor cells after retransfusion, and cytokine concentrations, ex vivo culture conditions and, importantly, the patient selection (hematopoietic disorders versus patients with solid tumors) differed markedly from our study, these observations indicate that a procedure which allows expansion of committed hematopoietic progenitors but not of more early cells such as LTC-IC might not be suitable to supply sufficient numbers of cells that provide long-term hematopoiesis after myeloablative conditioning. Thus any ex vivo expansion approach to be used in a myeloablative setting should also expand more primitive cells.

For example, *Connie Eaves's* group recently reported that it is indeed possible to generate an expanded population of LTC-IC (30- to 50-fold) starting from CD34$^+$CD38$^-$ steady-state bone marrow cells by using high concentrations of SCF and Flt-3 ligand (Flt-3L) and, importantly, low concentrations of IL-3 [7]. Furthermore, *B. Ziegler* from our group was able to demonstrate an about 10-fold LTC-IC amplification in a serum-free liquid phase system using SCF, Flt-3L, IL-3 (low-dose), IL-6 and thrombopoietin (TPO) (unpublished). Before starting a clinical transplantation trial utilizing such an ex vivo-generated population of early hematopoietic cells after myeloablative conditioning, we are currently testing the in vivo-repopulating capacity of these expanded cells in the nonobese diabetic/severe-combined immunodeficiency (NOD/SCID) mouse system (*T. Bock,* unpublished).

In this context it might be helpful to summarize existing published data with regard to the effect of colony-stimulating factors on long-term repopulating stem cells in animal models. Experiments by *P. Quesenberry's* group have shown in the murine system that stimulation of hematopoietic progenitor cells with SCF, IL-3, IL-6 and IL-11 with consecutive transplantation of these cells resulted in short-term reconstitution; however, long-term engraftment was substantially impaired [11]. *M. Ogawa* furthermore demonstrated that cells stimulated with SCF, IL-6, IL-11 and EPO mediated long-term engraftment in mice whereas the addition of IL-3 and IL-1 in the ex vivo culture system prohibited sustained engraftment [12]. Moreover, transplantation experiments performed by *C. Dunbar* and co-workers in monkeys showed that retrovirally marker gene-labeled cells expanded in SCF, IL-3 and IL-6 disappeared in animals following transplantation in addition to unmanipulated cells [13]. Thus the use of IL-3 has to be cautiously evaluated in attempts to expand early hematopoietic cells for use in a myeloablative clinical setting.

Meanwhile there are other reports indicating that defined culture conditions, specifically not those including IL-3 at higher doses, allow both short-term as well as long-term reconstitution or even the ability to serially transplant these cells [14]. The recent ex vivo expansion studies using human cells by *R. Hoffmann's, C. Eaves's* and *J. Dick's* groups [14], show hematopoietic reconstitution in the SCID system following transplantation of those cells. However, as reported by *J. Dick,* the duration of ex vivo cultures, in their nine-day versus four-day experiments, might be critical for the maintenance of primitive, repopulating cells [15].

UNSOLVED ISSUES IN THE EX VIVO EXPANSION OF CD34⁺ PBPC

Many unsolved issues remain. The first question surrounds the problem of defining which functional classes of stem and progenitor cells do contribute to early versus late recovery [16, 17]; this question has fundamental implications for the quality assessment of ex vivo-manipulated cell preparations. Meanwhile experiments reported by the groups of *Weismann, Fibbe* and *Deisseroth* indicate that committed progenitor cells are unlikely to generate enough mature end cells to explain recovery around 10 days post-transplant, and that primitive cells contribute to both short- and long-term recovery [14].

Another question relates to the efficiency of homing of ex vivo-manipulated cells to the bone marrow after retransfusion because changes in the expression of cytoadhesive proteins might influence engraftment [18]. Moreover, because it is possible that cytokines used for ex vivo expansion might also increase the clonogenic growth of tumor cells, monitoring of expanded cell preparations for the presence of residual tumor cells is mandatory. Finally, the answer to the question whether ex vivo expansion results in a loss of stem cell properties will only be definitively answered by appropriate clinical trials.

GENERATION OF MYELOID AND MEGAKARYOCYTIC POST-PROGENITOR CELLS

Transplantation of hematopoietic post-progenitor cells in addition to progenitor cells might help to further shorten or even abrogate the nadir period for neutrophils and platelets. Recently, *Williams et al.* reported that the additional transplantation of myeloid post-progenitor cells (MPPC) generated ex vivo in cultures stimulated by PIXY321 in nine patients was possible and safe [19]. However, no significant acceleration of neutrophil recovery was observed when compared to patients receiving only unmanipulated PBPC. One possible explanation for this observation might be that the number of transplanted MPPC was not large enough. Interestingly, we have recently shown by computer simulation of hematopoietic recovery after PBPC transplantation that amelioration of neutropenia can only be achieved when the additional MPPC graft consists of very high numbers of immature granulocytic cells, particularly myelocytes (at least 5.7×10^8 MPPC/kg) [20]. Based on these theoretical results it is not surprising that no effect on neutrophils was observed in the above-cited clinical study. Preclinical experimental ex vivo MPPC expansion studies furthermore indicate that successful MPPC transplantation might be feasible when starting from large numbers of CD34$^+$ cells (at least 5.5×10^6 CD34$^+$ cells per kg) and utilizing an optimum cytokine combination in view of an effective MPPC generation [21-22].

Similar expansion experiments can be done in order to induce megakaryocytic post-progenitor cells. Using a combination of early acting hematopoietic growth factors plus TPO it is possible to induce both committed megakaryocytic progenitor cells and a high yield of CD61$^+$ immature megakaryocytic cells out of CD34$^+$ cells in the starting population [23]. So far, only one clinical trial has been reported on the additional transplantation of ex vivo-generated megakaryocytic cells [24]. Here, megakaryocytic cells were generated ex vivo by liquid cultures in the presence of TPO as well as additional cytokines, and 10 cancer patients received expanded cells together with unmanipulated PBPC following high-dose therapy. Interestingly, although overall CD61$^+$ cell yield was not exceedingly high, platelet transfusions were not necessary for two out of four patients receiving the highest doses of cultured cells.

Whether ex vivo-generated post-progenitor cells are able to home in vivo and whether those ex vivo-activated cells are functionally active in vivo is currently not known. Based on our preclinical experiments demonstrating the feasibility of generating large numbers of myeloid and megakaryocytic cells from CD34$^+$ PBPC utilizing appropriate culture conditions for clinical use, clinical post-progenitor transplantation trials are now ready to be launched at our institution.

GENERATION OF IMMUNE EFFECTOR CELLS

There is growing interest to generate professional antigen-presenting dendritic cells that might be used for adoptive immunotherapy approaches after recovery from high-dose chemotherapy.

Two strategies to generate these cells are currently being pursued: A) Generation of dendritic cells can be derived from peripheral blood monocytes as well from CD34$^+$ PBPC cells. Several groups have clearly demonstrated that high numbers of functionally active dendritic cells can be generated using either approach (Table 2). B) Our group is particularly trying to compare the potential of peripheral blood monocyte-derived and CD34-derived dendritic cells as to their potential to prime a cytotoxic T lymphocyte response against breast cancer-associated antigens.

Table 2. Summary of selected references on the ex vivo generation of dendritic cells from human CD34$^+$ cord blood, bone marrow and PBPC

CD34$^+$ source	Author	Reference	Culture conditions	Cytokines
Cord blood	*Caux et al.* 1992	[25, 26]	RPMI + 10% FBS	GM-CSF ± TNF-α ± IL-3
	Santiago-Schwarz et al. 1992	[27]	RPMI + 5% NHS	GM-CSF, TNF-α
	Strobl et al. 1996	[28]	X-vivo15 ± CBP	GM-CSF, TNF-α, SCF ± TGF-β1
	Flores-Romo et al. 1997	[29]	RPMI + 10% FCS	CD40-ligand
Bone marrow	*Szabolcs et al.* 1995	[30]	IMDM + 20% FCS	TNF-α, GM-CSF ± SCF
	Young et al. 1995	[31]	IMDM + 20% FCS	GM-CSF, TNF-α, SCF
PBPC	*Siena et al.* 1995	[32]	IMDM + FCS/AS/HS	GM-CSF, TNF-α ± SCF ± Flt-3L
	Mackensen et al. 1995	[33]	RPMI + 10% FCS	SCF, EPO, IL-1, IL-3, IL-4, IL-6, GM-CSF
	Scheding et al. 1996	[34, 35]	RPMI + 10% FCS, X-vivo 10	SCF, EPO, IL-1, IL-3, IL-4, IL-6, GM-CSF ± Flt-3L

Abbreviations: CB= cord blood; BM= bone marrow; PB= peripheral blood; PBPC= peripheral blood progenitor cells; FCS= fetal calf serum; FBS= fetal bovine serum; AS= autologous serum; CBP= cord blood plasma; IMDM= Iscove's modified Dulbecco's medium.

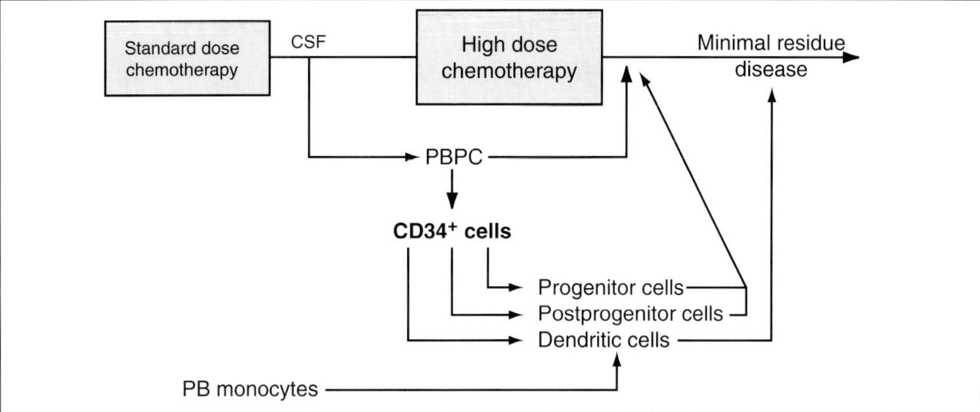

Figure 1. Ex vivo manipulation of PBPC.

CONCLUSION

Ex vivo manipulation of PBPC not only allows more advanced features for stem cell transplantation such as tumor cell depletion by CD34 selection, expansion of progenitor cells and induction of post-progenitor cells for possible abrogation of the nadir period, but also the generation of dendritic cells with the potential to treat minimal residual disease remaining after high-dose chemotherapy of malignancies (Fig. 1).

ACKNOWLEDGMENT

Supported in part by the Deutsche Forschungsgemeinschaft, Sonderforschungsbereich 510.

REFERENCES

1 Aversa F, Tabilio A, Terenzi A et al. Successful engraftment of T-cell-depleted haploidentical "three-loci" incompatible transplants in leukemia patients by addition of recombinant human granulocyte colony-stimulating factor-mobilized peripheral blood progenitor cells to bone marrow inoculum. Blood 1994;84:3948-3955.

2 Bachar LE, Rachamim N, Li HW et al. Megadose of T cell-depleted bone marrow overcomes MHC barriers in sublethally irradiated mice. Nat Med 1995;1:1268-1273.

3 Reisner Y, Martelli MF. Bone marrow transplantation across HLA barriers by increasing the number of transplanted cells. Immunol Today 1995;16:437-440.

4 Brugger W, Heimfeld S, Berenson RJ et al. Reconstitution of hematopoiesis after high-dose chemotherapy by autologous progenitor cells generated ex vivo (Comments). N Engl J Med 1995;333:283-287.

5 Barnett MJ, Eaves CJ, Phillips GL et al. Autografting with cultured marrow in chronic myeloid leukemia: results of a pilot study (Comments). Blood 1994;84:724-732.

6 Dexter TM, Chang J. New strategies for the treatment of chronic myeloid leukemia (Editorial, Comment). Blood 1994;84:673-675.

7 Petzer AL, Eaves CJ, Barnett MJ et al. Selective expansion of primitive normal hematopoietic cells in cytokine-supplemented cultures of purified cells from patients with chronic myeloid leukemia. Blood 1997;90:64-69.

8 Brugger W, Mocklin W, Heimfeld S et al. Ex vivo expansion of enriched peripheral blood CD34+ progenitor cells by stem cell factor, interleukin-1 beta (IL-1 beta), IL-6, IL-3, interferon-gamma, and erythropoietin. Blood 1993;81:2579-2584.

9 Henschler R, Brugger W, Luft T et al. Maintenance of transplantation potential in ex vivo expanded CD34(+)-selected human peripheral blood progenitor cells. Blood 1994;84:2898-2903.

10 Holyoake TL, Alcorn MJ, Richmond L et al. CD34 positive PBPC expanded ex vivo may not provide durable engraftment following myeloablative chemoradiotherapy regimens. Bone Marrow Transplant 1997;19:1095-1101.

11 Peters SO, Kittler EL, Ramshaw HS et al. Ex vivo expansion of murine marrow cells with interleukin-3 (IL-3), IL-6, IL-11, and stem cell factor leads to impaired engraftment in irradiated hosts. Blood 1996;87:30-37.

12 Yonemura Y, Hirayama F, Souza L et al. Interleukin 3 or interleukin 1 abrogates the reconstitution ability of hematopoietic stem cells. Proc Natl Acad Sci USA 1996;93:4040-4044.

13 Tisdale JF, Sellers DE, Agricola BA et al. Gene marking studies indicate that ex-vivo expansion of mobilized peripheral blood cells results in rapid initial engraftment but diminished long-term repopulating ability. Blood 1996;88:300a.

14 Kanz L, Brugger W. Mobilization and ex vivo manipulation of peripheral blood progenitor cells for support of high-dose cancer therapy. In: Blume KG, Thomas ED, eds. Hematopoietic Cell Transplantation. 2nd Edition. Boston: Blackwell Scientific Publications; 1998 (in press).

15 Bhalia M, Bonnet D, Knapp U et al. Quantitative analysis reveals expansion of human hematopoietic repopulating cells after short-term ex vivo culture. J Exp Med 1997;186:619-624.

16 McCulloch EA. Stem cell renewal and determination during clonal expansion in normal and leukaemic haemopoiesis. Cell Prolif 1993;26:399-425.

17 Jones RJ, Celano P, Sharkis SJ et al. Two phases of engraftment established by serial bone marrow transplantation in mice. Blood 1989;73:397-401.

18 Mielcarek M, Torok-Storb B. Modulation of adhesion receptor expression during ex vivo expansion of CD34$^+$ peripheral blood progenitor cells. Blood 1996;88:107a.

19 Williams SF, Lee WJ, Bender JG et al. Selection and expansion of peripheral blood CD34$^+$ cells in autologous stem cell transplantation for breast cancer. Blood 1996;87:1687-1691.

20 Scheding S, Franke H, Brugger W et al. How many myeloid post-progenitor cells have to be transplanted to completely abrogate neutropenia after high-dose chemotherapy and peripheral blood progenitor cell transplantation? Blood 1995;86:224a.

21 Scheding S, Meister B, Baum C et al. Flt-3 ligand promotes the ex-vivo generation of granulopoietic post-progenitor cells for clinical use after peripheral blood progenitor transplantation. Exp Hematol 1997;25:8a.

22 Scheding S, Buhring HJ, Ziegler B et al. Ex-vivo generation of myeloid post-progenitor cells from mobilized peripheral blood CD34$^+$ cells. Blood 1995;86:231a.

23 Kratz-Albers K, Scheding S, Mohle R et al. Large-scale generation of megakaryocytic cells from CD34$^+$ peripheral blood progenitors for clinical use after high-dose chemotherapy. Blood 1997;90:536a.

24 Bertolini F, Battaglia M, Pedrazzoli P et al. Megakaryocytic progenitors can be generated ex vivo and safely administered to autologous peripheral blood progenitor cell transplant recipients. Blood 1997;89:2679-2688.

25 Caux C, Dezutter-Dambuyant C, Schmitt D et al. GM-CSF and TNF-alpha cooperate in the generation of dendritic Langerhans cells. Nature 1992;360:258-261.

26 Caux C, Vanbervliet B, Massacrier C et al. Interleukin-3 cooperates with tumor necrosis factor alpha for the development of human dendritic/Langerhans cells from cord blood CD34$^+$ hematopoietic progenitor cells. Blood 1996;87:2376-2385.

27 Santiago-Schwarz F, Belilos E, Diamond B et al. TNF in combination with GM-CSF enhances the differentiation of neonatal cord blood stem cells into dendritic cells and macrophages. J Leukoc Biol 1992;52:274.

28 Strobl H, Riedl E, Scheinecker C et al. TGF-beta 1 promotes in vitro development of dendritic cells from CD34$^+$ hemopoietic progenitors. J Immunol 1996;157:1499-1507.

29 Flores-Romo L, Bjorck P, Duvert V et al. CD40 ligation on human cord blood CD34$^+$ hematopoietic progenitors induces their proliferation and differentiation into functional dendritic cells. J Exp Med 1997;185:341-349.

30 Szabolcs P, Moore MA, Young JW. Expansion of immunostimulatory dendritic cells among the myeloid progeny of human CD34$^+$ bone marrow precursors cultured with c-kit ligand, granulocyte-macrophage colony-stimulating factor, and TNF-alpha. J Immunol 1995;154:5851-5861.

31 Young JW, Szabolcs P, Moore MA. Identification of dendritic cell colony-forming units among normal human CD34$^+$ bone marrow progenitors that are expanded by c-kit-ligand and yield pure dendritic cell colonies in the presence of granulocyte/macrophage colony-stimulating factor and tumor necrosis factor alpha. J Exp Med 1995;182:1111-1119.

32 Siena S, Di NM, Bregni M et al. Massive ex vivo generation of functional dendritic cells from mobilized CD34$^+$ blood progenitors for anticancer therapy. Exp Hematol 1995;23:1463-1471.

33 Mackensen A, Herbst B, Kohler G et al. Delineation of the dendritic cell lineage by generating large numbers of Birbeck granule-positive Langerhans cells from human peripheral blood progenitor cells in vitro. Blood 1995;86:2699-2707.

34 Scheding S, Gruber I, Wirths S et al. FLT-3 ligand promotes the development and function of CD1a$^+$ cells generated ex-vivo from CD34$^+$ peripheral blood progenitor cells. Blood 1996;88:299a.

35 Scheding S, Wirths S, Buhring HJ et al. FLT-3 ligand, TGF-ß, and GM-CSF/IL-4 are critical growth factors for the induction of CD1a$^+$/CD14$^-$/CD80$^+$ dendritic cell (DC) development from CD34$^+$ PBPC in serum-free medium. Blood 1997;90:478a.

T Lymphocytes Determine the Development of Xeno GVHD and of Human Hemopoiesis in NOD/SCID Mice Following Human Umbilical Cord Blood Transplantation

Stefan F.F. Verlinden,[a,b] Andries H. Mulder,[c]
Johannes P. de Leeuw,[d] Dirk W. van Bekkum[a]

[a]Introgene BV, Leiden, The Netherlands; [b]Gene Therapy Section of the Department of
Molecular Biology Medical Faculty, Leiden University, The Netherlands;
[c]Pathologisch Laboratorium, Dordrecht, The Netherlands; [d]Department of Gynaecology,
Rijnland Hospital, Leiderdorp, The Netherlands

Key Words. *Xenogenic GVHD · Human stem cell transplantation · NOD/SCID mice · Human NOD/SCID chimera
· Human umbilical cord blood · T lymphocytes/monocytes/megakaryocytes*

Abstract

Over the past decade the human-immunodeficient mouse chimera has become a well-established in vivo model for studying the human immune system and/or hemopoiesis. Under certain experimental conditions and depending on the composition of the human cell graft, the recipient mice may develop a fatal disease, designated as discordant xenogenic graft-versus-host-disease (GVHD), which differs in target tissues and histopathology from allogenic GVHD. Experimental evidence is presented that immunodeficient mice are equally susceptible to allogenic GVHD as normal immunocompetent mice.

Whole human cord blood and distinct cellular subpopulations from a single cord blood harvest were transplanted in NOD/severe combined immunodeficient mice and the repopulation of human cells was monitored over time.

Depending on the ratio of lymphocytes to hemopoietic stem cells, proliferation of human T cells, hemopoiesis or a combination of the two is observed in widely varying proportions. When the graft contains a preponderance of lymphocytes, fatal protracted discordant xenogenic GVHD develops. Mice receiving purified CD34 cells survived up to 207 days in good health with more than 95% human cells in the bone marrow. In those mice all lineages (B and T lymphocytes, monocytes, granulocytes, erythrocytes and thrombocytes) were demonstrated in the bone marrow and peripheral blood. *Stem Cells 1998;16(suppl 1):205-217*

Introduction

Persistent engraftment leading to human lymphocyte proliferation and/or hemopoiesis can be obtained by grafting human peripheral blood (PB) [1], bone marrow (BM) [2], umbilical cord blood (CB) [3] or mobilized peripheral blood (MPB) [4] mononuclear cells (MNC) into hereditary immunodeficient mice. However, the take rate and level of engraftment varies considerably This variation can be ascribed to the various strains of immunodeficient mice employed by various groups. Within one

Characteristics and Potentials of Blood Stem Cells
Stem Cells **1998;16(suppl 1):205-217**

strain, engraftment can be improved by conditioning the recipients with high dose TBI or cyclophosphamide [5]. Other important determinants for engraftment are the cellular composition of the graft and the number of cells transplanted. These parameters also influence the composition of the human cells populating the recipient mice. If the graft contains predominantly lymphocytes, as is the case with (nonmobilized) PB MNC grafts, T and B lymphocytes proliferate in the recipient and infiltrate many tissues including the BM [1, 5-7]. When grafting BM, MPB or CB cells which contain both large numbers of lymphocytes and hematopoietic stem cells (HSC), the mice are repopulated by both human hematopoietic cells and lymphocytes in varying proportions [2, 3]. When transplanting T cell depleted or purified CD34 cells with or without [8] human cytokine support, human hemopoietic cells are dominating the blood forming tissues of the chimeric mice.

The engraftment barrier from human to mouse is much more pronounced than in some other xenogenic donor-host combinations, e.g., from rat to mouse or from Syrian hamster to mouse. These xenogenic combinations are categorized as discordant and concordant, respectively. With concordant combinations, heavy immunosuppression, as provided by a lethal dose of TBI as well as a certain minimal number of cells in the graft, is the main requirement for engraftment [9, 10]. In the case of discordance, an additional barrier is the presence of natural serum antibodies (Ab) which opsonize the donor cells. These Ab are absent in certain immunodeficient mouse strains, which explains their improved acceptance of human hemopoietic cell grafts. In normal mice the titers of the natural Ab against different donor blood groups vary, being highest for antihuman blood group A Ab [11]. Using grafts of human PB MNC, very large numbers of cells (1-2 $\times$ 10^7 per g body weight) can overcome the anti-B and anti-O natural Ab barrier probably by depletion of the Ab. Additional conditioning with cobra venom factor (to eliminate the third factor of complement) and with dichloromethylene diphosphate liposomes (to deplete the monocyte/macrophage system) is needed to abrogate the barrier against human blood group A cells. Furthermore, natural Ab titers are absent or minimal in newborn mice: in CBA/N mice (B cell deficient) until about three weeks of age and in normal mice which have been treated with anti-IgM Ab from birth. Such recipients were also shown to accept human cell grafts.

Interestingly, successful engraftment of human MNC resulting in large numbers of human lymphocytes in the recipient does not induce characteristic graft-versus-host-disease (GVHD) as seen following allogenic transplants (allo GVHD). Some, but not all authors have reported the occurrence of wasting and mortality in severe combined immunodeficiency syndrome (SCID) or BNX mice with human cell grafts and ascribed this to a GVH reaction [4, 6, 7, 12]. One of us has described the acute human versus mouse GVHD as a distinct histopathological entity, characteristic of discordant xenografts [5]. The main distinction of this syndrome, which we designated as disconcordant xeno GVHD (dx GVHD), from allo GVHD is the absence of lesions in the skin and the intestine, and the destruction of the BM of the host (mouse) by infiltrating human lymphocytes. As this novel form of GVHD was described in BNX, SCID and CBA/N mice, it had to be ascertained that the different manifestations of dx GVHD were not due to an inherent defect in the target tissues of the immunodeficient mice. In this paper we present evidence that BNX and SCID mice indeed develop the characteristic lesions of allo GVHD following irradiation and grafting with allogenic mouse BM and spleen cells.

We also describe a more protracted fatal syndrome that occurred in NOD/SCID mice after grafting of human whole CB and the post Ficoll (PF) fraction of CB cells. The histopathology of this syndrome closely resembles that described previously for acute dx GVHD. Evidence is presented that protracted dx GVHD is similarly induced by human T lymphocytes. It can be prevented by T cell depletion of the graft, in this case grafting of purified CD34^{bright} cells. Our data suggest that in these mice long-term repopulation with human hematopoietic cells of all lineages in both BM and PB is accompanied by a generation of human T lymphocytes which is no longer reacting against mouse tissues.

MATERIALS AND METHODS

Mice and Transplantation Procedures

Inbred CBA/Rij, C57BL/Rij, BCBA (C57BL×CBA F1 hybrid), CB17- and Balb/c SCID/SCID (SCID) and NOD/LtSz-SCID/SCID (NOD/SCID, Jackson Laboratories; Bar Harbor, ME) as well as random bred CBA/N (XID) and Bg/Nu/XID (BNX, stock kindly provided by *Dr. Sebesteny*, Imperial Cancer Research Fund; London, UK) were bred and kept under specific pathogen-free conditions in our own breeding colony. Animals of both sexes were used at the age of 4-30 weeks. Immunodeficient mice in experiments were housed in filter top cages which were kept and handled in sterile laminar cross flows. The immunodeficient mice were provided with acidified drinking water containing Polymyxin B 100 mg/l, Amphotericin B 200 mg/l, Ciproxin 100 mg/l and sugar 40 g/l. The normal mice received acidified water.

All mice were fed standard autoclaved pellets (AM2 Hope Farms; Woerden, The Netherlands) ad libitum.

TBI was performed with type 20 Gamma Cell (Atomic Energy of Canada; Ottawa, Canada), equipped with two opposing ^{137}Cs gamma ray sources providing a homogenous dose distribution. The dose rate at the position of the mice was 0.9 Gy/min. Cells were transplanted by i.v. injection in a volume of 0.5-1.0 ml within two h after TBI. No human cytokines were administered to the mice.

Murine Donor Cell Preparations

Mouse BM was collected by flushing the femurs of sacrificed mice with RPMI 1640 medium. A monocellular suspension was prepared by passing the samples through a filter consisting of four layers of 100 micron nylon gauze. Spleens were cut with scissors in RPMI medium into small pieces and the resulting mash was gently rubbed with a spatula and medium through a similar filter. Viable cells were counted in a hemocytometer in 0.4% trypan blue or 0.2% eosin.

CB Collection

CB was obtained from uncomplicated full term deliveries after clamping and cutting of the umbilical cord by using protocols approved by the Medical Ethical Committee of the Rijnland Hospital (Leiderdorp, The Netherlands). Collections were made while the placenta was still in utero. The blood was collected in a blood bag containing 13 ml CPDA-1 (NPBI; Emmer-Compascuum, The Netherlands) by inserting the 16-gauge needle into an umbilical vein and placing the bag below the needle point allowing the blood to flow by gravity.

Separation of CB Cells

Whole CB was used without lysis of the red cells. To obtain PF and purified CD34^{bright} cells one volume of hydroxyethyl starch 6% (w/v) (Sigma-Aldrich; Steinheim, Germany) was added to eight volumes of CB. The bag was stored for 30 min at 37°C. Next the contents of the bag were mixed and portions of 15 ml were layered onto 10 ml Ficoll-Paque (Pharmacia Biotech; Uppsala, Sweden). After 20 min centrifugation at 800 g, the layer of light density cells was collected, washed in phosphate buffered saline and resuspended in MACS buffer (phosphate-buffered saline containing 0.5% [w/v] bovine serum albumin [Sigma-Aldrich] and 2 mM EDTA).

CD34^{bright} cells were purified from the PF fraction by magnetic cell sorting (MACS, Miltenyi Biotec; Bergisch Gladbach, Germany) according to the manufacturer's protocol. Purity of the CD34^{bright} cell fraction was at least 90%.

Cell Preparation for Flow Cytometric Analyses

Mouse BM was either harvested from the femurs of sacrificed mice or from living mice by femur puncture as described elsewhere [13]. By this technique on the average $\pm 1.6 \times 10^6$ (range 0.1-3.6) nucleated cells (NC) can be collected. PB blood was collected also under anesthesia, by retro orbital puncture.

PB samples were diluted in a 10-fold volume of lysis buffer (NH_4CL 8.32 g/l, $NaHCO_3$ 1.04 g/l, Na_2EDTA 0.037 g/l).

Flow Cytometric (FACS) Determination of Chimerism and Phenotype of Human Cells

The analysis of BM and PB cells of the mice transplanted with human cells was performed on a FACSort machine (Becton-Dickinson; San Jose, CA). The following monoclonal antibodies (mAb) were used: antihuman CD45 fluorescein isothiocyanate (FITC) or PerCP, antihuman CD34 phycoery-thrin (PE), antihuman CD2 FITC, antihuman CD3 biotin, antihuman CD4 PE, antihuman CD8 FITC, antihuman CD11b PE, antihuman CD15 FITC, antihuman CD20 PE, antihuman CD33 FITC, antihuman CD56 PE, antihuman CD61 FITC, antihuman CD71 FITC, murine IgG1 isotype control FITC, murine IgG1 isotype control PE, strepavidin PE or PerCP (all from Becton-Dickinson), antihuman CD64 FITC (Medarex; Annadale, NJ), antihuman glycophorin A PE (DAKO; Glostrup, Denmark), antihuman CD38 FITC (Pharmingen; Hamburg, Germany) and antimurine CD11a PE (Caltag Laboratories, San Francisco, CA).

To determine the percentage of human NC in the BM of chimeric mice each sample (10^5 NC) was stained with 5 µl antihuman CD45 FITC and 5 µl antimurine CD11a PE. The percentage human NC ($CD45^+$) was calculated by dividing the number of human NC by the total number of NC ($CD45^+$ and $CD11a^+$) and multiplying this by 100 (Fig. 1). Phenotype of the human NC was determined by three color flow cytometric analysis. In all cocktails of mAb, CD45 PerCP or FITC was always present. One mAb combination called lineage marker (lin) is a mixture of antihuman CD33, 38 and 71 all labeled with FITC. By gating out $CD45^+$ cells all human NC are detected. Subsequently the phenotype is presented as percentage of human NC. All mAb used, except for CD11b are species specific, as verified in BM from normal mice and in fresh CB. Human and murine CD11b cells are distinguished by CD45; only human cells are $CD45^+CD11^+$.

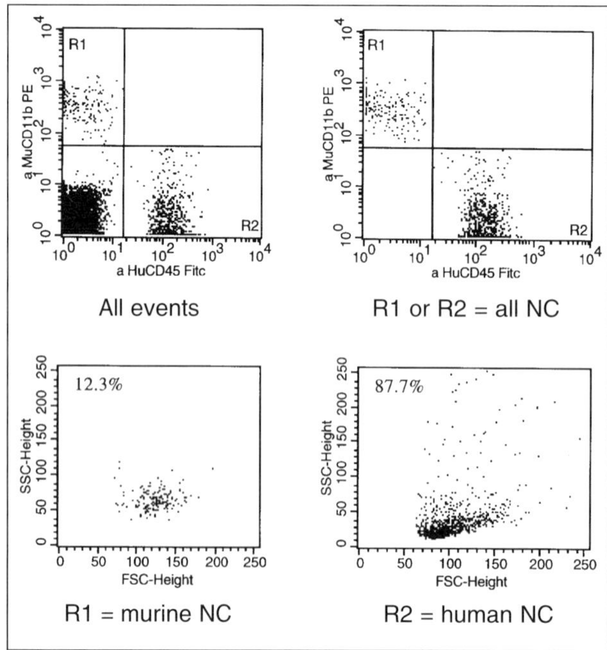

Figure 1. Flow cytometric analysis of a BM sample obtained by puncture of a chimeric mouse at day 31 after transplanting 10^6 CD34^{bright} cells. This representative sample contains 12.3% murine NC and 87.7% human NC.

Histopathology

Following gross necropsy, tissue samples were fixed in 4% phosphate buffered formalin for routine processing in paraffin and staining with hematoxylin and eosin. Specific immunohistochemistry was performed on five micron thick paraffin sections using the following primary mouse mAb: antihuman CD45, antihuman CD45RO, antihuman CD20 (BioGenex; San Ramon, CA), antihuman CD20 (DAKO), and antihuman CD3 (Novacastra Laboratories; Newcastle, UK). To visualize the cells a secondary labeling was performed with an antimouse mAb labeled with peroxidase. An enzymatic reaction with DAP H_2O_2 stained the labeled cells brown in a blue background.

Human granulocytes were detected by staining with napthol AS-D chloroacetate esterase (Leder).

RESULTS

Induction of Allo GVHD in BNX and SCID Mice

In pilot experiments groups of BNX mice were exposed to graded doses of radiation and BM or BM plus spleen cells to establish conditions for clinical GVHD to develop and sufficient survival to perform histology at various time points. This resulted in a regimen for BNX mice of 8.5 Gy TBI and 10^6 BM cells or 10^6 BM and 5×10^6 spleen cells from C57BL donor mice. Normal control CBA mice received 10 Gy TBI, 10^7 BM cells and 10^6 spleen cells from C57BL donors. One to four animals (usually two) were sacrificed at the time points shown in Table 1. At each time point mice with overt symptoms of GVHD were selected, if present. Otherwise, mice were picked at random. Characteristic lesions were observed in the three main target tissues of allo GVHD. There was no difference between the incidence of the lesions in BNX mice and CBA mice treated with BM and spleen cells. There were fewer mice with lesions, in particular of the intestines, among BNX mice treated with BM only, as compared to the BNX mice grafted with BM and spleen, which is to be expected from the established GVHD initiating role of T lymphocytes. In mouse BM the percentage of T lymphocytes is no more than a few percent.

The lesions observed in the BNX tissues did not differ from those seen in the CBA mice, both showing the classical picture of crypt necrosis in the colon, acanthosis, dyskeratosis and hyperkeratosis in the epidermis and periportal mononuclear cell infiltration with scattered parenchymal cell necrosis in the liver.

SCID mice are known to be much more radiosensitive than normal mice. They were subjected to graded sublethal doses of TBI and grafted with a fixed number of 10^6 BM cells and graded numbers of spleen cells from CBA donors (Table 2). In most groups the mice died after a relatively short interval with severe diarrhea and emaciation. As autolysis sets in shortly after death in mice,

Table 1. Histological lesions characteristic for allo GVHD after transplantation of allogenic BM and spleen

Recipients	Graft	5	9	15	20	26	30	58
					Intestines			
BNX	BM	00	00	00	00	01	01	02
						23		
	BM + spl	01	11	01	12	02	22	02
CBA	BM + spl	02	11	00	00		02	23
					Liver			
BNX	BM		00	02	22	12	00	1
	BM + spl	00	02	22	02	22	22	22
CBA	BM + spl	00	00	22	22		22	22
					Skin			
BNX	BM	01	22	01	01	01	00	0
	BM + spl	00	2	01	11	11	12	12
CBA	BM + spl	00	11	22	22		22	22

Severity of lesions indicated by single digit figures, one for each mouse analyzed as follows: 0 = normal, 1 = slight, 2 = moderate, 3 = widespread and severe.
BNX mice were conditioned with 8.5 Gy TBI and grafted with 10^6 BM cells with or without 5×10^6 spleen cell (spl).
CBA mice were conditioned with 10 Gy and grafted with 10^7 BM cells and 10^6 spleen cells.
Donors were C57BL mice.

we sacrificed some of the animals when moribund and thus obtained evaluable tissues from several mice in each group. These showed the characteristic colitis and dermatitis. The liver lesions, however, were dominated by widespread necrosis of the parenchyma and in some cases infiltration of biliary ducts with mononuclear cells. This pronounced affection of the liver has been described in all species in cases of severe hyperacute GVHD [9]. Nontransplanted mice did not die. Some of the latter were sacrificed between 5 and 10 days after irradiation (two Gy). These mice did not show any of the lesions described above.

It is apparent from these findings that SCID mice are as sensitive as, if not more sensitive to allogenic T lymphocytes than normal mouse strains. We also observed moderate nonfatal GVHD dominated by diarrhea in nonirradiated SCID mice after grafting with 5×10^6 spleen cells from BCBA mice. These lesions of allo GVHD are easily distinguished from those found in both BNX and SCID mice after transplantation with large numbers of human PBC [5].

Engraftment of Human CB Fractions and Phenotype of Human Cells

Groups of three NOD/SCID mice were sublethally irradiated (2.5 Gy) and injected i.v. with either 2×0.5 ml (one h interval) whole CB containing a total number of 10^7 NC, 10^7 PF NC in 0.5 ml, 10^5 CD34^{bright} cells in 0.5 ml or 10^6 CD34^{bright} cells in 0.5 ml, all from a single CB collection.

At day 31 post-transplantation, BM and PB of the mice were obtained by femur and retro-orbital puncture. The cell content of the BM sample of one NOD/SCID grafted with PF cells was too low ($<10^5$ NC) for a complete FACS analysis; it was used to determine chimerism only. Figure 2 shows that all mice except those grafted with 10^5 CD34^{bright} cells acquired high levels of chimerism in both BM (21%-91%) and PB (9%-70%) at day 31 after transplantation. The three mice that did not graft were used as negative controls. There was no significant difference ($p > 0.5$ Student's t test) in the level of chimerism in the BM between the groups that showed engraftment. In the PB however, the level of engraftment in mice transplanted with 10^6 CD34^{bright} cells is significantly higher ($p < 0.01$ Student's t test) than those transplanted with whole CB.

Table 2. Survival time (days) of SCID mice after TBI and grafting of CBA spleen and BM (10^6) cells[1]

TBI dose	—	10^6	2×10^6	3×10^6	5×10^6
		Number of spleen cells			
2 Gy				4.6	
3 Gy		$>70^2$	5.4		5.0
4 Gy	6.7				4.0^3

[1]Mean, $n = 10$ per group except for [3]$n = 20$.
[2]All mice showed pronounced GVHD, 50% mortality.

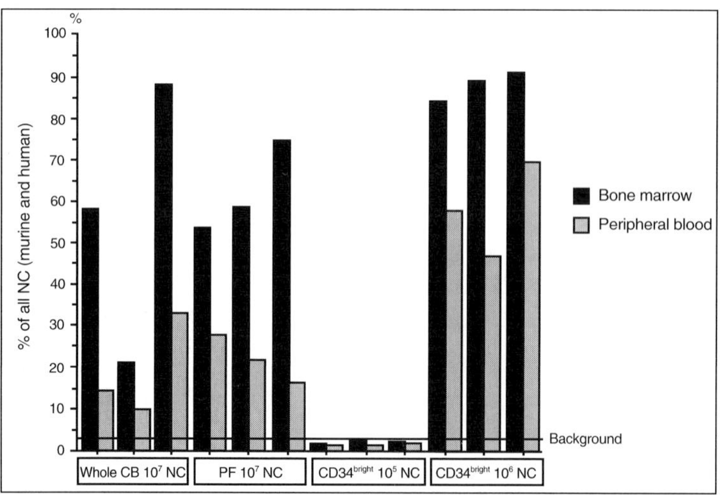

Figure 2. Human CD45⁺ NC in human-NOD/SCID mice BM and PB at 31 days after transplantation. *Four groups of three mice were transplanted with whole CB, PF, 10^5 CD34^{bright} and 10^6 CD34^{bright} cells, respectively.*

Between 4-12 weeks after the grafting of whole CB or PF cells the condition of the mice deteriorated; they became anemic and failed to gain weight. All mice, except one, died without symptoms of classical GVHD, i.e., diarrhea and skin lesions. Mice in the groups grafted with sufficient (10^6) or insufficient (10^5) numbers of CD34^{bright} cells all survived for more than 142 days, in excellent condition. At day 142 BM was obtained from all mice by puncture; unfortunately, one mouse (mouse no. 1) died during anesthesia. FACS analyses revealed high levels of chimerism in the BM (>90%) and PB (>35%) of all mice transplanted with 10^6 CD34^{bright} cells. Of the human cells in the PB of mouse 1, 43% were CD20$^+$ (B cell), 9% CD11b$^+$ (myeloid), 43% CD2$^+$CD3$^+$CD4^{++} (T$_h$) and 5% CD2$^+$CD3$^+$CD8$^+$ (T$_c$) phenotype. Figure 3 shows FACS analyses results of mouse 1 and 2 PB cells stained with CD45 PerCP, CD3 PE and CD8 FITC or CD45 PerCP, CD2 FITC and CD4 PE. In the BM large numbers of cells with the B

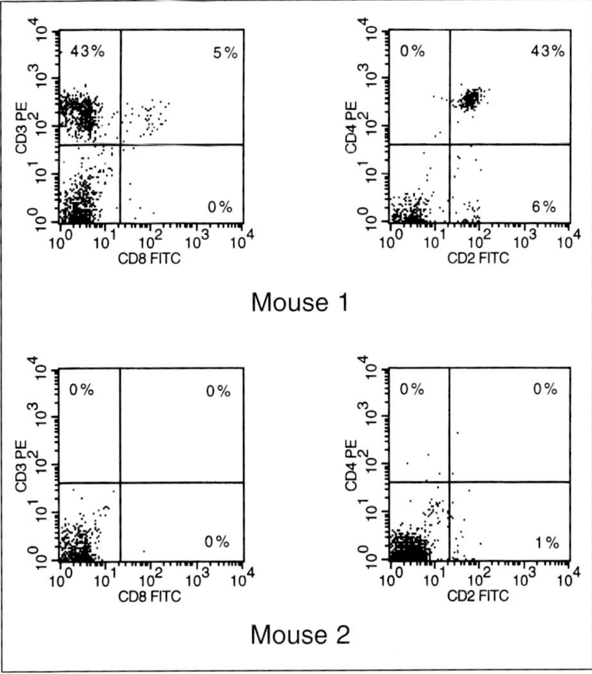

Figure 3. CD2$^+$CD3$^+$CD4^{++} and CD2$^+$CD3$^+$CD8$^+$ T lymphocytes in PB of human-NOD/SCID mouse 142 days after transplantation with 10^6 CD34^{bright} cells. Both mice nos. 1 and 2 are transplanted with similar numbers of CD34^{bright} cells from the same CB sample. PB of chimeric mice was stained with a cocktail of CD45 PerCP, CD3 PE and CD8 FITC or CD45 PerCP, CD2 FITC and CD4 PE. Mouse no. 1 showed high numbers of Th (43%) and Tc (5%) lymphocytes in the PB. In mice nos. 2 and 3 no such cells could be detected. Only mouse no. 2 is shown.

cell (>75%) and myeloid phenotype (>15%) were found, but the number of T cells was lower (<10%). The latter were exclusively CD2$^+$CD3$^+$CD4$^+$, a phenotype (CD4^{dim}) not found in the PB. The BM of the other two mice (mice nos. 2 and 3) grafted with 10^6 CD34^{bright} cells contained only 5% T lymphocytes, also expressing the CD4^{dim} phenotype. In the PB only 1% CD2$^+$CD4$^-$ cells and no CD4^{bright} cells could be detected (Fig. 3, mouse no. 2). At day 207 similar results were obtained with mouse no. 2.

The survival time of the chimeras in the various groups was found to be inversely related to the frequency of distinct mature human cell populations. Mice with the highest numbers of T lymphocytes and monocytes in the PB and/or BM, at day 31, had the shortest life span (Table 3). On the contrary, mice with the lowest frequency of human T lymphocytes and a high frequency of B lymphocytes or mice which did not take the graft, all survived for more than 140 days.

Histology

In the group grafted with whole CB the first mouse died at day 42; only the skin and intestines were examined and showed no pathology. The second mouse was sacrificed on day 48 in very poor condition. Large numbers of activated human T cells were found in the spleen, lungs, BM and, to a lesser extent, in the kidneys and liver (Fig. 4). In the spleen the T lymphocytes were predominantly present in the white pulpa as dense periarteriolar sheets. Aggregates of B lymphocytes were also

Table 3. Survival of chimeras versus frequency of mature human cells in BM and PB at 31 days after transplantation

Graft	Survival in days	% in BM			% in PB		
		T lymphocytes	B lymphocytes	Monocytes/macrophages	T lymphocytes	B lymphocytes	Monocytes/macrophages
Whole CB	52	12.7	36.6	29.3	38.9	9.5	ND
PF	82	1.8	59.4	13.8	12.6	35.1	ND
10^6 CD34^{++}	>140	0.5	54.3	5.4	1.7	56.0	ND

present intermingled with small numbers of T cells. The red pulpa contained moderate numbers of diffusely spread T lymphocytes. In the lungs, the alveolar interstitium was heavily infiltrated with activated human T cells, the picture resembling that of an interstitial pneumonitis. There was also infiltration of human T lymphocytes in the wall of the larger vessels of the lungs; B lymphocytes were present in small clusters adjacent to bronchi. In sections of the skin and the intestines no human T cells were seen, except for an occasional T lymphocyte in a vessel wall. These tissues showed no abnormalities (Fig. 4).

The BM was poorly populated with hemopoietic cells and in some sites even aplastic (Fig. 5). Activated human T cells were abundantly present, suggesting ongoing destruction of mouse BM similar to that described previously by one of us in the BM of immunodeficient mice grafted with large numbers of normal human PB leukocytes [5]. Previous FACS analysis of BM of the same mouse on day 31 also revealed large numbers of human T lymphocytes and, additionally, 30% human monocytes. The mice grafted with PF cells died on days 47, 66 and 131, respectively (average survival was 82 days). Unfortunately, all three cadavers were found when already autolytic.

The two mice of the group grafted with CD34^{bright} cells that were autopsied on day 142 (mouse no. 1) and 207 (mouse no. 2), respectively did not show histological abnormalities. Specifically, T cell infiltrates were not present in the lungs and the BM. Furthermore, the BM which contained more than 90% human cells by FACS showed abundant myelopoietic and erythropoietic activity as well as many human megakaryocytes. In the spleen, extensive murine hemopoiesis was present, with large numbers of human B cells in the white pulpa. In mouse no. 1 moderate numbers of activated T lymphocytes were found with a normal distribution pattern in the white pulpa. In mouse no. 2, autopsied on day 207, few human T lymphocytes were observed in all organs.

One control mouse, grafted with 10^5 CD34^{bright} cells was also sacrificed at day 207. The tissues of this mouse were normal, except for some infiltrates of MNC in the lungs and the kidney possibly due to early stage lymphoma. Human cells were not present in the tissues of this mouse, which is in concordance with the FACS results.

Human CD34^{bright}lin$^+$ and CD34^{bright}lin$^-$ in Chimeric Mice

In the groups grafted with whole CB, PF cells or purified CD34 cells, 1/3, 2/2 and 3/3 mice, respectively, showed levels of CD34^{bright} cells of more than 1% above background and detectable levels of CD34^{bright}lin$^-$ cells (Fig. 6). Only small differences were found in the percentage of CD34^{bright} cells in the BM of mice grafted with whole CB (1.6), PF cells (1.7) and 10^6 CD34^{bright} cells (2.8) which is surprising in view of the widely different numbers of CD34^{bright} cells grafted: 5×10^4, 10^5 and 10^6, respectively. It can be calculated that in mice grafted with whole CB or PF cells a 48-96-fold expansion of CD34^{bright} cells had occurred by day 31, whereas in mice grafted with CD34 cells the expansion was only eightfold (Table 4). The same calculations for CD34^{bright}lin$^-$ cells yield an expansion of 600-2,400-fold for mice transplanted with PF cells and whole CB and only 90-fold for those transplanted with 10^6 CD34^{bright} cells.

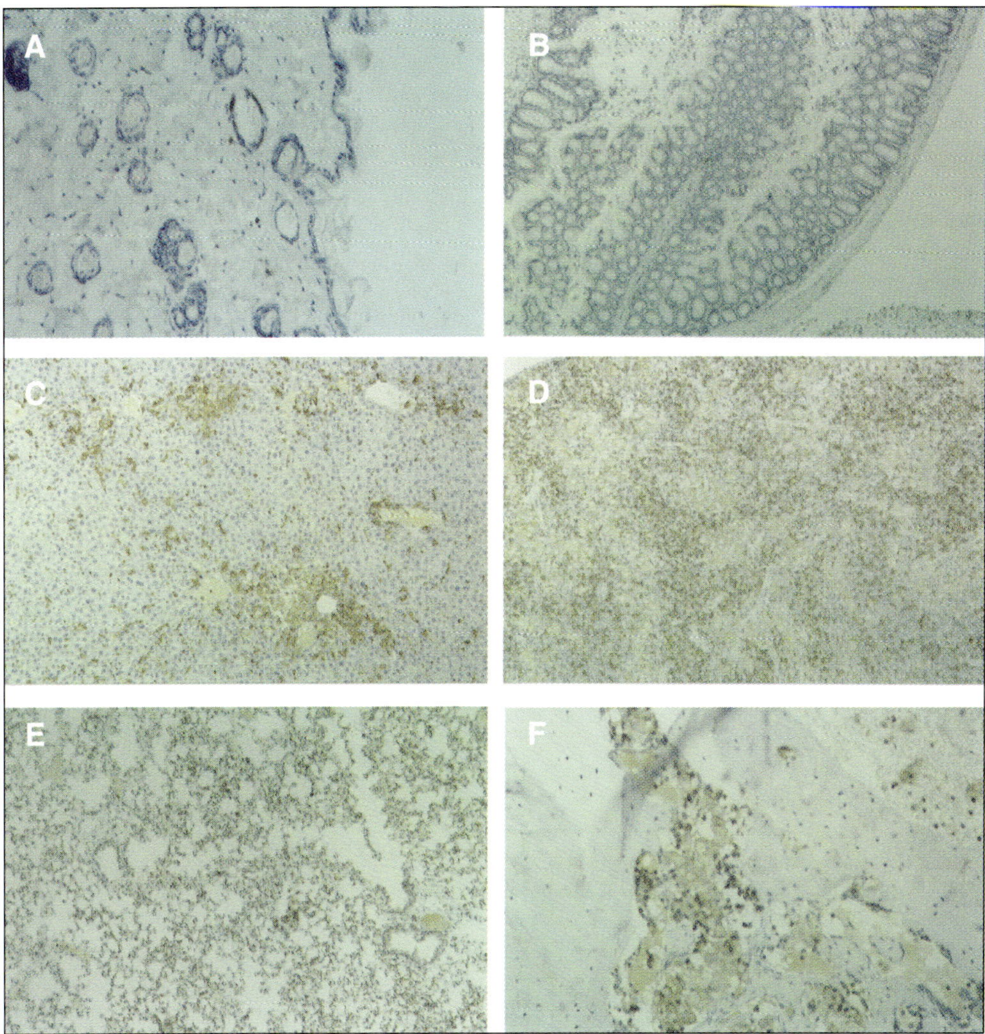

Figure 4. Immunohistopathology at day 48 of mouse transplanted with whole CB. *Sections of the skin (A), intestine (B), liver (C), spleen (D), lungs (E) and BM (F). Activated T lymphocytes were detected in paraffin sections by labeling with an antihuman CD45 RO mAb followed by an immunoperoxidase reaction which stains labeled cells brown. Nonlabeled cells are blue. Typically no signs of allo GVHD are found in the skin and intestine. The liver shows moderate and the spleen, BM and lungs show heavy infiltration with activated T cells. Infiltrated T cells cause aplasia in the BM and interstitial pneumonitis in the lungs.*

DISCUSSION

The absence of characteristic lesions of classical GVHD in the gut and the skin as well as of the related clinical symptoms of diarrhea and dermatitis in human-(immunodeficient) mice chimeras raised the question whether some host components required for the development of the allo GVH reaction might be missing. After all, the delayed form of allo GVHD which occurs after grafting of moderate numbers of allogenic major histocompatibility complex disparate BM cells is largely prevented by thymectomy of the recipients, in contrast to the acute form of GVHD [14, 15].

Our results leave no doubt that hereditary immunodeficient mice develop similar lesions in the same target tissues as immunocompetent mice after transplantation of allogenic BM and/or spleen cells. The completely different disease pattern and histopathology that has been observed in mice following transplantation and engraftment of human cells from BM or PB must therefore be due to species barriers in this disconcordant xenogenic combination. Similar to allo GVHD the effector cells of dx GVHD are the T lymphocytes, and the more T lymphocytes administered the higher the morbidity and mortality and the more rapidly its development. However while allo GVHD is characterized by lymphatic atrophy and a relative scarcity of T lymphocytes even within the target tissues, in dx GVHD excessive proliferation of T lymphocytes occurs in a variety of tissues leading to their destruction. Among these locations are the alveolar septa in the lung, the vessel walls in many locations, and the BM. In contrast to allo GVHD the destructive process does not seem to be accompanied by an inflammatory reaction.

The most rapidly progressing fatal dx GVHD is induced with large numbers of T lymphocytes from normal human PB, as described previously, causing death between 6 and 12 days after transplantation [5].

A more protracted but not less fatal dx GVHD as occurred in our experiments with whole CB and FP CB cells, has been reported by others, after transplanting lower numbers of human cells of various sources into SCID mice. *Pflumio et al.* transplanted sublethally irradiated newborn SCID mice i.p. with $5\text{-}20 \times 10^6$ PB lymphocytes or BM MNC. Almost 50% of the highly engrafted mice became moribund and had to be killed for analysis four weeks after transplantation. At that time, these mice were anemic and weighed 50% less than their normal littermates. The deterioration was closely related to the numbers of human T lymphocytes in the BM. Microscopic examination and immunohistochemical staining showed abundant infiltration of human lymphocytes in the spleen, the lungs and the liver. No infiltration or necrosis was found in the intestines or the skin [6]. The BM was not examined microscopically. These authors pointed out some differences in the histopathology of their animals and those described by *Huppes et al.*, who grafted adult mice with large numbers of PB leukocytes, e.g., an atrophic spleen instead of an enlarged spleen, and peribronchial instead of perivascular infiltrates in the lungs. In our view these differences relate to a milder and more prolonged course of the dx GVHD in the experiments of

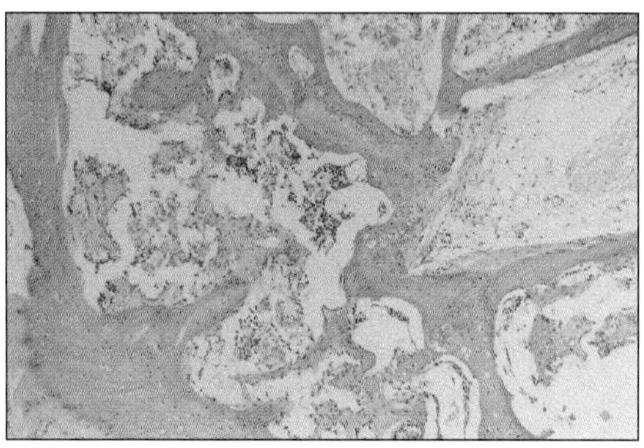

Figure 5. Hematoxylin and eosin staining at day 48 of mouse BM transplanted with whole CB. BM is poorly populated with hemopoietic cells.

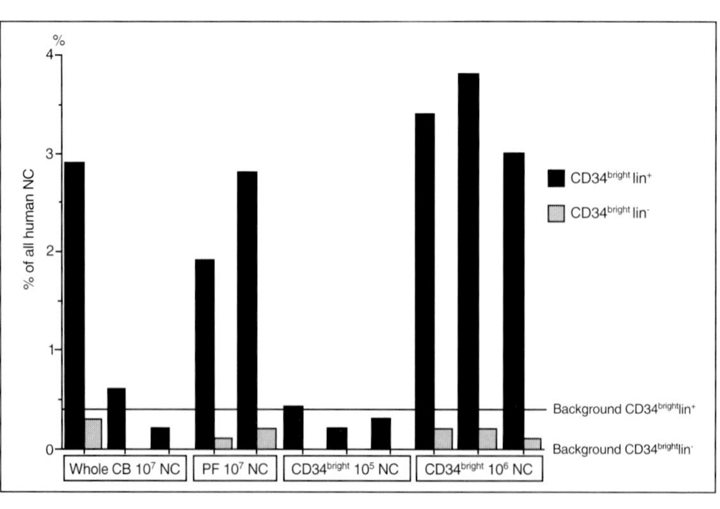

Figure 6. Human HSC in human-NOD/SCID mice BM 31 days after transplantation. Four groups of three mice were transplanted with whole CB, PF, 10^5 CD34^bright and 10^6 CD34^bright cells, respectively. Percentages of CD34^bright and CD34^bright lin^- cells are shown. Background is due to autofluorescence in some murine cells and is 0.4% in the CD34^bright fraction and 0.0% in the CD34^bright lin^- fraction.

Table 4. CD34^{bright}lin$^+$ and CD34^{bright}lin$^-$ cells in different human CB fractions

Cells transplanted

Fraction human CB	Total NC (10^6)	CD34^{bright}lin$^+$		CD34^{bright}lin$^-$	
		%	Total (10^4)	%	Total (10^2)
WB	10	0.5	5	0.005	5
PF	10	1.0	10	0.01	10
10^5 CD34	0.1	100	10	1	10
10^6 CD34	1	100	100	1	100

Cells recovered from chimera after grafting

Fraction human CB	Total NC (10^6)	CD34^{bright}lin$^+$		CD34^{bright}lin$^-$	
		%	Total (10^4)	%	Total (10^2)
WB	300*	1.6	480	0.4	12,000
PF	300	1.7	510	0.2	6,000
10^5 CD34	300	0.0	0	0.0	0
10^6 CD34	300	2.8	840	0.3	9,000

Expansion of human CB subsets in 31 days

Fraction human CB	CD34^{bright}lin$^+$ fold expansion	CD34^{bright}lin$^-$ fold expansion
WB	96	2,400
PF	48	600
10^5 CD34	0	0
10^6 CD34	8.4	90

*Total number of nucleated BM cells is 3×10^8 [9]. Cell numbers remain equal after grafting of human cells (data not shown).

Pflumio. Goan et al. grafted MPB cells in unirradiated SCID mice aged four to five weeks. After i.v. transplantation all animals died within nine weeks with symptoms of dx GVHD [4]. When the same numbers of cells were injected i.p. no symptoms of dx GVHD were observed for up to 24 weeks. Low levels (2%-20%) of human cells were found in the BM of the latter chimeras; phenotypically the human fraction consisted of B lymphocytes, myeloid cells and hemopoietic progenitor cells. T lymphocytes were present in the PB but not in the BM of these mice. The occurrence of dx GVHD after i.v. administration of cells and its absence after i.p. administration is consistent with our observations that 50 times more lymphocytes are required via the i.p. route than via the i.v. route for inducing allo GVHD in lethally irradiated mice [16].

Histological lesions consistent with protracted dx GVHD were observed in unirradiated NOD/SCID mice at eight weeks after i.p. administration of 2×10^7 PB MNC but not in similarly treated SCID mice [7]. Nearly all human cells detected in the spleen and the peripheral blood of the engrafted mice were activated T lymphocytes. The NOD/SCID mice had 10%-35% of these cells in the PB, against 1% in the SCID mice. This different engraftment must be explained by the fact that NOD/SCID mice have an extra defect in their innate immunity on top of an adaptive immune defect which both strains share [17].

Lowry et al. reported 27% mortality in sublethally irradiated NOD/SCID mice three to five weeks after the i.v. injection of 1 ml of whole CB. These animals suffered from runting, wasting and weight loss. The skin and intestines did not show allo GVHD lesions [12].

In our hands the NOD/SCID mice transplanted with whole CB or PF MNC died of dx GVHD on average after 52 and 82 days, respectively. The most notable pathological changes were infiltration with human T lymphocytes of the alveolar interstitium of the lungs and BM aplasia. The BM, which was heavily infiltrated with activated T cells, additionally contained many human (CD64$^+$) monocytes/macrophages (Table 3). Some of these mice showed significant human myelopoiesis. Human B lymphocytes were found in all animals. Proliferation of T lymphocytes and hemopoiesis seemed to be inversely related: more human hemopoiesis was seen in the animals grafted with PF cells than in those given whole CB.

The mice transplanted with T cell depleted grafts, i.e., CD34^{bright} cells, survived up to 207 days without signs of disease or histopathological evidence of dx GVHD. More than 95% of all BM cells were human and all lineages (B and T lymphocytes, monocytes, granulocytes, erythrocytes and thrombocytes) could be identified in both BM and PB. Two of the three mice had only less than 5% T cells in the BM and the PB. In the third mouse the numbers of T cells increased in the PB to reach 50%. Yet this mouse showed no signs of dx GVHD. Possibly, these late appearing T lymphocytes arise from primitive stem cells and acquire host tolerance in the process.

In conclusion, after transplanting immunodeficient mice with grafts containing high numbers of immunocompetent MNC and low numbers of HSC (PB MNC), T cell proliferation is predominant causing acute or more protracted lethal dx GVHD depending on the number of MNC grafted and the route of administration. Interestingly, myeloablation does not influence this process. When transplanting human cell populations with both high numbers of immunocompetent MNC and HSC (BM, MPB and CB) a similar pattern of dx GVHD is found accompanied by more profound hemopoiesis with high levels of B lymphocytes and myeloid cells in both BM and PB.

If high numbers of purified HSC (CB) are transplanted no dx GVHD is found, and nearly complete long-term repopulation of the mouse BM with human HSC accompanied by differentiation into all lineages takes place.

Similar levels of engrafted HSC were found in the three groups of mice grafted with whole CB, PF or 10^6 CD34^{bright} cells, although the absolute number of CD34^{bright} cells administered is only about 5 $\times$ 10^4 with whole CB and about 10^5 with PF cells. On the other hand, 10^5 purified CD34^{bright} cells did not engraft. We postulate that the coengraftment of T lymphocytes enhances the take of stem cells due to stimulation of their proliferation shortly after homing by the secretion of human specific hemopoietic growth factors. In fact, *Goan et al.* were able to demonstrate the presence of substantial levels of human interleukin 3, human interleukin 6 and human GM-CSF in the serum of unconditioned SCID mice for at least 12 weeks after i.p injection of fresh MPB MNC [4].

Furthermore, *Larochelle et al.* obtained long term engraftment with as few as 5 $\times$ 10^4 CD34^{bright} cells from CB provided the mice were treated with human hemopoietic growth factors [18].

Apparently, when human cytokine support is provided either by human lymphocytes in the graft or by injecting cytokines, 10 times less HSC is required for equivalent engraftment levels. Since our purified CD34^{bright} samples, in some cases, contained less than 3% contamination, it has to be concluded that stem cells can facilitate their own engraftment in a xenogenic environment provided at least 5 $\times$ 10^5 are grafted (data from our lab, not presented here). It remains to be established if this facilitating mechanism is based on the production of human cytokines. Further insight into the proliferation kinetics of the grafted stem cells, especially shortly after homing, would be valuable for improving present gene transfer protocols for hemopoietic stem cells.

ACKNOWLEDGMENTS

The authors' thanks are due to *Harry Brok* for his excellent technical assistance, the staff of the Department of Gynaecology, Rijnland Hospital, Leiderdorp, The Netherlands, for collecting the CB samples, *Dr. Shoshan Knaän-Shanzer* for critical reading of the manuscript, and *Professor Peter J. Heidt* of the Biomedical Primate Research Centre, Rijswijk, The Netherlands, who kindly advised us on the gnotobiological issues.

This study was supported by a grant from the Mercury Phoenix Trust.

REFERENCES

1 Mosier DE, Gulizia RJ, Baird SM et al. Transfer of a functional human immune system to mice with severe combined immunodeficiency. Nature 1988;335:257-259.

2 Kamel-Reid S, Dick JE. Engraftment of immune-deficient mice with human hematopoietic stem cells. Science 1988;242:1706-1709.

3 Vormoor J, Lapidot T, Pflumio F et al. Immature human cord blood progenitors engraft and proliferate to high levels in severe combined immunodeficient mice. Blood 1994;83:2489-2497.

4 Goan SR, Fichtner I, Just U et al. The severe combined immunodeficient-human peripheral blood stem cell (SCID-huPBSC) mouse: a xenotransplant model for huPBSC-initiated hematopoiesis. Blood 1995;86:89-100.

5 Huppes W, de Geus B, Zurcher C et al. Acute human vs. mouse graft vs. host disease in normal and immunodeficient mice. Eur J Immunol 1992;22:197-206.

6 Pflumio F, Lapidot T, Murdoch B et al. Engraftment of human lymphoid cells into newborn SCID mice leads to graft-versus-host disease. Int Immunol 1993;5:1509-1522.

7 Hesselton RM, Greiner DL, Mordes JP et al. High levels of human peripheral blood mononuclear cell engraftment and enhanced susceptibility to human immunodeficiency virus type 1 infection in NOD/LtSz-scid/scid mice. J Infect Dis 1995;172:974-982.

8 Verlinden SFF, Knaan-Shanzer S, Valerio D et al. Engraftment and hematopoiesis of purified human umbilical cord blood CD34+ cells in NOD-SCID mice. Blood 1996;88(suppl 1):45a.

9 van Bekkum DW, de Vries MJ. Radiation Chimeras. London and New York: Logos Press Limited, Academic Press, Inc., 1967:57-59

10 van Bekkum DW. A new heterologous radiation chimera. Nature 1964;202:1311-1312.

11 Huppes W, Paulonis J, Dijk H et al. The role of natural antibodies and ABO (H) blood groups in transplantation of human lymphoid cells into mice. Eur J Immunol 1993;23:26-32.

12 Lowry PA, Schultz LD, Greiner DL et al. Improved engraftment of human cord blood stem cells in NOD/LtSz-scid/scid mice after irradiation or multiple-day injection into unirradiated recipients. Biol Bone Marrow Transplant 1996;2:15-23.

13 Verlinden SFF, van Es HG, van Bekkum DW. Serial bone marrow sampling for long term follow up of human hemopoiesis in NOD/SCID mice. Exp Hematol (in press).

14 van Putten LM. Thymectomy: effect on secondary disease in radiation chimeras. Science 1964;145:935-937.

15 O'Kunewick JP, Meredith RF, Braunschweiger PG et al. Definition and prevention of GvH disease with the use of monoclonal antibodies. Exp Hematol 1982;10(suppl 12):12-16.

16 van Bekkum DW. Use and abuse of hemopoietic cell grafts in immune deficiency diseases. Transplant Rev 1972;9:3-53.

17 Schultz LD, Schweitzer PA, Christianson SW et al. Multiple defects in innate and adaptive immunologic function in NOD/LtSz-scid mice. J Immunol 1995;154:180-191.

18 Larochelle A, Vormoor J, Hanenberg H et al. Identification of primitive human hematopoietic cells capable of repopulating NOD/SCID mouse bone marrow: implications for gene therapy. Nat Med 1996;2:1329-1337.

Amplification of True Hemopoietic Stem Cells: Possibilities and Limitations

IRIS FRIESECKE,[a] GERARD WAGEMAKER[b]

[a]Institut für Arbeits- und Sozialmedizin, University of Ulm, Germany, and
[b]Institute of Hematology, Erasmus University, Rotterdam, The Netherlands

Panelists and contributors: Dirk W. van Bekkum, Hal E. Broxmeyer, Albert B. Deisseroth, Connie J. Eaves, Theodor M. Fliedner, Lothar Kanz, Philippe Hénon, Makio Ogawa, Peter J. Quesenberry, Gerard Wagemaker, Benedikt L. Ziegler.

The panel discussion was structured by sequentially discussing the validity and predictive value of stem cell assays and surface markers, the stromal and growth factor requirements for stem cell expansion and gene transfer, and the possibility of stem cell impairment due to in vitro or in vivo manipulation.

Stem Cell Assays and Surface Markers

There was a general consensus that the ultimate stem cell assay consists of a long-term, competitive repopulation assay, which is feasible in congenic mice donor/recipient pairs. It was also felt that the human/SCID chimeric mouse is the best alternative to monitor ex vivo manipulation of human stem cells. The latter assay, however, has limitations and quantitation is difficult to accomplish. Advocated were the use of the long-term culture initiating cells (LTC-IC) assay or its variant, the late-appearing cobblestone area forming cell (CAFC), and the high proliferative potential colony-forming cell (HPP-CFC) as in vitro read-outs for repopulating stem cells, insofar as the correlation is verified and holds up. There was a general agreement that, at present, enumeration of $CD34^+/CD38^-$ cells in humans correlates best with hemopoietic reconstitution following transplantation and it was postulated that $CD34^+/CD38^+$ cells do not contribute significantly to reconstitution. Consequently, ex vivo generation of $CD38^+$ progenitor cells could well prove to be of limited benefit.

Growth Factors and Stromal Elements Required for Stem Cell Amplification

The fields of ex vivo expansion of and gene transfer into hemopoietic cells are still in developmental stages and, consequently, there appeared to be no true consensus on protocols to stimulate the cell cycling, self-renewal and expansion of long-term repopulating stem cells. Data presented at the meeting were discussed, and it was felt that growth factors such as Flt-3 ligand, kit-ligand, IL-11, IL-3 (possibly at a low concentration), IL-6 and, initially unexpected, thrombopoietin, were growth factors to be further explored for their potential to stimulate long-term repopulating cells. Recent reports on specific stromal cell lines supporting long-term repopulating cells should also be further explored in conjunction with

---

Table 1. Assays for stem cells and progenitor cells

In vitro assays

▲ Colony assays in semisolid or viscous media

▲ HPP-CFC

▲ Blast cell colonies

▲ Long-term bone marrow cultures and quantitative variants:

    LTC-IC

    Early and late appearing CAFC

▲ Immunophenotyping, such as $CD34^+/Lin^-$, $CD34^+/CD38^-$, $CD34^+/HLA-DR^-$, $CD34^+/kit^{low}$

In vivo assays

▲ Early- and late-appearing CFU-S

▲ Competitive and/or long-term repopulation assays using congenic mice (LTRA)

▲ Marrow repopulating ability (MRA)

▲ Quantitation of short-term and long-term repopulation in large outbred animal models, using allogeneic or genetically marked cells

▲ Human/SCID chimeras, SCID-repopulating cells by limiting dilution

---

growth factors. It was pointed out that fetal liver, umbilical cord, peripheral blood and bone marrow stem cells may have important differences in cell cycle and reconstitution kinetics, which should be taken into account.

Quality of Expanded/Manipulated Stem Cells

Beginning with the general question of whether all manipulations of stem cells, including transplantation and ex vivo expansion of progenitor cells would result in a (relative) depletion of cells with long-term repopulating ability, it was pointed out that early serial transplantation experiments did not provide convincing evidence for stem cell exhaustion [1, 2]. Reference was also made to more recent work demonstrating full hemopoietic reconstitution of mice from very few to single stem cells. The rationale for ex vivo expansion of stem cells was questioned; in other words, is there a clinical need for ex vivo expansion of repopulating stem cells? There was a general consensus that the scientific basis for stem cell expansion, i.e., the regulatory mechanisms involved in stem cell self renewal, has not been resolved.

REFERENCES

1 Fliedner TM, Heit H. Alterungsvorgänge in Zellerneuerungssystemen. Verh.Dtsch.Ges.Path. 1975;59:71-77.

2 Lajtha LG, Schofield R. Regulation of stem cell renewal and differentiation: possible significance of aging. Adv Gerontol Res 1971;3:131-146.

CHAPTER VII

BLOOD STEM CELLS:
TARGETS FOR GENE TRANSFER

RETROVIRAL VECTORS CONTAINING A VARIANT DIHYDROFOLATE REDUCTASE GENE FOR DRUG PROTECTION AND IN VIVO SELECTION OF HEMATOPOIETIC CELLS

James A. Allay, Jacques Galipeau, Raymond L. Blakley, Brian P. Sorrentino

NEW VECTORS FOR GENE THERAPY

Manuel Grez, Harald von Melchner

ALPHA INTERFERON (IFN-α) GENE TRANSFER INTO HEMATOPOIETIC STEM CELLS (ABSTRACT)

N.G. Abraham, E. Feldman, T. Ahmed

RESULTS OF RETROVIRAL AND ADENOVIRAL APPROACHES TO CANCER GENE THERAPY

L.H. Yin, S.Q. Fu, T. Nanakorn, F. Garcia-Sanchez, I. Chung, R. Cote, G. Pizzorno, E. Hanania, S. Heimfeld, R. Crystal, A. Deisseroth

CYTOKINE GENE TRANSFER IN CANCER THERAPY

Lei Cao, Peter Kulmburg, Hendrik Veelken, Andreas Mackensen, Beata Mézes, Albrecht Lindemann, Roland Mertelsmann, Felicia M. Rosenthal

Retroviral Vectors Containing a Variant Dihydrofolate Reductase Gene for Drug Protection and In Vivo Selection of Hematopoietic Cells

JAMES A. ALLAY, JACQUES GALIPEAU, RAYMOND L. BLAKLEY, BRIAN P. SORRENTINO

Departments of Hematology and Oncology, Biochemistry, and Molecular Pharmacology, St. Jude Children's Research Hospital, Memphis, Tennessee, USA

Key Words. *Gene therapy · Dihydrofolate reductase · Trimetrexate · Nucleoside transport inhibitors · NBMPR · In vivo selection · Myelosuppression*

ABSTRACT

Transfer of drug resistance genes to hematopoietic cells is being studied as a means to protect against the myelosuppression associated with cancer chemotherapy and as a strategy for the in vivo selection and amplification of genetically modified cells. The goal of this study was to test if retroviral-mediated gene transfer of a dihydrofolate reductase (DHFR) variant (L22Y) could be used for in vivo selection of transduced myeloid cells and to determine what proportion of transduced cells was required for protection from myelosuppression. Based on previous work suggesting that selection with antifolates may also require inhibition of nucleoside transport mechanisms, mice transplanted with DHFR-transduced bone marrow cells were treated with trimetrexate and the nucleoside transport inhibitor prodrug nitrobenzylmercaptopurine riboside phosphate. In vivo selection of transduced myeloid progenitors was seen in the bone marrow and in circulating mature peripheral blood cells following drug treatment. These results show that the novel combination of the L22Y-DHFR cDNA, trimetrexate and nitrobenzylmercaptopurine riboside phosphate can be used to select for transduced myeloid cells, and that this approach warrants further study in large animal models. A bicistronic vector containing a human CD24 reporter gene was used to determine the number of modified cells needed for chemoprotection. Partial protection from neutropenia was seen when greater than 10% of myeloid cells expressed the vector, and high levels of protection were obtained when the proportion exceeded 30%. These results suggest that gene transfer may be useful for myeloprotection in certain pediatric cancers, but that more efficient gene transfer will be required to apply this approach to adult cancer patients. *Stem Cells 1998;16(suppl 1):223-233*

INTRODUCTION

In murine transplant models, transfer of drug resistance genes into hematopoietic cells provides significant protection from the myelosuppressive effects of many commonly used anticancer drugs.

Protection has been noted using retroviral vectors containing the human multidrug resistance 1 (MDR1) gene [1-3], various dihydrofolate reductase (DHFR) genes [4-6], and DNA alkyltransferase genes such as methylguanine methyltransferases [7-9]. Gene transfer offers several advantages over more commonly used modalities, including the elimination of hematopoietic nadirs, durable resistance to repeated treatment courses, and protection of multiple hematopoietic lineages [10]. Despite these attractive features, the low efficiency of gene transfer into repopulating primate hematopoietic cells has limited the clinical utility of this treatment strategy [11], as it has many other gene therapy approaches [12]. In the mouse models where chemoprotection has been demonstrated, the overall gene transfer efficiency was much higher than that currently achievable in clinical trials and in nonhuman primate experiments. Two important but unanswered questions are exactly how many resistant myeloid cells are required to protect against myelosuppression, and whether an adequate number of resistant cells can be achieved using current clinical gene transfer protocols.

One possibility for increasing the numbers of transduced hematopoietic cells is a process called in vivo selection. With this strategy, post-transplant treatment with a cytotoxic drug is used to enrich and amplify the number of hematopoietic cells that express a transferred drug resistance vector [10]. The feasibility of this approach has been demonstrated using taxol to select for murine hematopoietic cells that were transduced with MDR1 retroviral vectors [1, 3]. We have recently focused on DHFR vectors for in vivo selection based on a number of considerations. Relatively high levels of drug resistance can be obtained using variant DHFR cDNAs to protect against antifolates. We have recently identified a novel human DHFR mutant, containing a leucine to tyrosine substitution in codon 22 (L22Y) [13], that confers a 100-fold increase in resistance to the nonclassical antifolate trimetrexate (TMTX) [6]. Another advantage is the small size of the DHFR cDNA (690 bp), which allows easy incorporation of a second therapeutic gene into selectable bicistronic vectors [14]. Furthermore, antifolates such as methotrexate (MTX) are commonly used following bone marrow (BM) transplantation and for the treatment of nonmalignant diseases.

Despite these advantages, equivocal results have been obtained using MTX to select for DHFR-transduced cells in transplanted mice [5, 15]. One explanation for this lack of convincing selection is the fact that antifolates are not toxic to myeloid progenitor cells. In normal mice treated with either MTX or TMTX very little toxicity was seen in the colony forming unit culture (CFU-C) and CFU-spleen compartment [16]. The mechanism by which myeloid progenitors escape antifolate toxicity is cell cycle independent, given the lack of drug sensitization with stem cell factor-induced cycling [16]. As a result of this intrinsic resistance of unmodified cells, no survival advantage is expected for progenitor cells that express a DHFR resistance gene. We have recently shown that nucleotide salvage mechanisms are responsible for this sparing effect [17]. Myeloid progenitors and repopulating stem cells import thymidine and nucleobases from the serum and thereby overcome antifolate-induced inhibition of de novo nucleotide biosynthesis (Fig. 1). We have further demonstrated that this salvage process can be pharmacologically inhibited with drugs that block facilitative thymidine transport. Drugs such as nitrobenzylmercaptopurine riboside (NBMPR), which block the *es* nucleoside transporter [18], markedly sensitize both CFU-C and repopulating stem cells to the toxic effects of TMTX [17]. These observations predict that the combination of TMTX and nitrobenzylmercaptopurine riboside phosphate (NBMPR-P) should select for primitive myeloid cells that express resistance-conferring DHFR vectors in vivo.

To test this hypothesis, we transplanted mice with BM cells transduced with a vector expressing the L22Y DHFR variant. After reconstitution, mice were treated with TMTX and NBMPR-P and the numbers of transduced myeloid progenitors in the BM were determined immediately after treatment. Virtually every CFU-C analyzed contained the resistance vector in drug-treated mice. In contrast, untreated mice had much lower numbers of progenitors that contained the DHFR vector.

To determine if this enrichment in transduced BM progenitors would be reflected by an increase in vector-expressing cells in the peripheral blood, human CD24 was utilized as an in vivo reporter system [19]. A bicistronic vector expressing both the CD24 cDNA and the L22Y cDNA

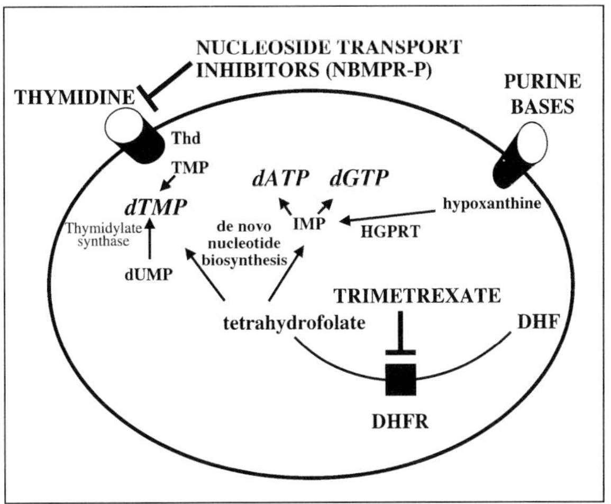

Figure 1. The effects of TMTX and nucleoside transport inhibitors on nucleotide metabolism in primitive myeloid cells. Reduced folate is a necessary cofactor for the de novo biosynthesis of dTTP, dATP, and dGTP. TMTX interrupts these de novo pathways by inhibiting DHFR function and thereby blocking production of reduced folates. Myeloid progenitors and repopulating stem cells can bypass the effects of DHFR blockade by importing thymidine and purine bases, normally present in the serum, to allow salvage synthesis of thymidylate and the purine nucleotides. In early myeloid cells, thymidine influx is mainly mediated by the es facilitative nucleoside transporter. Intracellular thymidine (Thd) is then converted through a series of steps to thymidylate. Purine bases such as hypoxanthine enter through different transport systems and are then processed via a number of enzymatic steps to generate dATP and dGTP. The net effect of these salvage pathways is to protect primitive myeloid cells from the toxic effects of antifolates. Cells can be sensitized to antifolates with drugs such as NBMPR which inhibit nucleoside transport. These drugs block importation of thymidine, thereby rendering cells susceptible to TMTX-induced inhibition of de novo thymidylate synthesis.

was transferred to mouse BM cells. After transplant, CD24 expression was detected in a subpopulation of peripheral RBCs and platelets in reconstituted mice. Treatment with TMTX and NBMPR-P increased the proportion of CD24-expressing cells in mice analyzed 45 days after drug treatment, demonstrating that this strategy can be used for the stable enrichment of genetically modified peripheral blood cells. The CD24 reporter system was also used to determine the proportion of modified cells required to protect against drug-induced neutropenia. Significant protection was seen when greater than 10% of peripheral blood myeloid cells expressed the resistance vector, with near complete protection when greater than 30% of myeloid cells scored positive for vector expression. These results suggest that, in the best of circumstances, current gene transfer protocols may be sufficient for conferring a protective effect.

MATERIALS AND METHODS

DHFR Vectors and Producer Cells

HaL22Y, containing the human DHFR variant leucine for tyrosine substitution at codon 22 (L22Y), and HaMDR, containing the human MDR cDNA, vectors and producers have previously been described [1, 6]. HaCID was constructed by cloning the full length human CD24 cDNA (kindly provided by *R. Keith Humphries,* Terry Fox Cancer Center; Vancouver, BC, Canada), an encephalomyocarditis virus internal ribosomal entry site (kindly provided by Genetic Therapy, Inc.; Gaithersburg, MD) and DHFR[L22Y] into a Harvey murine sarcoma retroviral vector using standard molecular biology techniques (Fig. 2). HaCID ecotropic producers were made in GP + E86 by previously described techniques [6]. A high titer polyclonal population was isolated that transmitted a full length vector genome to target cells and was free of detectable replication competent retrovirus as determined by a marker rescue assay.

Mice

Female mice purchased from Jackson Laboratories (Bar Harbor, ME) were used for experiments between 8 and 14 weeks of age.

Figure 2. DHFR retroviral vectors. Both vectors are based on the Harvey murine sarcoma virus (HaMSV) backbone. The HaL22Y vector contains a human DHFR cDNA encoding a leucine to tyrosine substitution in codon 22. Transcription of the L22Y-DHFR cDNA is controlled by the retroviral promoter located within the 5′ long terminal repeat. The HaCID vector expresses a bicistronic transcript encoding both the L22Y-DHFR gene as well as a gene for the human CD24 antigen. Cap 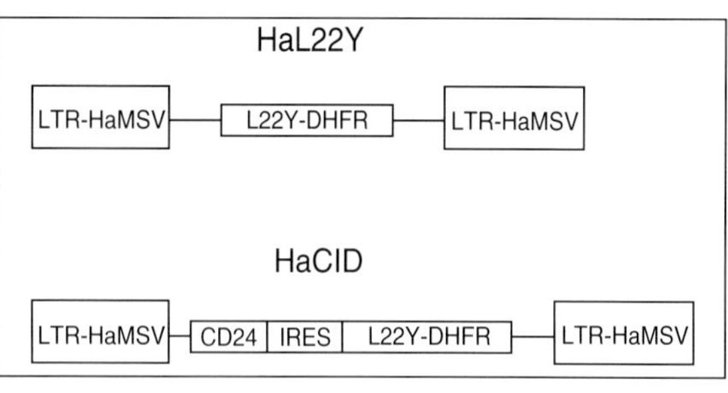

independent translation of the downstream DHFR gene is controlled by a viral internal ribosomal entry sequence isolated from the encephalomyocarditis virus [34].

Retroviral-Mediated BM Transduction and Transplantation

BM transduction was done as previously described [6]. Briefly, unseparated BM from C57Bl/6 donors treated 48 h previously with 150 mg/kg 5-fluorouracil was prestimulated for 48 h in Dulbecco's modified Eagle's medium containing 15% fetal bovine serum (FBS) plus 20 ng/ml murine interleukin 3 (IL-3), 50 ng/ml human IL-6 and 50 ng/ml rat stem cell factor (all kindly provided by Amgen; Thousand Oaks, CA) at 37°C, 5% CO_2. BM cells were harvested and placed in coculture with 1,000 rad irradiated HaL22Y, HaMDR, or HaCID GP + E86 ecotropic producer cells with the above cytokines and 6 μg/ml polybrene. Nonadherent cells were harvested 48 h later and 2×10^6 cells were transplanted into $WB/B6F_1$ W/Wv or $WB/B6F_1$ $^{+/+}$ mice irradiated with 900 rad one to three h previously. Mice were placed on chlorinated drinking water three days prior to and four weeks after transplantation.

Drug Treatment of Mice

TMTX base was received from the Drug Synthesis Chemistry Branch, Developmental Therapeutic Program, Division of Cancer Treatment, NCI and converted to the glucuronate salt as previously described [6]. Nitrobenzylmercaptopurine riboside 5′ monophosphate (NBMPR-P) was prepared as previously described [17], and the lyophilized powder was dissolved in sterile water immediately prior to use and administered as an i.p. injection. Transplanted mice were treated for five consecutive days with 130 mg/kg TMTX and 20 mg/kg NBMPR-P.

In Vivo Myeloid Progenitor Toxicity

BM was harvested from the femurs of untreated and TMTX + NBMPR-P treated mice 24 h following the final treatment and resuspended in equal volumes of phosphate-buffered saline (PBS) + 2% FBS. The volume equivalent of 1×10^5 BM cells from untreated mice was plated in 3 ml of methylcellulose-containing growth media (3430 media from Stem Cell Technologies; Vancouver, BC, Canada) and the number of myeloid progenitors was determined after 7-12 days of culture at 37°C, 5% CO_2.

Polymerase Chain Reaction (PCR) Analysis of Myeloid Progenitors Colonies

Individual myeloid progenitor colonies were isolated from methylcellulose plates and prepared for PCR as previously described [8]. Amplification of HaL22Y vector and beta-globin sequences were performed using previously described primers and conditions [6] except that 30 cycles of amplification were used for both the beta-globin and HaL22Y amplification reactions.

Hematology

Blood obtained from the retro-orbital sinus was used to determine standard hematological parameters. White blood cell counts were performed on erythrocyte-depleted blood diluted 1,000-fold in Isoton using a Coulter counter analyzer. The hematocrit was determined by manually reading the height of packed red cells. Differentials were performed manually on Wright Giemsa stained blood films.

CD24 Antibody Staining and Flow Cytometry of RBCs and Platelets

One μl of whole blood was resuspended in 1 μg phycoerythrin-conjugated anti-CD24 monoclonal antibody (Pharmingen; San Diego, CA) or 1 μg phycoerythrin-conjugated IgG2a isotypic control monoclonal antibody (Becton Dickinson; San José, CA) in PBS containing 2% FBS (PBS/2% FBS) and incubated on ice for 45 min. Cells were washed twice with 1 ml PBS/2% FBS, filtered and analyzed on a FACSCAN flow cytometer (Becton Dickinson). CD24 positivity was calculated by subtracting background as determined by isotype staining of experimental mice or CD24 staining of blood from a naive C57Bl/6 mouse, both giving identical histograms.

RESULTS

Protection of BM Cells from TMTX and NBMPR-P with a DHFR Vector

An ecotropic retroviral vector expressing the L22Y-DHFR variant (HaL22Y) was generated as previously described [6] (Fig. 2). Using a standard coculture transduction protocol [20], irradiated mice were transplanted with transduced BM cells. Twenty-four weeks after transplant, the mice were treated with a five-day course of TMTX (130 mg/kg/day) and NBMPR-P (20 mg/kg/day). Control animals transplanted with cells containing a MDR1 retroviral vector [1] were also treated with both drugs. Twenty-four h after the last drug dose, the mice were killed and BM cellularity was determined. Severe BM hypocellularity was seen in the MDR1 control mice, with the average BM cellularity reduced to 5% of the untreated controls (Fig. 3). In contrast, four out of five HaL22Y mice showed significant degrees of protection, with cellularities in animals L22Y-3, L22Y-4 and L22Y-13 approaching that seen in untreated controls. These results show that the HaL22Y vector can protect myelopoiesis against the toxic effects of TMTX and NBMPR-P.

To determine if protection was occurring at the level of clonogenic myeloid progenitors, BM cells from the treated mice were plated in a standard myeloid CFU-C assay to determine the

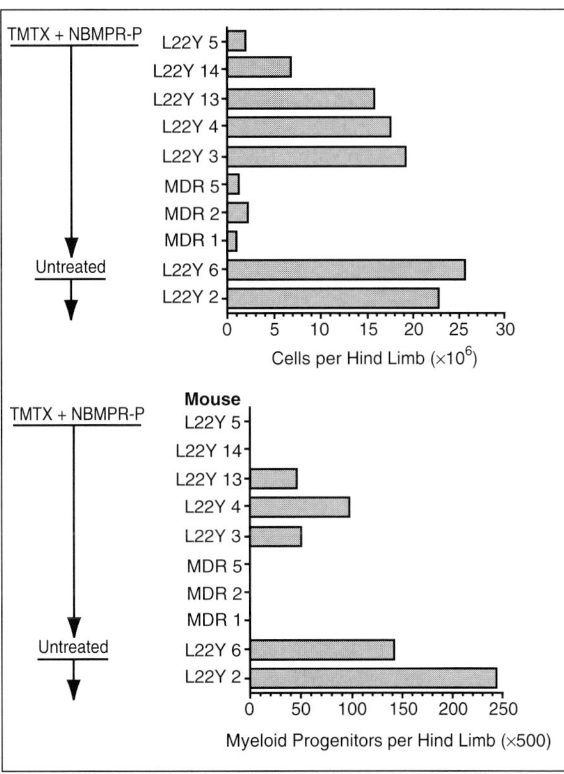

Figure 3. Effects of the HaL22Y vector on BM cellularity and myeloid progenitor content in mice treated with TMTX and NBMPR-P. *The top panel shows the total BM cellularity per hind limb and the bottom panel shows the progenitor content per hind limb volume for 10 mice containing the indicated vectors. Mice transplanted with either the HaL22Y vector (L22Y3-5, 13-14), or with a control MDR1 vector (MDR1, 2 and 5), were treated with both TMTX 130 mg/kd/day and NBMPR-P 20 mg/kg/day for five consecutive days. The mice were subsequently killed for BM analysis 24 h after the last treatment. Two HaL22Y mice (2 and 6) were left untreated and served as controls to define the normal BM cellularity and progenitor content. Mice received drug treatment six months after transplant.*

progenitor content per hind limb volume. As we have recently described [17], the combination of TMTX and NBMPR-P was extremely toxic to myeloid progenitors from control mice. No colonies were observed using BM obtained from treated MDR1 mice (Fig. 3). In contrast, significant numbers of myeloid colonies were noted from three of five treated L22Y mice. On average, these mice contained 33% of the progenitor content measured in untreated controls. These data show that the HaL22Y vector can protect myeloid progenitors in vivo from the toxic effects of TMTX and NBMPR-P. Two L22Y mice (L22Y-5 and 14) showed no protection of progenitors in the BM, presumably due to low levels of transduction or vector expression, commonly seen in mice analyzed for extended periods of time after transplant [21].

In Vivo Selection of HaL22Y-Transduced Myeloid Progenitors

We next tested if drug treatment resulted in enrichment of progenitors containing the HaL22Y vector. DNA prepared from seven day myeloid colonies was amplified using PCR primers specific for vector sequences, and primers for the endogenous murine beta-globin gene as internal controls for DNA loading. In the two HaL22Y controls that did not receive drug treatment (L22Y-2 and 6), the proportion of transduced myeloid colonies was 6% and 42%, respectively (Fig. 4). In contrast, vector sequences were detected in essentially all colonies from drug-treated HaL22Y mice. In animals L22Y-4 and -13, 100% of the colonies scored positive for DNA sequences from the HaL22Y vector. In the third treated animal (L22Y-3), 95% of the colonies were positive. These data show that TMTX and NBMPR-P can be used for in vivo selection of DHFR-transduced myeloid progenitors in the BM.

In Vivo Selection of Peripheral Blood Cells Expressing a Linked Reporter Gene

We next determined if selection at the level of progenitor cells would result in an increase in vector-expressing cells in the peripheral blood. To investigate this possibility, we generated a bicistronic vector (HaCID) expressing both the L22Y-DHFR cDNA and the human CD24 cell surface reporter cDNA [19] (Fig. 2). To construct the HaCID vector, the DHFR cDNA was inserted immediately downstream of a viral internal ribosomal entry sequence to direct cap-independent translation of the DHFR gene. This design was chosen to allow codominant expression of both linked genes from a single transcript, thereby ensuring that all cells scored as CD24+ would also express significant levels of the DHFR resistance gene. A polyclonal ecotropic producer cell population with a titer

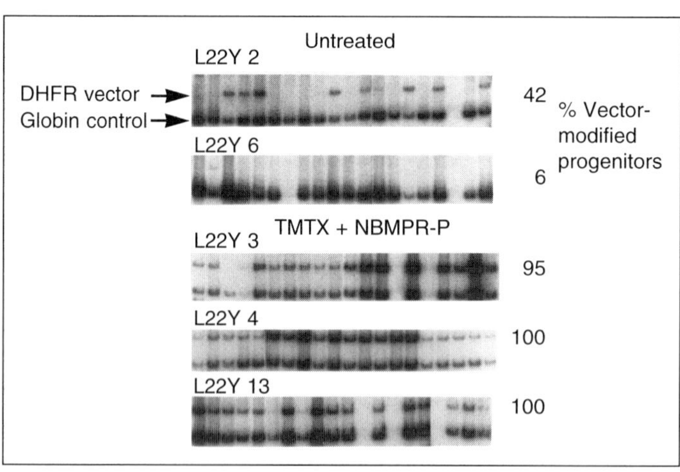

Figure 4. The prevalence of HaL22Y-transduced progenitors in BM samples from untreated and TMTX + NBMPR-P treated mice. Myeloid colonies were isolated from the BM of three drug-treated mice and two control mice as described in Figure 3. DNA prepared from these colonies was analyzed by PCR for the presence of HaL22Y vector sequences (upper band) and, as a positive control for DNA loading, sequences from the endogenous beta-globin locus (lower band). Each lane of the gels represents analysis of a single progenitor-derived colony. The first two rows show the results from two control animals which did not receive drug treatment (L22Y 2 and 6). The last three rows show the results from three mice which were treated with TMTX and NBMPR-P (L22Y 3, 4 and 13). The proportion of vector-modified progenitors seen in each animal is indicated on the right.

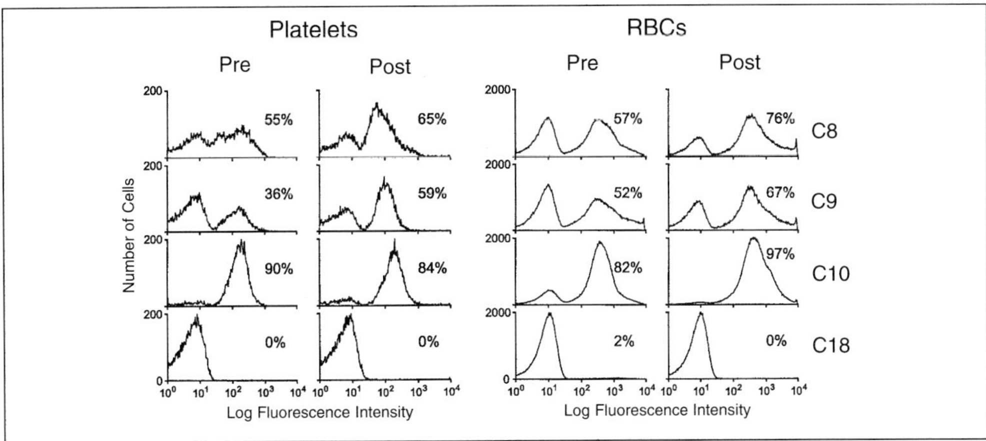

Figure 5. CD24 FACS analysis of platelets and RBCs obtained from HaCID-transduced mice both before and after treatment with TMTX and NBMPR-P. Peripheral blood was collected from four mice transplanted with HaCID-transduced cells (C8-10, 18). Samples were obtained both prior to a five-day treatment course with TMTX and NBMPR-P (Pre), or 45 days after the treatment (Post). Cells were stained with a phycoerythrin-conjugated monoclonal antiCD24 antibody, and gated populations of platelets (left panels) or RBCs (right panels) were analyzed for fluorescence. The number to the right of each FACS histogram indicates the percentage of cells that expressed the CD24 antigen, as defined by fluorescence greater than 98% than that seen with an isotype control antibody or with CD24 antibody staining of negative control C57Bl/6J mice.

of 1×10^6 pfu was used for transplant experiments.

Four mice were transplanted with BM cells transduced with the HaCID vector. Eight weeks after transplant, flow cytometry of peripheral blood cells was used to detect expression of the transferred CD24 gene. Forward and side scatter gates were used to separate erythrocyte and platelet populations for analysis. Three of the four HaCID mice (C8-10) showed high levels of CD24 expression in subpopulations of platelets and erythrocytes (Fig. 5). The proportion of vector-expressing cells ranged from 36% to 90% for platelets and from 52% to 82% for erythrocytes. These mice were then treated with a five-day course of TMTX and NBMPR-P and the CD24 analysis was repeated 45 days after the last dose (91 days after transplant). All three animals that were initially positive for marked cells showed increases in the proportion of CD24-expressing erythrocytes in the post-treatment sample. One animal (C10) showed near complete elimination of the untransduced population. Increases in CD24-expressing platelets were also noted in two of four cases. Although the increase in the proportion of marked cells was modest in most cases, we have noted that the number of vector-expressing cells naturally decreases over time (data not shown). Therefore, even modest increases in the proportion of CD24$^+$ cells over pretreatment levels represent significant enrichment.

The Proportion of Transduced Cells Required for Protection from Myelosuppression

A second set of mice was transplanted with HaCID-transduced BM cells to determine what proportion of transduced cells was required to protect against drug-induced myelosuppression. Twelve weeks after transplant, the number of vector-expressing myeloid cells was determined by CD24 expression analysis on peripheral blood platelets. The mice were then treated with a five-day course of TMTX and NBMPR-P, and the absolute neutrophil count nadir was measured 24 h after the last dose. In ten control mice transplanted with mock-transduced marrow, the ANC fell to 0 cells/μl on day 6 (Fig. 6). Very little protection was seen in another group of mice that contained between 0% and 10% transduced cells. In contrast, mice that contained between 10% and 30% CD24$^+$ cells demonstrated significant protection, with an increase in the neutrophil count nadir to 221 cells/μl. When the number of transduced cells

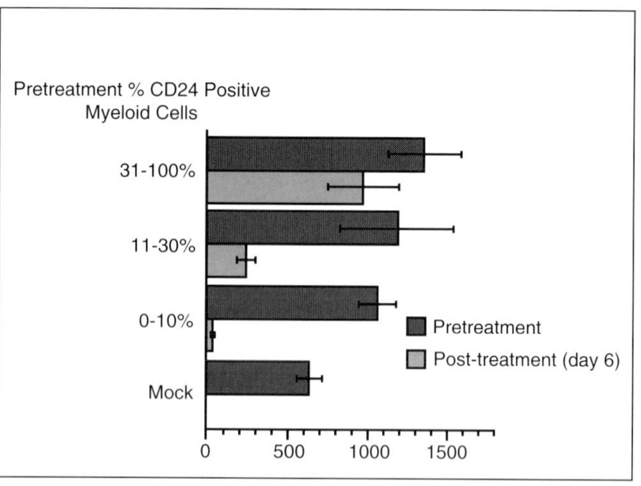

Figure 6. Neutrophil count nadirs in drug-treated mice containing varying proportions of HaCID-expressing myeloid cells. Mice were treated with a five-day course of TMTX (130 mg/kg/day) and NBMPR-P (20 mg/kg/day). The absolute neutrophil count was determined both before treatment (solid gray bars), and 24 h after the last dose (stippled bars). The percentage of platelets that expressed the transferred CD24 gene was determined immediately before treatment as shown in Figure 5. Based on these determinations, data were grouped from mock transplanted mice (n = 10), mice with between 0% and 10% CD24⁺ cells (n = 13), mice with between 11% and 30% CD24⁺ cells (n = 5), and mice with between 31% and 100% expressing cells (n = 5). The bars show the average neutrophil counts for these groups, and the error bars show one standard deviation of the mean.

exceeded 30%, hematopoietic protection was nearly absolute. In this group of five mice, the ANC on day 6 averaged 948 cells/μl: a value not significantly different from the pretreatment counts. These data show that greater than 10% transduced cells are required to protect myelopoiesis against the toxicity of TMTX and NBMPR-P and that high levels of protection can be obtained when greater than 30% of myeloid cells express the resistance vector. To determine to what degree in vivo selection has occurred in this cohort of animals, post-treatment analysis for CD24 expression is in progress and will be reported elsewhere.

DISCUSSION

Despite several attractive features of using DHFR variants for in vivo selection, antifolates alone cannot exert selective pressure at the level of myeloid progenitors and stem cells [16]. We have recently shown that this intrinsic antifolate resistance is due to nucleotide salvage mechanisms, and that these pathways can be pharmacologically blocked [17]. Our current working model shows the myelosuppressive effects of antifolates occurring relatively late in hematopoietic development, at a stage where the myeloid compartment size is dramatically expanding (Fig. 7). This toxicity profile can be modulated using nucleoside transport inhibitors such as NBMPR-P, which sensitize progenitor and stem cells to the cytotoxic effects of antifolates. This model predicts that treatment with TMTX and NBMPR-P should provide adequate selective pressure for multipotential cells that express resistance-conferring DHFR vectors. We have tested this prediction and now report that this strategy does result in in vivo selection in a mouse transplant model. Treatment with TMTX and NBMPR-P resulted in marked enrichment for BM-derived myeloid progenitors that contained the HaL22Y vector. Using a bicistronic vector expressing both the DHFR-L22Y gene and a linked CD24 reporter, we have further shown that drug treatment increased the number of vector-expressing erythrocytes and platelets circulating in the peripheral blood. These latter results suggest that this approach can be used as a generic strategy for enrichment and amplification of blood cells expressing a variety of linked therapeutic genes.

One potential application of this system is for the gene therapy of hemoglobinopathies. For diseases such as sickle cell anemia and thalassemia, an effective selection system would provide an important therapeutic advantage for obtaining the relatively high numbers of corrected RBCs needed to reverse the disease phenotype. Our data provide the first demonstration that in vivo selection can be used to increase the number of genetically modified erythrocytes that express a transferred gene. Advantages of the

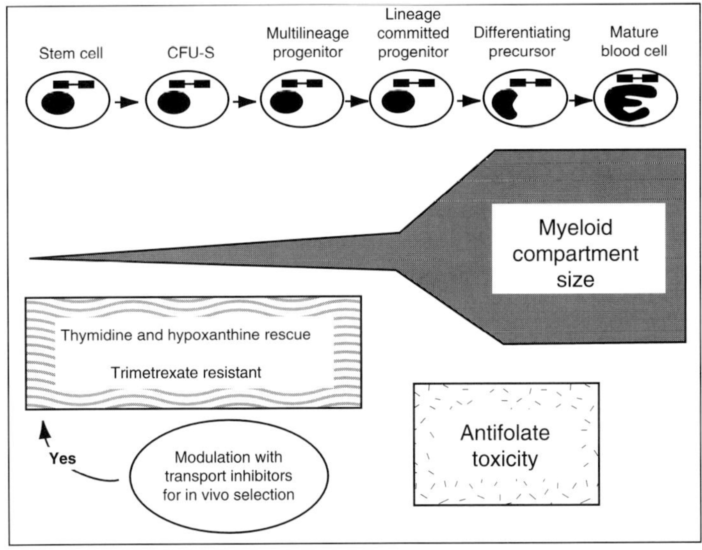

Figure 7. Working model for in vivo selection of primitive DHFR-transduced myeloid cells with trimetrexate and nucleoside transport inhibitors. The top row of cells depicts the progression of myeloid differentiation from stem cells through mature blood cells. The hatched area directly below the cells shows the relative contribution of cells at each differentiation stage to the total myeloid compartment size. The bracketed area indicates the stage of differentiation where antifolates normally exert their toxic effects. The rectangular area shows the more primitive cells where nucleotide salvage mechanisms confer relative antifolate resistance. Nucleoside transport inhibitors can sensitize this primitive compartment and thereby increase the selective advantage for stem cells and multilineage progenitors which express a transferred DHFR resistance gene.

DHFR/TMTX system for in vivo selection is that antifolates are not mutagenic, have been safely used in other nonmalignant diseases, and have no known long-term organ toxicity. Another advantage is the relatively small size of the DHFR cDNA, which should allow generation of high titer, selectable vectors that express other therapeutic genes. One remaining question is which genes will be best for correcting defects in globin structure or expression. Current progress in defining such therapeutic genes has offered several interesting candidates [22, 23].

There are several unanswered questions regarding the suitability of this approach for clinical application. One question is whether required doses of nucleoside transport inhibitors will have acceptable clinical toxicity. Because these drugs also block the transport of adenosine in endothelial cells, they can have potent vasodilatory effects including hypotension and tachycardia. These potential side effects can be inhibited by the commonly used adenosine receptor antagonists caffeine and theophylline [24], suggesting that these effects will not necessarily become dose-limiting toxicities for the in vivo selection approach. Although there is clinical experience with draflazine and dilazep as transport inhibitors, much less in known about the toxicity of NBMPR-P. Normal volunteers have been treated with the drug and experienced only mild nausea and headache (*Paterson*, personal communication). Another question is what is the minimum number of transduced cells necessary for selection and amplification. In our mouse model, the proportion of transduced peripheral blood cells prior to selection was relatively high compared to what has been obtained in primate models [25] or in clinical trials [26, 27]. Future experiments will be needed to determine if a threshold level of gene transfer is required for a selective effect. It is also not certain which vector will provide optimal expression of DHFR in early myeloid cells. We chose the Harvey vector based on data showing significant mRNA expression in primitive murine myeloid cells [28]. The recent description of retroviral vectors isolated for high level expression in stem cells [29-31] may offer even greater levels of stem cell expression and selection.

The other main use of drug resistance vectors is for chemoprotection of hematopoietic cells. Murine models provide clear evidence that gene transfer can be used for myeloprotection [10, 32, 33], but that degree of protection is directly related to the number of modified cells present at the time of drug treatment [6]. It is not known if a protective effect can be achieved at currently achievable levels of clinical gene transfer. Our data with the bicistronic DHFR vector show that partial protection can be obtained when the proportion of transduced cells exceeds 10%, and that high level protection is expected when the transduced population exceeds 30%. The fact that marking efficiencies of up to 15% have been obtained in pediatric marking trials [27] suggests that genetic myeloprotection may be feasible in the best of clinical circumstances. On the other hand, gene marking efficiencies have been much less in adult cancer patients [26], predicting that drug resistance gene transfer would not be effective in this patient population. This fact, taken together with the near absolute protection seen in our mouse model when the transduced cells exceeded 30% of the total population, makes it clear that the use of gene transfer for myeloprotection will be greatly enhanced by advances in gene therapy protocols leading to a higher proportion of modified cells in patients.

SUMMARY

In a mouse transplant model, treatment with NBMPR-P and TMTX led to in vivo selection of transduced hematopoietic cells which expressed a resistance-conferring variant of human DHFR. These results support the further study of this antifolate-based selection strategy as a means to enrich for genetically modified hematopoietic cells following transplant. Our results also show that protection from myelosuppression can be achieved when greater than 10% of myeloid cells expressed the resistance vector in vivo. This degree of gene transfer has been achieved in some but not all clinical protocols, suggesting that gene therapy-mediated chemoprotection may be feasible in the best of clinical circumstances. The future development of methods that achieve higher proportions of transduced cells could broaden the application of this approach for intensifying cancer chemotherapy.

ACKNOWLEDGMENTS

Supported in part by the National Heart, Lung, and Blood Institute Program Project Grant No. P01 53749-02 (*BPS*), The James S. McDonnell Foundation Grant No. 94-50 (*BPS*), The John H. Sununnu Postdoctoral Fellowship (*JAA*), US Public Health Service Grant No. P01 CA 31922 (*RLB*), Cancer Center Support Grant No. P30 CA 21765 (*BPS* and *RLB*), and by the American Lebanese Syrian Associated Charities (ALSAC).

REFERENCES

1 Sorrentino BP, Brandt SJ, Bodine D et al. Selection of drug-resistant bone marrow cells in vivo after retroviral transfer of human MDR1. Science 1992;257:99-103.

2 Hegewisch-Becker S, Hanania EG, Fu S et al. Transduction of MDR1 into human and mouse haemopoietic progenitor cells: use of rhodamine (Rh123) to determine transduction frequency and in vivo selection. Br J Haematol 1995;90:876-883.

3 Podda S, Ward M, Himelstein A et al. Transfer and expression of the human multiple drug resistance gene into live mice. Proc Natl Acad Sci USA 1992;89:9676-9680.

4 Williams DA, Hsieh K, DeSilva A et al. Protection of bone marrow transplant recipients from lethal doses of methotrexate by the generation of methotrexate-resistant bone marrow. J Exp Med 1987;166:210-218.

5 Zhao SC, Li MX, Banerjee D et al. Long-term protection of recipient mice from lethal doses of methotrexate by marrow infected with a double-copy vector retrovirus containing a mutant dihydrofolate reductase. Cancer Gene Ther 1994;1:27-33.

6 Spencer HT, Sleep SE, Rehg JE et al. A gene transfer strategy for making bone marrow cells resistant to trimetrexate. Blood 1996;87:2579-2587.

7 Moritz T, Mackay W, Glassner BJ et al. Retrovirus-mediated expression of a DNA repair protein in bone marrow protects hematopoietic cells from nitrosourea-induced toxicity in vitro and in vivo. Cancer Res 1995;55:2608-2614.

8 Allay JA, Dumenco LL, Koc ON et al. Retroviral transduction and expression of the human alkyltransferase cDNA provides nitrosourea resistance to hematopoietic cells. Blood 1995;85:3342-3351.

9 Harris LC, Marathi UK, Edwards CC et al. Retroviral transfer of a bacterial alkyltransferase gene into murine bone marrow protects against chloroethylnitrosourea cytotoxicity. Clin Cancer Res 1995;1:1359-1368.

10 Sorrentino BP. Drug Resistance Gene Therapy. In: Brenner MK, Moen RC, eds. Gene Therapy in Cancer. New York: Marcel Dekker, Inc., 1996:189-230.

11 Hanania EG, Giles RE, Kavanagh J et al. Results of MDR-1 vector modification trial indicate that granulocyte/macrophage colony-forming unit cells do not contribute to posttransplant hematopoietic recovery following intensive systemic therapy. Proc Natl Acad Sci USA 1996;93:15346-15351.

12 Karlsson S. Treatment of genetic defects in hematopoietic cell function by gene transfer. Blood 1991;78:2481-2492.

13 Lewis WS, Cody V, Galitsky N et al. Methotrexate-resistant variants of human dihydrofolate reductase with substitutions of leucine 22. Kinetics, crystallography, and potential as selectable markers. J Biol Chem 1995;270:5057-5064.

14 Galipeau J, Benaim E, Spencer HT et al. A bicistronic retroviral vector for protecting hematopoietic cells against antifolates and P-glycoprotein effluxed drugs. Hum Gene Ther 1997 (in press).

15 Corey CA, DeSilva AD, Holland CA et al. Serial transplantation of methotrexate-resistant bone marrow: protection of murine recipients from drug toxicity by progeny of transduced stem cells. Blood 1990;75:337-343.

16 Blau CA, Neff T, Papayannopoulou T. The hematologic effects of folate analogs: implications for using the dihydrofolate reductase gene for in vivo selection. Hum Gene Ther 1996;7:2069-2078.

17 Allay JA, Spencer HT, Wilkinson SL et al. Sensitization of hematopoietic stem and progenitor cells to trimetrexate using nucleoside transport inhibitors. Blood 1997 (in press).

18 Griffiths M, Beaumont N, Yao SY et al. Cloning of a human nucleoside transporter implicated in the cellular uptake of adenosine and chemotherapeutic drugs. Nat Med 1997;3:89-93.

19 Pawliuk R, Kay R, Lansdorp P et al. Selection of retrovirally transduced hematopoietic cells using CD24 as a marker of gene transfer. Blood 1994;84:2868-2877.

20 Bodine DM, McDonagh KT, Seidel NE et al. Survival and retrovirus infection of murine hematopoietic stem cells in vitro: effects of 5-FU and method of infection. Exp Hematol 1991;19:206-212.

21 Challita PM, Kohn DB. Lack of expression from a retroviral vector after transduction of murine hematopoietic stem cells is associated with methylation in vivo. Proc Natl Acad Sci USA 1994;91:2567-2571.

22 Donze D, Jeancake PH, Townes TM. Activation of delta-globin gene expression by erythroid Krupple-like factor: a potential approach for gene therapy of sickle cell disease. Blood 1996;88:4051-4057.

23 McCune SL, Reilly MP, Chomo MJ et al. Recombinant human hemoglobins designed for gene therapy of sickle cell disease. Proc Natl Acad Sci USA 1994;91:9852-9856.

24 Rongen GA, Smits P, Ver Donck K et al. Hemodynamic and neurohumoral effects of various grades of selective adenosine transport inhibition in humans. Implications for its future role in cardioprotection. J Clin Invest 1995;95:658-668.

25 Dunbar CE, Seidel NE, Doren S et al. Improved retroviral gene transfer into murine and rhesus peripheral blood or bone marrow repopulating cells primed in vivo with stem cell factor and granulocyte colony-stimulating factor. Proc Natl Acad Sci USA 1996;93:11871-11876.

26 Dunbar CE, Cottler-Fox M, O'Shaughnessy JA et al. Retrovirally marked CD34-enriched peripheral blood and bone marrow cells contribute to long-term engraftment after autologous transplantation. Blood 1995;85:3048-3057.

27 Brenner MK, Rill DR, Holladay MS et al. Gene marking to determine whether autologous marrow infusion restores long-term haemopoiesis in cancer patients. Lancet 1993;342:1134-1137.

28 Sorrentino BP, McDonagh KT, Woods D et al. Expression of retroviral vectors containing the human MDR1 cDNA in hematopoietic cells of transplanted mice. Blood 1995;86:491-501.

29 Baum C, Eckert HG, Stockschlader M et al. Improved retroviral vectors for hematopoietic stem cell protection and in vivo selection. J Hematother 1996;5:323-329.

30 Baum C, Hegewisch-Becker S, Eckert HG et al. Novel retroviral vectors for efficient expression of the multidrug resistance (mdr-1) gene in early hematopoietic cells. J Virol 1995;69:7541-7547.

31 Hawley RG, Lieu FH, Fong AZ et al. Versatile retroviral vectors for potential use in gene therapy. Gene Ther 1994;1:136-138.

32 Banerjee D, Zhao SC, Li MX et al. Gene therapy utilizing drug resistance genes: a review. STEM CELLS 1994;12:378-385.

33 Koc ON, Allay JA, Lee K et al. Transfer of drug resistance genes into hematopoietic progenitors to improve chemotherapy tolerance. Semin Oncol 1996;23:46-65.

New Vectors for Gene Therapy

MANUEL GREZ,[a] HARALD VON MELCHNER[b]

[a]Laboratory for Molecular Virology, Georg-Speyer-Haus, Frankfurt, Germany;
[b]Laboratory for Molecular Hematology, Department of Hematology,
University of Frankfurt Medical School, Frankfurt, Germany

Key Words. *Retroviruses · Cre/loxP recombination · Gene therapy · Gene expression*

ABSTRACT

Retrovirus-based vectors are presently the most efficient gene transfer vehicles for introducing genes into human hematopoietic stem and progenitor cells. However, their use for gene therapy is still problematic. A major obstacle is viral sequences such as the tRNA primer binding site or the dimerization and encapsidation signals that are not required for the expression of the therapeutic gene. These sequences can recombine with endogenous and/or exogenous retroviruses to generate new forms of unpredictable retroviruses. Moreover, these sequences are the targets for transcriptional repressors which inhibit the expression of the transduced genes. Therefore we have developed a new generation of retrovirus vectors which self-delete upon integration. The vectors are based on the natural life cycle of retroviruses, involving duplication of the terminal control regions U5 and U3 to generate long terminal repeats, and on the ability of the P1-phage site-specific recombinase (Cre) to excise any sequences positioned between two target sequences (*loxP*). Thus, while inserting a therapy gene into the genome, the vectors simultaneously excise most proviral sequences that are not required for gene expression. *Stem Cells 1998;16(suppl 1):235-243*

INTRODUCTION

Several viral and nonviral vectors have been employed to deliver genes to mammalian cells. However, the most widely used are retroviruses based on Moloney murine leukemia virus (MoMuLV), a retrovirus that normally infects mice [1-4]. These vectors are easy to make, and up to now the most efficient agents yet identified for transferring genes into human cells. Moreover, retroviruses have the unique advantage of integrating by a precise mechanism into the genome causing little if any damage to both transduced and target DNAs. Once integrated in the genome as proviruses, the transduced genes are transmitted to daughter cells which in principle, should ensure their long-term expression. For these reasons, retroviruses have been used in 63% of the human gene therapy trials approved to date [4-6].

Figure 1 shows the prototype of a conventional retrovirus vector used in most clinical trials. The therapy gene is typically inserted into the body of the virus between the long terminal repeats (LTRs). Transcripts initiate in the 5′LTR promoter and terminate in the polyadenylation sequence of the 3′LTR. In a short term this insures high levels of gene expression. However, in a long term, expression is repressed, particularly in primary cells, by mechanisms which involve at least in part retroviral sequences that are either not required for expression or can be exchanged with sequences that are less

Characteristics and Potentials of Blood Stem Cells
STEM CELLS **1998;16(suppl 1):235-243** ©AlphaMed Press. All rights reserved.

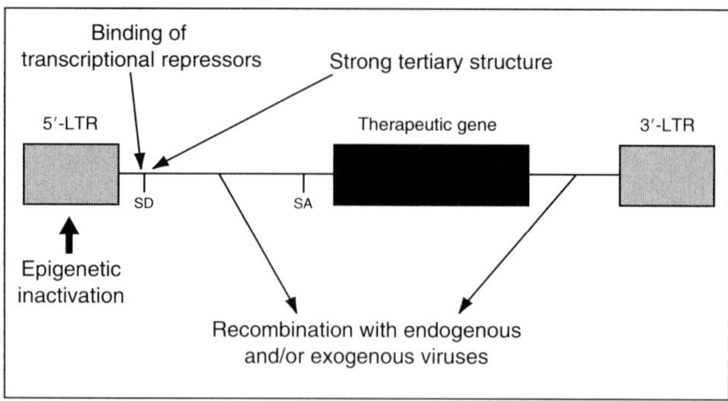

Figure 1. Viral elements involved in silencing of gene expression. The figure shows regions within conventional retroviral vectors which are detrimental for gene expression (epigenetic inactivation of the enhancer function in the LTR, binding of transcriptional repressors to the PBS region) or may contribute to mobilization of retroviral vector sequences (5'-leader region including part of gag, 3'-untranslated region including part of env).

susceptible to inactivation. Thus, LTRs are frequently inactivated by epigenetic mechanisms resulting in inadequate expression of the transgene [5-7], and 5' untranslated proviral sequences provide a target for gene inactivation through binding of cell-specific transcriptional repressors [8-10]. The latter region is usually co-expressed with the therapy gene and contains the viral dimerization and encapsidation signals which, albeit essential for viral replication, can cause mobilization of vector RNA in presence of helper virus (Fig. 1).

Some of these problems have been solved by using internal promoters for the expression of the transduced gene. Since in this case gene expression is independent of the retroviral LTR, vectors with deleted LTR enhancers have been developed and shown to perform reasonably well [11]. Enhancer deleted vectors are generally safer because they are less likely to activate adjacent genes. Such gene activation can result in cancer if integration occurs adjacent to a proto-oncogene [12-14]. In principle, such integrations cannot be avoided since retroviruses integrate randomly throughout the genome. However, oncogenic events are rare and thus far have not been observed in transduced human cells.

To improve transduction efficiencies, many protocols rely on the use of selectable marker genes. While such genes allow significant enrichment of transduced cells, they are also the source of additional problems. Besides interfering with cellular metabolism [15], marker proteins may elicit an immune response which could eliminate the transduced cells [16].

A final problem which is particularly relevant for the noncycling hematopoietic stem cells is the inability of MoMuLV based vectors to infect G_0 cells. Although lentiviral vectors that do infect nondividing cells could be an alternative, their potential use for gene therapy still raises serious safety concerns.

To address some of these issues, we have developed a new class of retroviral vectors that self-delete after inserting a gene into the genome. This was achieved by exploiting the natural life cycle of retroviruses, involving duplication of the terminal control regions U5 and U3 to generate LTRs [17] and the ability of the P1-phage site specific recombinase (Cre) to excise any sequences positioned between two target sequences (*loxP*) from the mammalian genome [18].

MATERIALS AND METHODS

Plasmids

The sequences for Cre recombinase and *loxP* were derived from pMCCre and pGEM30, respectively [19]. The mouse phosphoglycerate-kinase-promotor (pgk) was obtained from ppgkCat [20] and the SV40/puromycin-acetyltransferase cassette from pBABEpuro [21]. pggU3en(-) was derived from pggU3Neoen(-) [22] by deleting neo and subcloning the viral sequences as an SstI fragment into the backbone of pBABEpuro. pggSVCreU3lx was constructed by sequentially inserting the Cre region of MCCre, the SV40 promoter of pBABEpuro and the *loxP*-fragment of pGEM30 which includes a downstream HindIII site, as blunt-ended fragments into the BamHI, XhoI and Nhe I sites of pGgU3en(-), respectively. pggSVCreU3lxpgkpuro and pggSVCreU3lxSVpuro were obtained by ligating blunt-ended pgk-puro- or SV40-puro expression cassettes into the HindIII site of *loxP*.

Cells and Viruses

NIH3T3, 293T [23] and BOSC23 [16] cells were grown in Dulbecco's modified Eagle's medium (GIBCO; Grand Island, NY) supplemented with 10% fetal bovine serum (GIBCO). Helper virus-free recombinant retroviruses were obtained by transient transfection of BOSC23 cells as described by *Pear et al.* [16]. Infections were performed by incubating for 24 h 10^5 NIH3T3 cells with serial dilutions of filtered viral supernatants in the presence of 4 µg/ml polybrene (Aldrich; St. Louis, MO). Provirus expressing clones were isolated by selecting for seven days in medium containing 2 mg/ml puromycin (Sigma; St. Louis, MO) or 1 mg/ml G418 (GIBCO).

Analysis of Cre Activity

Analysis of Cre activity was performed by cotransfecting Cre-expressing plasmids with the reporter plasmid pAMA (10 µg of each) into 293T cells. pAMA (provided by *Dr. F. Sablitzky*) contains an *E. coli* β-galactosidase (lacZ) gene expressed from an MC promoter [29]. However, the lacZ coding sequence is interrupted by two *loxP* sites inserted immediately downstream of the LacZ- AUG. Additional in-frame stop codons and polyadenylation sequences inserted between the *loxP* sites prevent LacZ expression. By deleting the sequences flanked by *loxP*, Cre-mediated recombination fuses the AUG and the remaining *loxP* sequence to the LacZ reading frame thereby restoring LacZ function. Thus, β-galactosidase, translated as a *loxP*/LacZ fusion protein, can be readily detected by X-Gal staining. Accordingly, Cre activity in 293T cells was estimated 48 h after transfection by staining with X-Gal [24]. pMCCre and pBABEpuro were used as positive and negative controls, respectively.

DNA Hybridizations and Polymerase Chain Reaction (PCR)

DNA hybridizations were performed with ^{32}P-labeled probes as previously described [22]. Southern blots were scanned with a PhosphoImager (Molecular Dynamics; Sunnyvale, CA) and analyzed with ImageQuantNT software (Molecular Dynamics). For PCR assays, 150 ng of genomic DNAs were amplified for 40 cycles (94°C 30', 60°C 1', 72°C 2') using the Cre-specific primers 5'-TTAGCTAGCATGCCCAAGAAGAAGAAG-3' and 5'-GGAGCTAGCCTAATCGCCATCTTCCAG-3'. Control PCRs were performed under the same condition except for using actin-primers as previously described [25].

RESULTS

Self-deleting retroviral vectors were created by inserting a transcriptional unit consisting of the puromycin resistance gene controlled either by SV40 or pgk promoters into the 3'-U3 region of an enhancerless MoMuLV retrovirus vector [26]. A Cre-recombinase target sequence (*loxP*) was inserted upstream of the puromycin cassette (Fig. 2A). Since Cre requires two identically oriented *loxP* sites to mediate excision, only viral replication and LTR-mediated duplication create a valid recombination target. Thus, after virus integration most proviral sequences are placed between *loxP* sites and therefore become susceptible to excision by Cre-recombinase (Fig. 2B).

There are two ways to express Cre-recombinase in cells with *loxP* proviruses. The conventional method uses expression of Cre-recombinase in *trans*. Accordingly, Cre is introduced either as a protein or as cDNA cloned into an expression vector into cells infected with *loxP* retroviruses. However, for gene therapy the approach does not seem suitable because it involves additional cell manipulation which almost always reduces gene transduction efficiencies. The second approach in which Cre and *loxP* sequences reside on the same provirus seems far more promising. In this case Cre would be provided in *cis* and thus avoid a second transduction. Moreover, when Cre is expressed from within the provirus it would excise itself along with all the other viral or nonviral sequences placed between *loxP* sites (Figs. 2C and 2D).

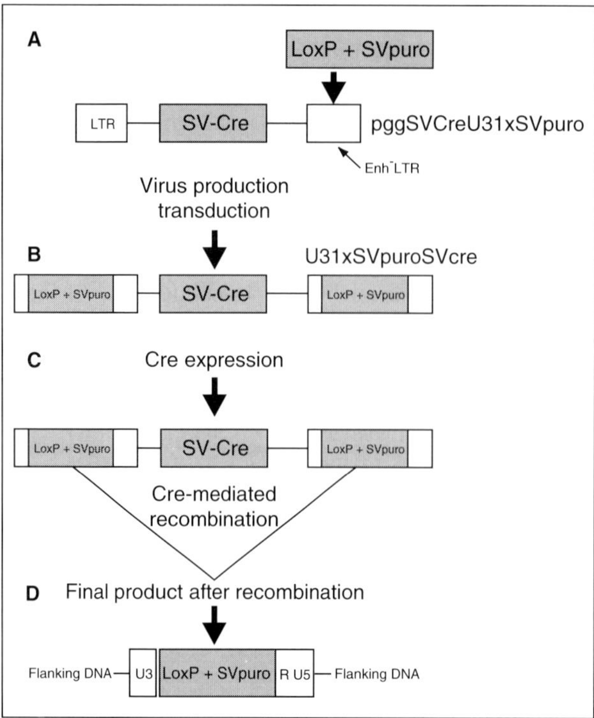

***Figure 2. Structure and excision mechanism of Cre/loxP retrovirus
vectors.*** *A) Structure of the Cre/loxP retroviral vector at the plasmid
stage; B) integrated provirus with duplicated and translocated U3-
regions; C) cre-mediated excision of sequences flanked by* loxP *elements; D) recombination product consisting of a single LTR with
inserted* loxP *and SVpuro sequences.*

Gene sequences present in the vector are labeled as follows: loxP,
*P1 phage site-specific recombination target; enh⁻ designates a 178 nt
deletion in the 3′ LTR encompassing the viral enhancer; Cre, P1
phage site specific recombinase; SV, Simian virus 40 promoter; Puro,
puromycin resistance gene.*

To generate a retroviral vector with these features, an SV40-Cre cassette was introduced into the body of the pggU3lxSVpuro retrovirus (Fig. 2). However, this turned out to be more difficult than initially anticipated. Recombination products obtained during the various cloning steps were often rearranged or contained deletions. Since these were most likely the result of Cre-mediated recombination between *loxP* site-containing plasmids, we screened for functional recombinase by cotransfecting candidate plasmids into 293T cells expressing the reporter plasmid pAMA. pAMA is an MC-promoter-controlled LacZ expression plasmid in which the LacZ gene is disrupted by two *loxP* sites inserted downstream of the LacZ-AUG. An in-frame stop codon and a polyadenylation sequence between the two *loxP* sites prevents LacZ expression in the absence of Cre-recombinase. By deleting the sequences flanked by *loxP*, Cre-mediated recombination fuses the AUG and the remaining *loxP* sequence to the LacZ reading frame thereby restoring LacZ function. Thus, an active Cre-recombinase can be readily detected by simple X-Gal staining. The few plasmids that were active in this assay were used to produce infectious virus.

A pggSVCreU3lxSVpuro construct with functional Cre-recombinase was transfected into BOSC23 helper cells [16] to obtain infectious virus (Fig. 3). Recovered viruses were titered on NIH3T3 cells by selecting in puromycin and counting colony forming units after seven days of incubation. Titers for U3lxSVpuroSVCre were high (1.5-3.7 × 10^5 colony forming units/ml/10^7 producer cells) and similar to what we and others have obtained with MoMuLV vectors carrying genes in U3 [11, 24, 26-28]. This indicated that inserting Cre into a vector with *loxP* sites in U3 does not markedly interfere with virus replication.

To analyze recombination, genomic DNA obtained from puromycin-resistant clones was analyzed by Southern blotting. Figure 4A shows the predicted structures of U3lxSVpuroSVCre proviruses in presence or absence of Cre-recombinase. LTR-mediated duplication includes a unique proviral HindIII site located in U3 (Fig. 4A). Thus, genomic DNA containing nonrecombined proviruses will generate an internal proviral fragment of 4.5 kb when cleaved with HindIII which hybridizes to both SV40 and puromycin specific probes. Since the second HindIII site is excised by Cre, recombined proviruses will lack this internal fragment. Accordingly, each puromycin resistant clone generates unique hybridizing bands reflecting fragments extending from the HindIII site of the 3′LTR, to sites in the 5′ flanking cellular DNA (Fig. 4A, + Cre). The pattern obtained on Southern blots suggested that all sequences between the *loxP* sites have been deleted

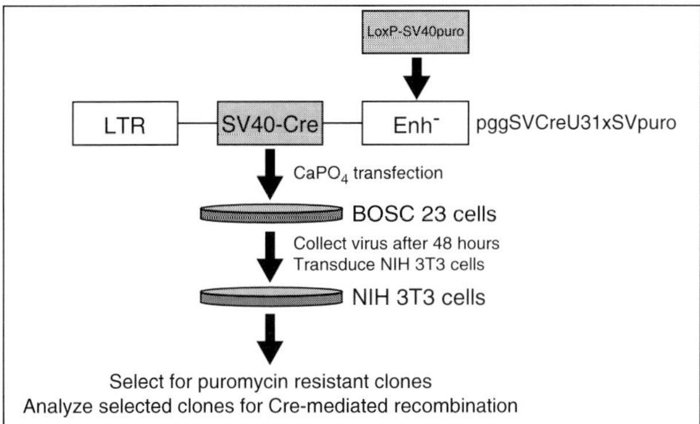

Figure 3. Transient generation of Cre/loxP viral particles and transduction of target cells. *The plasmid pggSVCreU3lxSVpuro was transfected into BOSC 23 cells using calcium phosphate precipitation. The BOSC23 is a packaging cell line expressing the proteins required for encapsidation dimerization. Target cells were infected by incubating with virus containing supernatants. Puromycin resistant clones were isolated for further analysis following selection for seven days.*

by Cre-recombinase (Fig. 4B). Furthermore, PCR analysis indicated that most clones with recombined hybridization patterns failed to generate Cre-specific amplification products when subjected to PCR (Fig. 4C). However, 3 out of 12 clones generated faint Cre-specific amplification products, indicating incomplete recombination (clones 7, 10 and 11 in Fig. 4C).

To determine the minimum number of cells required to generate a Cre-specific signal, serial dilutions of DNA derived from a single copy clone expressing a mutationally inactivated Cre provirus were mixed

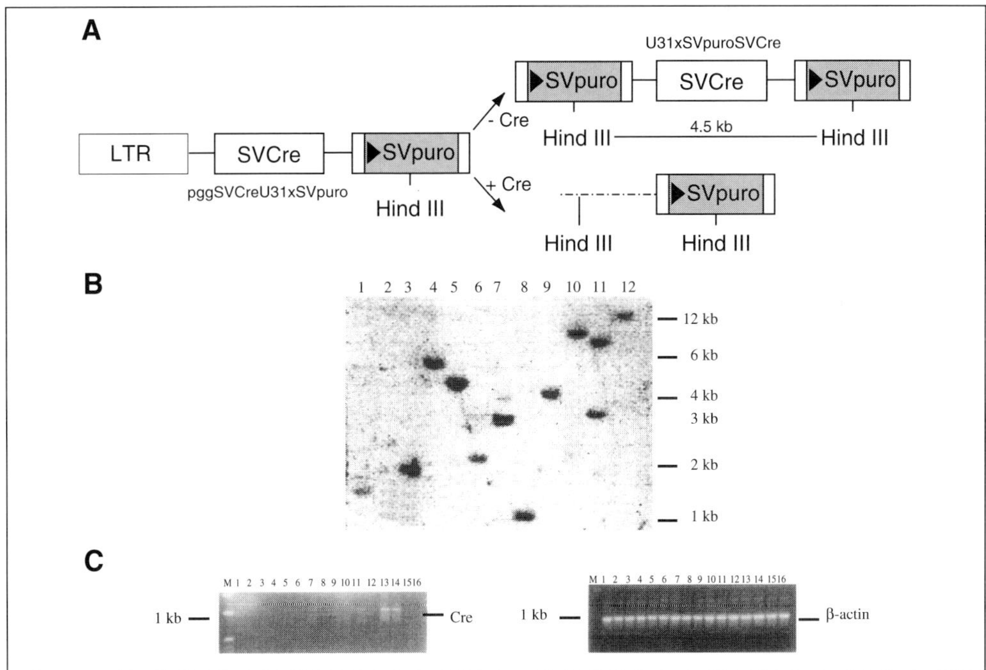

Figure 4. Recombination of U3lxSVPuroSVCre proviruses in NIH3T3 cells. A) Structure of the Cre/loxP vector at the plasmid DNA stage (left) and predicted structures of proviruses in presence or absence of Cre-recombinase. B) Southern blot analysis of U3lxSVPuroSVCre proviruses. Cell DNAs were cleaved with Hind III, processed as described in **Materials and Methods** and hybridized to a ^{32}P-labeled SV40 probe. Lanes 1-12, U3lxSVPuroSVCre expressing clones 1-12. C) PCR analysis of U3lxSVPuroSVCre expressing clones. Genomic DNA was amplified using Cre- (left) or β-actin- (right) specific primers. Amplification products were resolved in 1% agarose gels and visualized by ethidium-bromide staining in lanes as follows: M, molecular weight standards (BRL 1 kb ladder); 1-12, U3lxSVPuroSVCre expressing clones 1-12; 13-14, single copy U3pgklxtkneoMCCre expressing clones (positive controls); 15-16, single copy U3pgklxtkneo expressing clones (negative controls). The Southern blot and the PCR-results are reprinted with permission from [29] (Fig. 5).

with DNA of uninfected cells and subjected to PCR with Cre-specific primers. No signal was obtained with dilutions up to 1:625, indicating that in clones with no detectable signal more than 99.8% of the cells have undergone recombination.

The high recombination frequency achieved by U3lxSVpuroSVCre virus was not completely reproducible with a second retroviral construct in which the SV40puro-casette was replaced with a pgkpuro-casette (U3lxpgkpuroSVCre). In this case, Southern analysis showed that 2 out of 14 puromycin resistant clones failed to recombine. Moreover, all clones, including those that appeared recombined on Southern blots, generated Cre-specific amplification products when analyzed by PCR [29]. Although in some cases the levels of amplification products were 10- to 50-fold lower than in nonrecombined clones, the results suggest that the recombinase did not uniformly achieve the threshold levels required for recombination. This is most likely caused by integration-specific repression of gene expression. Interestingly, in spite of sharing all components except for pgk, U3lxSVpuroSVCre recombined more efficiently than U3lxpgkpuroSVCre. Although the mechanisms are not known, the difference may reflect suppression of the SV40 promoter by the upstream pgk promoter, not unlike promoter interference described elsewhere [28, 30, 31]. However, despite the recorded differences, recombination frequencies for both vectors obtained without selection were high and comparable to other systems in which Cre and *loxP* were independently transduced and selection was applied [19].

Discussion

A major problem encountered with gene transduction, particularly into hematopoietic cells, is lack of gene expression. Although rates of transfer are relatively high with retroviruses (70%-90%), rates of gene expression are generally low (10%-30%) [32]. While the mechanisms of gene silencing are largely unknown, several observations suggest that methylation of viral sequences or binding of transcriptional repressors to the primer binding site is involved [5, 6, 9, 10]. For example, a fourfold reduction of transgene expression was observed in a murine pluripotent myeloid stem cell line (FDCP-mix) with a construct containing a viral LTR and the primer binding site of MoMuLV [10]. This observation suggested that transgene expression should improve considerably after eliminating the viral targets for methylation and repressor binding. However, since the sequences involved are essential for virus replication (e.g., LTRs and primer binding sites), their deletion is only conceivable following provirus integration. To achieve this, we have exploited the features of retroviral replication to duplicate a *loxP* target sequence inserted in the U3 region. In the integrated provirus, this places all viral and nonviral sequences inserted into the body of the virus between *loxP* sites and thus makes them susceptible to excision by Cre-recombinase.

By accommodating Cre and *loxP* sites in the same provirus, the vectors have several advantages over previously used Cre/*loxP* excision systems in which Cre and *loxP* were independently transduced [18, 33-35]. First, the vectors avoid additional cell manipulations imposed by separate Cre and *loxP* transductions. Second, the Cre sequences placed between *loxP* sites are eliminated from the provirus, ensuring that the recombinase is only transiently expressed. This reduces the risk of an immune response against the bacterial enzyme.

Proviral self-excision also would allow the safe use of selectable marker genes which, due to their immunogenicity, have become increasingly unpopular [16]. Nevertheless, in instances in which rates of gene transfer and expression are low and inconsistent (e.g., hematopoietic precursor cells), selectable marker genes are still highly desirable. Such genes enable safe selection and expansion of transduced cells which should have a higher therapeutic value. With the Cre/*loxP* vectors described here the advantages of selection can be maintained without risking an immune response by simply inserting a selectable marker gene into the body of the virus and by using an inducible Cre-recombinase. Thus, once selection is completed, the marker gene can be eliminated by activating the recombinase. We are presently testing several inducible Cre-recombinases where the C-terminus of Cre is fused to the hormone binding domain of a mutant mouse estrogen receptor gene. Enzyme activity is induced by treating with 4-hydroxy-tamoxifen which specifically binds the receptor [36].

Further improvements of the vectors would include a marker gene that would allow selection for recombination. For example, the HSV-TK co-expressed with Cre may be used to eliminate all cells with proviruses that have failed to recombine (Fig. 5). Since only these cells express HSV-TK, they will be killed selectively by ganciclovir (Fig. 5C).

In summary, Cre/*loxP* vectors seem to have clear advantages over conventional retroviral vectors not only in terms of safety but also in terms of gene transduction and expression. Still, like all other vectors used for gene therapy they have some limitations, most of which can be dealt with or are minor. For example, establishing stable producer cell lines with Cre/*loxP* vectors is difficult. The reason for this is presumably transrecombination between multiple copy plasmids resulting in aberrant structures that cannot be packaged into virions. Although single copy

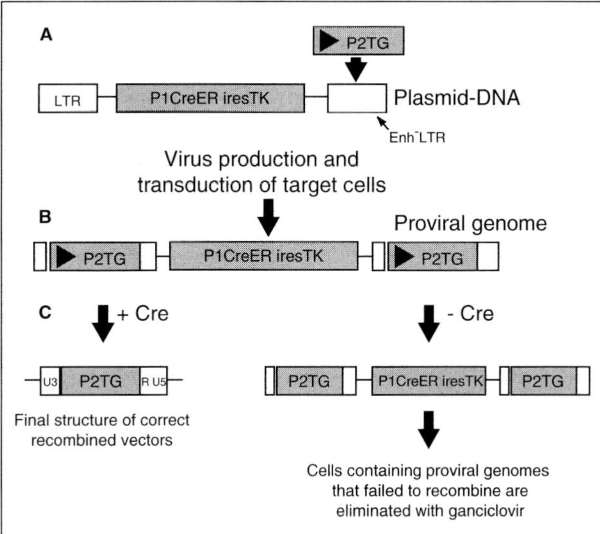

Figure 5. Future developments of Cre/loxP retroviruses. The inclusion of the herpes simplex thymidine kinase gene within the body of a Cre/loxP retrovirus enables selection for recombination, while the inclusion of a Cre gene fused to the hormone binding domain of the estrogen receptor (Cre/ER) enables its conditional expression. Moreover, a selectable marker can be included to select for transduced cells.

Gene sequences present in the vector are labeled as follows: loxP, *P1 phage site-specific recombination target; enh⁻ designates a 178 nt deletion in the 3´ LTR encompassing the viral enhancer; CreER, P1 phage site-specific recombinase fused to the coding region of the hormone binding domain of a mutant mouse estrogen receptor gene that binds 4-hydroxytamoxifen [36]; SV, Simian virus 40 promoter; Puro, puromycin resistance gene; P1/P2 promoter/enhancer elements; TG: therapy gene; ires: internal ribosome entry site; TK: herpes simplex thymidine kinase gene.*

producer cells would circumvent this problem, the viral titers of such cells are normally too low for therapeutic purposes. However, high titer Cre/*loxP* viruses can be produced by using the transient packaging lines based on human 293T cells [16]. Recombination between Cre/*loxP* plasmids can be avoided by using inducible Cre-recombinase as described above.

Transrecombination between *loxP* sites could in theory produce chromosomal translocations in cells with two or more proviruses [37]. Although transrecombination is a rare event (1×10^{-8} for cells containing two or more *loxP* sites on separate chromosomes [25]), chromosomal translocations are highly undesirable since they may lead to cancer. In principle, translocations can be avoided by adjusting multiplicities of infection to obtain one provirus per cell. Ex vivo selection for recombination using HSV-Tk and Ganciclovir would also avoid this problem.

Finally, intrachromosomal recombination between two or more proviruses located on the same chromosome could result in chromosomal excisions with loss of genetic information. However, several considerations suggest that in a real therapy setting an intrachromosomal recombination between *loxP* sites is highly unlikely. First, the efficiency of excision is inversely related to the length of DNA flanked by site specific recombination targets. For example, a 300 nt segment is excised eight times more efficiently than a 3,000 nt fragment [38]. Second, recombination events increase with time and levels of Cre-expression [39]. Since retroviruses express Cre only transiently, recombination between the closely linked proviral sites should be strongly favored. Third, intrachromosomal recombination that may occur between adjacent proviruses that are closer to each other than the length of the proviral sequence flanked by *loxP* is also very unlikely. Assuming that the average length of this sequence is 3,000 nt, and retroviral integration is essentially random, approximately 10^6 independent integrations are required to obtain one provirus in every 3,000 nt of the genome (size of the haploid genome = 3×10^9 nt divided by 3,000 = 10^6). Thus, the probability of one retrovirus integrating into a given 3 kb genomic segment is 10^{-6} whereas that of a second retrovirus integrating into the same genomic site is 10^{-12}. Since most standard gene therapy approaches employ no more than 10^6-10^8 transduced cells, recombination between adjacent proviruses is probably negligible.

In conclusion, Cre/*loxP* vectors have several unique advantages over conventional retrovirus vectors which makes them likely candidates for future gene therapy trials. By eliminating most sequences that are not required for gene expression, the vectors should be both safer and more efficient transducers of therapy gene into the genome. In this context, we have recently observed that the level of expression of a cell surface marker gene transduced by Cre/*loxP* vectors into murine fibroblasts is between 5-10 times higher than that achieved with a conventional retroviral vector (*Kerstin Gotta, Harald von Melchner,* and *Manuel Grez,* unpublished results).

Acknowledgments

We wish to thank the members of our laboratories who have contributed to this work. This work was supported in part by grants from the Deutsche Forschungsgemeinschaft to *Manuel Grez* and *Harald von Melchner* and by a grant from the Deutsche Krebshilfe, Bonn, Germany to *Harald von Melchner.*

References

1 Crystal RG. Transfer of genes to humans: early lessons and obstacles to success. Science 1995;270:404-410.

2 Miller AD. Human gene therapy comes of age. Nature 1992;357:455-460.

3 Morgan RA, Anderson WF. Human gene therapy. Ann Rev Biochem 1993;62:191-217.

4 Nienhuis AW, Walsh CE, Liu J. Viruses as therapeutic gene transfer vectors. In: Young NS, ed. Viruses and Bone Marrow. New York: Marcel Dekker, 1993:353-414.

5 Akgün E, Ziegler M, Grez M. Determinant of retrovirus gene expression in embryonal carcinoma cells. J Virol 1991;65:382-388.

6 Challita PM, Kohn DB. Lack of expression from a retroviral vector after transduction of murine hematopoietic stem cells is associated with methylation in vivo. Proc Natl Acad Sci USA 1994;91:2267-2271.

7 Grez M, Akgün E, Hiberg F et al. Embryonic stem cell virus, a recombinant murine retrovirus with expression in embryonic stem cells. Proc Natl Acad Sci USA 1990;87:9202-9206.

8 Yamauchi M, Freitag B, Khan C et al. Stem cell factor binding to retrovirus primer binding site silencers. J Virol 1995;69:1142-1149.

9 Eckert HG, Stockschläder M, Just U et al. High-dose multidrug resistance in primary human hematopoietic progenitor cells transduced with optimized retroviral vectors. Blood 1996;88:3407-3415.

10 Baum C, Hegewisch-Becker S, Eckert HG et al. Novel retroviral vectors for efficient expression of the multidrug resistance (mdr-1) gene in early hematopoietic cells. J Virol 1995;69:7541-7546.

11 Bordignon C, Yu SF, Smith CA et al. Retroviral vector-mediated high-efficiency expression of adenosine deaminase (ADA) in hematopoietic long-term cultures of ADA-deficient marrow cells. Proc Natl Acad Sci USA 1989;86:6748-6752.

12 Donahue R, Kessler S, Bodine D et al. Helper virus induced T cell lymphoma in nonhuman primates after retroviral mediated gene transfer. J Exp Med 1992;176:1125-1135.

13 Vanin E, Kaloss M, Broscius C et al. Characterization of replication-competent retroviruses from nonhuman primates with virus-induced T-cell lymphomas and observations regarding the mechanism of oncogenesis. J Virol 1994;68:4241-4250.

14 van Lohuizen M, Berns A. Tumorogenesis by slow-transforming retroviruses—an update. Biochem Biophys Acta 1990;1032:213-235.

15 von Melchner H, Housman DE. The expression of the neomycin phosphotransferase in human

promyelocytic leukemia cells (HL-60) delays their differentiation. Oncogene 1988;2:137-140.

16 Pear WS, Nolan GP, Scott ML et al. Production of high-titer helper-free retroviruses by transient transfection. Proc Natl Acad Sci USA 1993;90:8392-8396.

17 Varmus H. Retroviruses. Science 1988;240:1427-1435.

18 Sauer B, Henderson N. Site-specific recombination in mammalian cells by the Cre recombinase of bacteriophage P1. Proc Natl Acad Sci USA 1988;85:5166-5170.

19 Gu H, Zou Y, Rajewsky K. Independent control of immunoglobulin switch recombination at individual switch regions evidenced through Cre-*loxP*-mediated gene targeting. Cell 1993;73:1155-1164.

20 von Melchner H, Ruley HE. Identification of cellular promoters by using a retrovirus promoter trap. J Virol 1989;63:3227-3233.

21 Morgenstern JP, Land H. Advanced mammalian gene transfer: high titer retroviral vectors with multiple drug selection markers and a complementary helper-free packaging cell line. Nucleic Acids Res 1990;18:3587-3596.

22 von Melchner H, Housman DE. The expression of the neomycin phosphotransferase in human promyelocytic leukemia cells (HL-60) delays their differentiation. Oncogene 1988;2:137-140.

23 DuBridge RB, Tang P, Hsia HC et al. Analysis of mutation in human cells by using an Epstein-Barr virus shuttle system. Mol Cell Biol 1987;7:379-387.

24 Reddy S, DeGregori JV, von Melchner H et al. Retrovirus promoter-trap vector to induce lacZ gene fusions in mammalian cells. J Virol 1991;65:1507-1515.

25 Smith AJH, De Sousa MA, Kwabi-Addo B et al. A site-directed chromosomal translocation induced in embryonic stem cells by Cre-*loxp* recombination. Nat Genet 1995;9:376-385.

26 von Melchner H, DeGregori JV, Rayburn H et al. Selective disruption of genes expressed in totipotent embryonic stem cells. Genes Dev 1992;6:919-927.

27 Stuhlmann H, Jaenisch R, Mulligan RC. Construction and properties of replication-competent murine retroviral vectors encoding methotrexate resistance. Mol Cell Biol 1989;9:100-108.

28 von Melchner H, Ruley HE. Retroviruses as genetic tools to isolate transcriptionally active chromosomal regions. Environ Health Perspect 1989;88:141-148.

29 Russ AP, Friedel C, Grez M et al. Self-deleting retrovirus vectors for gene therapy. J Virol 1996;70:4927-4932.

30 Emerman M, Temin HM. Genes with promoters in retrovirus vectors can be independently suppressed by an epigenetic mechanism. Cell 1984;39:459-467.

31 Emerman M, Temin HM. Quantitative analysis of gene suppression in integrated retrovirus vectors. Mol Cell Biol 1986;6:792-800.

32 Kohn D, Weinberg K, Nolta J et al. Engraftment of gene-modified umbilical cord blood cells in neonates with adenosine deaminase deficiency. Nat Med 1995;1:1017-1023.

33 Araki K, Araki M, Miyazaki J et al. Site-specific recombination of a transgene in fertilized eggs by transient expression of Cre recombinase. Proc Natl Acad Sci USA 1995;92:160-164.

34 Logie C, Stewart A. Ligand-regulated site-specific recombination. Proc Natl Acad Sci USA 1995;92:5940-5944.

35 Metzger D, Clifford J, Chiba H et al. Conditional site-specific recombination in mammalian cells using a ligand-dependent chimeric Cre recombinase. Proc Natl Acad Sci USA 1995;92:6991-6995.

36 Littlewood TD, Hancock DC, Danielian PS et al. A modified estrogen receptor ligand-binding domain as an improved switch for the regulation of heterologous proteins. Nucleic Acids Res 1995;23:1686-1690.

37 Baubonis W, Sauer B. Genomic targeting with purified Cre recombinase. Nucleic Acids Res 1993;21:2025-2029.

38 Gronostajski RM, Sadowski PD. The FLP protein of the 2-micron plasmid of yeast. J Biol Chem 1985;260:12328-12335.

39 Sauer B. Manipulation of transgenes by site-specific recombination: use of Cre recombinase. Methods Enzymol 1993;225:890-900.

Results of Retroviral and Adenoviral Approaches to Cancer Gene Therapy

L.H. Yin,[a] S.Q. Fu,[a] T. Nanakorn,[a] F. Garcia-Sanchez,[a] I. Chung,[a] R. Cote,[b] G. Pizzorno,[a] E. Hanania,[a] S. Heimfeld,[c] R. Crystal,[d] A. Deisseroth[a]

[a]Genetic Therapy Program of the Yale Cancer Center, and the Medical Oncology Section of the Department of Internal Medicine of the Yale University School of Medicine, New Haven, Connecticut, USA; [b]Cotton Norris Cancer Center, Los Angeles, California, USA; [c]CellPro. Inc., Bothell, Washington, USA; and [d]Cornell Medical School, New York, New York, USA.

Key Words. *Adenovirus · Retrovirus · Breast cancer · Cytosine deaminase · Multidrug resistance gene*

ABSTRACT

Genetic modification for cancer treatment has involved the introduction of chemotherapy protection and sensitization genes into normal and tumor cells, respectively, for the purpose of improving the outcome of conventional approaches to the treatment of solid tumor neoplasms. This paper will review the use of multidrug resistance-1 retroviral vectors and cytosine deaminase adenoviral prodrug activation vectors for this purpose. *Stem Cells* 1998;16 (suppl 1):247-250

METHODS AND RESULTS

MDR-1A, Retroviral Vectors for Chemoprotection

Michael Gottesman and his coworkers had first created transgenic mice carrying the multidrug resistance-1 (MDR-1) cDNA driven by a Harvey Sarcoma Virus long-terminal repeat [1]. This promoter is active in the more mature cells of the bone marrow, in contrast to the endogenous promoter, which is downregulated during myeloid maturation [2]. *Gottesman*'s data showed that the bone marrow cells in MDR-1 transgenic mice exhibited high levels of p-glycoprotein, and that these cells were resistant to the toxic effects of drugs recognized and transported by the p-glycoprotein transporter [1]. *Sorrentino et al.* [3], *Podda et al.* [4] and *Hanania et al.* [5] all reported that transplantation of MDR-1 vector-modified marrow cells into lethally irradiated mice resulted in marrow cells which were resistant to drugs recognized by the p-glycoprotein [3-5] in vivo selection of the MDR-1 vector-modified cells with post-transplant chemotherapy [3, 4]. These studies showed sufficient self-renewal capabilities in the MDR-1 vector-modified cells to sustain six serial transplants [5], and persistant expression of the human MDR-1 gene in the mouse marrow cells over 17 months of continuous in vivo passage [5]. These animal model data formed the basis for the information upon which four different institutions launched retroviral MDR-1 vector-mediated genetic chemoprotection trials in New York, Houston, Washington D.C., and Rotterdam.

The following were the goals of these trials: A) to test for toxicity of the vector modification; B) to test for resistance phenotypes post-transplant, and C) to determine if the post-transplant adminstration of 12 cycles of chemotherapy (taxol) would provide additional responsiveness of the tumors in these patients, above and beyond that which was achievable with the single adminstration of intensive therapy pretransplant. In our own trial [6], bone marrow or peripheral blood hematopoietic cells were collected from patients with carcinomas of the ovary or breast, respectively, whose disease had recurred following surgery, and was only partially responsive to conventional-dose chemotherapy. Following CD34 selection of these cells, two vector transduction procedures were used: A) suspension of the CD34-selected cells in the MDR-1 retroviral supernatant and B) innoculation of the CD34-selected cells on preformed irradiated autologous stromal monolayers in the presence of low doses of interleukin 3 (IL-3) and IL-6 (10 units/cc). This was repeated every 12 h for four feedings and the cells were then incubated an additional 24 h in the absence of the retroviral supernatant, following which the cells were cryopreserved.

Following the adminstration of intensive systemic chemotherapy, which was designed to destroy systemic disease, the MDR-1-transduced bone marrow or peripheral blood cells were transplanted into the patients and G-CSF was administered at a dose of 5 μg/day s.c., until hematopoietic recovery had occurred. In a dose escalation schedule, taxol was administered every three weeks until 12 courses were completed at a maximum dose of 275 mg/M^2 or until relapse or unacceptable levels of toxicity occurred. Ten patients with ovarian cancer and 10 patients with breast cancer were so treated. The results of this trial have been previously reported [6].

The results of the trials are as follows:

A) Toxicity of retroviral transduction: hematopoietic recovery occurred to an absolute neutrophil count of 500/cu mm within 9-14 days post-transplantion suggesting that the retroviral transduction did not reduce the short-term reconstitution capability of the CD34$^+$ cells.

B) Post-transplant response of the breast or ovarian cancer to the post-transplant taxol: the post-transplant taxol resulted in conversion of minimal responses to the pretransplant chemotherapy to complete responses in four patients and a conversion of a minimal response to a partial response in one additional patient. These data suggested that the post-transplant chemotherapy (the first time this has ever been done) was effective in completing the induction of remission in these patients.

C) Resistance phenotype post-transplant: there were three patterns of resistance or sensitivity post-transplant during the administration of the post-transplant taxol: 1) Sensitive: each cycle of taxol resulted in very low day 8 post-taxol neutrophil nadirs throughout the 12 cycles of post-transplant taxol; 2) Primary Resistant: the day 8 post-taxol neutrophil nadirs were high (above 2,000) right from the start of post-transplant taxol, a time at which only 5% of the cells were modifed with the MDR-1 vector (at most). This suggested that endogenous MDR-1 gene activation, rather than vector MDR-1 gene expression, was responsible for the resistance phenotype; 3) Evolution of resistance: these patients were sensitive immediately post-transplant but evolved resistance phenotypes to taxol during the 12 cycles of post-transplant taxol. Since the vector MDR-1-positive cells were detectable post-transplant for only one to two months, it is possible that again the endogenous MDR-1 genes were being induced by the chemotherapy, or that other mechanisms of resistance are responsible for this evolution in these patients.

D) Vector-positive cells pretransplant: DNA polymerase chain reaction of methylcellulose cultures (grown in medium supplemented with taxol), was used pretransplant and post-transduction to show that the transduction frequency pretransplant was 1%-20% and that there was no difference between the results obtained pretransplant with the two transduction protocols used (the suspension method in which the CD34-selected cells were suspended in retroviral supernatant for four h and then frozen, and the monolayer method, in which the CD34-selected cells were inoculated on preformed irradiated autologous stromal monolayers in the presence of low doses of IL-3 and IL-6 (10 units/cc).

E) Vector-positive cells post-transplant: vector-positive cells were detectable in none of the patients transplanted with cells transduced by suspending the cells in retroviral supernatant for four h. In contrast, five of eight of the patients transplanted with cells transduced on preformed irradiated stromal monolayers were positive post-transplant, but as noted, these vector-positive cells persisted only for one to two months post-translant. This short-term engraftment of the MDR-1 vector-modified cells was attributed to the following possible factors: 1) the low multiplicity of infection (0.5) used for the transduction; 2) the low-dose of post-transplant taxol during the time that the vector MDR-1-positive cells were circulating in the patient, immediately following recovery from the transplant, which was below the dose at which a selective advantage could accrue from the presence of the vector MDR-1 transgene; 3) the heavy prior chemotherapy exposure of the patients' hematopoietic cells to chemotherapy, which might have resulted in high levels of endogenous MDR-1 gene-mediated resistance to the taxol, and 4) the use in the transduction protocol of serum and IL-3 in the medium for the incubation of the CD34 cells during four days on stromal monolayers. Work in other laboratories has suggested that IL-3 and serum, both in the mouse and the primate model, especially if the IL-3 is high-dose, can induce differentiation of the early cells, thereby limiting their proliferative potential post-transplant.

Adenoviral Vectors for Chemotherapy Sensitization of Breast Cancer Cells in Collections of Marrow or Peripheral Blood from Ovarian Cancer or Breast Cancer, Respectively

An adenoviral vector carrying the cytosine deaminase or beta galactosidase gene was used to study the feasibility of selectively sensitizing breast cancer cells to the effects of chemotherapy. Cytosine deaminase sensitizes cells by converting a non-toxic prodrug, 5-fluorocytosine, into a toxic drug, 5-fluorouracil (5-FU). The following discoveries were made: A) The early hematopoietic cells are not infectable (<1%) by the adenoviral vector if they are not induced to differentiate by growth factors, whereas the breast cancer cells are infectable; B) the level of orotate phosphoribosyl transferase, which is necessary for the phosphorylation of 5-FU, in the hematopoietic cells is 1/50th of that in epithelial neoplastic cells, thus further protecting the hematopoietic cells; C) exposure of a mixture of MCF-7 breast cancer cells and hematopoietic cells to the cytosine deaminase adenoviral vector (which deaminates 5-fluorocytosine thus converting it to 5-FU), results in at least a millionfold reduction in the level of MCF-7 breast cancer cells in a mixture of MCF-7 cells with hematopoietic cells (HL60 cells). No significant reduction in the level of colony-forming units-granulocyte-macrophage from the hematopoietic population was seen when these cells were exposed to the identical conditions of the cytosine deaminase adenoviral vector and 5-fluorocytosine.

SUMMARY

A trial using MDR-1 retroviral vector-mediated modification to make safe post-transplant chemotherapy (taxol) has been completed. The results of this trial suggest that post-transplant chemotherapy generates responses above and beyond that generated by a single exposure to intensive systemic chemotherapy. A trial using adenoviral vectors carrying the cytosine deaminase gene to sensitize breast cancer cells is being prepared at Yale to purge the collections of hematopoietic CD34$^+$ cells of contaminating breast cancer cells.

ACKNOWLEDGMENT

A. Deisseroth acknowledges support from the Anderson Chair for Cancer Research and the Bush Leukemia Research Fund of the University of Texas MD Anderson Cancer Center; the Hull Development Fund of the Yale Cancer Center; the Ensign Professorship of the Yale University School of Medicine; the Susan Komen Foundation, and support from NIH grants NIH P01 CA49269 and NIH P01 CA55164.

REFERENCES

1 Gottesman MM, Ambudkar SV, Ni B et al. Exploiting multidrug resistance to treat cancer. Cold Spring Harb Symp Quant Biol 1994;59:677-683.

2 Chaudhary PM, Roninson I. Expression and activity of p-glycoprotein, a multidrug efflux pump, in human hematopoietic stem cells. Cell 1992;66:85-94.

3 Sorrentino BP, Brandt SJ, Bodine D et al. Selection of drug-resistant bone marrow cells in vivo after retroviral transfer of human MDR-1. Science 1992;257:99-101.

4 Podda S, Ward M, Himelstein A et al. Transfer and expression of the human multiple drug resistance gene into live mice. Proc Natl Acad Sci USA 1992;89:9676-9680.

5 Hanania EG, Fu S, Roninson I et al. Resistance to taxol chemotherapy produced in mouse marrow cells by safety-modified retrovirus containing a human MDR-1 transcription unit. Gene Ther 1995;2:279-284.

6 Hanania EG, Giles RE, Kavanagh J et al. Results of MDR-1 vector modification trial indicate that granulocyte/macrophage colony-forming unit cells do not contribute to post-transplant hematopoietic recovery following intensive systemic therapy. Proc Natl Acad Sci USA 1996;93:15346-15351.

Cytokine Gene Transfer in Cancer Therapy

Lei Cao, Peter Kulmburg, Hendrik Veelken, Andreas Mackensen,
Beata Mézes, Albrecht Lindemann, Roland Mertelsmann,
Felicia M. Rosenthal

Department of Internal Medicine I (Hematology/Oncology),
University Medical Center Freiburg, Freiburg, Germany

Key Words. *Gene transfer · Cytokines · Tumor cells · Immunity · Vaccine*

Abstract

New strategies based on gene transfer technology are employed in cancer therapy. Cytokines are polypeptides involved in immunity and inflammation, and essentially control the magnitute of the immune response. Genetically modified tumor cells releasing various cytokines have been shown to enhance tumor immunogenicity and to induce the regression of preexisting tumors. In some instances, immunological memory has been generated to resist the subsequent challenge with unmodified, parental tumor cells. Cytokine gene transfer into antitumor effector cells, as well as antigen presenting cells, is also being investigated to augment antitumor immune responses. *Stem Cells 1998;16:(suppl 1):251-260*

Introduction

Important advances in recombinant DNA technology and cell biology over the past decade, as well as the identification of factors that regulate gene expression, have led to a better understanding of diseases at the molecular and cellular levels, and notable progress in the field of gene therapy. Gene therapy is defined as the introduction of an exogenous gene into a host cell to achieve a therapeutic benefit [1]. Although initially regarded as primarily treatment for inherited disorders, this approach is now also being applied to a wide variety of acquired diseases ranging from cancer to degenerative diseases [1, 2]. Different from somatic gene therapy, gene transfer to sperm, ova or embryonal stem cells would aim to prevent the transmission of defective genes to subsequent generations. However, germ line therapy in humans is far from clinical application because it is facing many technical and ethical problems. Yet, whereas practical gene therapy is still facing significant problems, various protocols have been proposed and approved for clinical trials with surprising rapidity. The initial clinical trials have demonstrated that gene transfer in human subjects can be performed safely and with public acceptance. Most of these protocols require an ex vivo approach; i.e., somatic cells are cultured and transfected in vitro, then genetically modified cells are returned to the body. However, in certain clinical situations, it would be advantageous to develop in vivo gene therapeutic approaches. Therefore, gene transfer techniques that can achieve targeted in vivo transfection are currently under intense investigation.

Gene transfer into cells can be accomplished by viral and nonviral, i.e., chemical, physical and receptor-mediated means [3] (Table 1). Murine retroviral vectors have been the most extensively studied [4]. Retroviruses are modified to be nonpathogenic and replication-defective by deleting structural

Characteristics and Potentials of Blood Stem Cells
STEM CELLS 1998;16(suppl 1):251-260

Table 1. Gene transfer techniques

Nonviral methods

Physical methods

Electroporation

Particle bombardment

Microinjection

Lipofection

Chemical methods

Calcium phosphate coprecipitation

Receptor-mediated transfer

DNA/protein complexes

DNA/virus complexes

Viral vectors

Retrovirus

Adenovirus

Adeno-associated virus

Herpes simplex virus

Other: Epstein-Barr virus, HIV, vaccina virus, poliovirus,
SV40 virus

Bacterial vectors

Salmonella, listeria

genes from the virus genome. These genes coding for capsid proteins (gag), reverse transcriptase (pol) and envelope glycoproteins (env) which are essential for the virus life cycle are provided *in trans* by packaging cell lines in which the structural viral genes have been introduced. Packaging cell lines, when transfected with recombinant viral backbone DNA, produce infectious but replication-defective viruses. The primary advantages of retroviral vectors are their high efficiency of gene transfer and stable integration of proviral sequences into the host cell genome. Their main disadvantages are the size constraint (up to 9kb of foreign DNA) and the dependence on active DNA replication for efficient integration [5]. Adeno-associated viruses (AAVs) and adenoviruses represent two additional viral vectors. AAVs are single-stranded DNA parvoviruses that are not pathogenic in humans. AAV wild-type virus has been demonstrated to integrate into the host genome at specific regions of chromosome 19 [6]. Adenovirus vectors are currently being applied for many in vivo gene transfer efforts because they combine the characteristics of a high titer and the ability to infect nondividing cells with a broad host range and a tropism for epithelial tissue [7]. However, the properties of current generation adenoviral vectors may result in only transient gene expression due to residual expression of viral genes leading to immune reactivity [8]. Nonviral gene transfer methods (e.g., electroporation, microinjection, particle bombardment, lipofection) are less efficient with regard to integration of the exogenous gene into the host cell genome and therefore often only lead to transient expression. For several therapeutic situations, however, such as vaccine approaches for cancer using genetically modified cells, short-term expression of the transgene might be sufficient or even more desirable [9]. Direct injection of "naked" plasmid DNA, liposome-encapsulated DNA, as well as DNA-protein conjugates into various tissues has also been described [10, 11].

Besides the genes coding for therapeutic molecules, the transfer of marker genes (e.g., neomycin resistance gene) allows investigation of the trafficking, survival and functional properties of the marked cell following adoptive transfer in vivo. Although without a direct therapeutic goal, gene marking can help to study several aspects of pathogenesis and the biology of a disease as well as physiological aspects of hematopoiesis or the immune system in vivo. This approach is currently used in several clinical trials of autologous bone marrow (BM) transplantation or peripheral stem cell transplantation after high-dose chemotherapy to investigate the efficacy of purging, the mechanism of relapse and the biology of marrow reconstitution [12, 13].

Cytokines are a group of hormone-like polypeptides that play important regulatory roles either under normal or pathological conditions, and modulate the functional activities of a variety of individual cells and tissues. Because of their broad spectrum of activity, cytokines have been used in various therapeutic settings including both infectious diseases and neoplasia [14]. While systemic administration of hematopoietic cytokines like G-CSF, GM-CSF or erythropoietin (EPO) is routinely used in the prevention or treatment of chemotherapy-induced cytopenias with minimal side effects, systemic therapies with immunomodulatory cytokines like interleukin 2 (IL-2) are limited by important systemic and often life-threatening toxicities. Complete remissions of up to 20% in patients with malignant melanoma and renal cell carcinoma, however, have suggested the potential of IL-2-based immunotherapeutic approaches in cancer therapy. To circumvent the problems associated with systemic injection of immunomodulatory cytokines and to mimic the physiological release of cytokines at the effector-target sites, efforts to deliver cytokines by genetically modified cells have been stimulated. The following chapter will focus on the use of cytokine gene transfer for the modulation of the immune and hematopoietic systems.

Cytokine Gene Transfer to Modulate the Immune System

In the tumor-bearing host, the lack of an effective tumor-specific immune response may be due to weak tumor antigenicity or a tumor-immunosuppressive environment [15, 16]. The goal of cytokine-mediated cancer therapy is to alter the tumor-host relationship and to facilitate the recognition and destruction of malignant cells. Cytokines can influence the immune responses at two different levels. They may modulate the afferent arm of the immune response by direct actions on target cells. Certain cytokines may enhance tumor cell immunogenicity by increasing the expression of tumor-associated antigens, major histocompatibility complex (MHC) molecules (e.g., interferon-γ [IFN-γ]) and costimulatory or accessory signals which enhance the ability of lymphocytes to respond to mitogenic stimuli (e.g., IL-1, -6, -7, -12 and tumor necrosis factor [TNF]). The absence of such accessory signals involved in antigen processing and presentation may lead to immunological anergy [17-19]. On the other hand, cytokines can modulate the efferent arm of the immune response by activating effector cells of the immune system. IL-2 and IL-4, for example, can augment T cell proliferation and overcome the requirement for helper T cell cooperation in the generation of cytotoxic T cell responses [20, 21]. Some proinflammatory cytokines can directly activate cells to become cytotoxic for tumor cells. Therefore, the initial attempts to provide cytokines for the stimulation of cell-mediated immunity focused on the systemic administration of IL-2 and IFN-γ [22, 23]. Toxicity and variability in effectiveness of systemic administration have promoted the search for local delivery systems that provide cytokines in the microenvironment of the tumor and thus circumvent systemic side effects. This can be accomplished by the transfer of certain cytokine genes into tumor cells (autocrine secretion) or fibroblasts coinjected with tumor cells (paracrine secretion). Moreover, gene transfer into cytotoxic antitumor effector cells as well as antigen presenting cells (APC) is also being investigated.

Cytokine Gene Transfer into Tumor Cells

One approach to genetic immunomodulation in cancer is the introduction of cytokine genes into tumor cells with the aim to induce an immune reaction against both modified and unmodified tumor cells. The underlying assumption of such genetically modified tumor vaccines is that tumor cells might encode tumor-specific antigens, but they seem unable to elicit an adequate antitumor response due to a number of factors such as deficient antigen presentation, lack of immune costimulation and insufficient help from CD4$^+$ helper T cells. To overcome these deficiencies tumor cells have been genetically engineered with cytokine genes or costimulatory molecules to induce an effective immune reaction against both modified and unmodified tumor cells [24]. To date a wide variety of cytokines have been studied in many different tumor models using a range of different approaches like autologous versus allogeneic, irradiated verus unirradiated or in vitro versus in vivo gene transfer. Tumor cells engineered to release several different cytokines have been rejected when implanted into syngeneic animals. The magnitude of the antineoplastic response has been demonstrated to be dependent on the particular cytokine used, the level of cytokine expression, the inherent biological properties of the tumor, the number of injected tumor cells, the site of immunization and challenge, and the immunological status of the host.

Tumor cells transfected with IL-1 [25], IL-2 [26, 27], IL-4 [21], IL-6 [28, 29], IL-7 [4], IFN-α [30], IFN-γ [31, 32], TNF-α [33], G-CSF [34] and GM-CSF [35, 36] have been shown to be less tumorigenic in mice than the parental tumor cells, whereas transfection of the genes for IL-5, IL-10 and M-CSF does not alter tumor immunogenicity [37, 38]. Transfection of the gene for the immunosuppressive cytokine transforming growth factor-ß (TGF-ß) even increases tumorigenicity [39]. In several of these experimental models, injection of a mixture of cytokine-secreting and parental tumor cells results in killing of both populations, and generates a tumor-specific immunity that is capable of protecting the animal from a second challenge with parental, unmodified tumor cells [38].

The effector cells mediating or contributing to primary tumor rejection and immunity have been investigated by histological and immunohistological examinations of the tumor inoculation site, as well as by in vivo depletion of effector cell subpopulations with antibodies or experiments in effector cell-deficient mouse strains (nude, severe combined immunodeficiency or beige mice). Depending on the transfected cytokine genes, cellular infiltrates predominantly consist of nonspecific inflammatory cells such as macrophages, eosinophils, neutrophils and natural killer (NK) cells or of specific immune effector cells like T lymphocytes. The initial response to tumor inoculation in several models is largely due to a nonspecific inflammatory immune response, both in immunocompetent and in immunodeficient animals [33, 40, 41]. However, the establishment of a long-term protective immune response requires the presence of CD8$^+$ and/or CD4$^+$ MHC-restricted T cells. The exact mechanism of this "cross talk" between nonspecific and specific cellular elements has not been clearly elucidated but presumably relates to the processing and presentation of antigens [40]. This "cross talk" might explain the unexpected results that hematopoietic cytokines of the granulocyte/macrophage lineage (G-CSF, GM-CSF) are particularly effective in inducing specific antitumor immunity. In contrast, at high concentration, IL-2, a potent lymphocyte stimulator, appears to generate nonspecific lymphokine-activated killer, macrophage and NK cell cytotoxicity and its induction of T cell memory is not very efficient [42, 43]. To be optimally effective in stimulating a specific immune response, the level of IL-2 secreted locally by genetically modified cells seems to be crucial. Other cytokines may also share such dose-dependent phenotypic effects.

In most tumor systems, it has been difficult to demonstrate regression of preestablished lesions. This in part may be due to the rapid growth of transplanted murine tumors providing little time for immunotherapeutic intervention. However, in some animal models, certain cytokine-producing tumor cells (IL-2, IL-4, IL-6, IFN-α and GM-CSF) have also shown to be effective in the treatment of existing tumors as well as distant metastasis [35, 44-48]. Particularly in the Lewis lung carcinoma model, genetically modified tumor cells used in a postsurgical setting have shown their efficacy against metastatic growth of residual tumors [29, 32]. Those studies which have used irradiated tumor cell preparations as vaccines and which have shown the efficacy of genetically modified tumor cells in animals bearing nonimmunogenic tumors represent the most convincing demonstration of the potential of genetically modified tumor vaccines [49].

In addition, cytokine gene transfer into tumor cells may cause other phenotypic changes. An autocrine loop of certain cytokines may have influence on cell growth, secondary production of cytokines and adhesion molecules. For example, IFN-γ upregulates the expression of MHC antigens. Because MHC molecules are necessary for the stimulation of specific helper (MHC II) and cytotoxic (MHC I) T cell responses, their increase of expression in IFN-γ gene-transfected tumor cells could be important. The interaction in the complex network of cytokines may also contribute to the enhanced immunogenicity of cytokine gene-transfected tumors. TGF-ß has been shown to promote tumor growth and contribute to tumor escape from immune surveillance mechanisms. IL-7 production on the other hand can lead to downregulation of TGF-ß expression and therefore may result in an increase of tumor immunogenicity.

While in most studies, cytokine gene-transfected tumor vaccines have shown modest effects on preexisting tumors, one may expect that further optimization of protocols using genetically engineered vaccines will improve their potency. Understanding the mechanisms underlying the stimulation of the antitumor response provides valuable guidance for the design of further studies. Choosing more potent cytokines for particular tumor-type and therapeutic settings, or various combinations, such as the cotransfection of two cytokine genes [50] or the combination of cytokine gene transfer with the introduction of tumor-associated antigens, MHC molecules [46], foreign antigens and cell adhesion proteins or costimulatory molecules such as ICAM-1 [51] and B7 [18, 19] may improve therapeutic effects. For example it is thought that an effective antitumor response is generated through two distinct phases. First is the induction phase during which the naive T cells encounter for the first time tumor antigen and are activated. The tumor antigen is presented by professional APCs which pick up the tumor antigen released from the degraded tumor cells during an inflammatory reaction. There are also experimental data demonstrating that tumor cells themselves can contribute to the presentation of tumor antigens. In the second phase, the expansion phase, the newly activated tumor-specific T cells emigrate from the lymph node to the periphery where they encounter tumor cells, further proliferate and exert their effector functions by secreting cytokines or killing the tumor cells [49]. Some experiments suggest that different cytokines (e.g., GM-CSF or IL-2) or B7 gene-transfected tumor cells can mainly enhance the induction phase or the expansion phase of newly activated T cells [52, 53]. Therefore, a combination of cytokines (e.g., GM-CSF or IL-2) and B7 gene-modified tumor vaccines may have synergistic effects [18, 54].

Currently, most studies of tumor vaccination use an ex vivo strategy employing the removal of autologous tumor from the host, the genetic manipulation of the tumor cells with suitable genes in vitro and the reinjection of the modified cells into the host. This ex vivo strategy has the advantages of allowing clonal selection, expansion of clones expressing high levels of the transgenes in vitro and thorough characterization of the cell population which will be reinjected into the patient. However, the requirement of obtaining sufficient autologous tumor tissue for vaccine preparation and genetic manipulation limits its clinical application. A modified approach is to use cytokine gene-transfected, HLA-matched allogeneic tumor vaccines because human melanoma cells, and to some extent also other tumors, have been shown to present shared tumor-associated antigens that can be recognized by MHC-restricted T cells. Another alternative and considerably simpler approach is to genetically modify the tumor cells in situ. Such approaches require developing efficient gene transfer methods that are capable of transfecting a sufficient number of tumor cells in vivo. Intratumoral delivery of various viral vectors such as retrovirus [55], adenovirus [56] and vaccinia virus [57] vectors has been shown to retardate tumor growth and in some murine models generate long-lasting immunity against subsequent challenges with parental tumor cells. In vivo gene transfer with nonviral methods which are simpler, equally if not more efficient than viral vectors, such as lipofection [11, 58], receptor-mediated naked DNA gene trasfer [59] and particle bombardment [60] has also been investigated.

Whereas recent animal studies have attempted to mimic as closely as possible the clinical situations, animal models are unable to accurately reproduce the complexity and variability exhibited among cancer patients. However, such studies provide valuable information for planning clinical studies. A multitude of vaccine trials using cytokine gene-transfected tumor cells are currently underway in human patients with different types of cancers. So far no severe toxicities have been reported; the therapeutic efficacy of these approaches, however, remains to be demonstrated.

Cytokine Gene Transfer into Effector Cells of the Immune System

Another approach to genetic immunomodulation in cancer is based on gene transfer into antitumor immune cells to boost their killer activity. Adoptive immunotherapy of cancer has been attempted with ex vivo expanded tumor-infiltrating lymphocytes (TIL) in conjunction with IL-2 [61]. Regression of the tumor has been reported in patients with metastatic malignant melanoma. The first approved human gene transfer trial using retrovirally marked TIL in patients with advanced melanoma [61] has shown that genetically marked TIL can localize to the tumor site and thus may provide a vehicle for local delivery of therapeutic molecules to the tumor. Attempts were made to increase the antitumor activity of TIL by transfer of cytokine genes with cytotoxic activity like TNF [62-64]. A low transfection efficiency into TIL as well as a rapid decline of cytokine expression have hampered the progress of these clinical trials

[65]. Subsequently, TNF secretion was increased several-fold compared to the initial vector construct by modifying the TNF construct. In the new vector, the TNF transmembranous region was replaced with the IFN-γ signal peptide so that the smaller secreted form of TNF is directly transcribed and the membrane-bound TNF form is bypassed. Additional cytokines that have been studied for insertion into TIL include IFN-γ, IL-2 and IL-6 [61].

Cytokine Gene Transfer into APC or Bystander Cells

Given the difficulty in the culture and transfection of autologous tumor cells, bystander cells (e.g., fibroblasts) may be used as a vehicle for local cytokine production [9, 66, 67]. The paracrine secretion of cytokines by genetically engineered fibroblasts mixed with irradiated unmodified tumor cells also can induce systemic antitumor immunity. Our clinical trial using this approach attempts to induce antitumor immunity by stimulating tumor-specific cytotoxic T lymphocytes (CTL) with a genetically engineered vaccine. The vaccine is composed of autologous tumor cells, presumably carrying tumor-associated antigens, mixed with IL-2 secreting allogeneic fibroblasts as a paracrine source of IL-2 to provide an efficient costimulatory signal for activation of CTL [68]. In this phase I study, no toxicities were shown and tumor-specific CTLs were demonstrated in two patients [69, 70].

As tumor cells often appear to be defective in antigen processing and antigen presentation, the modulation of professional APCs such as dendritic cells by transfection of tumor-associated antigen genes might circumvent this problem [71]. Transfection of the elements involved in the generation or amplification of the immune responses such as cytokines or accessory molecules could enhance the function of APC and thus possibly improve the quality and nature of the resultant antitumor immune response. The establishment of protocols to generate sufficient highly purified human dendritic and Langerhans cells from peripheral blood hematopoietic stem cells will promote the clinical application of this approach [72].

Cytokine Gene Transfer to Modulate Hematopoiesis

Besides genetic immunopotentiation, gene transfer with hematopoietic cytokines has also been investigated after myelosuppressive chemo- or radiotherapy. Hematopoietic cytokines are a family of glycoprotein hormones which regulate the survival, proliferation and differentiation of hematopoietic progenitor cells as well as the function of mature cells [73]. G-CSF, GM-CSF and EPO have already been approved for human use, others are under investigations in clinical trials as treatment for hematopoietic deficiencies. Some disorders are characterized by a permanent deficiency of certain hematopoietic growth factors (e.g., EPO-deficiency in patients with renal failure), other clinical situations only require a transient supply of cytokines such as for the acceleration of hematopoietic recovery with G-CSF/GM-CSF after myelosuppressive therapy.

The reduction of hematopoietic precursors in the bone marrow (BM) associated with chemotherapy or irradiation results in hemorrhagic and infectious complications. These hematotoxicities are often dose-limiting in cancer therapy. Systemic administration of certain hematopoietic cytokines is widely used to accelerate BM recovery [74]. G-CSF and GM-CSF are often used to shorten the phase of neutropenia after cytotoxic therapy and BM or peripheral blood stem cell (PBSC) transplantation. In a preclinical murine model, a single injection of irradiated GM-CSF-transduced fibrosarcoma cells was shown to be equally efficacious as twice daily s.c. injections for seven days of the recombinant protein [75]. A single injection of irradiated G-CSF-secreting fibroblasts also leads to accelerated hematopoietic recovery as well as a mobilization of hematopoietic progenitor cells into the peripheral blood [76]. These results indicate that irradiated cytokine gene-transfected cells which have lost proliferation capability in vivo, retain the ability to secrete biologically active levels of cytokines over several days to weeks, periods sufficient for many clinical applications. Moreover, irradiation would be a precaution when cells are injected in vivo, since malignant transformation of genetically engineered fibroblasts has been described after in vivo transplantation in mice [77]. In vivo strategies are also investigated to deliver cytokines systemically. In an animal model, a single administration of an adenovirus vector encoding thrombopoietin (TPO) cDNA has been shown to abrogate thrombocytopenia induced by intensive chemotherapy [78]. Futhermore, the combined use of hematopoietic cytokines may act synergistically to reduce pancytopenia associated with myelosuppressive chemotherapy. TPO exhibits lineage-specific effects on platelet counts in normal animals, but in myelosuppressed animals, it cannot only reduce the time to platelet recovery, but also shorten the time to red blood cell and neutrophil recovery [79, 80]. It also shows synergistic effects with G-CSF on neutrophil recovery in myelosuppressed mice [81]. We are currently investigating whether the combination of genetically modified cells producing different hematopoietic cytokines can obtain synergistic effects on thrombocytopenia, anemia, and/or neutropenia after myelosuppressive therapy and BM or PBSC transplantation.

CONCLUSION

The last years have seen important advances in understanding diseases at the molecular and cellular levels. This knowledge may help to expand the application of somatic gene therapy to a wide variety of genetic and acquired diseases. As multifunctional regulators of cellular proliferation, differentiation, activation and motility, cytokines have been used in a variety of gene therapy settings, ranging from the modulation of immunity or hematopoiesis to wound healing [82]. In cancer therapy, cytokine gene transfer may stimulate antitumor immunity and protect the hematopoietic system so as to support high-dose chemotherapy. It is likely that the combined use of these promising novel approaches with more traditional forms of therapy will achieve better therapeutic efficacy in different clinical settings. Currently, gene therapy focuses on ex vivo manipulation of cultured cells. However, in certain situations, direct in vivo transfection appears beneficial as it would eliminate the requirement of isolation, transfection and implantation of modified cells. Thus, highly efficient and target-directed gene delivery systems have to be developed. At present, promising gene therapy strategies have been evaluated experimentally, and approved clinical protocols worldwide have continued to increase dramatically. Analysis of the 1996 data indicates that 75% of the 232 approved protocols have been initiated and at least 1,573 patients (some investigators did not provide a number) have been enrolled [83]. Although it remains difficult to predict the time point when gene therapy can be widely applied as a routine treatment, the era of gene therapy is surely coming.

REFERENCES

1 Morgan RA, Anderson WF. Human gene therapy. Annu Rev Biochem 1993;62:191-217.

2 Cao L, Zheng ZC, Zhao YC et al. Gene therapy of Parkinson disease model rat by direct injection of plasmid DNA-lipofectin complex. Hum Gene Ther 1995;6:1497-1501.

3 Yang NS. Gene transfer into mammalian somatic cells in vivo. Crit Rev Biotechnol 1992;12:335-356.

4 McLachlin JR, Cornetta K, Eglitis MA et al. Retroviral-mediated gene transfer. Prog Nucleic Acid Res Mol Biol 1990;38:91-133.

5 Miller DG, Adam MA, Miller AD. Gene transfer by retrovirus vectors occurs only in cells that are actively replicating at the time of infection. Mol Cell Biol 1990;10:4239-4242.

6 Kotin RM, Siniscalco M, Samulski RJ et al. Site-specific integration by adeno-associated virus. Proc Natl Acad Sci USA 1990;87:2211-2215.

7 Berkner KL Development of adenovirus vectors for the expression of heterologous genes. Biothechniques 1988;6:616-629.

8 Yang Y, Li Q, Ertl HC et al. Cellular and humoral immune responses to viral antigens create barriers to lung-directed gene therapy with recombinant adenoviruses. J Virol 1995;69:2004-2015.

9 Veelken H, Jesuiter H, Mackensen A et al. Primary fibroblasts from human adults as targets cells for ex vivo transfection and gene therapy. Hum Gene Ther 1994;5:1205-1212.

10 Liu Y, Liggitt D, Zhong W et al. Cationic liposome-mediated intravenous gene delivery. J Biol Chem 1995; 270:24864-24870.

11 Nabel GJ, Gordon D, Bishop K et al. Immune response in human melanoma after transfer of an allogeneic class I major histocompatibility complex gene with DNA-liposome complexes. Proc Natl Acad Sci USA 1996;93:15388-15393.

12 Brenner MK, Rill DR, Moen RC et al. Gene marking to trace origin of relapse after autologous bone marrow transplantation. Lancet 1993;341:85-86.

13 Dunbar CE, Cottler-Fox M, O'Shaughnessy JA et al. Retrovirally marked CD34-enriched peripheral blood and bone marrow cells contribute to long-term engraftment after autologous transplantation. Blood 1995;11:3048-3057.

14 Cohen MC, Cohen S. Cytokine function: a study in biologic diversity. Am J Clin Pathol 1996;105:589-598.

15 Bast RC Jr. Principles of cancer biology: tumor immunology. In: DeVita VT, Hellman S Jr, Rosenberg SA, eds. Cancer Principles and Practice of Oncology. Philadelphia, PA: JB Lippincott, 1985:125-150.

16 Wheelock EF. An overview of mechanisms responsible for tumor dormancy. In: Wheelock EF, ed. Cellular Immune Mechanisms and Tumor Dormancy. Boca Raton: CRC Press, 1992:1-13.

17 Allison JP, Hurwitz AA, Leach DR. Manipulation of costimulatory signals to enhance antitumor T-cell responses. Curr Opin Immunol 1995;7:682-686.

18 Cayeux S, Beck C, Aicher A et al. Tumor cells cotransfected with interleukin-7 and B7.1 genes induce CD25 and CD28 on tumor-infiltrating T lymphocytes and are strong vaccines. Eur J Immunol 1995;25:2325-2331.

19 Fenton RT, Sznol M, Luster DG et al. A phase I trial of B7-transfected or parental lethally irradiated allogeneic melanoma cell lines to induce cell-mediated immunity against tumor-associated antigen presented by HLA-A2 or HLA-A1 in patients with stage IV melanoma. Hum Gene Ther 1995;6:87-106.

20 Fearon ER, Pardoll DM, Itaya T et al. Interleukin-2 production by tumor cells bypasses T helper function in the generation of an antitumor response. Cell 1990;60:397-403.

21 Golumbek PT, Lazenby AJ, Levitzky HI et al. Treatment of established renal cancer engineered to secrete interleukin-4. Science 1991;254:713-716.

22 Rosenberg SA, Lotze MT, Yang JC et al. Experience with the use of high-dose interleukin-2 in the treatment of 652 cancer patients. Ann Surg 1989;210:474-484.

23 Veelken H, Rosenthal FM, Schneller F et al. Combination of interleukin-2 and interferon-α in renal cell carcinoma and malignant melanoma: a phase II clinical trial. Biotechnol Ther 1992;3:1-14.

24 Rosenfeld ME, Curiel DT. Gene therapy strategies for novel cancer therapeutics. Curr Opin Oncol 1996;8:72-77.

25 Douvdevani A, Huleihel M, Zoller M et al. Reduced tumorigenicity of fibrosarcomas which constitutively generate IL-1α either spontaneously or following IL-1α gene transfer. Int J Cancer 1992;51:822-830.

26 Gansbacher B, Zier K, Daniels B et al. Interleukin 2 gene transfer into tumor cells abrogates tumorigenicity and induces protective immunity. J Exp Med 1990;172:1217-1224.

27 Rosenthal FM, Cronin K, Bannerji R et al. Augmentation of antitumor immunity by tumor cells transduced with a retroviral vector carrying the interleukin-2 and interferon gamma cDNA. Blood 1994;83:1289-1298.

28 Mullen CA, Coale MM, Levy AT et al. Fibrosarcoma cells transduced with the IL-6 gene exhibit reduced tumorigenicity, increased immunogenicity, and decreased metastatic potential. Cancer Res 1992;52:6020-6024.

29 Porgador A, Tzehoval E, Katz A et al. Interleukin-6 gene transfection into Lewis lung carcinoma tumor cells suppresses the malignant phenotype and confers immunotherapeutic competence against parental metastatic cells. Cancer Res 1992;52:3679-3686.

30 Ferrantini M, Proietti E, Santodonato L et al. Alpha 1-Interferon gene transfer into metastatic friend leukemia cells abrogated tumorigenicity in immunocompetent mice: antitumor therapy by means of interferon-producing cells. Cancer Res 1993;53:1107-1112.

31 Gansbacher B, Bannerji R, Daniels B et al. Retroviral vector-mediated gamma-interferon gene transfer into tumor cells generates potent and long lasting antitumor immunity. Cancer Res 1990;50:7820-7825.

32 Porgador A, Bannerji R, Watanabe Y et al. Anti-metastatic vaccination of tumor-bearing mice with two types of gamma-interferon gene inserted tumor cells. J Immunol 1993;150:1458-1463.

33 Blankenstein T, Qin Z, Überla K et al. Tumor suppression after tumor cell-targeted tumor necrosis factor α gene transfer. J Exp Med 1991;173:1047-1052.

34 Colombo MP, Ferrari G, Stoppacciaro A et al. Granulocyte colony-stimulating factor gene transfer suppresses tumorigenicity of a murine adenocarcinoma in vivo. J Exp Med 1991;173:889-897.

35 Dranoff G, Jaffee E, Lazenby A et al. Vaccination with irradiated tumor cells engineered to secrete

murine granulocyte-macrophage colony-stimulating factor stimulates potent, specific, and long-lasting anti-tumor immunity. Proc Natl Acad Sci USA 1993;90:3539-3543.

36 Saito S, Bannerji R, Gansbacher B et al. Immunotherapy of bladder cancer with cytokine gene-modified tumor vaccines. Cancer Res 1994;54:3516-3520.

37 Allione A, Consalvo M, Nanni P et al. Immunizing and curative potential of replicating and nonreplicating murine mammary adenocarcinoma cells engineered with interleukin (IL)-2, IL-4, IL-6, IL-7, IL-10, tumor necrosis factor α, granulocyte-macrophage colony-stimulating factor, and -interferon gene or admixed with conventional adjuvants. Cancer Res 1994;54:6022-6026.

38 Tepper RI, Mule J. Experimental and clinical studies of cytokine gene-modified tumor cells. Hum Gene Ther 1994;5:153-164.

39 Torre-Amione G, Beauchamp RD, Koeppen et al. A highly immunogenic tumor transfected with a murine transforming growth factor type beta1 cDNA escapes immune surveillance. Proc Natl Acad Sci USA 1990;87:1486-1490.

40 Colombo MP, Modesti A, Parmiani G et al. Local cytokine availability elicits tumor rejection and systemic immunity through granulocyte-T-lymphocyte cross-talk. Cancer Res 1992;52:4853-4857.

41 Tepper RI, Coffman RL, Leder P. An eosinophil-dependent mechanism for the antitumor effect of interleukin-4. Science 1992;257:548-551.

42 Cavallo F, Giovarell M, Gulino A et al. Role of neutrophils and CD4+ T lymphocytes in the primary and memory response to nonimmunogenic murine mammary adenocarcinoma made immunogenic by IL-2 gene. J Immunol 1992;149:3627-3635.

43 Schmidt W, Schweighoffer T, Herbst E et al. Cancer vaccines: the interleukin 2 dosage effect. Proc Natl Acad Sci USA 1995;92:4711-4714.

44 Connor J, Bannerji R, Saito S et al. Regression of bladder tumors in mice treated with interleukin 2 gene-modified tumor cells. J Exp Med 1993;177:1127-1134.

45 Cao X, Zhang W, Gu S et al. Induction of antitumor immunity and treatment of preestablished tumor by interleukin-6-gene-transfected melanoma cells combined with low-dose interleukin-2. J Cancer Res Clin Oncol 1995;121:721-728.

46 Porgador A, Tzehoval E, Vadai E et al. Combined vaccination with major histocompatibility class I and interleukin 2 gene-transduced melanoma cells synergizes the cure of postsurgical established lung metastases. Cancer Res 1995;55:4941-4949.

47 Zitvogel L, Tahara H, Robbins P et al. Cancer immunotherapy of established tumors with IL-12: effective delivery by genetically engineered fibroblasts. J Immunol 1995;155:1393-1403.

48 Yu JS, Burwick JA, Dranoff G et al. Gene therapy for metastatic brain tumors by vaccination with granulocyte-macrophage colony-stimulating factor-transduced tumor cells. Hum Gene Ther 1997;8:1065-1072.

49 Gilboa E. Immunotherapy of cancer with genetically modified tumor vaccines. Semin Oncol 1996;23:101-107.

50 Rosenthal FM, Zier KS, Gansbacher B. Human tumor vaccines: genetic engineering of tumors with cytokine and histocompatibility genes to enhance immunogenicity. Curr Opin Oncol 1994;6:611-615.

51 Sartor WM, Kyprianou N, Fabian DF et al. Enhanced expression of ICAM-1 in a murine fibrosarcoma reduces tumor growth rate. J Surg Res 1995;59:66-74.

52 Bannerji R, Arroyo CD, Cordon-Cardo C et al. The role of IL-2 secreted from genetically modified tumor cells in the establishment of antitumor immunity. J Immunol 1994;152:2324-2332.

53 Huang AYC, Golumbek P, Ahmadzadeh M et al. Role of bone marrow-derived cells in presenting MHC Class I-restricted tumor antigens. Science 1994;264:961-965.

54 Parney IF, Petruk KC, Zhang C et al. Granulocyte-macrophage colony-stimulating factor and B7-2 combination immunogene therapy in an allogeneic Hu-PBL-SCID/Beige mouse-human glioblastoma multiform model. Hum Gene Ther 1997;8:1073-1085.

55 Wie MX, Tamiya T, Hurford RK Jr et al. Enhancement of interleukin-4 mediated tumor regression in athymic mice by in situ retroviral gene transfer. Hum Gene Ther 1995;6:437-443.

56 Cordier L, Duffour MT, Sabourin JC et al. Complete recovery of mice from a pre-established tumor by direct intratumoral delivery of an adenovirus vector harboring the murine IL-2 gene. Gene Ther 1995;2:16-21.

57 Elkins KL, Ennist DL, Winegar RK et al. In vivo delivery of interleukin-4 by a recombinant vaccinia virus prevents tumor development in mice. Hum Gene Ther 1994;5:809-820.

58 Vieweg J, Boczkowski D, Roberson KM et al. Efficient gene transfer with adeno-associated virus-based plasmids complexed with cationic liposomes for gene therapy of human prostate cancer. Cancer Res 1995;55:2366-2372.

59 Zatloukal K, Schneeberger A, Berger M et al. Elicitation of a systemic and protective anti melanoma immune

response by an IL-2-based vaccine. J Immunol 1995;154:3406-3419.

60 Sun WH, Burkhoder JK, Sun J et al. In vivo cytokine gene transfer by gene gun reduces tumor growth in mice. Proc Natl Acad Sci USA 1995;92:2889-2893.

61 Rosenberg SA. Immunotherapy and gene therapy of cancer. Cancer Res 1991;51:5074-5079.

62 Rosenberg SA, Aebersold P, Cornetta K et al. Gene transfer into humans: immunotherapy of patients with advanced melanoma using tumor infiltrating lymphocytes modified by retroviral gene transduction. N Engl J Med 1990;323:570-578.

63 Rosenberg SA. TNF/TIL human gene therapy clinical protocol. Hum Gene Ther 1990;1:443-462.

64 Cournoyer D, Caskey CT. Gene transfer into humans: a first step. N Engl J Med 1990;323:601-603.

65 Hwu P, Yannelli J, Kriegler M et al. Functional and molecular characterization of tumor-infiltrating lymphocytes transduced with tumor necrosis factor-alpha cDNA for the gene therapy of cancer in humans. J Immunol 1993;150:4104-4115.

66 Lotze MT, Rubin JT, Carty S et al. Gene therapy of cancer: a pilot study of IL-4-gene-modified fibroblasts admixed with autologous tumor to elicit an immune response. Hum Gene Ther 1994;5:41-55.

67 Fakhrai H, Shawler DL, Gjerset R et al. Cytokine gene therapy with interleukin 2-transduced fibroblasts: effect of IL-2 dose on anti-tumor immunity. Hum Gene Ther 1995;6:591-601.

68 Mertelsmann R, Lindemann A, Boehm T et al. Pilot study for the evaluation of T-cell mediated tumor immunotherapy by cytokine gene transfer in patients with malignant tumors. J Mol Med 1995;73:205-206.

69 Mackensen A, Veelken H, Lahn M et al. Amplification of tumor specific cytotoxic T-lymphocytes by immunization with autologous tumor cells and interleukin-2 gene transfected fibroblasts. J Mol Med 1997 (in press).

70 Veelken H, Mackensen A, Lahn M et al. A phase I clinical study of autologous tumor cells plus interleukin-2-gene-transfected allogeneic fibroblasts as a vaccine in patients with cancer. Int J Cancer 1997;70:269-277.

71 Henderson RA, Nimgaonkar MT, Watkins SC et al. Human dendritic cells genetically engineered to expression high levels of the human epithelial tumor antigen mucin (MUC-1). Cancer Res 1996;56:3763-3770.

72 Mackensen A, Herbst B, Koehler G et al. Delineation of the dendritic cell lineage by generating large numbers of Birbeck granule-positive Langerhans cells from human peripheral blood in vitro. Blood 1995;86:2699-2707.

73 Nicola NA. Why do hematopoietic growth factor receptors interact with each other? Immunol Today 1987;8:134-139.

74 Mertelsmann R, Rosenthal FM, Lindemann A et al. Cytokines and hematopoietins: physiology, pathophysiology, and potentials as therapeutic agents. Recent Results Cancer Res 1991;121:121-140.

75 Rosenthal FM, Früh R, Henschler R et al. Cytokine therapy with gene transfected cells: single injection of irradiated granulocyte-macrophage colony-stimulating factor-transduced cells accelerates hematopoietic recovery after cytotoxic chemotherapy in mice. Blood 1994;84:2960-2965.

76 Rosenthal FM, Kulmburg P, Früh R et al. Systemic hematological effects of granulocyte colony-stimulating factor produced by irradiated gene transfected fibroblasts. Hum Gene Ther 1996;7:2147-2156.

77 Tani K, Ozawa K, Ogura H et al. Implantation of fibroblasts transfected with human granulocyte colony-stimulating factor cDNA into mice as a model of cytokine-supplement gene therapy. Blood 1989;74:1274-1280.

78 Ohwada A, Rafii S, Moore MAS et al. In vivo adenovirus vector-mediated transfer of the human thrombopoietin cDNA maintains platelet levels during radiation- and chemotherapy-induced bone marrow suppression. Blood 1996;88:778-784.

79 Kaushansky K, Broudy VC, Grossmann A et al. Thrombopoietin expands erythroid progenitors, increases red cell production, and enhances erythroid recovery after myelosuppressive therapy. J Clin Invest 1995;96:1683-1687.

80 Ulich TR, del Castillo J, Yin S et al. Megakaryocyte growth and development factor ameliorates carboplatin-induced thrombopenia in mice. Blood 1995;3:971-976.

81 Grossmann A, Lenox J, Deisher TA et al. Synergistic effects of thrombopoietin and granulocyte colony-stimulating factor on neutrophil recovery in myelosuppressed mice. Blood 1996;88:3363-3370.

82 Rosenthal FM, Cao L, Tanczos E et al. Paracrine stimulation of keratinocytes in vitro and continuous delivery of epidermal growth factor to wounds in vivo by genetically modified fibroblasts transfected with a novel chimeric construct. In Vivo 1996 (in press).

83 Anderson WF. End-of-the-year potpourri—1996. Hum Gene Ther 1996;7:2201-2202.

Complete Bibliography of
Professor Dr. med. Dr. h. c. mult. Theodor M. Fliedner

1954

Stodtmeister, R. und FLIEDNER, T.M.: Zur Pathogenese der Knochenmarkschädigung bei Ratten nach Totalbestrahlung mit schnellen Elektronen (15 Me V Siemens Betatron, Heidelberg), Schweiz. Med. Wochenschr. 84. Jahrgang (1954), Nr. 39, 1113-1116.

Stodtmeister, R. and FLIEDNER, T.M.: Structural alterations and blood cell regeneration in bone marrow of rats following single dose irradiation with fast electrons from 15 MeV Siemens betatron. Heidelberg, Rev. d'Hémat. 9:586-588,1954.

1955

FLIEDNER, T.M., Sandkühler, S. und Stodtmeister, R.: Die Knochenmarkstruktur bei Ratten nach Bestrahlung mit schnellen Elektronen. Ztschr. für Zellforschung 43 (1955) 195-205.

Stodtmeister, R., Sandkühler, St. und FLIEDNER, T.M.: Die Bedeutung der Sinuswand für regressive und regeneratorische Prozesse des Knochenmarkes. Schweiz. Med. Wochenschrift, 85. Jahrg. 38/39 (1955) 942-945.

1956

Becker, J., Stodtmeister, R., FLIEDNER, T.M. und Kuttig, H.: Experimentelle Untersuchungen zur Frage der Gitterbestrahlung. Strahlentherapie 101 (1956) 272-277.

FLIEDNER, T.M. und Stodtmeister, R.: Zur Knochenmarkwirkung von Radio-Gold (Au198). Strahlentherapie 101 (1956) 289-295.

FLIEDNER, T.M., Sandkühler, St. und Stodtmeister, R.: Untersuchungen zur normalen feingeweblichen Struktur des Knochenmarkes bei Ratten. Schweiz. Med. Wochenschrift, 86. Jahrg. 51/52 (1956) 1448-1452.

FLIEDNER, T.M., Sandkühler, St. und Stodtmeister, R.: Untersuchungen über die Gefäßarchitektonik des Knochenmarkes der Ratte. Zeitschr. für Zellforschung 45 (1956) 328-338.

Stodtmeister, R., Sandkühler, S. und FLIEDNER, T.M.: Zum Problem der Wirkungsspezifität ionisierender Strahlen auf das Knochenmark. In: V. Kongress der Europäischen Gesellschaft für Hämatologie in Freiburg vom 20-24. 9. 1955, Springer Verlag Berlin 1956.

Stodtmeister, R., Sandkühler, St. und FLIEDNER, T.M.: Zur Pathogenese der akuten Knochenmarkatrophie. Dtsch. Med. Wschrf. 81 (1956) 964-965.

Stodtmeister, R., Scheer, K.E., Sandkühler, St., und FLIEDNER, T.M.: Vergleichende Untersuchungen über die Einwirkung von Radiogold und Radioyttrium auf das Knochenmark. Schweiz. Med. Wochenschrift, 86. Jahrg. 51/52 (1956) 1450-1453.

Stodtmeister, R., FLIEDNER, T.M. und Sandkühler, S.: Die hämatologischen Grundlagen für die Beurteilung von Strahlenschutzmaßnahmen. Strahlentherapie 101 (1956) 296-307.

Stodtmeister, R., Sandkühler, S. und FLIEDNER, T.M.: Die Bedeutung von Gefäßwandschäden für die Pathogenese der Blutbildungsstörung bei Ratten nach Ganzkörperbestrahlung mit 15 Me V-Elektronen. Strahlentherapie 101 (1956) 308-318.

Stodtmeister, R., Sandkühler, S. und FLIEDNER, T.M.: Über die Pathogenese akuter Knochenmarkatrophie bei Ratten nach Ganzkörperbestrahlung mit schnellen Elektronen. Folia Haematologica, 3 (1956) 303-345.

1957

Becker, J. und FLIEDNER, T.M.: Aufgaben und Erkenntnisse der Strahlenhämatologie. Med. Klinik, Nr. 7 (1957) 264-273.

Becker, J. und FLIEDNER, T.M.: Voraussetzungen und Möglichkeiten der Therapie von Strahlenschäden. Med. Klinik, Nr. 34 (1957) 1456-1468.

Becker, J. und FLIEDNER, T.M.: Über die Voraussetzungen der Regeneration des Knochenmarks nach ionisierender Ganzkörperbestrahlung. In: Proceedings of the Conference Internationale sur l'Influence des Conditions de Vie et de Travail sur la Sante. Cannes. S. 3-18, 1957.

FLIEDNER, T.M., Sandkühler, St. und Stodtmeister, R.: Über die Voraussetzungen der Markregeneration nach Schädigung durch radioaktives Goldkolloid (Au 198). Schweiz. Med. Wschr., 87. Jahrg. 39/40 (1957) 1225-1227.

Stodtmeister, R., Sandkühler, St. und FLIEDNER, T.M.: Über die Beziehungen des Ausschwemmungsmechanismus zur Sinusfunktion im Knochenmark. Schweiz. Med. Wschr., 87. Jahrg. 39/40 (1957) 1225-1226.

Stodtmeister, R. und FLIEDNER, T.M.: Die akute Stress-Situation des Knochenmarkes. Med. Klinik 52 (1957) 2225-2227.

1958

Becker, J. and FLIEDNER, T.M.: Hämatologische Untersuchungen bei der klinischen Anwendung von radioaktivem Goldkolloid. In: Radioaktive Isotope in Klinik und Forschung. Int. Symposium Bad Gastein 1958. Urban & Schwarzenberg München 1958.

Becker, J. and FLIEDNER, T.M.: Premesse della rigenerazione del midollo osseo dopo radiazione ionizzante su tutto il corpo. Minerva Medica 49 (1958) 714-717.

Bond, V.P. and FLIEDNER, T.M.: DNA-Synthesis in Irradiated Bone Marrow and Peripheral Blood Cells Studied by in vitro Incorporation of H3-Thymidine. Rad. Res., Vol. 9 (1958).

Bond, V.P., Cronkite, E.P., FLIEDNER, T.M., and P. Schork: Deoxyribonucleic Acid Synthesizing Cells in Peripheral Blood of Normal Human Beings. Science, 128 (1958) 202-203.

Cronkite, E.P., FLIEDNER, T.M., Bond, V.P., Andrews, G.A. and A.M. Johnson: Special Hematologic Studies on Radiation Casualties in the Y-12 Accident. In: The Acute Radiation Syndrome, compiled by M. Brucer, U.S. Atomic Energy Commission, ORINS report 25 (1958).

Cronkite, E.P., FLIEDNER, T.M., Rubini, J.R., Bond, V.P. and W.L. Hughes: Dynamics of Proliferation Cell Systems of Man Studied with Tritiated Thymidine. J. Clin. Invest. 37 (1958) 887.

Cronkite, E.P., FLIEDNER, T.M., Bond, V.P., Rubini, J.R. and G. Brecher: The Implications of Deoxyribonucleic Acid (DNA) Synthesis by Marrow, Spleen and Lymph Node "Primitive Mesenchymal Cells". Abstract Nr. 444, VII. Congresso della Societa Intern. di Ematologia, Roma 1958.

FLIEDNER, T.M.: Zur Beeinflussung leukopenischer Zustände bei Bestrahlungspatienten. Med. Klinik, 53. Jhrg. 28 (1958) 1223-1224.

FLIEDNER, T.M., Sorensen, D.K., Bond, V.P., Cronkite, E.P., Jackson, D.P. and E. Adamik: Comparative Effectiveness of Fresh and Lyophilized Platelets in Controlling Irradiation Hemorrhage in the Rat. Proc. Soc. Exp. Biol. a. Med. 99 (1958) 731-733.

FLIEDNER, T.M.: Markzell-Suspensionen bei strahlenbedingter Knochenmarkschädigung. Strahlentherapie, Band 106, Heft 2, 212-222. Urban & Schwarzenberg München 1958.

FLIEDNER, T.M., Cronkite, E.P. and V.P. Bond: Autoradiographic and Cytologic Studies Using H3-Thymidine on the Proliferative Capacity of Bone Marrow in Total-Body Irradiated Mammals. Rad. Res., Vol. 9 (1958).

FLIEDNER, T.M.: Relations between the Architecture of the Marrow Circulation and Functions. Fed. Proc., Vol 17 (1958).

Rubini, J.R., Cronkite, E.P., Bond, V.P., FLIEDNER, T.M. and W.O. Hughes: Metabolism of Tritiated Thymidine in Man. Clin. Res. 6 (1958) 267.

Stodtmeister, R., Sandkühler, S. and FLIEDNER, T.M.: Dysreglatoric and Cytostatic Factors in the Initial Phase of Bone Marrow Destruction by Ionizing Radiation. Their Differential Role for the Possibilities of Therapy. In: II. UN Int. Conf. on the Peaceful Uses of Atomic Energy. Pergammon Press Genf 1958.

1959

Bond, V.P., FLIEDNER, T.M., Cronkite, E.P., Rubini, J.R., Brecher, G. and P.K. Schork: Autoradiographic Studies on DNA Synthesizing Cells in the Peripheral Blood. Haemat. Latina 2 (1959) 103-114.

Bond, V.P., FLIEDNER, T.M., Cronkite, E.P., Rubini, J.R., Brecher, G. and P.K. Schork: Proliferative Potentials of Bone Marrow and Blood Cells Studied by in vitro Uptake of H3-Thymidine. Acta Haemat. 21 (1959) 1-15.

Bond, V.P., FLIEDNER, T.M., Cronkite, E.P., Rubini, J.R. and Robertson, .S.: Cell Turnover in Blood and Blood-Forming Tissues Studied With Tritiated Thymidine. In: F. Stohlman (Ed.): The Kinetics of Cellular Proliferation, 188-200, Grune & Stratton, New York 1959.

Cronkite, E.P., Bond, V.P., FLIEDNER, T.M. and J.R. Rubini: The Use of Tritiated Thymidine in the Study of DNA Synthesis and Cell Turnover in Hemopoietic Tissues. Laboratory Investigation, No. 1 (1959) 263-277.

Cronkite, E.P., FLIEDNER, T.M., Bond, V.P. and J.S. Robertson: Anatomic and Physiologic Facts and Hypotheses About Hemopoietic Proliferating Systems. In: F. Stohlman (Ed.): The Kinetics of Cellular Proliferation, 7-14, Grune & Stratton, New York 1959.

Cronkite, E.P., FLIEDNER, T.M. Bond, V.P. and J.R. Rubini: Dynamics of Hemopoietic Proliferation in Man and Mice Studied by H3-Thymidine Incorporation into DNA. Annals New York Acad. Science 77 (1959) 803-820.

FLIEDNER, T.M., Cronkite, E.P., Bond, V.P., Rubini, J.R. and A. Gould: The Mitotic Index of Human Bone Marrow in Healthy Individuals and Irradiated Human Beings. Acta Haematologica, Int. J. Hemat. 22 (1959) 65-78.

FLIEDNER, T.M., Cronkite, E.P. and V.P. Bond: Die Proliferationsdynamik der Blutzellbildung, autoradiographisch untersucht mit tritiummarkiertem Thymidin. Schweiz. Med. Wsch., 89. Jhrg. 41 (1959) 1061-1081.

Jackson, D.P., Sorensen, D.K., Cronkite, E.P., Bond, V.P., and FLIEDNER, T.M.: Effectiveness of Transfusions of Fresh and Lyophilized Platelets in Controling Bleeding Due to Thrombocytopenia. J. Clin. Invest. 38 (1959) 1689-1697.

Killmann, S.A., Rubini, J.R., Cronkite, EP. FLIEDNER, T.M. and V.P. Bond: Urinary Excretion of β-Aminoisobutyric Acid in Chronic Myelogenous and Lymphocytic Leukemia. Fed. Proc., Vol. 18 (1959) 1026.

Killmann, S.A., Rubini, J.R., Cronkite, E.P., FLIEDNER, T.M. and V.P. Bond: Urinary Excretion of Beta-Aminoisobutyric Acid in Chronic Myelogenous and Lymphocytic Leukemia. Fed. Proc., 18 (1959).

Rubini, J.R., Cronkite, E.P., Bond, V.P. and FLIEDNER, T.M.: Urinary Excretion of Beta Aminoisobutyric Acid (BAIBA) in Irradiated Human Beings. Proc. of the Soc. f. Exp. Biol. a. Med. 100 (1959) 130-133.

Stodtmeister, R. and FLIEDNER, T.M.: Der Eisenstoffwechsel bei aplastischer Anämie. In: W. Keiderling (Ed.): Eisenstoffwechsel - Beiträge zur Forschung und Klinik. 221-225. Georg Thieme Stuttgart 1959.

1960

Bond, V.P., FLIEDNER, T.M. and E.P. Cronkite: Evaluation and Management of the Heavily Irradiated Individual. Journ. Nuclear Med., Vol. 1 (1960) 221-238.

Bond, V.P., Shellabarger, C.J., Cronkite, E.P. and FLIEDNER, T.M.: Studies on Radiation-Induced Mammary Gland Neoplasia in the Rat. Rad. Res. Vol. 13 (1960) 318-328.

Cronkite, E.P., Bond, V.P., FLIEDNER, T.M. and S.A. Killmann: The Use of Tritiated Thymidine in the Study of Haemopoietic Cell Proliferation. In: G.E.W. Wolstenholm and M. O'Connor (Ed.): CIBA Foundation Symposium on Haemopoiesis, 70-92, J. & A. Churchill Ltd. London 1960.

Cronkite, E.P., Bond, V.P., FLIEDNER, T.M., Rubini, J.R. and S.A. Killmann: Studies on the Life Cycle of Normal and Neoplastic Leukocytes by Labeling DNA with Tritiated Thymidine. In: B. Rajewsky (Ed.): IX. International Congress of Radiology, 25.7.-30.7.1959 in München, S. 894-905, Georg Thieme Stuttgart 1960.

FLIEDNER, T.M., Bond, V.P. and E.P. Cronkite: The Effect of Total Body Irradiation on 3H-Thymidine Incorporation into DNA of Rat Bone Marrow Cells. In: B. Rajewsky (Ed.): IX. International Congress of Radiology, 25.7.-30.7.1959 in München. S922-S926, Georg Thieme Stuttgart 1960.

FLIEDNER, T.M.: Zur Hämatologie des akuten Strahlensyndroms. In: Strahlentherapie, Band 112, Heft 4, Urban & SchwarzenbergMünchen und Berlin 1960.

FLIEDNER, T.M.: Die Transfusion von 3H-Thymidin-markierten homologen Knochenmarkzellen in ganzkörperbestrahlte Ratten. Nuclear-Medizin, Vol. 1 (1960) 299-313.

FLIEDNER, T.M. and H.G. Frischbier: Incorporation of Tritiated Thymidine into Neoplastic and Non-Neoplastic Cells of Human Effusions. Clin. Res. 8 (1960) 826.

FLIEDNER, T.M.: Hämatologische Untersuchungen bei einem Strahlenunfall im mittleren Letalbereich. In: Verhandl. der Deutschen Ges. für Innere Med., 66. Kongreß 1960, 943-949, J.F. Bergmann München 1960.

FLIEDNER, T.M., Cronkite, E.P., Bond, V.P. and G. Andrews: Mitotic Activity and Cytology of Human Bone Marrow After Accidental Exposure to Ionizing Radiation. In: E. Neumark (Ed.): Proc. of the 7th Congress of the European Society of Haematology, London 1959, 458-467, S. Karger, Basel, New York (1960).

Johnson, H.A., Haymaker, W.E., Rubini, J.R., FLIEDNER, T.M., Bond, V.P., Cronkite, E.P. and W.L. Hughes: A Radioautographic Study of a Human Brain and Glioblastoma Multiforme After the in vivo Uptake of Tritiated Thymidine. Cancer, Vol. 13 (1960) 636-642.

Rubini, J.R., Cronkite, E.P., Bond, V.P. and FLIEDNER, T.M.: The Metabolism and Fate of Tritiated Thymidine in Man. Journ. Clin. Invest., Vol. 39 6 (1960) 909-918.

1961

Bond, V.P., FLIEDNER, T.M., Cronkite, E.P. and G. Andrews: Deoxyribonucleic Acid Synthesizing Cells in the Blood of Man and Dog Exposed to Total Body Radiation. Journ. Lab. and Clin. Med., Vol. 57 (1961) 711-717.

Cronkite, E.P. Bond, V.P., FLIEDNER, T.M., Paglia, D.A. and E.R. Adamik: Studies on the Origin, Production and Destruction of Platelets. In: S.A. Johnson et al. (Ed.): Blood Platelets. 595-609, Little Brown and Co., Boston, Mass. 1961.

FLIEDNER, T.M.: Strahlenwirkung und Hämopoese. In: J. Becker und G. Schubert (Hrsg.): Die Supervolttherapie. 209-224, Georg Thieme Stuttgart 1961.

FLIEDNER, T.M., Cronkite, E.P. und V.P. Bond: Das Studium der Proliferationsdynamik der Myelopoese unter Verwendung der Einzelzellautoradiographie. Folia haematol., 6 (1961) 210-228.

FLIEDNER, T.M., Bond, V.P. and E.P. Cronkite: Structural, Cytologic and Autoradiographic (3H-Thymidine) Changes in the Bone Marrow Following Total Body Irradiation. Am. Journ. Path., Vol. 38 (1961) 599-623.

Killmann, S.A., Cronkite, E.P., Bond, V.P. and FLIEDNER, T.M.: Acute Radiation Effects on Man Revealed by Unexpected Exposures. In: WHO (Hrsg.): Diagnosis and Treatment of Acute Radiation Injury, 151-164, WHO Genf 1961.

Rubini, J.R., Bond, V.P., Keller, S., FLIEDNER, T.M. and E.P. Cronkite: DNA Synthesis in Circulating Blood Leukocytes Labeled in vitro with 3H-Thymidine. Journ. of Lab. and Clin. Med., Vol. 58 5 (1961) 751-762.

Stodtmeister, R., FLIEDNER, T.M. und M. Dietrich: Das Verhalten der 59Fe-Plasma-Clearance im Initialstadium der Knochenmarkschädigung nach subletaler Ganzkörperbestrahlung. Folia haemat. 6 (1961) 252-255.

Tsuya, A., Bond, V.P., FLIEDNER, T.M. and L.E. Feinendegen: Cellularity and Deoxyribonucleic Acid Synthesis in Bone Marrow after Total- and Partial-Body Irradiation. Rad. Res., Vol. 14 (1961) 618-632.

1962

Bond, V.P., FLIEDNER, T.M. and E. Usenik: Early Bone Marrow Hemorrhage in the Irradiated Dog. Arch. of Path., 73 (1962) 13-29.

Bond, V.P., Rubini, J.R., FLIEDNER, T.M. and E.P. Cronkite: Study of the Effect of Therapy on Cells in the Blood of Leukemic Patients Capable of Incorporating H3-Thymidine. J. Labor. Clin. Med., Vol. 59 3 (1962) 412-418.

Cronkite, E.P., FLIEDNER, T.M., Killmann, S.A. and J.R. Rubini: Tritium-Labeled Thymidine (H3-TDR): Its Somatic Toxicity and Use in the Study of Growth Rates and Potentials in Normal and Malignant Tissue of Man and Animals. In: Tritium in the Physical and Biological Sciences. Int. Atom. Energ. Agenc. Vienna 1962.

FLIEDNER, T.M., Cronkite, E.P. and V.P. Bond: Pathogenesis and Regeneration of Radiation Induced Bone Marrow Injury, and Therapeutic Implications. In: H. Fritz Niggli (Ed.): Strahlenwirkung und Milieu, Sonderbände zur Strahlentherapie, Bd. 51, 263-278, Urban & Schwarzenberg München und Berlin 1962.

FLIEDNER, T.M. und R. Stodtmeister: Experimentelle und klinische Strahlenhämatologie. In: W. Stich und G. Ruhenstroth-Bauer (Hrsg.): Hämatologie und Bluttransfusion, Band 1, Sonderband zu Blut. J.F. Lehmanns München 1962.

FLIEDNER, T.M., Cronkite, E.P. and V.P. Bond: Potentialities and Limitations of 3H-Thymidine Labeling of Hemopoietic Cell Systems in the Study of their Dynamics of Proliferation. In: Proc. VIII. Congr. Europ. Soc. Haemat., Vienna 1961, S. Karger, Basel, New York 1962.

Killmann, S.A., Cronkite, E.P., Bond, V.P. and FLIEDNER, T.M.: Proliferation of Human Leukemic Cells Studies with Tritiated Thymidine in vivo. In: Proc. VIII. Cong. Europ. Soc. Hematol, Wien 1961. S. Karger Basel-New York 1962.

Killmann, S.A., Cronkite, E.P., FLIEDNER, T.M. and V.P. Bond: Cell Proliferation in Multiple Myeloma Studied with Tritiated Thymidine in Vivo. Lab. Invest., Vol. 11 (1962) 845-853.

Killmann, S.A., Cronkite, E.P. FLIEDNER, T.M. and V.P. Bond: Mitotic Indices of Human Bone Marrow Cells. Blood, Vol. 19 (1962) 743-750.

1963

Cronkite, E.P., Jansen, C.R., Rai, K., Cottier, H. and FLIEDNER, T.M.: The Combined Application of Lymph Duct Drainage and Extracorporeal Irradiation of the Blood in the Study of Lymphopoiesis. In: Cell Proliferation - A Guinness Symposium. Blackwell Scientific Publications Oxford 1963, 126-156.

FLIEDNER, T.M., Cronkite, E.P. ad V.P. Bond: Studies on Myelocytic Cell Turnover in Bone Marrow and Blood. In: W. Keiderlin, G. Hofmann (Ed.): Nuclear-Medizin : Radio-Isotope in der Hämatologie: I. Int. Symp. Freiburg 1.-3.März 1962, Suppl. 1 and Vol. II. Schattauer Stuttgart 1963.

FLIEDNER, T.M. Stodtmeister R., Meyer, L. and E.P. Cronkite: Problems of Bone Marrow Cell Transfusions: Radiation Induced Bone Marrow Failure and Forms of Therapy. In: Nuclear-Medizin. Sympos. on Radioact. Isotopes in Haem. Freiburg, 1962, Suppl. 1, 262-270. Schattauer Stuttgart 1963.

Killmann, S.A., Cronkite, E.P., Robertson, J.S., FLIEDNER, T.M. and V.P. Bond: Estimation of Phases of the Life Cycle of Leukemic Cells from Labeling in Human Beings in vivo with Tritiated Thymidine. Lab. Invest., Vol. 12 (1963) 671-684.

Killmann, S.A., Cronkite, E.P., FLIEDNER, T.M., Bond, V.P. and G. Brecher: Mitotic Indices of Human Bone Marrow Cells. II. The Use of Mitotic Indices for Estimation of Time Parameters of Proliferation in Serially Connected Multiplicative Cellular Compartments. Blood, Vol. 21 (1963) 141-163.

Stodtmeister, R., und FLIEDNER, T.M.: Grundlagen, klinische Möglichkeiten und Grenzen der Knochenmarkzelltransfusion. In: H.J. Melching et al. (Edit): Strahlenschutz in Forschung und Praxis, Band 2, 187-199. Rombach Freiburg 1963.

1964

Cronkite, E.P. and FLIEDNER, T.M.: Granulocytopoiesis. New Engl. Journ. Med. 270 (1964) 1347-1352.

FLIEDNER, T.M.: Der Lebenszyklus neutrophiler Granulozyten. Verhandl. der Deutsch. Gesellsch. für Innere Medizin, 70. Kongress April 1964, 452-453.

FLIEDNER, T.M., Kesse, M., Cronkite, E.P., and J.S. Robertson: Cell Proliferation in Germinal Centers of the Rat Spleen. Ann. New York Acad. Scien., Vol. 113 (1964) 578-594.

FLIEDNER, T.M., Andrews, G.A., Cronkite E.P. and V.P. Bond: Early and Late Cytologic Effects of Whole Body Irradiation on Human Marrow. Blood, Vol. 23 (1964) 471-487.

FLIEDNER, T.M., Thomas, E.D., Meyer, L.M. and E.P. Cronkite: The Fate of Transfused H3-Thymidine-Labeled Bone-Marrow Cells in Irradiated Recipients. Ann. New York Acad. Scien., Vol. 114 (1964) 510-526.

FLIEDNER, T.M., Cronkite, E.P. and J.S. Robertson: Granulocytopoiesis. I. Senescence and Random Loss of Neutrophilic Granulocytes in Human Beings. Blood, Vol. 24 (1964) 402-414.

FLIEDNER, T.M. und E.P. Cronkite: Reifung, Lebenserwartung und Schicksal neutrophiler Granulozyten. Die Med. Welt 1964, 466-472.

FLIEDNER, T.M.: Hämatologische Befunde beim akuten Strahlensyndrom. In: Deutscher Röntgenkongreß 1963, Teil B. Sonderbände zur Strahlentherapie, Band 56. Urban & Schwarzenberg München-Berlin 1964.

FLIEDNER, T.M., Cronkite, E.P., Killmann, S.A. and V.P. Bond: Granulocytopoiesis. II. Emergence and Pattern of Labeling of Neutrophilic Granulocytes in Human. Blood Vol. 24 (1964) 683-699.

Killmann, S.A. Cronkite, E.P., FLIEDNER, T.M. and V.P. Bond: Mitotic Indices of Human Bone Marrow Cells. III. Duration of Some Phases of Erythrocytic and Granulocytic Proliferation Computed from Mitotic Indices. Blood, Vol. 24 (1964) 267-280.

Meyer, L.M., FLIEDNER, T.M. and E.P. Cronkite: Autologous Bone-Marrow Transfusion Following Chemotherapy. Ann. New York Acad. Scien., Vol. 114 (1964) 499-508.

Stodtmeister, R. and FLIEDNER, T.M.: Granulozytenanomalien als Ausruck destruktiver und regeneratorischer Phasen der strahleninduzierten Knochenmarkschädigung. Schweiz. med. Wschr., 94 (1964) 1401-1402.

1965

Bond, V.P., FLIEDNER, T.M. and J.O. Archambeau (Eds.): Mammalian Radiation Lethality: A Disturbance in Cellular Kinetics. Academic Press New York, London 1965.

Burrichter, M., FLIEDNER, T.M., Stodtmeister, R. und I. Fache: Verkürzung der Segmentierungszeit neutrophler Granulozyten. Schweiz. Med. Wschr. 95 (1965) 1520-1523.

Cronkite, E.P., FLIEDNER, T.M., Stryckmans, P., Chanana, A.D., Cuttner, J. and J. Ramos: Flow Patterns and Rates of Human Erythropoiesis and Granulocytopoiesis. Selected Papers from the Xth Congress of the Int. Soc. of Haematology, Stockholm 1964. Series Hematologica 5 (1965) 51-63.

FLIEDNER, T.M., Thomas, E.D., Fache, I., Thomas, D. and E.P. Cronkite: Pattern of Regeneration of Nitrogen-Mustard Treated Marrow after Transfusion into Lethally Irradiated Homologous Recipients. In: La Greffe des Cellules Hematopoietiques Allogeniques. Centre Nat. de la Recherche Scientifique. Centre Nat. Rech. Scient. Paris 1965.

FLIEDNER, T.M., Kretschmer, V., Hillen, M. und F. Wendt: DNA- und RNA-Synthese in mit Phytohäagglutinin stimulierten Lymphozyten. Schweiz. Med. Wschr. 95 (1965) 1499-1505.

Stodtmeister, R., Burrichter, M. und FLIEDNER, T.M.: Das morphologische Bild von ineffektiver neutrophiler Granulozytopoese bei Knochenmarkregeneration nach subletaler Ganzörperbestrahlung von Ratten. Schweiz. Med. Wschr. 95 (1965) 1490-1492.

Thomas, E.D., FLIEDNER, T.M., Thomas D. and E.P. Cronkite: The Problem of the Stem Cell: Observations in Dogs Following Nitrogen Mustard. Jour. Lab. a. Clin. Med., Vol. 65 (1965) 794-803.

Wendt, F., Doyen, A., Schoop, W., Schubothe, H., Hunstein, W., FLIEDNER, T.M. und .W. Wedler: Erythroblastophthise bei Thymom. Schweiz. Med. Wschr., 95 (1965) 1494-1499.

1966

FLIEDNER, T.M.: Zytokinetische Grndlagen der Wirkungen von zytostatischen Substanzen. Therapiewoche, 17 (1966) 1977-1980.

FLIEDNER, T.M.: Attitudes and Outlook in Haematology as Seen by A Continental European. New Zealand Med. Journ., Suppl. 65 (1966) 913-920.

FLIEDNER, T.M., Fache, I. und C. Adolphi: Über die Umsatzkinetik der Leukozyten bei keimfreien Mäusen. Schweiz. Med. Wschr., 96 (1966) 1236-1238.

FLIEDNER, T.M.: Grundlagen von Diagnostik und Therapie bei Strahlenunfällen. In: H.R. Beck et al. (Eds.): Strahlenschutz in Forschung und Praxis, Band 6, 245-259. Rombach Freiburg 1966.

Stodtmeister, R. und FLIEDNER, T.M.: Entstehungsweise und Ablauf einer erythropoetischen Phase in der Rattenmilz nach Ganzkörperbestrahlung. Schweiz. Med. Wschr. 96 (1966) 1280-1282.

Stryckmans, P., Cronkite, E.P. and FLIEDNER, T.M.: DNA Synthesis Time of Erythropoietic and Granulopoietic Cells in Human Beings. Schweiz. Med. Wschr., 96 (1966) 1278-1279 und Nature 1966, Aug. 13, 211 (50) 717-720.

1967

Boll, I., Kretschmer, V. und FLIEDNER, T.M.: Kinematographische Dokumentation einer amitotischen Zellteilung. Zschr. f. Zellforsch. 83 (1967) 1-7.

FLIEDNER, T.M.: Experimental Studies on PHA-Stimulated Lymphocytes and Auto transfusion of 3H-Cytidine Labeled Lymphocytes in Chronic Lymphocytic Leukaemia. In: E. Arnold (Ed.): The Lymphocyte in Immunology a. Haemopoiesis. Symp. Bristol 1966, 198-207. W. Clowes & Sons London and Becles 1967.

FLIEDNER, T.M.: On the Origin of Tingible Bodies in Germinal Centers. In: Germinal Centers in Immune Responses. Proc. of a Symposium, Bern, June 1966, 218-222. Springer Verlag Berlin 1967.

FLIEDNER, T.M. und W. Hauger (Hrsg.): Ärztliche Maßnahmen bei außergewöhnlicher Strahlenbelastung. Georg Thieme Verlag, Stuttgart 1967.

FLIEDNER T.M.: Der Strahlenunfall als Aufgabe für ärztliche Gruppenarbeit. In: FLIEDNER, T.M. und W. Hauger (Hrsg.): Ärztliche Maßnahmen bei außergewöhnlicher Strahlenbelastung. Informationstag. d. Ges. für Strahlenforschung mbH, Freiburg 1966, 1-9. Georg Thieme Stuttgart 1967.

FLIEDNER, T.M.: Cytokinetic Basis for the Action of Cytostatic Agents. Therapiewoche 17 (48), 1977-1980, 1967.

FLIEDNER, T.M.: Zytokinetische Grundlagen der Wirkungen von zytostatischen Substanzen. Therapiewoche 48 (1967) 1977-1980.

FLIEDNER, T.M., Laeger, F. und E.P. Cronkite: Zytokinetische Untersuchungen an menschlichen Blutmonozyten. In: H. Brücher (Ed.): Der Monozyt, Blut-Suppl.-Band., 39-51. J.F. Lehmanns München 1967.

FLIEDNER, T.M.: Regeneration von bestrahlten Geweben aus zellphysiologischer Sicht. In: Deutscher Röntgenkongreß 1967, Teil B, Strahlebehandlung und Strahlenbiologie (Sonderbände zur Strahlentherapie) Bd. 66, 301-315. Urban & Schwarzenberg. München, Berlin 1967.

FLIEDNER, T.M.: The Consequences of the Radiosensitivity of Hemopoiesis for the Evaluation of Radiation Injury. In: Proceedings of the Int. Symp. on Accidental Irradiation at Place of Work. Nice, April 1966, 105-131. EURATOM 1967.

Haas, R., Stehle, H. und FLIEDNER, T.M.: Autoradiographische Untersuchungen über schnell und langsam proliferierende Zellsysteme des neonatalen Knochenmarkes. Schweiz. med. Wschr. 97 (1967) 1472-1473.

Haas, R.J., Stehle, H. and FLIEDNER, T.M.: Autoradiographic Studies on Rapidly and Slowly Proliferating Cell Systems in Neonatal Bone Marrow. Helv. Med. Acta, Vol. 34 (1967) 54-56.

1968

Binet, J.L., Cottier, H., Cronkite, E.P., Dausset, J., Field, E.O., FLIEDNER, T.M. et al.: Discussion générale. Nouvelle Revue Francaise d'Hematologie 8 (5) 1968, 745-758.

FLIEDNER, T.M., Becker, H., Cronkite, E.P. and H. Messner: Myelofibrosis in Irradiated Rats after Bone-Marrow Transfusion - an Immunological Rejection Phenomenon? In: Radiation and the Control of Immune Response, 85-89. Int. Atomic Energy Agency Wien 1968.

FLIEDNER, T.M., Bremer, K., Pretorius, F., Drücke, G., Cronkite, E.P. and I. Fache: Utilisation de la Thymidine et de la Cytidine Tritiees pour l'Etude du Turnover et du Metabolisme des Lymphocytes Chez l'Homme. Nouv. Rev. Franc. d'Hemat., 8 (1968) 613-624.

FLIEDNER, T.M., Haas, R.J. und H. Stehle: Die 3H-Tymidinmarkierung aller Zellkerne neugeborener Ratten In: H. Zimmermann und J. Fautrez (Hrsg.): Autoradiographie, Acta histochemica, Suppl. VIII (Verh. der Ges. f. Histochem. XII. Symp. Genf, September 1967), 231-256. Gustav Fischer Jena 1968.

FLIEDNER, T.M., Haas, R.J., Stehle, H. and A. Adams: Complete Labeling of All Cell Nuclei in Newborn Rats with H3-Thymidine. A Tool for the Evaluation of Rapidly and Slowly Proliferating Cell Systems. Lab. Invest. 18 (1968) 249-259.

Haas, R., FLIEDNER, T.M. and H. Stehle: Cytokinetic Analysis of Slowly Renewing Bone Marrow Cells after Administration of Nitrogen Mustard. In: Doyle, E. (Ed.): Effects of Radiation on Cellular Proliferation and Differentiation. IAEA, Wien, 1968. Unipub, New York, 1968, 205-220.

Stecher, G., Kubanek, B., Zahnert, R., FLIEDNER, T.M. und K. Burckhardt: Über die Wirkung von Thorotrast auf das Knochenmark. Blut, XVI (1968) 328-332.

Stodtmeister, R., Becker, H., Cronkite, E.P., FLIEDNER, T.M. und H. Messner: Experimentelle Knochenmarkfibrose in Ratten nach subletaler Ganzkörper-Röntgenbestrahlung und Knochenmarktransfusion als Modell der menschlichen Myelofibrose. Schweiz. Med. Wschr., 98 (1968) 1671-1673.

1969

Dietrich, M., FLIEDNER, T.M. und H Heimpel: Die Verwendung eines Isolierbettsystems bei der intensiven Chemotherapie von akuten Leukämien. Verh. der Deutsch. Ges. für Innere Medizin 75 (1969) 914-916.

Dietrich, M., FLIEDNER, T.M. und H. Heimpel: Isolierbett-System zur Infektionsprophylaxe bei verminderter Resistenz. Dtsch. Med. Wschr., 94. Jg. 19 (1969) 1003-1012.

FLIEDNER, T.M.: Viability Tests for Fresh and Stored Haemopoietic Cells In: Bone-Marrow Conservation, Culture and Transplantation, 95 106. Int. Atomic Energ. Agency Wien 1969.

FLIEDNER, T.M. und H. Heit: Hematopoietic Death in Conventional and Germfree Mice. In: V.P. Bond and T. Sugahara (Eds.): Comparative Cellular and Species Radiosensitivity, 220-232. Igaku Shoin Ltd. Tokyo 1969.

FLIEDNER, T.M.: Viability Tests for Fresh and Stored Haemopoietic Cells. In: Bone-Marrow Conservation, Culture and Transplantation. Proc. of Panel on Current Problems of Bone-Marrow Cell Transplant. in Moscow, July 1968, 95-106. Int. Atomic Energy Agenc. Wien 1969.

FLIEDNER, T.M., Messner, H., und B. Kubanek: Neuere Erkenntnisse zur Physiologie und Pathophysiologie der Erythropoese. In: Hämatologie und Bluttransfusion, Band 8, 1-15. J.F. Lehmans München 1969.

FLIEDNER, T.M.: A Cytokinetic Comparison of Hematological Consequences of Radiation Exposure in Different Mammalian Species. In: V.P. Bond and T. Sugahara (Eds.): Comparative Cellular and Species Radiosensitivity, 89-102. Igaku Shoin Ltd. Tokyo 1969.

FLIEDNER, T.M. und W. Calvo: Orthologie und Pathologie der Knochenmarkregeneration. In: H.-W. Altman et al. (Hrsg.): Handbuch der Allgemeinen Pathologie, 6. Band, 2. Teil, 375-495. Springer Verlag Berlin 1969.

FLIEDNER, T.M., Haas, R., Bohne, F. and E.B. Harriss: Radiation Effects Produced in Pregnant Rats and Their Offspring by Continuous Infusion of Tritiated Thymidine. In: M.R. Sikov and D.D. Mahlum (Eds.): Radiation Biology of the Fetal and Juvenile Mammal. US Atomic Energy Comm. 1969.

FLIEDNER, T.M. und W. Adam: Leukämie durch Röntgenstrahlen. Deutsch. Med. Wochenschr. 94 (27) 1969, 1425-1426.

FLIEDNER, T.M., Laeger, F. und E.P. Cronkite: Zytokinetische Untersuchungen an menschlichen Blutmonozyten. Hämatologie und Bluttransfusion 7 (1969) 39-51.

Haas, R.J., FLIEDNER, T.M. und E. Sparrer: Autoradiographische Untersuchungen zur zytokinetischen Analyse der neonatalen Erythropoese bei Ratten. In: Hämatologie und Bluttransfusion, Band 8. J.F. Lehmanns München 1969.

Haas, R.J., Bohne, F. and FLIEDNER, T.M.: On the Development of Slowly-Turning-Over Cell Types in Neonatal Rat Bone Marrow (Studies Utilizing the Complete Tritiated Thymidine Labeling Method Complemented by C-14 Thymidine Administration) Blood, Vol. 34 (1969) 791-805.

Messner, H., FLIEDNER, T.M. and E.P. Cronkite: Kinetics of Erythropoietic Cell Proliferation in Pernicious Anemia. Ser. Haemat., Vol. II, 4 (1969) 44-64.

Meuret, G. Schütz, W., Harriss, E.B., FLIEDNER, T.M., Hoelzer, D. Afkam, J., Obrecht, P., Musshoff, K., Heinze, V. et al.: Die Behandlung der chronisch-lymphatischen Leukämie durch extrakorporale Blutbestrahlung unter Verwendung konventioneller Strahlentherapiegeräte. Strahlentherapie 137, 1969, 429-441.

Meuret, G., Afkham, J., Schütz, W., Obrecht, P., FLIEDNER, T.M. und K. Musshoff: Behandlung der chronisch lymphatischen Leukämie durch extrakorporale Blutbestrahlung. Haematologica Latina, Vol. XII, 3-4 (1969) 531-537.

Storb, U., Bauer, W., Storb, R., FLIEDNER, T.M. and R.S. Weiser: Ultrastructure of Rosette-Forming Cells in the Mouse during the Antibody Response. Journ. Immunology, Vol. 102 (1969) 1474-1485.

1970

Bohne, F., Haas, R.J., FLIEDNER, T.M. und I. Fache: The Role of Slowly Proliferating Cells in Rat Bone Marrow During Regeneration Following Hydroxyurea. Brit. J. Haemat., Vol. 19 (1970) 533-542.

Flad, H.D., Hochapfel, G., FLIEDNER, T.M. und H. Heimpel: Blastentransformation und DNS-Synthese in Lymphozytenkulturen von Patienten mit aplastischer Anaemie (Panmyelopathie). Acta Haematologica 44 (1) 1970, 21-31.

FLIEDNER, T.M.: In memoriam: Ludwig Heilmeyer. Blood 35 (4) 1970, 558-560.

FLIEDNER, T.M., Calvo, W., Haas, R.J., Forteza, J. and F. Bohne: Morphologic and Cytokinetic Aspects of Bone Marrow Stroma. In: F. Stohlman (Ed.): Hemopoietic Cellular Proliferation, Grune & Stratton, New York 1970, 67-86.

Haas, R.J., Bohne, F. und FLIEDNER, T.M.: Die Wirkung kontinuierlicher intrazellulärer Bestrahlung durch 3H-Thymidin auf schwangere Ratten und auf die Entwicklung ihrer Nachkommenschaft. Strahlentherapie, 139 (1970) 571-586.

Haas, R.J., Kretschmer, V. and FLIEDNER, T.M.: Phytohämagglutinin-Stimulation von Lymphozyten bei Patienten mit aplastischer Anämie. Med. Klinik, 65. Jhrg. 15 (1970) 724-729.

Haas, R.J., Werner, J. and FLIEDNER, T.M.: Cytokinetics of Neonatal Brain Cell Development in Rats as studied by the Complete 3H-Thymidine Labeling Method. J. Anat. 107 (1970) 421-437.

Haas, R.J., Sparrer, E. und FLIEDNER, T.M.: Zur Proliferationskinetik der Lebererythropoese heranwachsender Ratten. Acta Haemat. 43 (1970) 232-241.

Heit, H., FLIEDNER, T.M., Fache, I. und G. Schnell: A Comparison of Radiation-Induced Bone Marrow Degeneration in Germfree and Conventional Mice. Rad. Res., Vol. 41 (1970) 163-182.

Meuret, G. und FLIEDNER, T.M.: Zellkinetik der Granulopoese und des Neutrophilensystems bei einem Fall von zyklischer Neutropenie. Acta Haemat., Vol. 43 (1970) 48-63.

Trepel, F., Fröhlich, D., und FLIEDNER, T.M.: Zytokinetische Untersuchungen der lymphatischen Ruhezellen bei einer immunologischen Primär- und Sekundärreaktion. Verh. der Deutsch. Ges. für Pathologie 54, 1970, 238-242.

1971

Bremer, K. and FLIEDNER, T.M.: Studies on the in vitro uptake of H3-cytidine in human blood lymphocytes. Revue Europenne d'Etudes Cliniques et Biologiques XVI (1) 1971, 19-26.

Bremer, K., Wack, O., Schick, P. and FLIEDNER, T.M.: Pools Sizes and Recirculation of Lymphocytes in Patients with Malignant Lymphoma. Abstract. Eur. Journ. of Clinical Investigation 1 (5) 1971, 364.

Bremer, K., and FLIEDNER, T.M.: RNA Metabolism of Circulating Lymphocytes Studied in Man After Autotransfusion and in-vitro 3-Cytidine Labeling. Acta Haemat. 45 (1971) 181-191.

Chaudhuri, J.P., Haas, R.J., Schreml, W., Knörr-Gärtner, H. and FLIEDNER, T.M.: Cytogenetic and Teratologic Studies on Rats Continuously Infused with Various Doses of Tritiated Thymidine during Pregnancy. Teratology, Vol. 4 (1971) 395-403.

Congdon, C.C. and FLIEDNER, T.M.: Morphological Aspects of Radiation Injury. IAEA Techn. Reports Ser. No. 123. Vienna, 1971, 85-88.

Flad, H.D., FLIEDNER, T.M. and H. Heimpel: Blast Transformation and DNA Synthesis in Lymphocyte Cultures from Patients with Aplastic Anaemia. Bibl. Haemat., No. 38, part II, 447-450, Karger Basel 1971.

Flad, H.D., Genscher, U., Dietrich, M., Krieger, D., Trepel, F.W., Hochapfel, G., Teller, W. und FLIEDNER, T.M.: Immunological Deficiency Syndrome in Non-identical Twins: Maintenance in a Gnotobiotic State and Attempts at Treatment with Transplants of Bone Marrow and Foetal Thymus. Eur. J. Clin. a. Biol. Res., Vol. XVI, 4 (1971) 328-334.

FLIEDNER, T.M.: Clinical Recommendations. IAEA Techn. Reports Series No. 123, Manual on Radiation Haematology. Vienna, 1971, 333-338.

FLIEDNER, T.M.: Erkennung und Behandlung von Strahlenschäden beim Menschen. In: Kommission der Europäischen Gemeinschaften, EURATOM 4732d Bundesanzeiger Köln 1971.

FLIEDNER, T.M.: Seminar on Cell and Cell System Ecology. Abstract. Paris June 1969. Government Reports Announcements, 71 (9) 1971, 40.

FLIEDNER, T.M., Chaudhuri, J., Haas, R.J., Knörr-Gärtner, H. und W. Schreml: Radiation Aspects of Tritiated Thymidine Studied in Pregnant Rats and Their Offspring. In: IAEA (Hrsg.): Biophysical Aspects of Radiation Quality, 355-368, Int. Atomic Energy Agency Wien 1971.

FLIEDNER, T.M. and G. Meuret: Die extrakorporale Blutbestrahlung. Klin. Wschr. 49 (1971) 895-899.

Genscher, U., Dietrich, M., Krieger, D., Teller, W., Flad, H.D. Hochapfel, G. Trepel, F. and FLIEDNER, T.M.: Lymphopenische Hypogammaglobulinaemie bei zweieiigen Zwillingen: Aufzucht während des ersten Lebensjahres unter keimfreien, gnotobiotischen Bedingungen. Monatsschrift für Kinderheilkunde, 119 (7) 1971, 421-422.

Haas, R.J., Fache, I., Bohne, F. and FLIEDNER, T.M.: Die Wirkung von Hydroxyharnstoff auf die Haemopoese der Ratte nach einmaliger oder fraktionierter Gabe. Arzneimittel-Forschung 21 (7) 1971, 974-978.

Haas, R.J., Bohne, F. and FLIEDNER, T.M.: Cytokinetic Analysis of Slowly Proliferating Bone Marrow Cells during Recovery from Radiation Injury. Cell and Tissue Kinetics, Vol. 4 (1971) 31-45.

Haas, R.J. and FLIEDNER, T.M.: The Effect of Tritiated Thymidine on the Oocytes of Foetal Rats Following Maternal Infusion in Pregnancy. Int. J. Radiat. Biol. , Vol. 19 (1971) 197-200.

Hoelzer, D., FLIEDNER, T.M., and E.B. Harriss: Turnover of Blast Cells in Acute Leukemia Auto Transfusion Studies after In-Vitro Labeling with Tritiated Cytidine. Abstract. Eur. Journ. of Clin. Invest. 1 (5) 1971, 376.

Meuret, G., FLIEDNER, T.M., Schütz, W., Öhl, N., Afkha, J., Obrecht, P. und K. Musshoff: Erfahrungen mit der extrakorporalen Blutbestrahlung bei der Behandlung der chronisch lymphatischen Leukämie. Klin. Wschr. 49 (1971) 899-904.

Meyer-Hamme, K., Haas, R.J. and FLIEDNER, T.M.: Cytokinetics of Bone Marrow Stroma Cells after Stimulation by Partial Depletion of the Medullary Cavity. Acta Haem. 46 (1971) 349-361.

Stodtmeister, R., Becker, H. und FLIEDNER, T.M.: Experimentelle Beobachtungen zum Verlauf einer Myelofibroseentstehung. Schweiz. med. Wschr. 101 (1971) 1775-1777

1972

Cronkite, E.P. and FLIEDNER, T.M.: The Radiation Syndromes. In: O. Hug und A. Zuppinger (Hrsg.): Strahlenbiologie. Handbuch der Medizinischen Radiologie, Band 2, Teil 3, 299-339, Springer Berlin 1972.

Dietrich, M., FLIEDNER, T.M., Kubanek, B. und H. Heimpel: Gnotobiotische Therapie als wirksame Infektionsprophylaxe bei der akuten Leukämie. In: R. Gross u. J.v.d. Loo (Eds.): Leukämie, 675-678, Springer Verlag Berlin 1972.

Dietrich, M., Meyer, H., Krieger, D., Genscher, U., FLIEDNER, T.M. und W. Teller: Development and Use of a Children Plastic Isolation System for Prevention of Infection. Eur. J. Clin. Bio. Res., Vol. XVII 3 (1972) 488-492.

FLIEDNER, T.M.: The Role of the University and of the Research Institute in the Scientific Training of Research Workers. In: Training of Research Workers in the Medical Sciences. Proc. of a Round Table Conf. of the CIOMS 1970, WHO Genf 1972.

FLIEDNER, T.M. und D. Hoelzer: Über die Dynamik leukämischer Zellspeicher. In: R. Gross und J.v.d. Loo (Eds.): Leukämie, 165-175, Springer Berlin 1972.

FLIEDNER, T.M.: Ärztliche Maßnahmen bei akuter Ganz- bzw. Teilkörperbestrahlung. In: G. Möhrle (Hrsg.): Erste Hilfe bei Strahlenunfällen, Band 47, 35-82, A.W. Gentner Stuttgart 1972.

FLIEDNER, T.M., Hoelzer, D., Seidel, H.J., Harriss, E.B. and B. Kuske: Kinetics of Erythropoiesis in Acute Leukaemia in Man, Rats and Mice. In: The Nature of Leukaemia, 279-288, V.C.N. Blight New South Wales 1972.

Haas, R.J., FLIEDNER, T.M.; and H.D. Flad: Fractionation of Rat Bone Marrow Cells. A Study Model for "Stem Cells". Abstract. Pediatric Res. 6 (1), 1972, 65.

Haas, R.J., Meyer-Hamme, K. and FLIEDNER, T.M.: The Role of Transplanted Slowly Proliferating Bone Marrow Cells for Regeneration of Lethally X-irradiated Rat Bone Marrow. Scand. J. Haemat. 9 (1972) 121-129.

Harriss, E.B. und FLIEDNER, T.M.: Hämatologische Strahlenwirkung als Folge der Strahlenempfindlichkeit der Stammzellen. In: O. Hug (Ed.): Beiheft zu Fortschritte auf dem Gebiet der Röntgenstrahlen und der Nuklearmedizin, 25-26, Georg Thieme Stuttgart 1972.

Heit, H., FLIEDNER, T.M. und I. Fache: Bone Marrow Regeneration in Germfree NO-2 Mice After 700 Rad Whole Body Irradiation. Rad. Res. , Vol. 51 (1972) 72-83.

Hoelzer, D., und FLIEDNER, T.M.: Quantitative und qualitative Veränderungen des Knochenmarkes nach Teilkörperbestrahlung in Abhängigkeit von der Dosis und der Zeit. In: Fortschritte auf dem Gebiete der Röntgenstrahlen und der Nuklearmedizin, Suppl. 26-28, 1972.

Hoelzer, D., Harriss, E.B., FLIEDNER, T.M. and H. Heimpel: The Turnover of Blast Cells in Peripheral Blood After in vitro 3H-Cytidine Labeling and Retransfusion in Human Acute Leukaemia. Euro. J. Clin. Invest. 2 (1972) 259-268.

Meuret, G., Hoffman, G., FLIEDNER, T.M., Rau, M., Oehl, S., Walz, R. and A.v. Klein-Wisenberg: Neutrophil Kinetics in Man. Studies using Autotransfusion of 3H-DFG Labeled Blood Cells as Autoradiography. Blut, Band XXVI 2 (1972) 97-109.

1973

Bremer, K., FLIEDNER, T.M. and P. Schick: Kinetic Differences of Autotransfused 3H-Cytidine Labeled Blood Lymphocytes in Leukemic and non-Leukemic Lymphoma Patients. Europ. J. Cancer 9 (1973) 113-124.

Bremer, K., Hollinger, R., Bock, O., Fröhlich, D., FLIEDNER, T.M. and H. Heimpel: Changes in the Lymphocyte Pools in the Course of Extracorporeal Irradiation of the Blood in Patients with Chronic Lymphocytic Leukemia. Abstract. Eur. J. of Clinical Investigation, 3 (3), 1973, 217.

Dietrich, M. and FLIEDNER, T.M.: Gnotobiotic Care of Patients with Immunologic Deficiency Diseases. Transplant. Proc. Vol. 3 (1973) 1271-1277.

Dietrich, M., FLIEDNER, T.M. and D. Krieger: Germ-Free Technology in Clinical Medicine: Production and Maintenance of Gnotobiotic States in Man. In: J.B. Heneghan (Ed.): Germfree Research. Biological Effect of Gnotobiotic Environments. Symposium, New Orleans, April 16-20, 1972. Academic Press. New York, 1973, 21-30.

Fischer, H., FLIEDNER, T.M., Haas, R., Koprowski, H., Pernis, B und G. Schwick: Gezielte Immunostimulation und Resistenzsteigerung. 2. Rundtischgespräch. Verh. der Deutsch. Gesellsch. für Innere Medizin. Med. Klinik 68 (1973) 8422-8423.

FLIEDNER, T.M., Haas, R.J., und H. Blattmann: The Significance of "Resting" Cell Populations for Hematopoietic Regeneration After Ionizing Radiation or Application of Radiomimetic Substances. In: J.F. Duplan, A. Chapiro (Eds.): Advances in Rad. Res., Vol. 2, 707-724, Gordon and Breach Science New York 1973.

FLIEDNER, T.M.: Pathophysiologie der Strahlenempfindlichkeit des Knochenmarkes. In: H. Braun et a.(Hrsg.): Strahlenempfindlichkeit von Organen und Organsystemen der Säugetiere und d. Menschen, Strahlenschutz in Forschung u. Praxis, Band XIII, 38-48 Georg Thieme Stuttgart 1973.

FLIEDNER, T.M.: Lymphocyt = Lymphocyt? In: Verhandlungen der Deutschen Gesellschaft für Innere Med., 79. Band, 129-138, J.F. Begmann München 1973.

FLIEDNER, T.M. und H.D. Flad: Therapiemodell der strahleninduzierten Knochenmarkinsuffizienz untr Verwendung tiefgekühlkonservierter Blutstammzellen. Wehrmed. Monatsschrift., 17. Jahrg. 10 (1973) 322-324.

FLIEDNER, T.M.: Pathophysiology of Radiation Effects in Different Species of Laboratory Animals as Compared to Man. In: 5th ICLA Symposium, Gustav Fischer Stuttgart 1973.

FLIEDNER, T.M., Bruch, CH., Calvo, W., Flad, H.D., Herbst, E., Hügl, E., Huget, R., Nelson, B. and H.P. Schnappauf: Pattern of Early Hemopoietic Regeneration in Lethally Irradiated Dogs after Transfusion of Fresh and Frozen Blood Leukocytes. Exp. Hematol. 1 (1973) 282.

FLIEDNER, T.M.: Pathophysiology of Radiation Effects in Different Species of Laboratory Animals as Compared to Man. In: A. Spiegel (Ed.): 5th Symposium of the Int. Comm. on Labor. Animals, Hannover 1972, 303-311, Gustav Fischer Stuttgart 1973.

FLIEDNER, T.M., Haas, R, Koprowski, H, Pernis, B. Schwick: Rundtischgespräch: Gezielte Immunstimulation und Resistenzsteigerung. Med. Klinik 68/25, 1973, 842-843.

FLIEDNER, T.M. und B. Kubanek: Umsatzkinetik und Regulation der Erythropoese bei hämolytischen Syndromen. In: L. Nowicke, H. Martin und J.C.F. Schubet (Eds.): Hämolyse - hämatologische Erkrankungen, 1 8, J.F. Lehmanns München 1973.

Haas, R.J., Schreml, W., FLIEDNER, T.M. and W. Calvo: The Effect of Tritiated Water on the Development of the Rat Oocyte after Maternal Infusion during Pregnancy. Int. J. Radiat. Biol., Vo. 23 (1973) 603-609.

Haas, R.J., Flad, H.D., FLIEDNER, T.M. und I. Fache: Correlation Between Cytokinetically Resting Lymphocytes and Bone Marrow Restoration. Experiments Using a Discontinuous Albumin Gradient. Blood, Vol. 42 (1973) 209-218.

Hohage, R., Meyer, H. and FLIEDNER, T.M.: Influence of Antibiotic Decontamination on Thrombocytopenic Bleeding in Irradiated Rats. In: J.B. Heneghan (Ed.): Germfree Research. Biological Effect of Gnotobiotic Environments. Symposium, New Orleans, April 16 - 20, 1972. Academic Press. New York, 1973, 465-469.

Heit, H. and FLIEDNER, T.M.: The Possible Role of the Gnotobiotic Status of Allogeneic Bone Marrow Recipients for the Clinical Course of Secondary Disease. Abstract. Exp. Hematology 1 (5) 1973, 290.

Heit, H., Wilson, R., FLIEDNER, T.M. and E. Kohne: Mortality of Secondary Disease in Antibiotic-Treated Mouse Radiation Chimeras. In: J. Heneghan (Ed.): Germfree Research, Biological Effect of Gnotobiotic Environments. Symposium, New Orleans, April 16 - 20, 1972. Academic Press New York 1973, 477-483.

Hoelzer, D. und FLIEDNER, T.M.: Umsatzkinetik der normalen und leukämischen Hämopoese bei akuten Leukämien. Wiener klin. Wschr. 85 (1973) 470-473.

Nelson, B. and FLIEDNER, T.M.: Lymphocytopoiesis after Irradiation. In: A. Breit und K.-H. Kärcher (Eds.): Gemeinsamer Kongreß der Deutsch. und der Österr. Röntgenges. 1973 in Wien. Beiheft der Zeits. Fortschritte auf dem Gebiet d. Röntgenstr. und Nuklearmed., 290-292, Georg Thieme Stuttgart 1973.

Nelson, B., Calvo, W., Herbst, E., Buch, Ch., Schnappauf, H.P. and FLIEDNER, T.M.: Repopulation of Dog Lymph Nodes after 1200 Rads Total Body Irradiation and I.V. Administration of Autologous Mononuclear Blood Cells. Abstract from the 2nd. Annual Conference. Exp. Hemat. 1 (1973) 282-283.

Schick, P., Trepel, F., Theml, H., Benedek, S., Trumpp, P., Kaboth, W., Begemann, H. and FLIEDNER, T.M.: Kinetics of Lymphocytes in Hodgkin's Disease. Blut, 27 (1973) 223-235.

Stodtmeister, R. and FLIEDNER, T.M.: Morphological Aspects of Myelofibrosis, Observed in Rats Following Sublethal Whole Body Irradiation and Subsequent Allogeneic Bone Marrow Cell Transfusion. Folia Haematol. 100, 1/2 (1973) 23-50.

Teller, W.M., Genscher, U., Flad, H.D., Hochapfel, G., Huget, R.P., Dietrich, M., Krieger, D., Wilson, R., Köhle, K., Simons, C., FLIEDNER, T.M., and F. Trepel: Rearing of Non-Identical Twins with Lymphopenic Hypogammaglobulinaemia under Gnotobiotic Conditions. Acta Paediatrica Scandinavica, Suppl. 240, 1973, 1-46.

1974

FLIEDNER, T.M.: Zell- und Organtransplantation: ihre strahlenbiologischen, pathophysiologischen und immunologischen Probleme. In: K.H. Kärcher und C. Streffer (Eds.): Die Strahlenwirkung auf das lymphatische System, 79-85, Springer Berlin 1974.

FLIEDNER, T.M.: Kinetik und Regulationsmechanismen des Granulozytenumsatzes. Schweiz. Med. Wschr., 104 (1974) 98-107.

FLIEDNER, T.M.: Funktionelle Struktur der Hämopoetischen Stammzellen-Speicher. Abstract. Blut 28 (3) 1974, 203.

Hoelzer, D., Harriss, E.B., Jäger, C., Haas, R.J. and FLIEDNER, T.M.: Effect of the Acute Rat Leukemia L5222 on Bone Marrow Stroma Cells. Cancer Res. 34 (1974) 1892-1897.

Hoelzer, D., Kurrle, E., Dietrich, M., Meyer-Hamme, K-D. and FLIEDNER, T.M.: The Effects of Continuous Cell Removal on Blast Cell Kinetics in Acute Leukaemia. Scand. J. Haemat. 29 (1974) 318-320.

Meuret, G. and FLIEDNER, T.M.: Neutrophil and Monocyte Kinetics in a Case of Cyclic Neutropenia. Blood, Vol. 43 (1974) 565-571.

Nelson, B. and FLIEDNER, T.M.: Lymphocytopoiesis after Irradiation. In: A. Breit und K.H. Kärcher (Eds.): Gemeinsamer Kongreß der Deutschen und der Österreichischen Röntgenges. 1973, Beiheft d. Zeitschr. Fortschr. auf dem Gebiet der Röntgenstrah. u.d. Nuklearmed.,290-292, Georg Thieme Stuttgart 1974.

Schreml, W., Haas, R.J. and FLIEDNER, T.M.: Radiotoxicity of Tritium on the Developing Rat: the Effectiveness of Tritiated Thymidine (3H-TdR) and Tritiated Water (HTO). Abstract. Radiation Research 59 (1) 1974, 62.

Theml, H., Schick, P., Trepel, F., Heltzel, U., Kaboth, W., FLIEDNER, T.M. and H. Begemann: Kinetik der nicht-lympatischen Leukozyten bei chronischer lymphatischer Leukämie. Abstract. Blut 28 (3) 1974, 217.

1975

Bremer, K. and FLIEDNER, T.M.: Impaired Exchange of Autotransfused Blood Lymphocytes between Intra- and Extravascular Pools in Patients with Untreated Chronic Lymphatic Leukemia. Biomed. Vol. 22 (1975) 404-410.

Calvo, W., FLIEDNER, T.M., Herbst, E.W. and I. Fache: Regeneration of Blood-Forming Organs after Autologous Leukocyte Transfusion in Lethally Irradiated Dogs. I. Distribution and Cellularity of the Bone Marrow in Normal Dogs. Blood, Vol. 46 (1975) 453-457.

Flad, H.D. and FLIEDNER, T.M.: Transplantation von Stammzellen: einige ethische Aspekte. In: H.G. Schwick (Hrsg.): Immunologie und Gesellschaft. Wissensch. Verlagsges. Stuttgart 1975, 231-234.

Flad, H.D, Goldmann, S.F., Huget, R.P., Krumbacher-von Loringhoven, K., Schnappauf, H.P., Bruch, C., FLIEDNER, T.M., et al: Die Bedeutung der Histokompatibilitätstestung für die Transfusion allogener Blutstammzellen bei Hunden. In: M. Matthes und V. Nagel (Eds.): Forschungsergebnisse der Transfusionsmed. & Immunhaematologie, Band 2, 843-854, Medicus Berlin 1975.

FLIEDNER, T.M.: Hämopoetische Stammzellen: Eine Teilpopulation der "Lymphozyten". In: H. Theml und H. Begemann (Eds.): Lymphozyt und klinische Immunologie, 63-77, Springer Berlin, 1975.

FLIEDNER, T.M.: Concluding Remarks. Advances in the Biosciences. 14, 1975, 605-606.

FLIEDNER, T.M.: In memoriam: Frederik Stohlman Jr. Blut 31 (3) 1975, 129-132.

FLIEDNER, T.M.: Funktionelle Struktur der hämopoetischen Stammzellen-Speicher: Ihre Relevanz für das Problem der Knochenmarkinsuffizienz. Hämat. und Bluttransfus.(Suppl. zu Blut) 16. (1975) 14-26

FLIEDNER, T.M.: Pathophysiologische Grundlagen der Transfusion hämopoetischer Stammzellen und Probleme ihrer Gewinnung. In: M. Matthes u. V. Nagel (Eds.): Forschungsergebnisse der Transfusionsmed. & Immunhaematologie, Band 2, 781-800, Medicus Berlin 1975.

FLIEDNER, T.M. und H. Heit: Alterungsvorgänge in Zellerneuerungssystemen. Verh. Dtsch. Ges. Path. 59 (1975) 71-77.

FLIEDNER, T.M., Hoelzer, D., Köbele, K. and K.H. Steinbach: Kinetic studies on Normal and Leukemic Cell Production in Acute Leukemia. In: FLIEDNER, T.M. and S. Perry (Eds.): Advances in the Biosciences 14. Workshop on Prognostic Factors in Human Acute Leukemia, Germany 1973, 361-376, Pergammon Press, Vieweg New York, Braunschweig 1975.

FLIEDNER, T.M., Hügl, E.H., Flad, H.D., Nothdurft, W.H., Calvo, W., Huget, R., Ross, W.M., Schnappauf, H.P. und I. Steinbach: Collection and Use of Blood Stem Cells for the Treatment of Bone Marrow Aplasia: A Canine Model. In: J.M. Goldman and R.M. Lowenthal (Eds.): Leukocytes: Separation, Collection and Transfusion, 271-275 Academic Press London 1975.

Herbst, E.W. FLIEDNER, T.M., Calvo, W., Schnappauf, H.P. and H. Meyer: Untersuchungen über die Gewinnung hämopoetischer Stammzellen aus dem peripheren Blut von Hunden und über ihre Fähigkeit, die Blutzellbildung zu regenerieren. Blut, Heft 6, 30 (1975) 265-276.

Hoelzer, D., Kurrle, E., Harriss, E.B., FLIEDNER, T.M. and R.J. Haas: Evidence for Stem Cell Function of Resting Bone Marrow Lymphocytes Identified by the Complete 3H-Thymidine Labeling Method. Biomedicine, Vol. 22 (1975) 285-290.

Hoelzer, D., Pflieger, H., Kurrle, E., Dictrich, M. and FLIEDNER, T.M.: Kinetic Aspects of Treatment of Acute Leukaemia by Leukapheresis. In: J.M. Goldman and R.M. Lowenthal (Eds.): Leukocytes Separation Collection and Transfusion, 487-496, Academic Press London 1975.

Lohrmann, H.P., Dietrich, M., Goldmann, S.F., Kristensen, T., FLIEDNER, T.M., Abt, C., Pflieger, H., Flad, H.D. et al.: Bone Marrow Transplantation for Aplastic Anaemia from a HL-A and MLC-Identical Unrelated Donor. Blut 31 (1975) 347-354.

Schick, P., Trepel, F., Eder, M., Matzner, M., Benedek, S., Theml, H., Kaboth, W., Begemann, H. and FLIEDNER, T.M.: Autotransfusion of 3H-Cytidine-Labeled Blood Lymphocytes in Patients with

Hodgkin's Disease and Non-Hodgkin Patients. II. Exchangeable lymphocyte pools. Acta Haematologica 53 (4) 1975, 206-218.

Schreml, W., FLIEDNER, T.M., und E. Ellwanger: Erfahrungen mit der Lehre des ökologischen Stoffgebietes nach der neuen Approbationsordnung an der Universität Ulm. Dtsch. Rentenversicherung 6 (1975) 372-374.

1976

Abt, C., Arnold, R., Dietrich, M., FLIEDNER, T.M., Goldmann, S.F., Haas, R.J., Heimpel, H., Kleihauer, E., Kubanek, B., Lohrmann, H.P., Niethammer, D. und H. Pflieger: Erfahrungen mit Knochenmarktransplantationen bei schweren Panmyelopathien. Verh. der Deutschen. Ges. für Innere Medizin 82, 1976, 1575-1579.

Calvo, W., FLIEDNER, T.M., Herbst, E., Hügl, E. and C. Bruch: Regeneration of Blood-Forming Organs After Autologous Leukocyte Transfusion in Lethally Irradiated Dogs. II. Distribution and Cellularity of the Marrow in Irradiated and Transfused Animals. Blood, Vol. 47 (1976) 593-601.

Flad, H.D., Krumbacher, K., Schnappauf, H.P., Nothdurft, W., Steinbach, I., Huget, R.P. and FLIED-NER, T.M.: Transplantation of Allogeneic Dog Leukocytes into Lethally Irradiated Matched or Mismatched Recipients. Zschr. f. Immunitätsforschung-Immunbiol. 152 (1976) 326-330.

FLIEDNER, T.M., Steinbach, K.H. und H. Raffler: Zellbiologische Grundlagen des Lebens eines Organismus im Strahlenfeld. Atomwirtschaft - Atomtechnik, Jrg. XXI 6 (1976) 292-297.

FLIEDNER, T.M., Flad, H.D., Bruch, C., Calvo, W., Goldmann, S.F., Herbst, E., Hügl, E., Huget, R., Körbling, M. et al.: Treatment of Aplastic anemia by Blood Stem Cell Transfusion: A Canine Model. Haematologica, Vol. 61 (1976) 141-156.

FLIEDNER, T.M., Steinbach, K.H. and D. Hoelzer: Adaptation to Environmental change: The Role of Cell-Renewal Systems. In: E.S. Finckh (Ed.): The Effects of Environment on Cells and Tissues. Proc. IX. World Congress of Anatomic and Clinical Pathology, Sydney, Oct. 1975, 20-38, Excerpta Medica Amsterdam 1976.

FLIEDNER, T.M.: Das granulozytäre Zellerneuerungssystem: Ein Regelkreis. In: A. Stacher und P. Höcker (Hrsg.): Erkrankungen der Myelopoese, 7-13, Urban & Schwarzenberg München 1976.

FLIEDNER, T.M.: Standardisierung und Koordinierung: Die interdisziplinäre Krebsbehandlung des Onkologischen Areitskreises Ulm. Ärztliche Praxis, Jhrg. XXVII 99 (1976) 3971-3972.

FLIEDNER, T.M.: Three "C": A Challenge (Presidential Address 1975 of the European Society for Clinical Investigation). Europ. J. Clin. Invest. 6 (1976) 1-5.

FLIEDNER, T.M., Hoelzer, D. and K.H. Steinbach: Productivity in Normal and Leukemic Granulocytopoiesis. In: W. Stich, G. Ruhenstroth-Bauer und H. Heimpel (Hrsg.): Hämatologie und Bluttransfusion. Sonderband zu Blut: Modern Trends in Human Leukemia II, 9-19, J.F. Lehmanns München 1976.

FLIEDNER, T.M.: Analyse und Behandlung von außergewöhnlichen Strahlenbelastungen. Atomkernenergie (ATKE), Lfg. 1 28 (1976) 39-47.

FLIEDNER, T.M.: Über den derzeitigen Stand der zellsystemphysiologischen Kenntnis der Leber. In: L. Wannagat (Ed.): Toxische Leberschäden. 8. Lebertagung der Sozialmediziner, 1973, 72-80, Georg Thieme Stuttgart 1976.

Heit, H. und FLIEDNER, T.M.: Einfluß humoraler Faktoren auf die Stammzelldifferenzierung nach Ganzkörperbestrahlung. Abstract. Blut, Vol. 33 (Vortrag 99), 1976, 226.

Heit, H., Heit, W. and FLIEDNER, T.M.: Allogeneic Bone Marrow Grafting in Radiation-Induced Aplastic Anemia in Mice: Significance of the Gnotobiotic State. In: Leukemia and Aplastic Anemia. Proc. Int. Conf. Naples, Sept. 1974, 70-75. Is Pensiero Scientifico Rom 1976.

Hoelzer, D. and FLIEDNER, T.M.: Pathophysiological Aspects of Haemopoietic Failure in Acute Leukemia.. Proc. of the Int. Meeting on Basic Advances in Leukemia and Biol. Bases of its Therapy, Rom 1973, 114-121 Accademia Naz. del Lincei Rom 1976.

Körbling, M., Ross, W.M., Nothdurft, W., Schnappauf, H.P., Steinbach, I. and FLIEDNER, T.M.: Die Behandlung der hämatopoetischen Insuffizienz im präklinischen Hundemodell durch Transfusion angereicherter Blutstammzellsuspensionen. Abstract. Blut, Vol. 33, 1976, 221.

Kovacs, P., Bruch, C. and FLIEDNER, T.M.: Colony Formation by Canine Hemopoietic Cells in vitro. Acta Haemat. 56 (1976) 107-115.

Nelson, B., Calvo, W., FLIEDNER, T.M., Herbst, E., Bruch, Ch., Schnappauf, H.P. and H.D. Flad: The Repopulation of Lymph Nodes of Dogs After 1200 R Whole- Body X-Irradiation and Intravenous Administration of Mononuclear Blood Leukocytes. Amer. J. of Pathology, Vol. 84 (1976) 259-282.

Niethammer, D., Goldmann, S.F., Haas, R.J., Dietrich, M., Flad, H.D., FLIEDNER, T.M. and E. Kleihauer: Bone Marrow Transplantation for Severe Combined Immunodeficiency with the HL-A-A-Incompatible but MLC- Identical Mother as a Donor. Transplant. Proceed., Vol. VIII 4 (1976) 623-628.

Nothdurft, W., Körbling, M., Ross, W.M., Steinbach, I., Schnappauf, H.P. and FLIEDNER, T.M.: Die myeloisch-determinierte Stammzelle (CFUc) als Indikator für die Regeneration der Hämopoese nach Transfusion von Blutstammzellen am präklinischen Hunde-Modell. Abstract. Blut Vol. 33 (Vortrag 100), 1976, 226-227.

Ross, W.M., FLIEDNER, T.M., Körbling, M. and W. Nothdurft: Mobilization of Hematopoietic Stem Cells by Dextran Sulfate into Peripheral Blood (Dogs). Abstract. Experimental Hematology, Vol. 4, 1976, 52.

Steinbach K.H., Raffler, H. and FLIEDNER, T.M.: Untersuchungen zur Simulation eines mathematischen Modells des granulozytären Zellerneuerungssystems. Abstract. Blut 33 (Vortrag 102) (1976) 227.

1977

FLIEDNER, T.M.: Organizational Aspects of the Handling of Radiation Accidents in the Federal Republic of Germany. In: IAEA (Ed.): Handling of Radiation Accidents 1977, 251-261, Int. Atom. Energ. Agency Wien 1977.

FLIEDNER, T.M.: Örtliche und überregionale ärztliche Maßnahmen bei Arbeitsunfällen infolge erhöhter Einwirkung ionisierender Strahlen. In: L. Rausch et al. (Hrsg.): Strahlenschutz in Forschung und Praxis, Band XVII, 21-35, Georg Thieme Stuttgart 1977.

FLIEDNER, T.M., Körbling, M., Calvo, W., Bruch, Ch. and E. Herbst : Cryopreservation of Blood Mononuclear Leukocytes and Stem Cells Suspended in a Large Fluid Volume. A Preclinical Model for a Blood Stem Cell Bank. Blut 35 (1977) 195-202.

FLIEDNER, T.M.: Hiroshia - damals und heute. Dtsch. med. Wschr. Jhrg. 102 (1977) 111-113.

FLIEDNER, T.M. and D. Hoelzer: The L 5222 Acute Leukemia in Rats: Observations on Cellular Characteristics and on its Influence on Normal Hematopoiesis. Blood Cells 3 (1977) 505-518.

FLIEDNER, T.M., Steinbach, K.H. und H. Raffler: Erholungsvorgänge im Stammzellenbereich des Knochenmarks nach Strahleneinwirkung. In: O. Messerschmidt, G. Möhrle, O. Zimmer (Hrsg.): Strahlenschutz in Forschung und Praxis, Band XVIII, 4-20, Georg Thieme Stuttgart 1977.

FLIEDNER, T.M. and G. Freriks: Concluding Remarks. Session III - Patterns of Distribution in vivo. Leukemia Res., Vol. 1, 2/3 (1977) 141-142.

FLIEDNER, T.M., Heeg, S. and S. Biefang: The Role of Research and Development in the Improvement of Health Conditions. In: A. Gelhorn, T. Fülöp and Z. Bankowski (Eds.): Health Needs of Society: A Challenge for Medical Education, 89-92, World Health Organz. Genf 1977.

FLIEDNER, T.M. and S. Biefang: Health and Disease in an Industrialized Country: Implications for Medical Education. In: A. Gelhorn, T. Fülöp and Z. Bankowski (Eds.): Health Needs of Society: A Challenge for Medical Education, 19-27, World Health Organ. Genf 1977.

Franz, H.E., Szemere, P., Franz, M. and FLIEDNER, T.M.: Behavior of Leukocytes and Colony-Forming Units (CFU-C) in Blood of Chronic Uremic Patients During Hemodialysis and Hemodiafiltration. Jour. of Dialysis, 1 (1977) 705-714.

Heit, H., Heit, W., Kohne, E. FLIEDNER, T.M. and P. Hughes: Allogeneic Bone Marrow Transplantation in Conventional Mice: I. Effect of Antibiotic Therapy on Long term Survival of Allogeneic Chimeras. Blut 35 (1977) 143-153.

Hoelzer, D. and FLIEDNER, T.M.: Studies on the regulation of Leukemic Cell Production in Human acute Leukemia. Blood Cells 3 (1977) 519-533.

Körbling, M., FLIEDNER, T.M. and W.M. Ross: Collection of Hemopoietic Stem-Cells from Peripheral Blood of Human Donors. Abstract. Experimental Hematology, Vol. 5, (Suppl. 2), 1977, 94.

Körbling, M., FLIEDNER, T.M., Calvo, W., Nothdurft, W. and W.M. Ross: In-vitro and In-Vivo Properties of Canine Blood Mononuclear Leukocytes Separated by Discontinuous Albumin Density Gradient Centrifugation. Biomedicine, Vol. 26 (1977) 275-283.

Körbling, M., Ross, W.R., Pflieger, H., Arnold, R. and FLIEDNER, T.M.: Procurement of Human Blood Stem Cells by Continuous-Flow centrifugation - Further Comment. Blood, Vol. 50 (1977) 753-754.

Lohrmann, H.P., Heimpel, H., FLIEDNER, T.M. and W. Schreml: Studies on Blood Granulocytic Precursor Cells (CFU-C) following High-Dose Chemotherapy in Man. Abstract. Experimental Hematology, Vol. 5 (Suppl. 2), 1977, 95.

Lohrmann, H.P., Heimpel, H., FLIEDNER, T.M., and W. Schreml: Adjuvante, intermittierende Chemo-/ Immunotherapie beim Mammakarzinom. II. Reaktion der Granulozytopoese auf intermittierende Chemotherapie. Abstract. Blut, Vol. 35, 1977, 351.

Nothdurft, W. and FLIEDNER, T.M.: Studies on the CFU-C Concentration in the Blood of Dogs and Their Response to Low Dose Whole-Body X-Irradiation. Exp. Hemat., Vol. 5 (1977) 31.

Nothdurft, W., Bruch, Ch., FLIEDNER, T.M. and E. Rüber: Studies on the Regeneration of the CFU-C Population in Blood and Bone Marrow of Lethally Irradiated Dogs after Autologous Transfusion of Cryopreserved Mononuclear Blood Cells. Scand. J. Haematol. 19 (1977) 470-481.

Rodt, H., Netzel, B., Niethammer, D., Körbling, M., Götze, D., Kolb, H.J., E. Thiel, Haas, R.J., FLIEDNER, T.M. et al.: Specific Absorbed Antithymocyte Globulin for Incubation Treatment in Human Marrow Transplantation. Transplant. Proc., Vol. IX 1 (1977) 187-191.

Ross, W.M., Calvo, S., Nothdurft, W., FLIEDNER, T.M. and M. Körbling: Hematopoietic Blood Stem-Cell Mobilization by Dextran Sulphate. Abstract. Experimental Hematology, Vol. 5 (Suppl. 2), 1977, 13.

Ross, W.M., Körbling, M., Nothdurft, W., Calvo, W. and FLIEDNER, T.M.: Characterization of Bone Marrow and Lymph Node Repopulating Cells by Transplanting Mononuclear Cells into Radiated Dogs. In: S.J. Baum, G.D. Ledney (Eds.): Experimental Hematology Today, 29-38 Springer Verlag New York 1977.

Schreml, W., and FLIEDNER, T.M.: Distribution of Tritiated Compounds (Tritiated Thymidine and tritiated Water) in the others-Fetus System and its Consequences for the Radiotoxic Effect of Tritium. Current Topic in Rad. Res. Quarterly 12 (1977) 255-277.

1978

Abt, C., Arnold, R., Flad, H.-D., FLIEDNER, T.M., Goldmann, S.F., Heimpel, H., Kleihauer, E., Körbling, M., Kubanek, M. et al.: Application of Gnotobiotic Techniques in Bone Marrow Transplantation for Aplastic Anaemia. Bone Marrow Transplant., Vol. 26 (1978) 56-58.

Abt, C., Arnold, R., Flad, H.D., FLIEDNER, T.M., Goldmann, S.F., Heimpel, H., Kleihauer, E., Körbling, M., Kubanek, B., Lohrmann, H.P., Niethammer, D. und H. Pflieger: Bone Marrow Transplantation for Severe Aplastic Anemia: Ulm Experience. Pathologie Biologie 26 (1), 1978, 40-41.

Bruch, Ch., Kovacs, P., Rüber, E. and FLIEDNER, T.M.: Studies on the Inhibitory Effect of Granulocytes on Human Granulocytopoiesis in Agar Cultures. Exp. Hemat. 6 (1978) 337-345.

Calvo, W., FLIEDNER T.M., Steinbach, I., Alcober, V., Nothdurft, W. and I. Fache: Development of Fibrosis in Dogs as a Late Consequence of Whole-Body X-Irradiation. In: IAEA (Hrsg.): Late Biological Effects of Ionizing Radiation, Vol. II, 127-136, Int. Atomic Energ. Agency Wien 1978.

FLIEDNER, T.M., Hoelzer, D., und K.H. Steinbach: Physiologische und pathophysiologische Regulation der Erythropoese. In: Verhandlungen der Detuschen Gesellschaft für Innere Medizin, 84. Band, 15-27, J.F. Bergmann München 1978.

FLIEDNER, T.M. and W. Calvo: Hematopoietic Stem-Cell Seeding of a Cellular Matrix: A Principle of Initiation and Regeneration of Hematopoiesis. In: Differentiation of Normal and Neoplastic Hematopoietic Cells, 757-773, Cold Spring Harbor Lab. 1978.

FLIEDNER, T.M.: Advances in Hemopoietic Stem-Cell Research: Their Significance for Clinical Hematology. In: Proc. of the XII. Congress of the Int. Soc. of Hematology, 63-68, 1978.

FLIEDNER, T.M.: A Commentary to: Gorin, N.C., Elgjo, R., Stout, R. and T. Knutsen: "Long-Term Preservation of Canine Bone Marrow: in vitro Studies" (in Blood Cells 4, 419-429, 1978). Blood Cells 4 (1978) 431-433.

FLIEDNER, T.M., Calvo, W., Körbling, M., Kreutzmann, H., Nothdurft, W., Ross, W.M. and D. Vassileva: Hematopoietic Stem Cells in Blood: Characteristics and Potentials. In: D.W. Golde, M.J. Cline, D. Metcalf, C.F. Fox (Eds.): Hematopoietic Cell Differentiation. ICN-UCLA Symp. on Molecular Biology, Vol. X, 193-212, Academic Press 1978.

Gratwohl, A.A., Deisseroth, A.B., Jackson, R.C., Boritzki, T.J., Weber, G., Schreml, W., Lohrmann, H.P., Heimpel, H., FLIEDNER, T.M. et al.: Methotrexate Rescue. In: Siegenthaler, W. and R. Luthy: 10th Intern. Congress of Chemotherapy, Zurich, Switzerland, Sept. 1977. Current Chemotherapy, Vols. 1 and 2, 1978, 1262-1272.

Körbling, M., FLIEDNER, T.M., Pflieger, H.., Vassileva, D. and H. Heimpel: Yield and Efficiency of Collecting and Cryopreserving Human Hematopoietic Blood Stem Cells (HBSC) by Means of Continuous Flow Centrifugation (CFC). Abstract. Experimental Hematology, Vol. 6, 1978, 95.

Kovacs, P., Bruch, C., Herbst, E.W. and FLIEDNER, T.M.: Collection of in vitro Colony-Forming Units from Dogs by Repeated Continuous Flow Leukaphereses. Acta Haemat. 60 (1978) 172-181.

Kreutzmann, H. and FLIEDNER, T.M.: Granulocytic progenitor cells (CFU-C) as normal elements of the blood leukocyte population. In: Abstract Book (II) of the XVII. Congress of the Intern. Society of Hematology, Paris, July 27-28, 1978, p. 659.

Kreutzmann, H., FLIEDNER, T.M., Galla, H.J. and E. Sackmann: Fluorescence-Polarization Change in Mononuclear Blood Leukocytes after PHA Incubation: Differences in Cells from Patients with and Without Neoplasia. Br. J. Cancer 37 (1978) 797-805.

Lohrmann, H-P, Schreml, W., FLIEDNER, T.M. und H. Heimpel: Früh- und Spätveränderungen der Granulozytopoese unter intermittierender adjuvanter Chemotherapie des Mamma-Karzinoms. In: H. Huber, H. Senn und M. Falkensammer (Hrsg.): Adjuvante zytost. Chemotherapie. Hämat. und Bluttransf. Band 22, 15-23, Springer Berlin 1978.

Lohrmann, H.P., Schreml, W., FLIEDNER, T.M. and H. Heimpel: Reaction of Human Granulopoiesis to High-Dose Cyclophosphamide Therapy. Abstract. Experimental Hematology, Vol. 6 (Suppl. 3), 1978, 49.

Lohrmann, H.P., Schreml, W., Lang, M., Betzler, M., FLIEDNER, T.M. and H. Heimpel: Changes of Granulopoiesis During and After Adjuvant Chemotherapy of Breast Cancer. Brit. Journ. of Haematology 40 (1978) 369-381.

Nothdurft, W., FLIEDNER, T.M., Weindler, M. and R. Wurzberger: Correlations of Blood Levels of CSA with Degenerative and Regenerative Changes of the Granulopoietic Cell Renewal System in 1200 R Whole-Body X-Irradiated Dogs given autologous Stem-Cell Transf. Abstract Book of the XVII Congr. ISH. Paris 1978.

Nothdurft, W., FLIEDNER, T.M., Calvo, W., Flad, H.D., Huget, R., Körbling, M., Krumbacher-v.Lorginghofen, K., Ross, W.M. et al :CFU-C Populations in Blood and Bone Marrow of Dogs after Lethal Irradiation and Allogeneic Transfusion with Cryopreserved Blood Mononuclear Cells. Scand. J. Haemat. 21, 2 (1978) 115-130.

Ross, W..M., FLIEDNER, T.M. and E.B. Harriss: Blood stem-Cell Mobilization as a Monitor of the Functional State of the Stem-Cell System: Studies in Mice Using Dextran Sulfate. Exp. Hematology 6 (1978) 81.

Ross, W.M., Calvo, W. and FLIEDNER, T.M.: Extramedullary Hemopoiesis Induced by Dextran Sulfate in the Dog Spleen. Exp. Hematology, Vol. 6 (1978) 20.

Ross, W.M., Körbling, M., Nothdurft, W. and FLIEDNER, T.M.: The Role of Dextran Sulfate in Increasing the CFU-C-Concentration in Dog Blood. Proc. of the Soc. f. Exp. Biol. and Med. 157 (1978) 301-305.

Schreml, W., Lohrmann, H.-P., Heimpel, H. and FLIEDNER, T.M.: Granulocyte Precursor Cells (CFUC) in Peripheral Blood and Bone Marrow During High-Dose Methotrexate with Citrovorum Factor Rescue. In: Siegenthaler, W. (Hrsg.): Current Chemotherapy. Vols. 1 + 2, 1978, 1266-1268.

Steinbach, K.-H., Raffler, H. und FLIEDNER, T.M.: Computersimulation der Granulozytopoese. In: K. Oeff, H.A.E. Schidt (Eds.): Nuklearmedizin, Nuklearmedizin und Biokybernetik, Band II, 140 - 149, Medico-Informationsdienst Berlin 1978.

1979

Bhaduri, S., Kubanek, B., Heit, W., Pflieger, H., Kurrle, E., FLIEDNER, T.M. and H. Heimpel: A Case of Preleukemia - Reconstitution of Normal Marrow Function after Bone Marrow Transplantation (BMT) from Identical Twin. Blut 38 (1979) 145-149.

Bremer, K. und FLIEDNER, T.M.: Kinetik normaler und pathologischer Lymphozyten. In: A. Stacher und P. Höcker (Hrsg.): Lymphknotentumoren - Pathophysiologie, Klinik und Therapie, 13 - 19 Urban & Schwarzenberg München 1979.

Calamine, E., Calvo, W. and FLIEDNER, T.M. (Eds.): Atlas of Human Hemopoietic Development. Springer Verlag, Berlin, 1979.

Calvo, W., FLIEDNER, T.M., Steinbach, I., Alcober, V., Nothdurft, W., and I. Fache: Morphologic Alterations in Canine Marrow of Long-Term Survivors After 1200 R Whole-Body X-Irradiation and Autologous Blood Leukocyte Engraftment. Am. J. Pathol. 95 (1979) 379-388.

Carbonell, F., FLIEDNER, T.M., Kratt, E., and K. Sauerwein: Crecimiento de las células leucémicas en cultivo: seleccion de clones citobeneticamente anormales. SNGRA, 24 (1979) 1057-1060.

Dietrich, M., Abt, C., Arnold, R., Pflicger, H., Hoelzer, D., Kurrle, E., Rasche, H., Kubanek, B., Heimpel und FLIEDNER, T.M.: Die Wirksamkeit gnotobiotischer Maßnahmen bei der Behandlung der akuten Leukämie: Ergebnisse einer prospektiv randomisierten klinischen Studie. Onkologie 2 (1979) 102-107.

Epstein, R. and FLIEDNER, T.M.: Peripheral Blood Stem Cells. Exp. Hemat., Vol. 7, Suppl. 5 (1979) 104b.

FLIEDNER, T.M.: Altern und Lebensqualität. In: V. Böhlau (Hrsg.): Altern und Balneologie. Schattauer Verlag Stuttgart 1979, 35-48.

FLIEDNER, T.M.: Pathophysiology and Clinical Physiology as a Part of Medical Teaching and Research. In: J. Vasku, K. Sulc, J. Erban (Eds.): Progress in pathophysiology. Proc. of the IInd Int. Cong. on Pathol. Physiology, Prague 1975, 66-70, Czech. Acad. of Sciences Prag 1979.

FLIEDNER, T.M.: Cellular Kinetics of Malignant Tumors. In: H.-D. Flad, Ch. Herfarth, M. Betler (Eds.): Immunodiagnosis and Immunotherapy of Malignant Tumors, 3 - 10, Springer Berlin 1979.

FLIEDNER, T.M., Calvo, W., Körbling, M., Nothdurft, W., Pflieger, H. and W. Ross: Collection, Storage and Transfusion of Blood Stem Cells for the Treatment of Hemopoietic Failure. Blood cells 5 (1979) 313-328.

FLIEDNER, T.M.: Physiologische und Pathophysiologische Aspekte der Blutzellbildung als Grundlage der Beurteilung von Strahlenwirkungen. In: F.-E. Stieve und G. Möhrle (Hrsg.): Strahlenschutzkurs für ermächt. Ärzte. Kurslehrbuch über die Aufgaben des erm. Arztes, 154-170. H. Hofmann Berlin 1979.

FLIEDNER, T.M.: Akute allgemeine Veränderungen bei Ganz- und Teilkörperbestrahlung und deren Behandlung. In: F.E. Stieve und G. Möhrle (Hrsg.): Strahlenschutzkurs für ermächt. Ärzte. Kurslehrbuch über die Aufgaben des erm. Arztes, 264-277. H. Hoffmann Berlin 1979.

FLIEDNER, T.M.: Diagnostik und Therapie des akuten Strahlensyndroms. Ärzteblatt Baden-Württemberg 9 (1979).

FLIEDNER, T.M.: Ärztliche Ausbildung in der Rehabilitationsmedizin: Chancen in Gegenwart und Zukunft. In: J.F. Scholz (Hrsg.): Rehabilitation als Schlüssel zum Dauerarbeitsplatz, 683-697, Springer Berlin 1979.

FLIEDNER, T.M.: Ärztliche Versorgung Strahlengeschädigter. In: R. Kirchhoff und H.-J. Linde (Eds.): Reaktorunfälle und nukleare Katastrophen, 43 - 69. Dr. med. D. Staube Erlangen 1979.

FLIEDNER, T.M.: Perspectives in Experimental and Clinical Gnotobiotics. In: FLIEDNER, T.M. et al. (Eds.): Clin. a. Experim. Gnotobiotics, Zbl. Bakt. Suppl. 7, 5-11. Gustav Fischer Stuttgart 1979.

FLIEDNER, T.M., Heit, H., Niethammer, D. and H. Pflieger (Eds.): Clinical and Experimental Gnotobiotics. Proc. of the VIth Intern. Symposium on Gnotobiology, Ulm, June 1978. Supplement zu Zentralblatt für Bakteriologie, Parasitenkunde, Infektionskrankheiten und Hygiene, I., Abt., Gustav Fischer Verlag, Stuttgart 1979.

FLIEDNER, T.M., Körbling, M., Arnold, R., Grilli, G., Haen, M., Kreutzmann, H. and H. Pflieger: Collection and Cryopreservation of Mononuclear Blood Leukocytes and of CFU-C in Man. Exp. Hemat. Vol. 7, Suppl. 5 (1979) 398-408.

FLIEDNER, T.M. and W. Nothdurft: Structure and Function of Stem Cell Pools in Mammalian Cell Renewal systems. In: S. Okada et al. (Eds.): Radiation Research, 640-647. Toppan Printing Co. Tokyo 1979.

Gerhartz, H.H., Nothdurft, W. and FLIEDNER, T.M.. Albumin Gradient Centrifugation: An Effective Method to Separate Hemopoietic Cells of the Peripheral Blood from Immunocompetent Cells. Abstract. Experimental Hematology Vol. 7 (Suppl. 6), 1979, 116.

Gerhartz, H.H. und FLIEDNER, T.M.: Granulozytär determinierte Stammzellen (CFU-C) aus Knochenmark und Blut: Größenunterschiede vor und nach Dextransulfat-Mobilisation. Blut 38 (1979) 161-164.

Goldmann, S.F., Niethammer, D., Flad, H.D., Belohradsky, B.H., Colobani, J., Dieterle, U., Dosch, H.M., FLIEDNER, T.M. et al: Hemopoietic and Lymphopoetic Split Chimerism in Severe Combined Immunodeficiency Disease (SCID). In: Transplant. Proceed. Vol. XI, No, 1, 225-229, 1979.

Haen, M., Grilli, G., Neuman, M., Martin, H., Körbling, M. and FLIEDNER, T.M.: Functional Characterization of Mononuclear Blood Leukocyte Populations in Man Using the Albumin Gradient Technique. Exp. Hematal. Vol. 7 (Suppl. 6), 1979, 116.

Heit, H., Heit, W., Byrne, P., Rodded, H. and FLIEDNER, T.M.: Protective Effect of the Gnotobiotic Environment in Experimental Allogeneic Bone Marrow Transplantation. In: FLIEDNER et al. (Hrsg.): Clinical and Experimental Gnotobiotics. Proc. VIth Int. Symp. on Gnotobiology, Ulm, 1978, 265-270. Gustav Fischer, Stuttgart 1979.

Körbling, M., FLIEDNER, T.M., Calvo, W., Ross, W.M., Nothdurft, W. and I. Steinbach: Albumin Density Gradient Purification of Canine Hemopoietic Blood Stem Cells (HBSC): Long-Term Allogeneic Engraftment Without GVH-Reaction. Exp. Hemat., Vol. 7 (1979) 277-288.

Körbling, M., FLIEDNER, T.M., Pflieger, H., Ross, W, Arnold, R., Rüber, E. and H. Heimpel: Collection and Cryopreservation of Human Blood Stem Cells (CFUc) in a Closed System. In: F. Mandelli (Ed.): Therapy of acute leukemias. Proc. of the 2nd. Int. Symp. Rome 1977, 601-607. Lombardo Roma 1979.

Kreutzmann, H. and FLIEDNER, T.M.: Studies on the Presence and Possible Oscillations of Granulocytic Progenitor Cells (CFU-C) in Human Blood. Scand. J. Haematol. 23 (1979) 360-366.

Kreutzmann, H., FLIEDNER, T.M., Galla, H.-J. and E. Sackmann: Fluorescence Polarization Changes in Mononuclear Blood Leukocytes after PHA-Incubation: Differences in Cells From Patients with and without Neoplasia. In: Verh. Deutsch. Kebsges. 2, 343-345. Gustav Fischer Stuttgart 1979.

Kurrle, E., Bhaduri, S., Heimpel, H., Hoelzer, D., Abt, C., Krieger, D., Vanek, E., FLIEDNER, T.M. and B. Kubanek: Effect of Gnotobiotic Care on Remission Induction Therapy in Acute Leukaemia. In: FLIEDNER et al. (Eds.): Clin. and Exp. Gnotobiotics, Zbl. Bakt. Suppl. 7, 383-388. Gustav Fischer Stuttgart 1979.

Lohrmann, H.P., Schreml, W., FLIEDNER, T.M. and H. Heimpel: Reaction of Human Granulopoiesis to High-Dose Cyclophosphamide Therapy. Blut 38 (1979) 9-16.

Müller-Nübling, J. und FLIEDNER, T.M.: Präklinische Untersuchungen über die Reaktion der Blut-CFU- c-Konzentration auf eine einmalige Applikation von Cyclophosphamid. Blut 38 (1979) 175-179.

Nothdurft, W. und FLIEDNER, T.M.: Blutstammzellen als Indikator der Hämopoese. In: Schutzkommission beim BM des Inneren in Zusammearb. mit dem BA für Zivilschutz, Bonn, 207-224. 1979.

Nothdurft, W., and FLIEDNER, T.M.: Stem Cell Migration After Irradiation. In: S. Okada et al. (Eds.): Radiation Research, 657-663. Toppan Printing Co. Tokyo 1979.

Nothdurft, W., Calvo, W., FLIEDNER, T.M., and H.H. Gerhartz: Quantitative and Qualitative Aspects of CFU-C Mobilization in Normal and Splenectomized Dogs. Abstract. Experimental Hematology, Vol. 7 (Suppl. 6), 1979, 117.

Steinbach, K.H., Schick, P., Trepel, F., Raffler, H., Döhrmann, J., Heilgeist, G., Heltzel, W., FLIEDNER, T.M. et al.: Schätzung kinetischer Parameter der neutrophilen, eosinophilen und basophilen Granulozyten im menschlichen Blut. Blut 39 (1979) 27-38.

1980

Carbonell, F., FLIEDNER, T.M., Kratt, E. und K. Sauerwein: Ventajas des uso de cultivos de corta duración en medio liquido para el estudio citogenético de las lecemias. SNGRA 25 (1) 1980 1-4.

Carbonell, F., Calvo, W., Nothdurft, W., Gerhartz, H., Körbling, M. and FLIEDNER, T.M.: Cytogenetic studies in Canine Radiation Chimeras after Allogeneic Blood Stem Cell Transfusion. Abstract. Exp. Hematal. Vol. 8, Suppl. 7 (1980) 136.

Dicke, K.A., Zander, A.R., Spitzer, G., Verma, D.S., Peters, L., Vellekoop, L., Thomson, S., Stewart, D., McCredie: Autologous Bone Marrow Transplantation in Relapsed Adult Acute Leukemia. Hämatologie und Bluttransfusion 25 (1980) 309-320.

FLIEDNER, T.M.: Belastung und Beanspruchung des Organismus durch Umweltfaktoren: Die Rolle der Zellsysteme. In: Jahrbuch der Heidelberger Akademie der Wissenschaften, 23-26, 1980.

FLIEDNER, T.M.: Peripheral Blood Leukocytes as a Source of Hematopoietic Stem Cells. Abstract. Journ. of Supramolecular Structure 9 (Suppl. 4) 1980, 13.

FLIEDNER, T.M., Grilli, G., Calvo, W., Nothdurft, W., Haen, M. and F. Carbonell: Fetal Liver as an Alternative Source of Stem Cells for Hemopoietic Reconstitution: A Canine Model. Abstract. Exp. Hematal. Vol. 8, Suppl. 7 (1980) 23.

FLIEDNER, T.M., Haen, M. und F. Carbonell: Pathogenese und Symptomatik des akuten Strahlensyndroms. In: O. Messerschmidt, L.E. Feinendegen, W. Hunzinger (Hrsg.): Industrielle Störfälle und Strahlenexposition. Strahlenschutz in Forschung und Praxis, Band XXI, 180-192, Georg Thieme Stuttgart 1980.

FLIEDNER, T.M., Calvo, W., Nothdurft, W. and G. Grilli: Fetal Liver: A Transitory Site for Hemopoietic Stem Cell Replication and selective Differentiation. In: G. Lucarelli, FLIEDNER, T.M. and R.P. Gale (Eds.): Fetal Liver Transplantation, Proc. Int. Symp. on Fetal Liver Transpl. Pesaro, 5-13. Excerpta Medica Amsterdam 1980.

FLIEDNER, T.M. and W. Calvo: Current Concepts and Future Directions of Fetal Liver Transplantation. In: G. Lucarelli, FLIEDNER, T.M. and R.P. Gale (Eds.): Fetal Liver Transplantation. Proc. 1st Annual Int. Symp. on Fetal Liver Transplant., Pesaro, 1979, 305-309, Excerpta Medica Amsterdam 1980.

FLIEDNER, T.M.: Collection, Cryopreservation and Transplantation of Blood Stem Cells in the treatment of Hemopoietic Failure. In: S. Thierfelder, H. Rodded and H.J. Kolb (Hrsg.): Immunobiology of Bone Marrow Transplantation, 53-60. Springer Verlag Berlin 1980.

FLIEDNER, T.M.: Collection, Cryopreservation and Transplantation of Blood Stem Cells in the Treatment of Hemopoietic Failure. Hämatologie und Bluttransfusion, 25 (1980) 53-60.

Gerhartz, H.H., Nothdurft, W. and FLIEDNER, T.M.: Transplantation of "Purified" Stem Cells to Allogeneic Hosts. Abstract. Exp. Hematal. Vol. 8, Suppl. 7 (1980) 23.

Gerhartz, H.H., Nothdurft, W. and FLIEDNER, T.M.: Collection, Characterization and Purification of CFUc from Peripheral Blood. In: S.J. Baum, G.D. Ledney, D.W. van Bekkum (Hrsg.): Experimental Hematology Today, 309-316. S. Karger Basel 1980.

Gerhartz, H.H. and FLIEDNER, T.M.: Velocity Sedimentation and Cell Cycle Characteristics of Granulopoietic Progenitor Cells (CFUC) in Canine Blood and Bone Marrow: Influence of Mobilization and CFUC Depletion. Exp. Hemat., Vol. 8 (1980) 209-218.

Grilli, G., Carbonell, F. and FLIEDNER, T.M.: Granulopoietic and Erythropoietic Progenitor Cells in Human Bone Marrow and Blood: Their Growth Characteristics, Concentrations and Correlations. Abstract. Exp. Hematal., Vol. 8, Suppl. 7 (1980) 42.

Grilli, G., Carbonell, F. and FLIEDNER, T.M.: Variations in Erythroid and Myeloid Progenitor Cell Numbers in Normal Human Peripheral Blood. Brit. Journ. of Haemat. 44 (1980) 679-681.

Haen, M., Grilli, G, Nothdurft, W., and FLIEDNER, T.M.: Studies on the Repopulating Ability of Blood Stem Cells of Dogs given a Single High Dose of Cyclophosphamide. Abstract. Exp. Hematal. Vol. 8, Suppl. 7 (1980) 26.

Hartmann, W., Sackmann, E., Eisert, W.G., Eisert, R. and FLIEDNER, T.M.: Detection of Lymphocyte Stimulation by Flow cytometry: Differences in Cells from Patients with and without Neoplasia. Biomedicine 32 (1980) 185-188.

Hoelzer, D., Harriss, E.B., Bültmann, B., FLIEDNER, T.M. and H. Heimpel: Differentiation into Granulopoiesis in Human Acute-Leukemia and Blast Crisis in Chronic Myelocytic Leukemia. In: Cronkite, E.P. and A.L. Carsten (Eds.): Diffusion Chamber Culture. Hemopoiesis, Cloning of Tumors, Cytogenetic and Carcinogenic Assays. Springer-Verlag, Berlin, 1980, 242-250.

Körbling, M., FLIEDNER, T.M., Rüber, E. and H. Pflieger: Description of a Closed Plastic Bag System for the Collection and Cryopreservation of Leukapheresis-Derived Blood Mononuclear Leukocytes and SFUc from Human Donors. Transfusion, 20 (1980) 293-300.

Körbling, M., FLIEDNER, T.M. and H. Pflieger: Collection of Large quantities of Granulocyte/Macrophage Progenitor Cells (CFUc) in Man by Means of Continuous-Flow Leukapheresis. Scand. J. Haematol. 24 (1980) 22-28.

Lucarelli, G., FLIEDNER, T.M. and R.P. Gale (Eds.): Fetal Liver Transplantation. International Congress Series Vol. 154, Proceedings of the First International Symposium on Fetal Liver Transplantation, Pesaro, Italien, September 1979. Excerpta Medica, Amsterdam 1980.

Niethamer, D., Goldmann, S.F., Flad, H.D., Wernet, P., Stursberg, G., Colombani, J., FLIEDNER, T.M. and E. Kleihauer: Split Chimerism in Three Patients Suffering from Severe Combined Immunodeficiency (SCID). In: S. Thierfelder, H. Rodded, and H.J. Kolb (Hrsg.): Immunbiology of Bone Marrow Transplantation. Haematology and Blood Transfusion, 391-401. Springer Berlin 1980.

Niethammer, D., Bienzle, U., Rodt, H., Goldmann, S.F., Körbling, M., Flad, H.D., Netzel, B., Haas, R.J., FLIEDNER, T.M. et al.: Rhesus Incompatibility and Aplastic Anemia as the Consequence of Split Chimerism after Bone-Marrow Transplantation for Severe Combined Immunodeficiency. Thymus 2 (1980) 75-82.

Nothdurft, W. and FLIEDNER, T.M.: Acute and Delayed Effects of Total-Body Irradiation on the Granulocytic Progenitor Cell Compartment in Dogs. Abstract. Radiat. Environ. Biophys. 17 (1980) 284-288.

Nothdurft, W., Calvo, W., FLIEDNER, T.M. and H.P. Schnappauf: Investigations on the Pool Size, Proliferative State and Differentiation Pattern of Splenic CFUc in Normal Dogs. Exp. Hematal. Vol. 8 (1980) 988-995.

Steinbach, K.H., Raffler, H., Pabst, G. and FLIEDNER, T.M.: A Mathematical Model of Canine Granulocytopoiesis. J. Math. Biology 10 (1980) 1-12.

1981

Carbonell, F., Grilli, G. and FLIEDNER, T.M.: Cytogenetic evidence for a clonal selection of leukemic cells in culture. Leukemia Research 5 (4-5) 1981, 395-398.

FLIEDNER, T.M.: Die fetale Leber als hämatopoetisches Organ. In: L. Wannagat (Hrsg.): Leber. Morphologie - Pathophysiologie - Klinik, 81-86. Georg Thieme Stuttgart 1981.

FLIEDNER, T.M.: Strategien zur strahlenschutzmedizinischen ambulanten Versorgung von "Betroffenen" bei kerntechnischen Unfällen. In: O. Messerschmidt, B. Betz, FLIEDNER, T.M. (Hrsg.): Med. Erstmaßnahmen bei kerntechnischen Unfällen. Band XXII, 71-82. Georg Thieme Stuttgart 1981.

FLIEDNER, T.M., Nothdurft, W., Grili, G. and K.H. Steinbach: Blood Bone Marrow and Fetal Liver Cell Transplantation in Dogs - Correlations Between Granulopoietic Progenitor Cells Number in the Transfusate and Regeneration of Progenitor and Blood Cell Compartments. Abstract. Exp. Hematology 9, Suppl. 9, 1981, 93.

FLIEDNER, T.M.: Das zweite Gedächtnis. In: Geo, Nr. 10/Oktober 1981, 95-102.

Gerhartz, H.H., Nothdurft, W., und FLIEDNER, T.M.: Granulozytär determinierte Vorläuferzellen (CFU-C) und hämopoetisches Potential: Eine Studie im Hundemodell. Blut 43 (1981) 89-92.

Grilli, G., Calvo, W., Carbonell, F., Haen, M. Nothdurft, W. and FLIEDNER, T.M.: Collection, Cryopreservation and Transfusion of Fetal Liver Cells for the Restoration of Hemopoiesis in Lethally Irradiated Dogs. In: F. Gavosto et al. (Eds.): Hemolymphopoiesis: Normal and Path. Cell Different., 193-197. Editrice Esculapio Bologny 1981.

Grilli, G., Calvo, W., Carbonell, F., FLIEDNER, T.M. and W. Nothdurft: Pattern of Early Reconstitution of Hemopoiesis in Irradiated Dogs given Transfusion of Stem Cells Obtained from Blood, Bone Marrow and Fetal Liver. Abstract. Exp. Hematal., Vol. 9, Suppl. 9 (1981) 66.

Grilli, G., Carbonell, F. and FLIEDNER, T.M.: Cytogenetical Studies on Erythropoietic and Myelopoietic Progenitor Cells in Vitro in Chronic Myelogenous Leukemia. Haematologica, Vol. 66 (1981) 733-739.

Issaragrisil S., Grilli, G. and FLIEDNER, T.M.: Studies on the Changes of Erythropoietic Burst Forming Cell and Granulopoietic Progenitor Cell Concentrations in Normal Human Peripheral blood as a Function of Time After Blood Sampling. Abstract. Experimental Hematal. 9 (Suppl. 9), 1981, 22.

Kurrle, E., Bhaduri, S., Gaus, W., Heimpel, H. and FLIEDNER, T.M.: Pathogenicity of Microorganisms for Oropharyngeal and Respiratory Tract Infections in Acute Leukaemia Patients under Total and Selective Decontamination. In: S. Sasaki et al. (Eds.): Recent Advances in Germfree Research, 693-696. Tokai University Press 1981.

Messerschmidt, O., Betz, B. und FLIEDNER, T.M. (Hrsg.): Medizinische Erstmaßnahmen bei kerntechnischen Unfällen. Strahlenschutz in Forschung und Praxis, Band XXII, Georg Thieme Stuttgart 1981.

Nothdurft, W., Braasch, E., Calvo, W., Carbonell, F., Grilli, G. and FLIEDNER, T.M.: Studies on Granulocyte/Macrophage Progenitor Cells (CFU-GM) in Different Organs of Dogs During Fetal development. Abstract. Exp. Hematal., Vol. 9, Suppl. 9 (1981) 163.

Pflieger, H., Wiesneth, M., Haem, M., Arnold, R., Steinbach, K.H. and FLIEDNER, T.M.: Granulocyte Regulation after Leukapheresis Cytomorphological Studies on the Peripheral Blood and Bone Marrow. Abstract. Experimental Hematology, Vol. 9, Suppl. 9, 1981, 199.

Raghavachar, A., Nothdurft, W., Grilli, G., Steinbach, K.-H. and FLIEDNER, T.M.: Kinetic Parameters of Circulating CFUC in the Dog Using Different Experimental approaches. Abstract. Exp. Hematal., Vol. 9, Suppl. 9 (1981) 53.

Ross, W.M., FLIEDNER, T.M. and E.B. Harriss: Influence of 80 Rad x-Radiation on Mobilization of Hemopoietic Stem Cells by Dextran Sulfate into Blood in Mice. Abstract. Rad. Res. 87 (2) 1981, 395-396.

1982

Carbonell, F, Calvo, W. and FLIEDNER, T.M.: Cellular Composition of Human Fetal Bone Marrow. Histologic study in Methacrylate Sections. Acta anat. 113 (1982) 371-375.

Carbonell, F., Ganser, A., Suhr, E., Wandl, U., Hauf, R. und FLIEDNER, T.M.: Chromosomenanalysen bei schadstoff-exponierten Personen: Möglichkeiten und Probleme am Beispiel von Toluolexposition. In: FLIEDNER, T.M. (Hrsg.): Verhandl. der Deutsch. Gesellsch. für Arbeitsmed., 22. Jahrestagung, Ulm/Neu-Ulm 1982,269-272. Gentner Stuttgart 1982.

FLIEDNER, T.M.: Late Consequences of Irradiation: Background and Purpose of this Symposium. In: FLIEDNER, T.M. et al. (Eds.): Radiation Protection. Proc. EULEP-Symposion München August 1981, Commission of the European Communities, Luxembourg 1982, 3-8.

FLIEDNER, T.M., Gössner, W., and G. Patrick: Late Effects after Therapeutic Whole-Body Irradiation. Vol. 1982. Eur. Late Effects Project Group Symposium on Late Effects after Therapeutic Whole-Body Irradiation. München August 1981. Commission of the European Communities, Luxembourg 1982.

FLIEDNER, T.M.: Medizinische Aspekte des Strahlenunfalles. In: FLIEDNER, T.M. (Hrsg.): Verhandlungen der Deutschen Gesellschaft für Arbeitsmedizin e.V., 22. Jahrestagung Ulm/Neu-Ulm, 1982, Gentner Stuttgart 1982, 17-28.

FLIEDNER, T.M. (Hrsg.): Bericht über die 22. Jahrestagung der Deutschen Gesellschaft für Arbeitsmedizin e.V. Ulm/Neu-Ulm, 27-30. April 1982. Gentner Stuttgart 1982.

FLIEDNER, T.M.: Entwicklung und Funktion der blutbildenden Gewebe. Therapiewoche 32 (1982) 2137-2146.

FLIEDNER, T.M., Calvo, W., Nothdurft, W., und G. Grilli: Die Stammzelltransfusion als hämopoetische Transplantation. In: Wilmanns, W. und R. Hartenstein (Hrsg.): Aktuelle Probleme der Hämatologie und Onkologie. Vol. 13. Beiträge zur Onkologie. S. Karger, Basel 1982, 54-69.

FLIEDNER, T.M., Wandl, U.B. and W. Calvo: Medulläre und extramedulläre Hämopoiese im Hund nach Ganzkörperbestrahlung und Transfusion von aus dem Blut gewonnenen Stammzellen. Schweiz. med. Wschr. 112 (1982) 1423-1429.

FLIEDNER, T.M., Calvo, W. and U. Wandl: Splenic Hemopoiesis in Dogs Subsequent to Whole Body Irradiation and Stem Cell Transplantation as a Model to Study Pathogenetic Mechanisms of Extramedullary Blood Cell Formation. Abstract. Exp. Hematal., Suppl. 10 (1982) 53.

FLIEDNER, T.M. und W. Calvo: Alterungsvorgänge in hämatopoetischen Zellerneuerungssysteme n. In: J. Böhnel, R. Heinz, A. Stacher (Hrsg.): Hämatologie im Alter, S. 8 - 12. Urban & Schwarzenberg 1982.

FLIEDNER, T.M., Wandl, U.B. and W. Calvo: Hemopoietic Proliferation and Differentiation in Bone Marrow and Spleen of Dogs after Whole Body Irradiation and Transfusion of Blood-Derived Autologous and Allogeneic Hemopoietic Progenitor Cells. Abstract. Stem Cells, 2 (1982) 361.

FLIEDNER, T.M., Hoelzer, D. und K.H. Steinbach: Blast Cell and Granulocyte Production in Human Leukemia: Pathophysiological Concepts Based on Computer Simulation Using Discrete Modeling Techniques. Blood Cells 8 (1982) 535-548.

FLIEDNER, T.M., Pabst, G. und U. Wandl: Pathophysiologie der Mehrfachbelastungen von Zellsystemen. In: FLIEDNER, T.M. (Hrsg.): Verhandlungen der Deutschen Gesellschaft für Arbeitsmedizin e.V., 22. Jahrestagung Ulm/ Neu-Ulm 1982, 82-98. Gentner Verlag Stuttgart 1982.

Ganser, A., Carbonell, F., FLIEDNER, T.M. and H. Heimpel: The Value of Cytogenetic Findings in Patients with Chronic Myeloproliferative Disorders. Abstract. Annual Congress of the Austrian and German Societies of Hematology and Oncology. Blut 45 (1982) 229.

Ganser, A., Carbonell, F., Semotan-Mass, S. und FLIEDNER, T.M.: Chromosomenaberrationen als biologischer Indikator für berufliche und therapeutische Strahlenexposition. In: FLIEDNER, T.M. (Hrsg.): Verhandl. der Deutschen Gesellschaft für Arbeitsmed., 22. Jahrestagung Ulm/Neu-Ulm, 1982. 535-539, Gentner Stuttgart 1982.

Gerhartz, H.H., Nothdurft, W., and FLIEDNER, T.M.: Effect of Low-Dose Whole-Body Irradiation on Granulopoietic Progenitor Cell Subpopulations: Implications for CFUc Release. Cell Tissue Kinet. 15 (1982) 371-379.

Grilli, G., Nothdurft, W., and FLIEDNER, T.M.: Radiation Sensitivity of Human Erythropoietic and Granulopoietic Progenitor Cells in the Blood and in the Bone Marrow. Int. J. Radiat. Biol., Vol. 41 6 (1982) 685-687.

Grilli, G., Rüber, E., Baur, B. und FLIEDNER, T.M.: Survival of Human Granulocyte-Macrophage Progenitor Cells (CFU-C) after Cryopreservation as a Function of the Time of Storage. Haematologica, Vol. 67 (1982) 517-521.

Haen, M., Grilli, G. and FLIEDNER, T.M.: Characterization of Blood and Bone Marrow Derived CFU-C after a Single High Dose of Cyclophosphamide. Abstract. Annual Congress of the Austrian and German Societies of Hematology and Oncology. Innsbruck, Oktober 1982. Blut 45 (1982).

Nothdurft, W., Faul, H. and FLIEDNER, T.M.: Short-Term and Long-Term effects of Total-body X-Irradiation of Dogs on the Granulocyte Macrophage Progenitor Cells GM-CFU in the Bone-Marrow - Kinetics in Suspension Culture and Determinations of the Mobilizable GM-CFU Reserve. Abstract. Experimental Hematology, Vol. 10, 1982, 176.

Nothdurft, W., Steinbach, K.H., Ross, W.M. and FLIEDNER, T.M.: Quantitative Aspects of Granulocytic Progenitor Cell (CFUc) Mobilization from Extravascular sites in Dogs using Dextran Sulphate (DS). Cell Tissue Kinet. 15 (1982) 331-340.

Nothdurft, W., and FLIEDNER, T.M.: The Response of the Granulocytic Progenitor Cells (CFU-C) of Blood and Bone Marrow in Dogs Exposed to Low Doses of X- Irradiation. Rad. Res. 89 (1982) 38-52.

Prümmer, O., Raghavachar and FLIEDNER, T.M.: Immunological Recovery after Autografts from Canine Blood and Bone Marrow. Abstract. Annual Congress of the Austrian and German Societies of Hematology and Oncology. Blut 45 (1982) 218.

Prümmer, O., Calvo, W., and FLIEDNER, T.M.: Development of Immunocompetence in the Fetal dog. Abstract. Annual Congress of the Austrian and German Societies of Hematology and Oncology. Insbruck, Oktober 1982. Blut 45 (1982) 217.

Raghavachar, A., Prümmer, O., and FLIEDNER, T.M.: A Comparative Study of the Repopulating Potential of Autografts from Canine Blood and Bone Marrow. Abstract. Annual Congress of the Austrian and German Societies of Hematology and Oncology. Innsbruck, Oktober 1982. Blut 45 (1982).

Raghavachar, A., Sulc, K. and FLIEDNER, T.M.: Granulocytic Progenitor Cells (CFU-C) in Canine Blood: Mobilization by Dexamethasone? Blut 44 (1982) 107-110.

Raghavachar, A., Prümmer, O. and FLIEDNER, T.M.: Blood stem Cell Mobilization as a Monitor of the Functional State of the Stem Cell System: Studies in Dogs Using Dextran Sulfate after Lethal Total Body Irradiation and Autologous Stem Cell Transplantation. Abstract. STEM CELLS 2 (1982) 371.

Szemere, P., FLIEDNER, T.M., Nothdurft, W. and D. Breitig: Extracorporeal Irradiation of Dog Blood: The Effects of a Radiostrontium Irradiator on Blood Stem Cells (CFU-C). Strahlentherapie, 158 (1982) 444-449.

Wiesneth, M., Pflieger, H., Arnold, R. and FLIEDNER, T.M.: Cytomorphological Studies on the Peripheral Blood and Bone Marrow in Persons Undergoing Leukapheresis. Abstract. Annual Congress of the Austrian and German Societies of Hematology and Oncology. Innsbruck, Oktober 1982. Blut 45 (1982) 231.

1983

Bittighofer, P.M., Zinser, D., FLIEDNER, T.M. und K. Reichenbach: Belastung und Beanspruchung von Arbeitern im Straßenbau durch Asphalt-Bitumen. Verh. Deutsch. Ges. f. Arbeitsmed. 23 (1983) 439-444.

Calvo, W., Ross, W.M. and FLIEDNER, T.M.: Stimulation of Extramedullary Hemopoiesis by Dextran Sulfate. Blut 46 (1983) 39-45.

Carbonell, F., Ganser, A., Arnold, R., Schmeiser, T., FLIEDNER, T.M., Heimpel, H. and B. Kubanek: Cytogenetic evidence for the Persistence of Host Lymphocytes after Total Body Irradiation and Bone Marrow Transplantation . Abstract. Exp. Hematol. Vol. 11, Suppl. 13 (1983) 15.

Carbonell, F., Ganser, A., FLIEDNER, T.M., Arnold, R. and B. Kubanek: The Fat of Cells with Chromosome Aberrations after Total- Body Irradiation and Bone Marrow Transplantation. Rad. Res. 93 (1983) 453-460.

Carbonell, F, Hoelzer, D., Grilli, G., Issaragrisil, S., Harriss, E.B. and FLIEDNER, T.M · Chronic Myelotic Leukaemia: Cytogenetical Studies on Haemopoietic Colonies and Diffusion Chamber Cultures. Scand. J. Haematol. 30 (1983) 891.

Carbonell, F., Hoelzer, D., Thiel, E., Ganser, A., Anger, B., Stötter, H. and FLIEDNER, T.M.: Philadelphia Chromosome Positive Acute Leukaemia: Heterogeneity of Cytogenetics, Immunological Diagnosis, Proliferation and Differentiation Patterns in Culture. Abstract. Exp. Hematal. Vol. 11, Suppl. 14 (1983) 169.

FLIEDNER, T.M. and W. Calvo: Stammzellreplikation und Differenzierung in ihrer Beziehung zur Mikroökologie des Knochenmarkes. Verh. Dtsch. Ges. Path. 67 (1983) 101-111.

FLIEDNER, T.M., Carbonell, F. and A. Ganser: Vergleichende Untersuchungen über die Verwendung biologischer Indikatoren zum Nachweis von Strahlenbelastung. In: K. Stalder (Hrsg.): Verhandlungen der Deutsch. Ges. für Arbeits med. 23. Jahrestagung Göttingen, 363-364. Gentner Stuttgart 1983.

FLIEDNER, T.M.: Erhaltung und Wiederherstellung der Gesundheit, eine Herausforderung an die Rehabilitationsmedizin der achtziger Jahre. Mitteilungen der LVA Württemberg 10 (1983) 230-235.

FLIEDNER, T.M., Calvo, W. and P.H. Tang: Realitäten in der Blutbildung am Beispiel des Megakaryozyten- Blutplättchen-Systems. In: R. Gross (Hrsg.): Modelle und Realitäten in der Medizin. Symp. der Med. Universitätsklinik Köln am 1.10.1982, 64-80. Schattauer Stuttgart 1983.

Heeg, S., und FLIEDNER, T.M.: Vorbereitung der Förderung von Therapiestudien als offener Planungsprozeß. Z. Rheumatol. 42 (1983) 370-375.

Körbling, M., Dörken, B., Tischbirek, K., Zipperle, G., Ho, A.D., FLIEDNER, T.M. and W. Hunstein: Autologous Transplantation of a Bone Marrow Graft Manipulated by Chemoseparation to Eliminate Residual Tumor Cells. Blut 46 (1983) 89-93.

Nothdurft, W., Steinbach, K.H. and FLIEDNER, T.M.: In vitro Studies on the Sensitivity of Canine Granulopoietic Progenitor Cells (GM-CFC) to Ionizing Radiation: Differences between Steady State GM-CFC from Blood and Bone Marrow. Int. J. Radiat. Biol., Vol. 43 (1983) 133-140.

Prümmer, O., Calvo, W., and FLIEDNER, T.M.: Development of Immunocompetence in the Fetal Dog. Abstract. J. Cell Biochem., Suppl. 71 (1983) 73.

Prümmer, O., Raghavachar, A., Calvo, W., Carbonell, F., Werner, Ch. und FLIEDNER, T.M.: Restauration der Hämopoese mittels kryopräservierter fötaler Leberzellen beim Hund. Abstract. Onkologie 6 (1983) 241.

Prümmer, O., Raghavachar, A., Calvo, W., Carbonell, F. and FLIEDNER, T.M.: Transplantation of Cryopreserved Fetal Liver cells in the Dog after Total Body Irradiation. Abstract. Exp. Hematal., Vol. 11, Suppl. 14 (1983) 97.

Prümmer, O., Calvo, W., FLIEDNER, T.M. and W. Nothdurft: Immunological Characterization of Canine Fetal Liver Cells. In: R.P. Gale (Ed.): Recent Advance in Bone Marrow Transplantation, 841-848. Alan R. Liss New York 1983.

Prümmer, O., Raghavachar, A., Calvo, W., Carbonell, F. and FLIEDNER, T.M.: Restoration of Hemopoiesis by Cryopreserved Fetal Liver Cells in a Canine Model. In: R.P. Gale (Ed.): Recent Advances in Bone Marrow Transplantation. 857-863. Alan R. Liss, New York 1983.

Raghavachar, A., Steinbach, K.., Prümmer, O., Grilli, G. and FLIEDNER, T.M.: Survival of Transfused Cryopreserved Granulocytic Progenitor Cells (CFU-C) in Recipient Circulation. Cell Tissue Kinet. 16 (1983) 303-311.

Raghavachar, A., Prümmer, O., FLIEDNER, T.M. and K.H. Steinbach: Functional Studies on Myeloid Progenitor Cell Reconstitution after Autologous Stcm Cell Transplantation. Abstract. Exp. Hematal. Vol. 11, Suppl. 14 (1983) 71.

Raghavachar, A., Prümmer, O., FLIEDNER, T.M., Calvo, W. and I. Steinbach: Stem Cells from Peripheral Blood and Bone Marrow: a Comparative Evaluation of the Hemopoietic Potential in the Dog. Int. J. of Cell Cloning 1 (1983) 191-205.

Raghavachar, A. Prümmer, O, FLIEDNER, T.M. und K.H. Steinbach: Physikalische Separation hämopoetischer Progenitorzellen (CFU-GM) und regeneratives Potential: Eine Studie im Hundemodell. Abstract. Onkologie 6 (1983) 241.

Raghavachar, A., Prümmer, O., FLIEDNER, T.M. und K.H. Steinbach: Progenitor Cell (CFUc) Reconstitution After Autologous Stem Cell Transfusion in Lethally Irradiated Dogs: Decreased CFUc Populations in Blood and Bone Marrow Correlate with the Fraction Mobilizable by Dextran Sulphate. Exp. Hematal., Vol. 11 (1983) 996-1004.

Raghavachar, A., Prübber, O., FLIEDNER, T.M. and K.H. Steinbach. Comparison of the Repopulating Potential of Stem Cells Derived from Blood and Bone Marrow: Autotransplants in Dogs. Abstract. Journ. of Cellular Biochemistry, Suppl. (7 Part A), 1983, 78.

Szemere, P., and FLIEDNER, T.M.: Blood Leukocyte Responses to Extracorporeal Circulation. II. Medium Term Extracorporeal Circulation without and with Extracorporeal Irradiation in Normal and Splenectomized Dogs. Folia Haematol. 10 (1983) 198-208.

Szemere, P. and FLIEDNER, T.M.: Blood Leukocyte Responses to Extracorporeal Circulation. III. Long Term Extracorporeal circulation without and with Irradiation in Normal and Splenectomized Dogs. Folia Haematol. 10 (1983) 209-217.

Szemere, P. and FLIEDNER, T.M.: Blood Leukocyte Responses to Extracorporeal Circulation. I. Short term Extracorporeal circulation in Dogs without and with Extracorporeal Irradiation. Folia Haematol. 10 (1983) 187-197.

Zinser, D., Bittighofcr, P.M., FLIEDNER, T.M. und R. Berz: Belastung und Beanspruchung von Xylol-exponierten Personen. In: H. Konietzko, F. Schuckmann (Hrsg.): Bericht über die 24. Jahrestagung der Dtsch. Ges. für Arbeitsmed., 263-266. Gentner Stuttgart 1983.

1984

Arnold, R., Schmeiser, T., Friedrich, W., Carbonell, F., Goldmann, S.F., Heit, W., Kohne, E., FLIEDNER, T.M. et al.: Knochenmarktransplantation bei Panmyelopathie, akuter Leukämie und chronisch myeloischer Leukämie: Ergebnisse der "Ulmer Transplantationsgruppe". Klin. Wschr. 62 (1984) 577-585.

Bittighofer, P.M., Peleschka, M., Carbonell, F., FLIEDNER, T.M. und K. Reichenbach: Untersuchungen der mutagenen Aktivitäten im Urin und Blut von Straßenbauarbeitern. In: H. Konietzko, F. Schuckmann (Hrsg.): Verhandlungen der Dtsch. Ges. für Arbeitsmed. e.V., 24. Jahrestagung in Mainz, Mai 1984, 389-395. Gentner Stuttgart 1984.

Bödey, B., Calvo, W., Prümmer, O., Carbonell, F. and FLIEDNER, T.M.: Regeneration of Thymus after Total Body Irradiation in Dogs Rescued by Transfusion of Fetal Liver Cells. Abstract. 1984 Annual Meeting. Int. Society for Exp. Hematology, August 1984 Atlanta Exp. Hematol., Vol. 12 (1984) 451.

Bödey, B., Calvo, W., Prümmer, O. and FLIEDNER, T.M.: Development of the Thymus in Dogs. Abstract. European Developmental Biology Congress. Journal of Embryology and Experimental Morphology. Southampton, September 1984. University of Cambridge, Cambridge 1984.

Carbonell, F., Binder, T., Ganser, A., FLIEDNER, T.M. and H. Heimpel: Cytogenetic Analysis of Malignant Lymphomas by Means of Fine-Needle Aspiration Biopsy. Abstract. Blut 49 (3) 1984, 284.

Carbonell, F., Calvo, W., FLIEDNER, T.M., Kratt, E., Gerhartz, H., Körbling, M., Nothdurft, W. and W.M. Ross: Cytogenetic Studies in Dogs after Total Body Irradiation and Allogeneic Transfusion with Cryopreserved Blood Mononuclear Cells: Observations in Long-Term Chimeras. Int. Journal of Cell Cloning 2 (1984) 81-88.

FLIEDNER, T.M.: Biologische Grenzwerte: Grundlagen, gegenwärtige Bedeutung, Perspektiven. Zbl. Arbeitsmed., 34 (1984) 322-328.

FLIEDNER, T.M.: Physiology and Pathophysiology of Migratory Blood Cells. In: G.F. Fueger (Ed.): Blood Cells in Nuclear Medicine, Part II. Migratory Blood Cells, 23-40. Martinus Nijhoff, The Hague 1984.

FLIEDNER, T.M.: Gedanken zur Physiologie und Pathophysiologie des Alterns. Onkologie 7 (1984) 68-81.

FLIEDNER, T.M.: Die Knochenmarktransplantation als Beispiel medizinischen Fortschritts duch interdisziplinäre Kooperation. Rektorats rede am 21.10.83. In: Sonderbroschüre Ulm Intern. Die Umschau Nr. 19, Mai 1984. Ulmer Forum Nr. 69, Frühjahr 1984. Ulm 1983/84.

FLIEDNER, T.M.: Gesundheit in hundert Jahren. Die Umschau 8 (1984) 241-242.

FLIEDNER, T.M.: Stammzellen der Blutbildung - Ein Beispiel für die Biologie des ewigen Lebens. In: Ministerium für Wissenschaft und Kunst (Hrsg.): Gründe und Hintergründe. Informatonsschrift für Studenten, S. 11. Min. für Wiss. u. Kunst Stuttgart 1984.

FLIEDNER, T.M.: Leukämie heilbar? Knochenmarktransplantation als Beispiel medizinischen Fortschritts duch interdisziplinäre Kooperation. Die Umschau, 84. Jhrg. 10 (1984) 308-311.

FLIEDNER, T.M., Becklake, et al.: Severe Exposure to Pollutants - Accidents in Industry. In: Dunn, C., Garnett, H.M. and P. Jacobs (Eds.): Environmental Pollution and Man. Immunology and Hematology Research Monographs, Vol. 3, 236-238, 1984.

FLIEDNER, T.M., Nothdurft, W., Calvo, W., Steinbach, K.H., Pabst, G. and P. Szemere: Possibilities and Limitations of Hematopoiesis to Tolerate Low-Level Exposure to cyto-toxic Agents and Ionizing Radiation. In: Dunn, C., Garnett, H.M. and P. Jacobs (Eds.): Environmental Pollution and Man. Immunology and Hematology Research Monographs .Vol. 3, 150-155, 1984.

FLIEDNER, T.M. and W. Calvo: Replication and Differentiation of Stem Cells in Relation to the Microenvironment of the Bone Marrow. In: K. Lennert (Ed.): Histopathology of the Bone Marrow, 54-63. Fischer Kiel 1984.

FLIEDNER, T.M., Nothdurft, W. and H. Heit: Biological Factors Affecting the Occurrence of Radiation Syndromes. In: J.J. Broerse, T.J. MacVittie (Eds.): Response of Different Species to Total Body Irradiation. 209-219. Martinus Nijhoff, The Hague 1984.

FLIEDNER, T.M., Thiess, Cronkite, E.P., Carsten, A.L., Latarjet, R., et al.: Environmental Pollution and Man - The Magnitude of the Problem - Historical Aspects and Definitions. In: Dunn, C., Garnett, H.M. and P. Jacobs (Eds.): Environmental Pollution and Man. Immunology and Hematology Research Monographs. Vol. 3, 16-21, 1984.

Friedrich, W., Vetter, U., Heymer, B., Reisner, Y., Goldmann, S.F., FLIEDNER, T.M., Peter, H.H. and E. Kleihauer: Immunoreconstitution in Severe Combined Immunodeficiency after Transplantation of HLA-Haploidentical, T-Cell-Depleted Bone Marrow. Abstract. The Lancet Apr. 7 (1984) 761.

Gerhartz, H.H. and FLIEDNER, T.M.: Physical Separation of Stem Cells from Immunocompetent Lymphocytes for Allogeneic Transplantation. In: S. Slavin (Ed.): Tolerance in Bone Marrow and Organ Transplantation., 309-323. Elsevier Amsterdam, New York, Oxford 1984.

Glatzel, M., Klauk, E., und FLIEDNER, T.M.: Belastung und Beanspruchung bei Kanalarbeitern. In: H. Konietzko, F. Schuckmann (Hrsg.) Verhandlungen der Dtsch. Gesellschaft für Arbeitsmedizin, Jahrestagung Mainz, Mai 1984, 249-252. Gentner Stuttgart 1984.

Issaragrisil, S., Grilli, G. and FLIEDNER, T.M.: Preservation of Haemopoietic Progenitor Cells. Brit. J. of Haemop. Progenitor Cells 55 (1984) 383-385.

Issaragrisil, S., Grilli, G., Nothdurft, W. and FLIEDNER, T.M.: Characterization of Erythroid and Granulocyte Monocyte Progenitors in Human Cord Blood. Scand. J. Haematol. 33 (1984) 317-322.

Kelemen, E., Janossa, M., Calvo, W. and FLIEDNER, T.M.: Developmental Age Estimated by Bone-Length Measurement in Human Fetuses. The Anatomical Record 209 (1984) 547-552.

Körbling, M. and FLIEDNER, T.M.: Autologous Transplantation of Blood Derived Hematopoietic Stem-Cells. In: Smit Sibinga, C.T., Das, P.C. and G. Opelz: Transplantation and Blood Transfusion. Vol. 10, 1984, 199-203.

Körbling, M., Hunstein, W. und FLIEDNER, T.M.: Die autologe Knochenmarktransplantation. Dtsch. Med. Wschr. 7 (1984) 265-271.

Körbling, M., FLIEDNER, T.M. and W. Hunstein: Elimination of Residual Tumor Cells from the Autologous Stem Cell Graft by Chemoseparation. In: J.G. MacVittie et al. (Eds.): Autologous Bone Marrow Transplantation and Solid Tumors. Mo. Ser. Eur. Org. f. Res. on Treat. of Cancer, Vol. 14, 29-32. Raven Press New York 1984.

Nothdurft, W., Braasch, E., Calvo, W., Prümmer, O., Carbonell, F. , Grilli, G. and FLIEDNER, T.M.: Ontogeny of the Granulocyte/Macrophage Progenitor Cell (GM-CFC) Pools in the Beagle. J. Embryol. exp. Morph. 80 (1984) 87-103.

Nothdurft, W., Steinbach, K.H. and FLIEDNER, T.M.: Dose and Time-Related Quantitative and Qualitative Alterations in the Granulocyte/Macrophage Progenitor Cell (GM-CFC) Compartment of Dogs After Total-Body Irradiation. Rad. Research 98 (1984) 332-344.

Prümmer, O, Raghavachar, A., Siebert, K. and FLIEDNER, T.M.: In Vitro Induction of B Cell Differentiation in Canine Mononuclear Blood Cells: Bacterial Lipopolysaccharide Modulates the Action of Pokeweed Mitogen. J. of Immunol. Methods 75 (1984) 193-199.

Prümmer, O., Raghavachar, A., Werner, C., Calvo, W., Carbonell, F. and FLIEDNER, T.M.: Recovery of Lymphopoiesis Following total Body Irradiation and Fetal Liver Transplantation in the Dog. Abstract. Thirteenth Annual Meeting Atlanta Georgia of the Internat. Soc. for Exp. Hematology. Exp. Hematology, Vol. 12 (1984) 467.

Prümmer, O., Werner, C., and FLIEDNER, T.M.: Reconstitution of the Granulocyte-Macrophage Progenitor Cell Compartment after Fetal Liver Transplantation in Dogs. Abstract. Blut 49 (3) 1984, 288.

Raghavachar, A., Prümmer, O. and FLIEDNER, T.M.: The Effect of Cyclophosphamide Treatment in Canine Long-Term Survivors after Autologous Bone Marrow Transplantation. Abstract. Thirteenth Annual Meeting Atlanta of the Intern. Society for Exp. Hematology. Exp. Hematol., Vol. 12 (1984) 439.

Raghavachar, A. and FLIEDNER, T.M.. Analysis of the Dynamics of Progenitor Cell Exchange Between Extravascular and Intravascular Sites after Autologous Bone Marrow Transplantation in the Dog. Abstract. Blut 49 (3) 1984, 287-288.

Werner, C., Prümmer, O., Nothdurft, W. and FLIEDNER, T.M.: Growth of Megakaryocytic Colonies from Normal Canine Bone Marrow in Semisolid Medium. Abstract. Thirteenth Annual Meeting Atlanta, August 1984 of the Intern. Society for Exp. Hematology. Exp. Hematol., Vol. 12 (1984) 444.

Zinser, D., Bittighofer, P.M., FLIEDNER, T.M., Weitbrecht, U. und A. Tenbaum: Belastung und Beanspruchung von Styrol-exponierten Personen. Arbeitsmed, Sozmed. Präventivmed., 19. Jrg 10 (1984) 238-242.

1985

Carbonell, F., Klinnert, V., Ganser, A., FLIEDNER, T.M., Heimpel, H. und D. Hoelzer: Cytogenetic Studies in Acute Leukemia and in the Blast Phase of the Chronic Myelocytic Leukemia. In: Büchner et al. (Eds.): Tumor Aneuplody, 1-11. Springer Berlin 1985.

Carbonell, F., Heimpel, H., Kubanek, B. and FLIEDNER, T.M.: Growth and Cytogenetic Characteristics of Bone Marrow Colonies from Patients with 5q-Syndrome. Blood, Vol. 66 (1985) 463-465.

Ebell, W., Friedrich, W., Blütters-Sawatzki, R., Goldmann, S.F., Raghavachar, A., Peter, H., Kleihauer, E. and FLIEDNER, T.M.: Immunoreconstitution Pattern in Various Subtypes of Severe Combined Immunodeficiency (SCID) Following HLA-Haploidentical Bone Marrow Transplantation (BMT). Abstract. Exp Hematol., Vol. 33 (1985) 345.

FLIEDNER, T.M.: Medical Research as an Instrument to Support the "Health for all" Concept of the World Health Organization. In: Intern. Colloquium, Medical Research in Europe: Present and Future. 1985.

FLIEDNER, T.M.: Einführung in die Thematik. In: LVA Württemberg (Hrsg.): Lehre und Forschung in der Rehabilitationsmedizin. Klausurtagung Juli 1984 Schloß Reisensburg. Schriftenreihe der LVA Württemberg 3 (1985) 1-3.

FLIEDNER, T.M. und W. Nothdurft: Pathopysiologie der chronischen Strahlenbelastung des Organismus. In: W. Leppin et al. (Hrsg.): Die Hypothesen im Strahlenschutz. 24. Jahrestag. der Vereinig. Deutsch. Strahlenschutzärzte, Strahlensch. in Forsch. u.Praxis, Band XXV, 102-9. Georg Thieme Stuttgart 1985.

FLIEDNER, T.M., Steinbach, K.H., Prümmer, O., and W. Calvo: Pathophysiological Mechanisms Responsible for Different Blood Cell Recoveries after Transfusion of Stem Cells from Various Sources. Abstract. Exp. Hematol., 13 (1985) 336.

FLIEDNER, T.M., Calvo, W., Klinnert, V., Nothdurft, W., Prümmer, O. and A. Raghavachar: Bone Marrow Structure and its Possible Significance for Hematopoietic Cell Renewal. In: V.P. Bond, P. Chandra, K.R. Rai (Eds.): Hematopoietic Cellular Prolif. An Int. Conf. in Honor of E.P. Cronkite, Annals of the N.Y. Acad. of Sc, 73-84. The N.Y. Acad. of Sci. New York 1985.

FLIEDNER, T.M., Knoerzer, J. und M. Glatzel: Hypertonie. In. H.M. Bolt, C. Piekarski, und J. Rutenfranz (Hrsg.) :Verh. Deutsch. Ges. für Arbeitsmed. 25. Jahrestagung Dortmund Mai 1985. Gentner Verlag Stuttgart (1985) 19-25.

Gerdes, K. und FLIEDNER, T.M.: Methodische Probleme bei der Erfolgsbeurteilung von Rehabilitationsmaßnahmen. In: LVA Württemberg (Hrsg.): Lehre und Forschung in der Reha-Medizin. Klausurtagung Juli 1984., Schriftenreihe der LVA Württemberg 3 (1985) 64-83.

Gerhartz, H.H., Nothdurft, W., Carbonell, F. and FLIEDNER, T.M.: Allogeneic Transplantation of Blood Stem Cells Concentrated by Density Gradients. Exp. Hematol. 13 (1985) 136-142.

Klinnert, V., Nothdurft, W. and FLIEDNER, T.M.: CFU-F from Dog Marrow: A Colony Assay and its Significance. Blut 50 (1985) 81-87.

Körbling, M., Dörken, B., Ho, A., Maier, W.D., Hunstein, W., and FLIEDNER, T.M.: Autologous Transplantation of Blood-Derived Hemopoietic Stem Cells After Myeloablative Treatment in a Patient with Burkitt's Lymphoma. Abstract. Int. J. of Cell Cloning 3 (41) 1985, 224-225.

Körbling, M., Ho, A., Doerken, B., Kiesel, S., Schwarz, C., Hunstein, W. and FLIEDNER, T.M.: Autologous Blood Stem Cell Transplantation Following Myeloablative Therapy in a Patient with Burkitt's Lymphoma. Abstract. Blut 51 (3) 1985, 219.

Martin, H., Neumann, M., Fache, I., FLIEDNER, T.M. and H. Pflieger: Gradient Separation of Granulocytic Progenitor Cells (CFUc) from Human Blood Mononuclear Leukocytes. Exp. Hematol. 13 (1985) 79-86.

Prümmer, O., Raghavachar, A., Werner, Ch., Calvo, W., Carbonell, F., Steinbach I. and FLIEDNER, T.M.: Fetal Liver Transplantation in the Dog. I. Restoration of Hemopoiesis with Cryopreserved Fetal Liver cells from DLA-Identical Siblings. Transplantation, Vol. 39 (1985).

Prümmer, O., Calvo, W., Werner, Ch., Carbonell, F. and FLIEDNER, T.M.: Hemopoiesis and Immune Functions in Dogs Following Fetal Liver Transplantation. In: Fetal Liver Transplantation, 175-194. Alan R. Liss 1985.

Prümmer, O., Werner, Ch., Raghavachar, A., Nothdurft, W., Calvo, W., Steinbach, K.H. and FLIEDNER, T.M.: Fetal Liver Transplantation in the Dog. II. Repopulation of the Granulocyte-Macrophage Progenitor Cell Compartment by Fetal Liver Cells from DLA Siblings. Transplantation, Vol. 40 (1985) 498-503.

Prümmer, O., Nothdurft, W., and FLIEDNER, T.M.: Canine Blood Mononuclear Cells Inhibit Granulocyte-Macrophage Colony Formation of Adult Bone Marrow and Fetal Liver Cells. Abstract. J. Exp. and Clin. Hematol, Vol. 51 (1985).

Prümmer, O., Nothdurft, W., FLIEDNER, T.M., Baur, G. and E. Rüber: Canine Blood Mononuclear Cells Mediate Contact-Dependent Impairment of Granulocyte-Macrophage Colony Formation by Bone Marrow Cells. Exp. Hematol. 13 (1985) 1033-1038.

Prümmer, O., Nothdurft, W. and FLIEDNER, T.M.: Contact-dependent Inhibition of Granulocyte-Macrophage Colony Formation Mediated by Canine Mononuclear Blood Cells. Abstract. Exp. Hematol., Vol. 13 (1985) 328.

Prümmer, O., Raghavachar, A. and FLIEDNER, T.M.: Recovery of Immune Functions in Dogs after Total Body Irradiation and Transplantation of Autologous Blood or Bone Marrow Cells. Exp. Hematol. 13 (1985) 891-898.

Raghavachar, A., Prümmer, O., Calvo, W., Nothdurft, W.,Steinbach, K.H. and FLIEDNER, T.M.: Repopulating Potential of Canine Bone Marrow Cells: Differences Between Large and Small Cells Separated by Velocity Sedimentation. British J. of Haematology 60 (1985) 33-40.

Seidel, H.J. und FLIEDNER, T.M.: Kinetik der myeloischen Leukämien. In: R. Gross und C.G. Schmidt (Hrsg.): KlinischeOnkologie, 10.1-10.16. Georg Thieme Stuttgart 1985.

Zinser, D. und FLIEDNER, T.M.: Zur Bezugsgrößen-Problematik von BAT-Werten im Urin. In: M. Bolt, C. Piekarski, J. Rutenfranz (Hrsg.): Verhandlungen d. Deutsch. Gesellschaft für Arbeitsmedizin, 27. Jahrestag. in Dortmund, Mai 1985, 167-170. Gentner Stuttgart 1985.

Zorn, H., Kittel, R., Seitz, J., Burk, C., Bittighofer, P. und FLIEDNER, T.M.: Vorbeugender Hautschutz-Praktische Erfahrungen mit einer neuen Hautschutzcreme. Arbeitsmed., Sozialmed., Präventivmed., 4 (1985) 91-94.

1986

Calvo, W., Prümmer, O., Carbonell, F. and FLIEDNER, T.M.: Reconstitution of the Lymph Nodes of Dogs after Fractionated Total Body Irradiation and Transfusion of Foetal Liver Cells. Abstract. Int. Journ. of Radiat. Biology and Related Studies in Physics, Chemistry and Medicine 49 (4) 1986, 720.

Carbonell, F. and FLIEDNER, T.M.: Radiation Induced chromosome Aberrations after Total body Irradiation and Bone Marrow Transplantation. In: A. Kaul et al. (Hrsg.) Biol. Indic. for Radiat. Dose Assessment, bga- Schriften 2/86, 255-260. Medizin München 1986.

Carbonell, F. and FLIEDNER, T.M.: Radiation Induced Chromosome Aberrations after Total Body Irradiation and Bone Marrow Transplantation. In. A. Kaul et al. (Hrsg.): Biological Indicators for Radiation Dose Assessment. bga-Schriften 2/86, 255-259. Medizin München 1986.

FLIEDNER, T.M. and W. Nothdurft: Hematopoetic Progenitor cell Changes in the Blood as Indicators of Radiation Damage to the Bone Marrow. In: A. Kaul et al. (Hrsg.): Biological Indicators for Radiation Dose Assessment, bga-Schriften 2/86, 270-273. Medizin München 1986.

FLIEDNER, T.M., Nothdurft, W., and W. Calvo: Bone Marrow Repopulation and Extramedullary Hemopoiesis in Dogs after Partial Body Irradiation. Abstract. Exp. Hematology, Vol. 14 (1986) 460.

FLIEDNER, T.M. and W. Nothdurft: Cytological Indicators: Hematopoietic Effects. In: A. Kaul et al. (Hrsg.): Biological Indicators for Radiation Dose Assessment. bga-Schriften 2/86, 123-127, Medizin München 1986.

FLIEDNER, T.M. and W. Nothdurft: Hematopoetic Progenitor Cell Changes in the Blood as Indicators of Radiation Damage to the Bone Marrow. In: A. Kaul et al. (Hrsg.): Biological Indicators for Rad. Dose Assessment. bga-Schriften, 270-273. Medizin München 1986.

FLIEDNER, T.M., Nothdurft, W. and W. Calvo: The Development of Radiation Late Effects to the Bone Marrow after Single and Chronic Exposure. Int. J. Radiat. Biol., Vol. 49, No. 1 (1986) 35-46.

FLIEDNER, T.M.: Pathophysiologische Konzepte des malignen Wachstums am Beispiel der Leukämien. In: L. Wanagat (Hrsg.): Onkologie, 1. Bad Mergenthemier Gespräch, 41-45. Georg Thieme Stuttgart 1986.

FLIEDNER, T.M.: Management of chemical risk: the need for international training in occupational risk. Medichem '86. Proceedings of the 14th Intern. Congress on Occupational Health in the Chemical Industry. Ludwigshafen, September 1986.

FLIEDNER, T.M., Nothdurft, W., Fritz, T., Calvo, W. and K.H. Steinbach: Concepts of Pathophysiological Mechanisms involved in the Development of Leukemia in Mammals after Exposure to Ionizing Radiation. Abstract. Leukemia Research, Vol. 10. 7 (1986) 867.

FLIEDNER, T.M., Nothdurft, W., Steinbach, K. and W. Calvo: Hemopoietic Stem Cells - Concepts and Realities. Serono Symposia Publications. Raven Press 34, 1986, 131-145.

FLIEDNER, T.M., Nothdurft, W., Steinbach, K.H. and W. Calvo: Pathophysiological Mechanisms of Tolerance of Hemopoietic Systems to Chronic Low Level Radiation Exposure. Abstract. Int. Jour. of Rad. Biol. and Related Studies in Physics, Chemistry and Medicine 49 (4) 1986, 720-721.

Halasy, K., Seitz, I., Hartmann, W., Gaedicke, G. and FLIEDNER, T.M.: Enrichment of Stem Cells from Bone Marrow and Peripheral Blood by Counterflow Centrifugation with the Beckman Elutriator System. Abstract. Blut, Vol. 53 (1986) 197.

Körbling, M., Dörken, B., Ho, A.D., Pezzutto, A., Hunstein, W. and FLIEDNER, T.M.: Autologous Transplantation of Blood-Derived Hemopoietic Stem Cells After Myeloablative Therapy in a Patient With Burkitt's Lymphoma. Blood, Vol.. 67 (1986) 529-532.

Michel, C., Calvo, W., Raghavachar, A. and FLIEDNER, T.M.: Histochemical Studies on the Effects of Lethal Total Body X-Irradiation on the Pancreas of Dogs Rescued by Autologous Bone Marrow Transplantation. Cellular and Molecular Biology, 32 (1986) 519-526.

Nothdurft, W., Calvo, W., Klinnert, V., Steinbach, K.H., Werner, C. and FLIEDNER, T.M.: Acute and Long-Term Alterations in the Granulocyte/Macrophage Progenitor Cell (GM-CFC) Compartment of Dogs after Partial-Body Irradiation: Irradiation of the Upper Body with a Single Myeloablative Dose. Int. J. Rad. Onc. Biol. Phys. 12 (1986) 949-957.

Prümmer, O., Calvo, W., Carbonell, F., Steinbach, I. and FLIEDNER, T.M.: Fetal Liver Transplantation in Dogs: A Model for Hemolymphopoietic Restoration with a T-Cell-Depleted Stem Cell Graft. Abstract. Annual Meeting of the German Society of Hematology and Oncology. Blut, Vol. 53, 3 (1986) 195.

Wurster, W.H., Zinser, D., FLIEDNER, T.M. und R. Benz: Untersuchung auf Schwermetalle (Cadmium, Blei und Quecksilber) bei Klärwerksarbeitern. In: E. Baumgartner et al. (Hrsg.): Industrieller Wandel - Arbeitsmedizin vor neuen Fragestellungen, Verh. Dtsch. Ges. für Arbeitsmed., 28. Jahrest. Innsbruck, Mai 1988, 237-241. Gentner Stuttgart 1988.

Zinser, D., Bittighofer, P.M. and FLIEDNER, T.M.: Biologisches Monitoring bei Styrol-exponierten Personen. In: E. Baumgartner et al. (Hsg.): Industrieller Wandel - Arbeitsmedizin vor neuen Fragestellungen. Verh. Dtsch. Ges. für Arbeitsmed., 28. Jahrest. Innsbruck, Mai 1988, 473-476. Gentner Stuttgart 1988.

1989

Baltschukat, K., FLIEDNER, T.M. und W. Nothdurft: Hematological Effects in Dogs after Irradiation of the Lower Part of the Body with a Single Myeloablative Dose. Radiotherapy and Oncology 14 (1989) 239-246.

FLIEDNER, T.M.: How I see it and what I would like to do in the future. In: H.J. Seidel (Hrsg.): The Hemopoietic Stem Cell. Universitätsverlag Ulm, 1990, 183-186.

Heeg, S., Biefang, S und FLIEDNER, T.M.: Arbeit und Gesundheit am Bau. Zusammenfassung einer Untersuchung zu Arbeitsbelastungen, berufstypischen Gesundheitsrisiken und Möglichkeiten der Prävention bei ausgewählten Bauberufen. Georg Thieme Stuttgart 1989.

Heinze, B., Arnold, R., Kratt, E., Bunes, D., Heit, W. and FLIEDNER, T.M.: Clonal Evolution of Chromosomal Anomalies in Leukemic Patients after Bone Marrow Transplantation. In: K.H. Chadwick, C. Seymour, B. Banhart (Eds.): Cell Transformation and Radiation-induced Cancer, 177-184. Adam Hilger Bristol, New York 1989.

Körbling, M., Hunstein, W., FLIEDNER, T.M., Cayeux, S., Dörken, B., Fehrentz, D., Hass, R., Ho, A.D., Keilholz, U. et al.: Disease-Free Survival After Autologous Bone Marrow Transplantation in Patients with Acute Myelogenous Leukemia. Blood, Vol. 74, No. 6 (1989) 1898-1904.

Körbling, M., Cayeux S., Baumann, M., FLIEDNER, T.M. et al.: Hemopoietic reconstitution and disease-free survival in a series of 45 patients with AML in first complete remission: A comparison between ABSCNT and ABMT. Bone Marrow Transplantation 4 (Suppl. 2) 49, 1989 (von Cronkite-Brief).

Nothdurft, W., Baltschukat, K. and FLIEDNER, T.M.: Hematological effects in dogs after sequential irradiation of the upper and lower part of the body with single myeloablative doses. Radiotherapy and Oncology 14 (1989) 247-259.

Szepesi, T. und FLIEDNER, T.M.: Reversible und irreversible Schädigung der Hämopoese nach unerwarteter Ganzkörperbestrahlung: Merkmale im peripheren Blut. Wiener Klin. Wochenschrift, Jg. 101 (1989) 309-314.

Szepesi, T. und FLIEDNER, T.M.: Dosis, Strahlenwirkung und Initialsymptomatik nach unerwarteter akuter Ganzkörperbestrahlung: eine Analyse von 19 Unfällen. Wiener klin. Wochenschrift, Jg 101 (1989) 305-309.

Weinsheimer, W., Nothdurft, W., Seifried, E. and FLIEDNER, T.M.: Stem Cell Mobilisation into the Peripheral Blood by Low Molecular Heparines - A Canine Study. Abstract. 34th Annual Congress of the German Society of Hematology and Oncology. Hannover October 1989. Blut, Vol. 59 (1989) 265.

1990

FLIEDNER, T.M., Heit, H. and G. Pabst: Evaluation and Prediction of Chemical Toxicity Using Haematopoietic Cell Renewal Systems. In: P. Bourdeau et al. (Eds.): Short-term Toxicity Tests for Non-genotoxic Effects (Scope 41). 177-192. John Wiley & Sons, Chichester, 1990.

FLIEDNER, T.M., Maiwald, M., Weinsheimer, W. and T. Szepesi: Prediction of Clinical Outcome of Radiation Accident Victims. In: The Biology of Hematopoiesis, 459-470. Wiley-Liss 1990.

FLIEDNER, T.M., Nothdurft, W. und W. Calvo: Das Stammzellsystem der Hämatopoese: physiologische und pathophysiologische Grundlagen. Verh. Dtsch. Ges. Path. 74 (1990) 1-18.

FLIEDNER, T.M.: Kurforschung 2000. Ztsch. d. Dtsch. Bäderverbandes, 42. Jg. 11 (1990) 365-370.

FLIEDNER, T.M.: Hematological Indicators to Predict Patient Recovery After Whole-Body Irradiation as a Basis for Clinical Management. In: R.C. Ricks, S.A. Fry (Eds.): The Medical Basis for Radiation Accident Preparedness, 445-460. Elsevier Oak Ridge, 1990.

Grüner, C., Bittighofer, P.M., Zinser, D. und FLIEDNER, T.M.: Crom-III-Belastung von Arbeitern bei der Chromgerbung. In:: F. Schuckann, S. Schopper-Jochum (IIrsg.): Berufskrankheiten - Krebserzeugende Areitsstoffe - Biological-Monitoring. Verh. der Dtsch. Ges. für Arbeitsmed., 38. Jtg., 295-299. Gentner Stuttgart 1990.

Heinze, B., Arnold, R., Kratt, E., Zick, L., Hertenstein, B., Heit, G., and FLIEDNER, T.M.: Cytogenetic Investigations of Radiation Induced Damage in Cells of Bone Marrow and Peripheral Blood in Leukemia Patients after Bone Marrow Transplantation. In: E. Riklis (Ed.): Frontiers in Radiation Biology, 111-124. Balaban Publ.,VCH Weinsheim 1990.

Körbling, M., Holle, R., Haas, R., Knauf, W., Dörksen, B., Ho, A.D., Kuse, R., Pralle, H., FLIEDNER, T.M. and W. Hunstein: Autologous Blood Stem-Cell Transplantation in Patients with Advanced Hodgkin's Disease and Prior Radiation to the Pelvic Site. J. of Clinical Oncology, Vol. 8, No. 6 (1990) 978-985.

Nothdurft, W., Baltschukat, K., FLIEDNER, T.M., Kreja, L., Krumwieh, D., Seiler, F.R. and W. Weinsheimer: Effects of Recombinant Human Granulocyte-Macrophage Colony Stimulating Factor on canine Bone Marrow Cells in Vitro and its in Vivo Effects in Normal Dogs and Dogs Receiving Sublethal Total Body Irradiation. Abstract. 208. Exp. Hematol. Vol. 18 (1990).

Szepesi, T. und FLIEDNER, T.M.: Konsequenzen aus Beobachtungen an 600 Patienten mit unfallbedingter Ganzkörperbestrahlung. In: G. Harrer und A. Zängl: 44. Österreichischer Ärztekongreß. Van Swieten-Tagung, Wien 22. -24. Oktober 1990. Verlag der Österreichischen Ärztekammer Wien 1990, 157-164.

Weinsheimer, W., Heinze., B., Rothenbach, D., Maiwald, M. und FLIEDNER, T.M.: Der Stellenwert der Chromosomenanalyse bei Verdacht auf Vorliegen einer strahleninduzierten Erkrankung. In: F. Schuckmann, S. Schopper-Jochum (Hrsg.): Berufskrankheiten, Krebserzeugende Arbeitsstoffe - Biologic. Monitoring, 331-334. Gentner Stuttgart 1990.

Ziegler, B., Kreja, L., Bunjes, D., Spiess, B., Seidel, H.J. and FLIEDNER, T.M.: Positive Selection of CD34-/HLA-Dr-Positive Bone Marrow (BM) Cells by Immunomagnetic Particles: Their Response to Hemopoietic Growths Factors. Abstract. Ann. Congr. of the German and Austrian Soc. of Hemat. and Oncology, 120. Blut, Vol. 61 2/3 (1990) 120.

Zinser, D., Weber, L., Mack, S. und FLIEDNER, T.M.: Aufnahme- und Wiederfindungsraten von Styrol bei verschied. Aktiv-Passiv-Sammelsystemen. In: F. Schuckmann, S. Schopper- Jochum (Hrsg.): Berufskrankheiten, Krebserz. Arbeitsstoffe - Biological-Monitoring, 38.Jtg. Dtsch. Ges. Arbeitsmed., 501-2. Gentner Stuttgart 1990.

1991

FLIEDNER, T.M.: Die Erhaltung der Integrität des menschlichen Organismus in einer belastenden Umwelt: Eine Herausforderung für die Forschung. In: Jahrbuch der Heidelberger Akademie der Wissenschaften für 1990, 53-62. 1991.

FLIEDNER, T.M., Kodym, R., Tibken, B., Hofer, E., Hunstein, W. and M. Körbling: Pathophysiology of Granulocyte Recovery in Patients after Total Body Irradiation with and without Autologous Stem Cell Transfusion: Evaluation of Remaining or Transfused Hematopoietic Stem Cell Function. Abstract. Exp. Hematology, Vol. 19 (6), 1991, 121.

Heinze, B., Arnold, R., Kratt, E., Bunjes, D., Reess, K., Plecity, P., Heimpel, H. and FLIEDNER, T.M.: Kinetics of Relapse of Leukemia after Bone Marrow Transplantation: cytogenetic Follow Up of Patients with Chronic Myelogenous Leukemia. Abstract. Bone Marrow Transplant. Vol. 7, Suppl. 2 (1991) 16.

Heinze, B., Arnold, R., Hertenstein, B. and FLIEDNER, T.M.: Development of Chromosomal Anomalies in Addition to the PH1-Chromosome During Cytogenetic Relapse after Bone Marrow Transplantation for Treatment of Chronic Myeloid Leukemia. Abstract no. 184. Onkologie, Suppl. 2 (1991).

Hofer, E.P., Tibken, B. and FLIEDNER, T.M.: Modern Control Theory as a Tool to Describe the Biomathematical Model of Granulocytopoiesis. In: Möller, D.P.F. und O. Richter (Hrsg.): Analyse dynamischer Systeme in Medizin, Biologie und Ökologie, Springer Verlag Berlin 1991.

Kodym, R. and FLIEDNER, T.M.: A Mathematical Model of the Thrombopoietic System in the Rat. Abstract. Exp. Hematology, Vol. 19 (1991) 492.

Körbling, M., FLIEDNER, T.M., Holle, R., Magrin, S., Baumann, S., Holdermann, E. and K. Eberhadt: Autologous Blood Stem Cell (ABSCT) versus Purged Bone Marrow Transplantation (pABMT) in

Standard Risk AML: Influence of Couce and Cell Composition of the Autograft on Hemopoietic Reconstitution and Disease-Free Survival. Bone Marrow Transplant. 7 (1991) 343-349.

Selig, C., Nothdurft, W., Kreja, L und FLIEDNER, T.M.: Influence of Combined Treatment with Interleukin 1 and Erythropoietin or GM-CSF and Erythropoietin on the Regeneration of Hemopoiesis in the Dog After Total Body Irradiation - A Preliminary Report. Boehring Inst. Mitt. 90 (1991) 86-92.

Weinsheimer, W., Szepesi, T. and FLIEDNER, T.M.: Early Indicators of Response to Accidental Radiation Exposure and the Relevance for Clinical Management Strategies. Prog. Clin. Biol. Res. 372 (1991) 155-165.

Weinsheimer, W., Kolb, H.J., Dull, T., and T.M. Fiedner: Late Effects in bone Marrow Transplanted Patients - a Multicenter Study Supported by EBMT and EULEP. Bone Marrow Transplant., 8 Suppl. 1 (1991) 25.

Ziegler, B.L., Lamping, C., Petri, J.B., Thomas, S., Kreja, L., Steinhoff, K., and FLIEDNER, T.M.: Effects of Il-3 and GM-CSF on CD34/HLA-DR-Positive Hemopoietic Progenitor Cells from Cord Blood Positively Selected by a Two-Step Immunomagnetic Cell Sorting Procedure. Abstract. Exp. Hematol., Vol. 19 (6), 1991, 470.

Ziegler, B., Thoma, S., Petri, B., Lamping, C. and FLIEDNER, T.M.: Amplification of C-DNA derived from M-RNA Transcripts in Small Numbers of Hemopoietic Cells by the Polymerase Chain Reaction. Abstract. Exp. Hematology, Vol. 19 (1991) 522.

1992

FLIEDNER, T.M.: Knochenmarktransplantation und ihre Problematik bei Strahlenunfällen. In: Strahlenschutz in Forschung und Praxis, Band 33, S. 185-191, 1992.

FLIEDNER, T.M.: Kontinuität und Wandel - das Spannungsfeld universitären Lebens. In: Uni Ulm (Hrsg.): ULMENSIEN, Band 5, 115-138. Universitätsverlag Ulm 1992.

FLIEDNER, T.M.: Lebendige Wissenschaft am Beispiel Ulm: Versuch einer Bilanz In: Uni Ulm (Hrsg.): ULMENSIEN, Band 5, 53-67 Universitätsverlag Ulm 1992.

FLIEDNER, T.M. Der Stellenwert der Reisensburg im regionalen und internationalen Wandel. In: D. Draf, K. Ackermann, R. Brunner, A. Spitzner, T. Waigel (Hrsg.): Schwaben - Bayern - Europa. Zukunftsperspektiven der bayerischen Bezirke. Festschrift für Dr. G. Simnacher. EOS Verlag Erzabtei St. Ottilien 1992, 41-48.

FLIEDNER, T.M., Heinze, B. und U. Plappert: Biologische Indikatoren zur Evaluation der Beanspruchung des Organisus durch ionisierende Strahlen. In: B. Kreutz und C. Piekarski (Hrsg.): 32. Jahrestagung der Deutschen Gesellschaft für Arbeitsmedizin in Köln 1992, 395-399. Gentner Stuttgart 1992.

FLIEDNER, T.M. und W. Nothdurft: Simulationsmodelle der Hämatopoese zur Abschätzung der Strahlenbeanspruchung bei fraktionierter oder chronischer Strahlenbelastung. In: B. Kreutz und C. Pierkarski (Hrsg.): 32. Jahrestagung der Dtsch. Ges. für Arbeitsmed., 400-406. Gentner Stuttgart 1992.

Kolb, H.J.,Guether, W., Duell, T., Socie, G., Schaeffer, E., Holler, E., Schumm, M., Horowitz, M.M., Gale, R.P. and FLIEDNER, T.M.: Cancer after Bone Marrow Transplantation, IBMTR and EBMT/ EULEP Study Group on Late Effects. Bone Marrow Transplant. 10, Suppl. 1 (1992) 135-138.

Nothdurft, W., Selig, C., FLIEDNER, T.M., Hintz-Obertreis, P., Kreja, L., Krumwieh, D, Kurrle, R. Seiler, F.R. et al.: Haematological Effects of rhGM-CSF in Dogs Exposed to Total- Body Irradiation with a Dose of 2.4 Gy. Int. J. Radiation Biology, Vol. 61 4 (1992) 519-531.

Petri, J.B., Thoma, S., Lamping, C., FLIEDNER, T.M., Peschle, C., Ziegler, B.L.: Retrovirus-mediated gene transfer into multipotent human hematopoietic progenitor cells. Abstract. Blood 80:179a (705) 1992.

Szepesi, T., FLIEDNER, T.M. und D. Densow: Entscheidungskriterien der medizinischen Erstversorgung nach nuklearen Unfällen in Notfallambulanzen. Beitr. Anaesth. Intens. Notfallmed. 41 (1992) 11-122.

Weinsheimer, M., Rothenbacher, D., Heinze, B. and FLIEDNER, T.M.: "Biologische Dosimetrie" am Beispiel der Srahlenexposition. In: Verh. der Deutsche Gesellschaft für Arbeitsmedizin, 31. Tagung in Berlin 1991, Genter Verlag Stuttgart 1992, 461-463.

Weinsheimer, C., Weinsheimer, W., Glatzel, M. und FLIEDNER, T.M.: Gesundheitsbeanspruchung von Klärwärtern. In: Verhandlungen der Deutschen Gesellschaft für Arbeitsmedizin, 31. Jahrestagung in Berlin 1991, Genter Verlag Stuttgart 1992, 133-134

Ziegler, B.L., Lamping, C., Petri, J.B., FLIEDNER, T.M., Thoma, S.: Phenotype analysis of umbilical cord blood (CB CD34+ cell subpopulations). Abstract. Blood 80:408a (1623) 1992.

1993

Calvo, W., Alabi, R., Nothdurft, W. and FLIEDNER, T.M.. Megakaryocyte Changes in the Marrow of Irradiated Dogs. Abstract. Experimental Hematology 21: 1040, 1993.

FLIEDNER, T.M.: Der Krebskranke in der Arbeitswelt: die Rolle der Rehabilitation. In: L. Wannagat (Hrsg.): Onkologie - der Krebskranke: sein Umfeld und sein Arzt. 4. Bad Mergentheimer Onkologisches Gespräch, Georg Thieme Stuttgart 1993, 72-78.

FLIEDNER, T.M.: Vom Muskel- ins Nervenzeitalter: Über den Wandel in der Arbeitswelt. In: Joachim Jungius Gesellschaft der Wissenschaften (Hrsg.): Jahresbericht 1993, 191-192.

FLIEDNER, T.M. und W. Nothdurft: Präklinische Untersuchungen zur Beschleunigung der Erholungsvorgänge in der Blutzellbildung nach Strahleneinwirkung durch Beeinflussung von Regulationsmechanismen. In. Bundesamt für Zivilschutz (Hrsg.): Beiträge zu Strahlenschäden und Strahlenkrankheiten. Max Schick GmbH München, 1993, 141-174.

FLIEDNER, T.M., Weiss, M., Hofer, E.P., Tibken, B. und Y. Fan: Blutzellveränderungen nach Strahleneinwirkung als Indikatoren für die ärztliche Versorgung von Strahlenunfallpatienten. In: F. Holeczke, Chr. Reiners, O. Messerschmidt: Strahlenexposition bei neuen diagnostischen Verfahren. Biologische Dosimetrie - 6 Jahre nach Tschernobyl. Strahlenschutz in Forschung und Praxis, Band 34, 137 - 154, Gustav Fischer Verlag Stuttgart, 1993.

Plappert, U., Radatz, K., Kreja, L, Barthel, E. and FLIEDNER, T.M.. The Comet Assay - useful tool for detection of DNA damage in mammalian cells. Abstract. Mutagenesis 8 (1993) 476-477.

Plappert, U., Barthel, E., Seidel, H.J. and FLIEDNER, T.M.. Rapid Detection of Benzene Toxicity in Mice Using the Comet Assay. Abstract 121. Experimental Hematology, vol 21 (1993) 1042.

Selig, C., Nothdurft, W. and FLIEDNER, T.M.: Radioprotective Effect of N-Acetylcysteine on Granulocyte/ Macrophage Colony-Forming Cells of Human Bone Marrow. J. Cancer Res. Clin. Oncol., 119 (1993) 346-349.

Stadtmüller, K., und FLIEDNER, T.M.: Berufsbedingte degenerative Diskopathien im Lendenwirbelsäulenbereich. Arbeitsmed. Sozialmed. Umweltmed. 28 (1993) 297-300.

Ziegler, B.L., Thoma, S., Lamping, C., Gause, H., Werner, A.K., FLIEDNER, T.M.: Identification of CD34$^+$ cell subsets from cord blood by flow cytometry and cDNA-PCR. Abstract. Experimental Hematology 21:1136,1993.

1994

Brusis, J., Gerdes, N., Pollack, H. und FLIEDNER, T.M.: Die "Multizentrische Reha-Studie 1992/93". Erste Ergebnisse aus der Gesamtstichprobe und aus der Stoffwechselklinik Bad Mergentheim. Z. Gastroenterol. (Suppl. 1) 1994;32:26-30.

Calvo, W., Alabi, R., Nothdurft, W. and FLIEDNER, T.M.: Cytotoxic Immigration of Granulocytes into Megakaryocytes as a Late Consequence of Irradiation. Radiat. Res. 138 (1994) 260-265.

Densow, FLIEDNER, T.M. und D. Arndt: Übersicht und Kategorisierung von Strahlenunfällen und - katastrophen als Grundlage medizinischer Maßnahmen.. In: Bundesminister für Umwelt, Naturschutz und Reaktorsicherheit (Hrsg.): Medizinische Maßnahmen bei Strahlenunfällen. Veröffentl. der Strahlenschutzkommission, Band 27, 9-50, Gustav Fischer, Stuttgart 1994.

FLIEDNER, T.M.: Strahlenwirkungen bei externer Ganz- und Teilkörperbestrahlung. In: Bundesminister für Umwelt, Naturschutz und Reaktorsicherheit (Hrsg.): Medizinische Maßnahmen bei Strahlenunfällen. Veröffentl. der Strahlenschutzkommission, Band 27, 65-84, Gustav Fischer, Stuttgart 1994.

FLIEDNER, T.M.: Blutstammzelltransplantation. In: Bundesminister für Umwelt, Naturschutz und Reaktorsicherheit (Hrsg.): Medizinische Maßnahmen bei Strahlenunfällen. Veröffentl. der Strahlenschutzkommission, Band 27, 241- 250, Gustav Fischer, Stuttgart 1994.

FLIEDNER, T.M.: Überblick über medizinische Maßnahmen beim Strahlenunfall. In: Bundesminister für Umwelt, Naturschutz und Reaktorsicherheit (Hrsg.): Medizinische Maßnahmen bei Strahlenunfällen. Veröffentl. der Strahlenschutzkommission, Band 27, 251-264, Gustav Fischer, Stuttgart 1994.

FLIEDNER, T.M., Greiner, C. and F.J. Radermacher: Reliable Predictions Concerning Human Health and Factors of the Living conditions of Human Beings. Abstracts of the 1st Intern. Symposium on Ecosystem Health & Medicine. June 19-23, 1994 Ottawa, Ontario, Canada, 33.

FLIEDNER, T.M.: Man-Made Environment and Health Development: A Challenge for the Scientific Community. In: WHO (Ed.): The impact of scientific advances on future health. Report of a WHO-CIOMS Colloquium, Charlottesville, Virginia, 20-24 June 1994, WHO/RPS/ACHR-CIOMS/95, 89-100.

FLIEDNER, T.M.: Fort- und Weiterbildung der Ärzte zur ärztlichen Versorgung von Strahlenunfallpatienten. In: Bundesminister für Umwelt, Naturschutz und Reaktorsicherheit (Hrsg.): Medizinische Maßnahmen bei Strahlenunfällen. Veröffentl. der Strahlenschutzkommission, Band 27, 327- 338, Gustav Fischer, Stuttgart 1994.

FLIEDNER, T.M., Nothdurft, W., Tibken, B., Hofer, E., Weiss, M. and H. Kindler: Haemopoietic Cell Renewal in Radiation Fields. Adv. Space Res. Vol. 14, No. 10, (10)541-(10)554, 1994.

FLIEDNER, T.M., Kindler, H., Densow, D, Baranov, A.E., Guskova, A- and T. Szepesi: The Moscow-Ulm Radiation Accident Clinical History Data Base. Advances in the Biosciences, Vol. 94,1994:271-279.

Greiner, C., Radermacher, F.J., Edrich, J. and FLIEDNER, T.M.: Monotonic Structures as Basis for Reliable Predictions Concerning Factors of the Human Habitat. In: L.M. Hilty, A. Jaeschke, B. Page und A. Schwabl: Informatik für den Umweltschutz. 8. Symposium, Hamburg 1994, Band I. Metropolis-Verlag, Marburg 1994, 435-442.

Hofer, E.P., Tibken, B. and FLIEDNER, T.M.: Modeling of the chronically irradiated hemopoietic system. In: Proceedings of the First Asian Control Conference (ASCC), Tokyo, July 27-30, 1994, Vol. 2, 173-175.

Körbling, M. and FLIEDNER, T.M.: History of blood stem cell transplants. In: R.P. Gale, Ch. Juttner and P. Henon (Eds.): Blood Stem Cell Transplants. Cambridge University Press 1994, 9-19.

Plappert, U., Barthel, E., Seidel, H.J. and FLIEDNER, T.M.: Early effects of benzene exposure in mice. Hematological versus genotoxic effects. Arch. Toxicol. 68 (1994) 284-290.

Szepesi, T. and FLIEDNER, T.M.: Evaluation of Accidental Acute Irradiated Persons with Respect to Therapeutic Measures. Izotoptechnika, Diagnosztika, Vol. 37, Suppl. 1994, 5-15.

WHO-Collaborating Centre for Radiation Emergency Medical Preparedness and Assistance: A.E. Baranov, D. Densow, FLIEDNER, T.M., H. Kindler: Clinical Pre Computer Proforma for the International Computer Database for Radiation Exposure Case Histories. Springer Verlag Berlin, Heidelberg 1994.

Ziegler, B.L., Thoma, S., Lamping, C., Treffler, B., Meier, T., Weber, L. and FLIEDNER, T.M.: A model for virus spread through laser application. In: L. Weber (Ed.): Indoor Air Pollution, Innenraumschadstoffbelastung. Indoor Air Intern. Rothenfluh Schweiz, 1994, 382-388.

Ziegler, B.L., Lamping, C., Thoma, S. und FLIEDNER, T.M.. Possible biological hazards through recombinant amphotropic retroviruses used for transduction of human cells. In: L. Weber (Ed.): Indoor Air Pollution, Innenraumschadstoffbelastung. Indoor Air Intern. Rothenfluh Schweiz, 1994, 389-405.

Ziegler, B.L., Lamping, C., Thoma, S., Peschle, C., FLIEDNER, T.M.: Single-cell RT-PCR: Isolation of mRNA from single hemopoietic cells allows detection of multiple mRNA species. Abstract. Blood 84 (suppl. 1): 1272 (1074) 1994.

Ziegler, B.L., Thoma, S., Lamping, C., Peschle, C., FLIEDNER, T.M.: A panel of monoclonal antibodies identifies chymopapain-resistant epitopes of antigens coexpressed on CD34$^+$ hemopoietic progenitor cells. Abstract. Blood 84 (suppl. 1) 272a (1075) 1994.

1995

Enderle, G., Friedrich, K., Plappert, U., Wüstermann, P.-R., Hagenmaier, A., Ziegler, B. and FLIEDNER, T.M.: East German Uranium Miners: The Risk of late Effects From Exposure to a Complex Physical and Chemical Environment. In: U. Hagen et al. (Eds.): Radiation Research 1895 - 1995. Congress proceedings, Volume 2. Würzburg: Stürtz 1995, 1207-1210.

Enderle, G., Hagenmaier A., Plappert, U., Wüstermann, P-R., Ziegler, B. and FLIEDNER, T.M.: Uranium Miners: The Risk of Late Effects from Exposure to a Complex Physical and Chemical Environment. In: Hagen, U., Jung, H. and C. Streffer (Eds.): Radiation Research 1895 - 1995. Vol. 1: Congress Abstracts. Congress Proceedings of the Tenth Intern. Congress of Radiation Research Würzburg, Germany 1995, 60.

FLIEDNER, T.M., Wüstermann, OP.-R., Tibken, B. and E.P. Hofer: Structure and Function of the Immune System under Influence of Ionizing Radiation: New Approaches of Biomathematical Modeling. In: Hagen, U., Jung, H. and C. Streffer (Eds.): Radiation Research 1895 - 1995. Vol. 1: Congress Abstracts. Congress Proceedings of the Tenth Intern. Congress of Radiation Research Würzburg, Germany 1995, 700-704.

FLIEDNER, T.M., Cronkite, E.P. and V.P. Bond (Eds.): Assessment of Radiation Effects by Molecular and Cellular Approaches. STEM CELLS, Vol. 13, Suppl. 1, May 1995, AlphaMed Press, Dayton, Ohio.

FLIEDNER, T.M.: The Need for an Expanded Protocol for the Medica Examination of Radiation-Exposed Persons. In: FLIEDNER, T.M., Cronkite, E.P. and V.P. Bond (Eds.): Assessment of Radiation Effects by Molecular and Cellular Approaches. STEM CELLS, Vol. 13, Suppl. 1, May 1995, AlphaMed Press, Dayton, Ohio, 1-6.

FLIEDNER, T.M.: Blood Stem Cell Transplantation: From Preclinical to Clinical Models. STEM CELLS, Vol. 13 (suppl. 3) 1995: 1-12.

Heinze, B., Arnold, R., Rutzen-Loesevitz, L. and FLIEDNER, T.M.: The Role of Stable Chromosome Aberrations as Biological Indicators of Radiation Effect: Studies in Patients after Total Body Irradiation and Bone Marrow Transplantation. In: FLIEDNER, T.M., Cronkite, E.P. and V.P. Bond (Eds.): Assessment of Radiation Effects by Molecular and Cellular Approaches. STEM CELLS, Vol. 13, Suppl. 1, May 1995, AlphaMed Press, Dayton, Ohio, 191-198.

Heinze, B. und FLIEDNER, T.M.: Was wissen wir über das Schicksal von bestrahlten Zellen der Blutbildung? Zeitschr. für Strahlenforschung (ZSF) NF, Vol. 17, 147-170, 1995.

Heinze, B., Bink, K., Bunjes, D., Rutzen-Loesevitz, L., Zick, L. and FLIEDNER, T.M.: Stable Chromosome Aberrations: Involvement of Special Chromosomes or of Specific Chromosome Break Points? In: Hagen, U., Jung, H. and C. Streffer (Eds.): Radiation Research 1895 - 1995. Vol. 1: Congress Abstracts. Congress Proceedings of the Tenth Intern. Congress of Radiation Research Würzburg, Germany 1995, 377.

Nadejina, N.M., Galstian, I.A., Weiss, M., Fischer, B., Suvorova, L.N., Pokrovskaya, V.N. and FLIEDNER, T.M.: Late Consequences Analysis in Chernobyl Accident Acute Radiation Disease Survivors. In: Hagen, U., Jung, H. and C. Streffer (Eds.): Radiation Research 1895 - 1995. Vol. 1: Congress Abstracts. Congress Proceedings of the Tenth Intern. Congress of Radiation Research Würzburg, Germany 1995, 331.

Nothdurft, W., FLIEDNER, T.M., Fritz, T.E. and T.M. Seed: Response of Hemopoiesis in Dogs to Continuous Low Dose Rate Total Body Irradiation. In: FLIEDNER, T.M., Cronkite, E.P. and V.P. Bond (Eds.): Assessment of Radiation Effects by Molecular and Cellular Approaches. STEM CELLS, Vol. 13, Suppl. 1, May 1995, AlphaMed Press, Dayton, Ohio, 261-267.

Plappert, U., Molt, S., Roth, S. and FLIEDNER, T.M.: DNA-Damage Detection in Man after Radioiodine Therapy. In: Hagen, U., Jung, H. and C. Streffer (Eds.): Radiation Research 1895 - 1995. Vol. 1: Congress Abstracts. Congress Proceedings of the Tenth Intern. Congress of Radiation Research Würzburg, Germany 1995, 209.

Plappert, U., Raddatz, K., Molt, S., Rieth, W., FLIEDNER, T.M.: Der Comet Assay - ein neuer Indikatortest zum Nachweis genotoxischer Beanspruchung. Arbeitsmed. Sozialmed., Umweltmed. 1995: 30, 60-65.

Plappert, U., Raddatz, K., Roth, S. and FLIEDNER, T.M.: DNA-Damage Detection in Man after Radiation Exposure - The Comet Assay - Its Possible Application for Human Biomonitoring. In: FLIEDNER, T.M., Cronkite, E.P. and V.P. Bond (Eds.): Assessment of Radiation Effects by Molecular and Cellular Approaches. STEM CELLS, Vol. 13, Suppl. 1, May 1995, AlphaMed Press, Dayton, Ohio, 215-222.

Plappert, U., Raddatz, K., Seidel, H.J. and FLIEDNER, T.M.: Does toluene reduce the genotoxicity of benzene? Abstract. Mutation Res. 335 (1995) 104.

Selig, C., Kreja, L., FLIEDNER, T.M. and W. Nothdurft: Influence of G-CSF and GM-CSF on Cycling Characteristics of Hematopoietic Cells at Different Sites of Canine Bone Marrow After Partial Body Irradiation. In: Hagen, U., Jung, H. and C. Streffer (Eds.): Radiation Research 1895 - 1995. Vol. 1: Congress Abstracts. Congress Proceedings of the Tenth Intern. Congress of Radiation Research Würzburg, Germany 1995, 235.

Weiss, M., Bebeshko, V.A., Belyi, D., Fischer, B. and FLIEDNER, T.M.: Late Effects, Clinical and Social Performance of Long Term Survivors after the Chernobyl Accident. In: Hagen, U., Jung, H. and C. Streffer (Eds.): Radiation Research 1895 - 1995. Vol. 1: Congress Abstracts. Congress Proceedings of the Tenth Intern. Congress of Radiation Research Würzburg, Germany 1995, 331.

Wüstermann, P.R., Tibken, B., Brücher, S., Mehr, K., FLIEDNER, T.M. and E. Hofer: Biomathematical Modeling of Lymphocyte Responses After Whole Body Irradiation to Assess the Degree of Damage to the Immune System. In: Hagen, U., Jung, H. and C. Streffer (Eds.): Radiation Research 1895 - 1995. Vol. 1: Congress Abstracts. Congress Proceedings of the Tenth Intern. Congress of Radiation Research Würzburg, Germany 1995, 265.

Ziegler, B.L, Lamping, C.P., Thoma, S.J. and FLIEDNER, T.M.: Analysis of Gene Expression in Small Numbers of Purified Hemopoietic Progenitor Cells by RT-PCR. In: FLIEDNER, T.M., Cronkite, E.P. and V.P. Bond (Eds.): Assessment of Radiation Effects by Molecular and Cellular Approaches. STEM CELLS, Vol. 13, Suppl. 1, May 1995, AlphaMed Press, Dayton, Ohio, 106-116.

Ziegler, B.L., Weiss, M., Thoma, S., Lamping, C. and FLIEDNER, T.M.: Biologic Indicators of Exposure: Are Markers Associated with Oncogenesis Useful as Biologic Markers of Effect? In: FLIEDNER, T.M., Cronkite, E.P. and V.P. Bond (Eds.): Assessment of Radiation Effects by Molecular and Cellular Approaches. STEM CELLS, Vol. 13, Suppl. 1, May 1995, AlphaMed Press, Dayton, Ohio, 326-338.

Ziegler, B.L, Lamping, C.P., Thoma, S.J., Thomas, C.A. and FLIEDNER, T.M.: Single-Cell cDNA-PCR. In: G. Sarkar (Ed.): Methods in Neurosciences. Vol. 26: PCR in Neuroscience, Academic Press, San Diego 1995, 62-74.

1996

Arndt, V., Rothenbacher, D., Brenner, H., Fraisse, E., Zschenderlein, B., Daniel, U., Schuberth, S. and FLIEDNER, T.M.: Older workers in the construction industry: results of a routine health examination and a five year follow up. Occupat. and Environm. Medicine 1996;53:686-691.

Densow, D., Kindler, H., and FLIEDNER, T.M.: Developing diagnostic guidelines for the acute radiation syndrome. In: A. Karaoglou, G. Desmet, G.N. Kelly and H.G. Menzel (Eds.): The radiological consequences of the Chernobyl accident. Proceedings of the first international conference Minsk, Belarus, March 1996. Office for Official Publications of the European Communities, Brussels, Luxembourg, 1996, 621-624.

Fischer, B., Belyi, D.A., Weiss, M., Nadejina, N.M., Galstian, L.A., Kovalenko, A.N., Bebeshko, V.G. and FLIEDNER, T.M.: A multi-centre clinical follow-up database as a systematic approach to the evaluation of mid- and long-term health consequences in Chernobyl acute radiation syndrome patients. In: A. Karaoglou, G. Desmet, G.N. Kelly and H.G. Menzel (Eds.): The radiological consequences of the Chernobyl accident. Proceedings of the first international conference Minsk, Belarus, March 1996. Office for Official Publications of the European Communities, Brussels, Luxembourg, 1996, 625-628.

FLIEDNER, T.M. Medizinische Maßnahmen bei externer Bestrahlung. Strahlenschutz in Forschung und Praxis, Band 38, Stuttgart, Jena, Lübeck, Ulm: Fischer 1996, 89-103.

FLIEDNER, T.M.: Methods for Assessing the Extent of Acute Radiation Injury. In: A. Karaoglou, G. Desmet, G.N. Kelly and H.G. Menzel (Eds.): The radiological consequences of the Chernobyl accident. Proceedings of the first international conference Minsk, Belarus, March 1996. Office for Official Publications of the European Communities, Brussels, Luxembourg, 1996, 569-581.

FLIEDNER, T.M., Tibken, B., Hofer, E.P. and W. Paul: Stem Cell Responses after Radiation Exposure: A Key to the Evaluation and Prediction of its Effects. Health Physics, June 1996, Vol. 70, No. 6, 787-797.

Frickhofen, N., Körbling, M. and FLIEDNER, T.M.: Is blood a better source of allogeneic hematopoietic stem cells for use after radiation accidents? Bone Marrow Transplantation, (1996) 17, 131-135.

Greiner, C., I.T., Hawryszkiewycz, I.T., Rose, T. and FLIEDNER, T.M.: Supporting Health Research Strategy Planning Processes of WHO with Information Technology. In: K. Sandkuhl, H. Weber (Eds.): ISST-Report "Tele-Cooperation Systems in Decentralized Organizations", Berlin 1996, ISSN 09433-1624, 121-145.

Greiner, C., Radermacher, F.J. and FLIEDNER, T.M.: Standard reference data and policy assistance systems for global health evolution. In: W. Schröder, O. Fränzle, H. Keune and P. Mandry (Eds.): Global Monitoring of Terrestrial Ecosystems. Ernst & Sohn, Berlin, 1996, 159-164.

Körbling, M. and FLIEDNER, T.M.: Historical Perspective: The evolution of clinical peripheral blood stem cell transplantation. Bone Marrow Transplantation (1996) 17, 675-678.

Radermacher, F.J., Benking, H., Brauer, G.W., FLIEDNER, T.M., Greiner, C., Malaska, P., Morath, K. and R. Pestel: Robust paths to global stability: Tough but feasible. People and Work - Research Report 8. Finnish Inst. of Occupational Health, Helsinki 1996, 13-40.

Rothenbacher, D., Arndt, V., Brenner, H., Fraisse, E., FLIEDNER, T.M., Zschenderlein, B., Daniel, U. und S. Schuberth: Bronchopulmonale Morbidität und deren prognostische Bedeutung für die Gesamtmortalität bei 4958 Beschäftigten der Bauindustrie. Pneumologie 1996; 50 (1. Sonderheft): 124 (abstract).

Rothenbacher, D., Brenner, H., Arndt, V., Fraisse, E., Zschenderlein, B. and FLIEDNER, T.M.: Smoking patterns and mortality attributable to smoking in a cohort of 3528 construction workers. Europ. Journal of Epidemiology 12:335-340, 1996.

Weiss, M., Bebeshko, V.G., Nadejina, N.M., Galstian, I.A., Belyi, D.A., Kovalenko, A.N., Fischer, B. and FLIEDNER, T.M.: Evaluation of mid- and long-term consequences, clinical and social performance in Chernobyl acute radiation syndrome patients in a multi-centre clinical follow-up study. In: A. Karaoglou, G. Desmet, G.N. Kelly and H.G. Menzel (Eds.): The radiological consequences of the Chernobyl accident. Proceedings of the first international conference Minsk, Belarus, March 1996. Office for Official Publications of the European Communities, Brussels, Luxembourg, 1996, 629-632.

Weiss, M., Klier, F., Fischer, B., FLIEDNER, T.M., Pieper, B., Wedel, R., Grossmann, H.P. and A.V. Akleyev: Telemedicine project RATEMA - radiation accident telecommunication medical assistance system. Journal of Telemedicine and Telecare 1996; 2 (Suppl. 1) 9-12.

Ziegler, B.L., S.J. Thoma, C. P. Lamping, M. Valtieri, R. Müller, P. Samoggia, H.J. Bühring, C. Peschle and FLIEDNER, T.M.: Surface Antigen Expression on CD34$^+$ Cord Blood Cells: Comparative Analysis by Flow Cytometry and Limiting Dilution (LD) RT-PCR of Chymopapain-Treated or Untreated Cells. Cytometry 25:46-57 (1996).

1997

Beyrer, K., Braur, G.W., FLIEDNER, T.M., Greiner, C., and U. Reischl: Visual Health Information profile (VHIP): A Quantitative Approach for Analysing the Health Status of a Population. In. Pappas, C., Maglaveras, N. and J.R. Scherrer: Medical Informatics Europe '97, IOS-Press, Amsterdam, Berlin, Oxford 1997, 874-878.

Brenner, H., Arndt, V., Rothenbacher, D., Schuberth, S., Fraisse, E. and FLIEDNER, T.M.: The Association between Alcohol Consumption and All-Cause Mortality in a Cohort of Male Employees in the German Construction Industry. Int. Journ. of Epidemiology, Vol. 26, No. 1, 1997, 85-91.

Heinze, B., Bink, K., Griesshammer, M., FLIEDNER, T.M. and R. Hehlmann: Cytogenetic response to therapy and the clonal evolution of additional chromosome aberrations in Ph-positive CML: results of cytogenetic analyses for the German multicenter study. Journ. of Molecular Med., Vol. 75, No. 7, 1997, B151.

Rothenbacher, D., Arndt, V, Fraisse, E., Daniel, U., FLIEDNER, T.M. and H. Brenner: Chronic respiratory disease morbidity in construction workers: patterns and prognostic significance for permanent disability and overall mortality. Eur. Respir. J. 1997;10:1093-1099.

Sayers, B. McA., Bailey, N.T.J., FLIEDNER, T.M., Jablensky, A., Karczewski, W. and M. Manciaux: Letter to the Editor: The disability adjusted life year concept: a comment. Eur. J. of Public Health., Vol. 7, 1997, No. 1, 113.

Weber, L.W., Sato, N., Zimmermann, C. and FLIEDNER, T.M.: Untersuchungen zur Dichtigkeit von medizinischen Schutzhandschuhen nach Gebrauch am Patienten bzw. im Labor. Krankenh.-Hyg. + Infekt.verh. 19, Heft 2 (1997) 52-59.

Contributors

Dr. Nader G. Abraham
New York Medical College
Department of Pharmacology
Valhalla, NY 10595, USA
Tel: 914-594-4132
Fax: 914-594-4119
e-mail: nader_abraham@NYMC.edu

Dr. Hal E. Broxmeyer
Department of Microbiology/Immunology
Walther Oncology Center
Indiana University School of Medicine
1044 W. Walnut Street, Room 302
Indianapolis, IN 46202, USA
Tel: 317-274-7510
Fax: 317-274-7592
e-mail: hal_broxmeyer@iucc.iupui.edu

Dr. Albert Deisseroth
Yale University
School of Medicine
333 Cedar Street
P.O. Box 208032
New Haven, CT 06520-8032, USA
Tel: 203-737-5608
Fax: 203-737-5698
e-mail: deisseroab@maspo2.mas.yale.edu

Dr. Allen C. Eaves
Terry Fox Laboratory
601 West 10th Avenue
Vancouver, BC
V5Z 1L3, Canada
Tel: 604-877-6070 x3112
Fax: 604-877-0712
e-mail: allen@terryfox.ubc.ca

Dr. Connie J. Eaves
Terry Fox Laboratory
601 West 10th Avenue
Vancouver, BC
V5Z 1L3, Canada
Tel: 604-877-6070 x3146
Fax: 604-877-0712
e-mail: connie@terryfox.ubc.ca

Dr. Theodor M. Fliedner
Department of Clinical Physiology,
Occupational and Social Medicine
University of Ulm
Albert-Einstein-Allee 11
D-89081 Ulm, Germany
Tel: 49-731-502-2900
Fax: 49-731-502-2902
e-mail: theodor.fliedner@medizin.uni-ulm.de

Dr. Julia Gidáli
National Institute of Haematology
  and Immunology, Budapest
P. O. Box 424
H-1519, Budapest,
Hungary
Tel: 36-1-166-5822
Fax: 36-1-166-6004

Dr. Philippe Hénon
Institut de Recherche en Hématologie et Transfusion
Hôpital du Hasenrain
87, rue d'Altkirch
68051 Mulhouse
Cédex, France
Tel: 33-3-89-64-74-18
Fax: 33-3-89-64-78-87

Dr. Dieter Hoelzer
Klinikum der Johann Wolfgang Goethe-Universität
Frankfurt am Main
Zentrum der Inneren Medizin
Medizinische Klinik III
60590 Frankfurt
Theodor-Stern-Kai 7, Germany
Tel: 49-69-6301-5194
Fax: 49-69-6301-7326
e-mail: hoelzer@em.uni-frankfurt.de

Dr. Surapol Issaragrisil
Division of Hematology
Siriraj Hospital
Bangkok 10700, Thailand
Tel: 66-2-4337110-1
Fax: 66-2-4337083

Dr. Lothar Kanz
University of Tübingen
Otfried-Müller-Straße 10
D-72076 Tübingen, Germany
Tel: 49-7071-2982726
Fax: 49-7071-293671
e-mail: lothar.kanz@uni-tuebingen.de

Dr. Anne Kessinger
University of Nebraska Medical Center
600 S. 42nd Street
Omaha, NE 68198-3330, USA
Tel: 402-559-7511
Fax: 402-559-6520

Dr. Martin Körbling
University of Texas
M.D. Anderson Cancer Center
Department of Hematology, Box 24
1515 Holcombe Boulevard
Houston, TX 77030, USA
Tel: 713-792-8750
Fax: 713-794-4902
e-mail: korblin@notes.mdacc.tmc.edu@internet

Dr. Bob Löwenberg
Daniel den Hoed Cancer Center
Groene Hilledijk 301
3075 EA Rotterdam
The Netherlands
Tel: 31-10-4391-598
Fax: 31-10-4842-008
e-mail: lowenberg@haed.azr.nl

Dr. Hans A. Messner
Princess Margaret Hospital
610 University Avenue
Toronto, Ontario
M5G 2A9 Canada
Tel: 416-946-2266
Fax: 416-946-6585

Dr. Donald Metcalf
The Walter and Eliza Hall Institute of Medical Research
P. O. Royal Melbourne Hospital
3050 Victoria, Australia
Tel: 61-3-9345-2555
Fax: 61-3-9347-0852

Dr. Robert Möhle
Department of Medicine II
University of Tübingen
Otfried-Müller-Str. 10
72076 Tübingen, Germany
Tel: 49-7071-2982726
Fax: 49-7071-293671
e-mail: rtmoehle@med.uni-tuebingen.de

Dr. Wilhelm Nothdurft
Department of Radiotherapy
University of Ulm
Robert - Koch - Straße 6
D-89081 Ulm, Germany
Tel: 49-731-502-4966
Fax: 49-731-502-4969

Dr. Makio Ogawa
VA Medical Center
109 Bee Street
Charleston, SC 29401-5799, USA
Tel: 803-577-5011, x6712
Fax: 803-953-6433

Dr. Cesare Peschle
Thomas Jefferson University
Kimmel Cancer Center
Bluemle Life Sciences Building
Room 528
233 South 10th Street
Philadelphia, PA 19107-5541, USA
Tel: 215-503-1763
Fax: 215-923-4153

Dr. Peter J. Quesenberry
Cancer Center
University of Massachusetts Medical Center
373 Plantation Street - Suite 202
Worcester, MA 01605, USA
Tel: 508-856-6956
Fax: 508-856-1310
e-mail: peter.quesenberry@banyan.UMMED.edu

Dr. Felicia Rosenthal
University Medical Center Freiburg
Department of Internal Medicine I
Hugstetter Straße 55
79106 Freiburg, Germany
Tel: 49-761-270-7200
Fax: 49-761-270-7210

Dr. Richard K. Shadduck
The Western Pennsylvania Hospital
4800 Friendship Avenue, Suite 2303
Pittsburgh, PA 15224, USA
Tel: 412-578-4355
Fax: 412-578-4391

Dr. Brian P. Sorrentino
Division of Experimental Hematology
St. Jude Children's Research Hospital
332 N. Lauderdale
Memphis, TN 38101, USA
Tel: 901-495-2727
Fax: 901-495-2176

Dr. Stefan F.F. Verlinden
IntroGene BV
P.O. Box 208
2301 CA, Leiden,
The Netherlands
Tel: 317-152-719-11
Fax: 317-152-719-01
e-mail: introgen@knoware.nl

Dr. Harald von Melchner
Laboratory for Molecular Hematology
Department of Hematology
University of Frankfurt Medical School
Theodor-Stern-Kai 7
60590 Frankfurt am Main, Germany

Tel: 069-6301-6696
Fax: 069-6301-7463
e-mail: melchner@em.uni-frankfurt.de

Dr. Gerard Wagemaker
Erasmus Universiteit Rotterdam
Institute of Hematology

H Ee 1314
P. O. Box 1738
3000 DR Rotterdam
The Netherlands
Tel: 31-10-4087766
Fax: 31-10-4362315
e-mail: wagemaker@hema.fgg.eur.nl

KEY WORD INDEX